The Nursing Assistant

ESSENTIALS OF HOLISTIC CARE

Second Edition

BRIEF EDITION

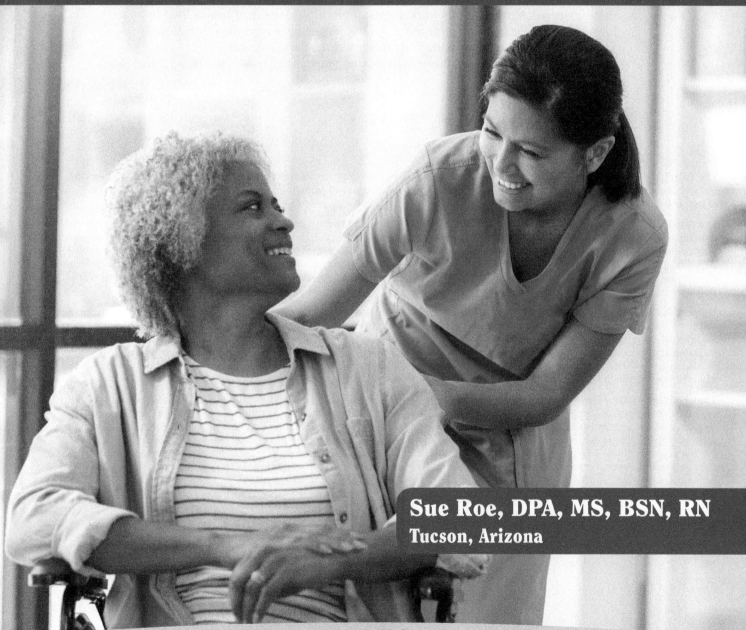

Sue Roe, DPA, MS, BSN, RN
Tucson, Arizona

Publisher
The Goodheart-Willcox Company, Inc.
Tinley Park, IL
www.g-w.com

About the Author

Dr. Sue Roe has extensive experience in healthcare, nursing, and education. She has worked in and has been an administrator of several clinical and educational settings. Dr. Roe has taught and designed academic courses and training programs in nursing, allied health, holistic health and wellness, leadership, and administration and has been consulting as The Roe Group Enterprises, LLC, for over 25 years.

Dr. Roe is the author of *The Nursing Assistant: Essentials of Holistic Care*, coauthor of *Health Science: Concepts and Applications,* and *Life by Personal Design: Realizing Your Dream.* She is the executive editor of *Wholistic NOW!*, an online briefing whose focus is holistic/integrative nursing, health and wellness, and caring for self and others, and she is also the leader of the Arizona chapter of the American Holistic Nurses Association.

Dr. Roe has a doctorate in public administration, with an emphasis in administration and health policy. She completed graduate-level work in educational administration and instructional development and holds a master of science degree and a bachelor of science degree in nursing.

New to This Edition

The second edition of *The Nursing Assistant, Brief Edition* has been revised and updated to reflect current practice. Information formerly included in Chapter 8 has been absorbed into other chapters to provide a more streamlined learning experience. Also, a new Building Math Skill problem has been added at the end of every chapter. In addition, content in individual chapters has been updated as follows:

- **Chapter 1 The Holistic Nursing Assistant** includes more information about professionalism and honoring resident rights.

- **Chapter 3 Legal and Ethical Practice** emphasizes resident rights and includes information about confidentiality in social media.

- **Chapter 4 Safe Practice** has been revised to increase clarity on the use of gloves in various situations.

- **Chapter 5 Emergencies and Disasters** includes information about climate change and pandemics.

- **Chapter 7 Human Behavior, Needs, and Work-Life Balance** includes information about stress and the importance of work-life balance.

- **Chapter 8 Infection Prevention and Control** includes SARS-COV-2, the virus that causes COVID-19, and includes expanded coverage of PPE.

- **Chapter 15 Vital Signs, Height, and Weight** includes updated information on CPR techniques.

- **Chapter 20 Hydration and Elimination** includes information about NPO status.

Reviewers

Goodheart-Willcox Publisher would like to thank the following instructors who reviewed selected chapters and provided valuable input into the development of this textbook program.

Shelia Adams
Program Coordinator, Department Chair
Richmond Community College
Hamlet, NC

Beth Batturs Martin
Assistant Dean
Anne Arundel Community College
Arnold, MD

Janette Beckley
Instructor
Columbus State Community College
Columbus, OH

Lynne Brodeur
Professor
Bristol Community College
Fall River, MA

Heather Brown
Nurse Aide Program Chair
Aims Community College
Greeley, CO

Kimberly Byron-Barnes
Program Chair/Clinical Coordinator
Edgecombe Community College
Rocky Mount, NC

Diane Cardamone
Department Head
Wake Technical Community College
Raleigh, NC

Lisa Cork
Director Nurse Assistant Program
San Diego Continuing Education
San Diego, CA

Dana E. Craven
Nurse Aide Program Coordinator
Stanly Community College
Peachland, NC

Victoria DeGuia
CNA Instructor
Harper College
Palatine, IL

Donna Dickson
Associate Professor
Oakton Community College
Skokie, IL

Jane Fritz
Professor and Nurse Aid Program Director
Trinity Valley Community College
Athens, TX

Shari Gould
Director, Allied Health CE
Victoria College
Victoria, TX

Jo Hart
Nursing Assistant Instructor
Gateway Technical College
Elkhorn, WI

Mia Jones
Nurse LVN
Lone Star College
Tomball, TX

Elaine Kafle
CNA/HHA Program Director/Faculty
Evergreen Valley College
San Jose, CA

Sharon Logsdon
Instructor CNA/GNA
Allegany College of Maryland
Cumberland, MD

Deborah Lord
Lead Nursing Instructor
Delaware Technical Community College
Dover, DE

Beverly Marquez
Director of Health Information Technology/Medical
    Coding Program, Health Occupations Certificate
    Programs and Medical Laboratory
State Fair Community College
Sedalia, MO

Alisa Montgomery
Dean, Health Sciences
Piedmont Community College
Roxboro, NC

Jamie O'Connor Florez
Professor CNA Program
Southwestern College
San Diego, CA

Kristi Shultz
Director of Nursing Home Training
Paris Junior College
Paris, TX

Jill Stonecliffe
Instructor
McHenry County College
Crystal Lake, IL

Linda Sulkowski
Program Director, Nurse Aide Training
Lorain County Community College
Elyria, OH

Candice Williams
Assistant Professor/Program Coordinator
Salt Lake Community College
West Jordan, UT

Rosa Wilson
Associate Professor/Nurse Aide Program Director
Danville Community College
Danville, VA

Dan Wojnicki
CNA Instructor
College of DuPage
Glen Ellyn, IL

Kristen Woods
Nursing Assistant Program Coordinator
Gateway Community College
Phoenix, AZ

Acknowledgments

Goodheart-Willcox Publisher and the author would like to thank Bev Riege and Emily Kroemer of Kirkwood Community College for class testing the materials with their students. We would also like to thank Rasmussen University for the use of their simulation lab for a photoshoot. The author would also like to thank Dina J. Capek, RN, MSN, LNHA, Director of Health Services, Royal Oaks Retirement Community, in Sun City, Arizona, who generously shared her expertise and experience with long-term care and at-risk geriatric populations and provided some needed supplies for the photoshoot. The author is also grateful to Sherry Zumbrunnen, BSN, MN, RN, HNBC, Certified Yoga Instructor, and Reiki Master, for her helpful insights and perspectives about holistic nursing care.

Guided Tour

The second edition of *The Nursing Assistant: Essentials of Holistic Care, Brief Edition* presents all of the key knowledge and skills you need to succeed when taking the certification competency exam in your state and begin your nursing assistant career. The text and its supplements also include abundant reinforcement opportunities and practice questions for the certification competency examination, challenging you to apply what you have learned and preparing you for success when taking the exam.

Emphasis on Holistic Care

The Nursing Assistant: Essentials of Holistic Care, Brief Edition takes a holistic approach to nursing assistant information, skills, and procedures. At the beginning of each chapter, a *Providing Holistic Care Framework* helps you visualize the aspects of holistic care and identify the concepts described in the chapter. *Becoming a Holistic Nursing Assistant* features also introduce important skills and knowledge needed to deliver holistic care. These features cover topics such as providing care in isolation, answering call lights, and the effects of aging.

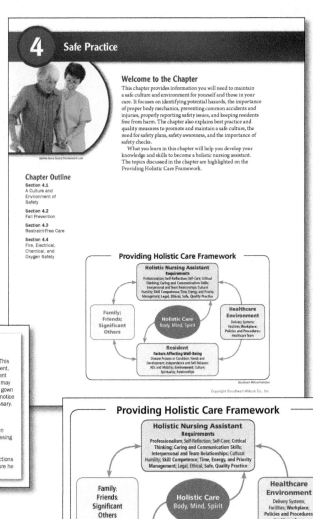

BECOMING A HOLISTIC NURSING ASSISTANT
Caring for Residents with Infections

When caring for residents with infections, holistic nursing assistants must remember several important things. Often, the focus of care is stopping the infection as quickly as possible. It is also important, however, to consider the psychosocial aspects of care.

When providing holistic care, be aware of and sensitive to the resident's fear or guilt surrounding an infection. Perhaps the resident knew someone who died from an infection; perhaps the resident did not keep a wound clean enough. It is important to recognize pain that can occur with an infection. Being sensitive to, observing, and reporting levels of pain will help relieve pain and promote healing.

Some people may be embarrassed by the odor associated from wound seepage (discharge) or rashes. As a holistic nursing assistant, help maintain good hygiene and keep any dressings clean and fresh. This will help eliminate the smell and any embarrassment.

Finally, realize that personal protective equipment (PPE) and the processes used in infection control may be frightening to residents. The sight of a mask and gown can be upsetting for older adults. Provide advance notice about the use of PPE and explain why PPE is necessary. You will learn more about PPE in the next section.

Apply It

1. Think back to a time when you were sick with an infection. Did you find your symptoms embarrassing or painful? What made you feel more at ease?
2. Some people find caring for a resident with an infection difficult, fearful, or unpleasant. What actions might a holistic nursing assistant take to be sure he or she feels able to provide this care?

Assessment and Practice Questions for the Certification Competency Examination

After studying this text, you will be prepared to take the certification competency examination in your state. At the end of each section, reinforcement, application, and critical thinking questions, as well as math problems, help solidify your learning of critical skills and knowledge. Each chapter assessment includes practice test questions similar to those found on certification competency examinations across the United States. These tests provide an opportunity to practice answering exam questions and apply test-taking skills. Exam questions are presented in a multiple-choice format and assess your understanding of the topics covered in each chapter. Two full practice exams are also provided in the Study Guide that accompanies this text.

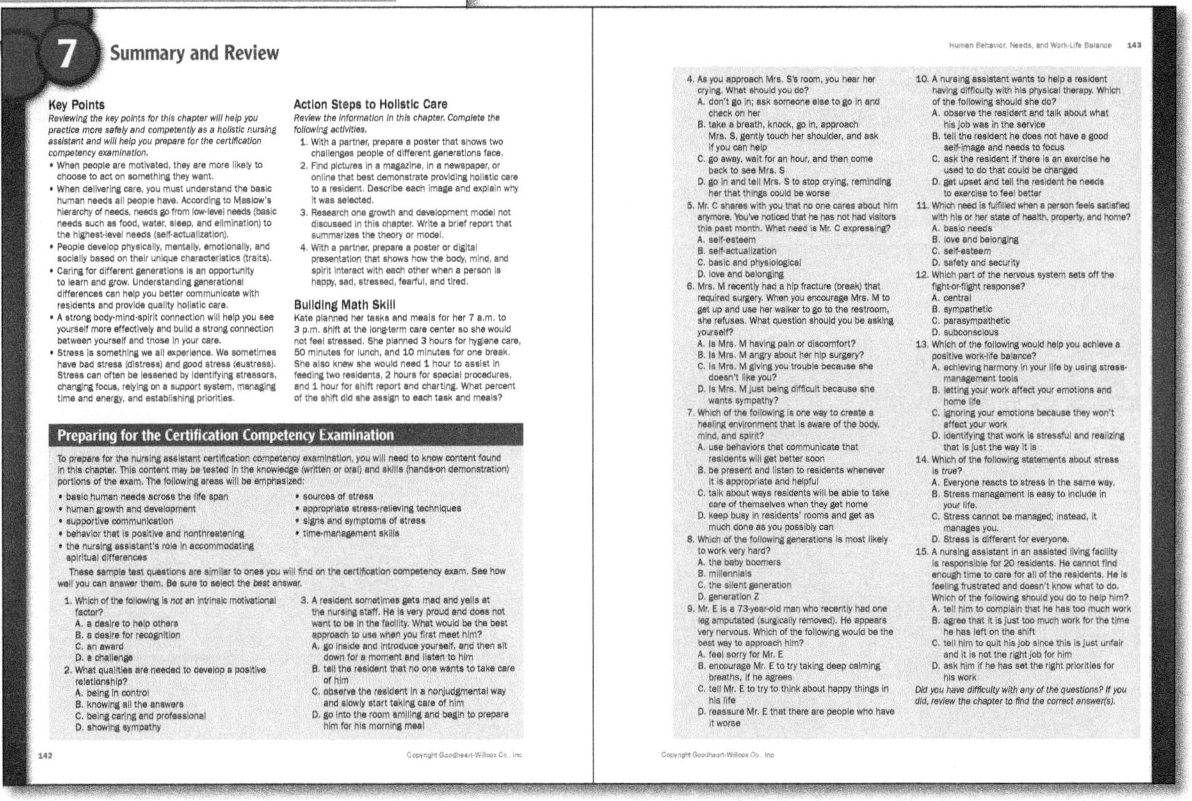

SECTION 5.1 Review and Assessment

Key Terms Mini Glossary

abdominal thrusts an emergency procedure in which a person places his or her fist just above the navel of a choking person, covers his or her fist with the other hand, and performs quick inward and upward thrusts.

allergen any substance that the body perceives as a threat, causing an allergic reaction.

anaphylaxis a severe allergic reaction that can affect the whole body; may cause skin reactions, swelling, trouble breathing, rapid pulse, nausea, and dizziness.

angina chest pain or discomfort; there may be a sensation of squeezing, pressure, heaviness, or tightness in the center of the chest.

asphyxia a lack of oxygen in the body; may be caused when breathing stops due to a blockage or swelling in the trachea.

automated external defibrillator (AED) a medical device that gives an electric shock to the heart to stop irregular heart rhythm and allow normal heart rhythm to begin.

basic life support (BLS) care given to a person experiencing respiratory arrest, cardiac arrest, or airway blockage.

includes giving cardiopulmonary resuscitation (CPR), using an automated external defibrillator (AED), and relieving a blocked airway.

cardiopulmonary resuscitation (CPR) an emergency procedure in which air is breathed into a person's mouth or nose to provide ventilation; external chest compressions help oxygenate blood flow to the brain and heart.

diabetes mellitus a disorder in which there are excessive amounts of glucose (sugar) in a person's blood due to insufficient production of insulin (the hormone that regulates glucose) or insulin resistance; commonly referred to as diabetes.

fibrillation an irregular heart rhythm.

grand mal seizure a generalized seizure in which a person may experience loss of consciousness and violent muscle contractions; caused by abnormal electrical activity in the brain.

Hands-Only™ CPR an emergency procedure in which uninterrupted chest compressions restore heartbeat and promote blood circulation; is a procedure for those not trained in conventional CPR.

hemorrhage the excessive loss of blood over a short period of time due to internal or external injury.

myocardial infarction a sudden medical emergency that occurs when blood flow to part of the heart muscle is blocked, causing the heart muscle to become severely damaged and die; can cause loss of heart function, or cardiac arrest; also known as a heart attack.

petit mal seizure a generalized seizure in which a person has no or lessened awareness and responsiveness and may lose consciousness; caused by abnormal electrical activity in the brain.

pulse the beat of the heart measured through the walls of a peripheral artery.

rule of nines a method of determining the surface area of the body affected by burns.

seizures sudden changes in the brain's normal electrical activity; cause a change in or loss of consciousness.

shock a condition in which the organs and tissues of the body do not have sufficient oxygen.

stroke a sudden blockage or rupture of a blood vessel in the brain; can cause a loss of consciousness, partial loss of movement, and speech impairment; also called a cerebrovascular accident (CVA).

Apply the Key Terms
Write a sentence using each key term properly.
1. anaphylaxis
2. angina
3. hemorrhage
4. seizure
5. shock

Know and Understand the Facts
1. What are three responsibilities nursing assistants have during medical emergencies?
2. Describe the role of the first responder.
3. What specific actions should you take to help someone who is in anaphylaxis?
4. How can you tell if someone has been poisoned?
5. What should you do if a person has a second-degree burn?

Analyze and Apply Concepts
1. Explain the importance of following Hands-Only™ CPR guidelines.
2. List the steps required to effectively use an AED.

3. Explain the procedures for responding to choking in adults and children over one year of age.
4. Describe the actions a nursing assistant should take if a resident has a seizure.

Think Critically
Read the following care situation. Then answer the questions that follow.

Jean, your best friend's grandmother, became very pale, clutched her chest, and started to collapse like she was fainting while she was making you and your friend lunch. You know that Jean had been sick last month and that she takes medication. She had been fine just a few minutes before and had been laughing and telling a great story. You are sitting closest to Jean.

1. What signs should you look for to tell if Jean might be having a heart attack?
2. What is the first action you should take?
3. What should you do to keep Jean safe?

Key Points
Reviewing the key points for this chapter will help you practice more safely and competently as a holistic nursing assistant and will help you prepare for the certification competency examination.
- When people are motivated, they are more likely to choose to act on something they want.
- When delivering care, you must understand the basic human needs all people have. According to Maslow's hierarchy of needs, needs go from low-level needs (basic needs such as food, water, sleep, and elimination) to the highest-level needs (self-actualization).
- People develop physically, mentally, emotionally, and socially based on their unique characteristics (traits).
- Caring for different generations is an opportunity to learn and grow. Understanding generational differences can help you better communicate with residents and provide quality holistic care.
- A strong body-mind-spirit connection will help you see yourself more effectively and build a strong connection between yourself and those in your care.
- Stress is something we all experience. We sometimes have bad stress (distress) and good stress (eustress). Stress can often be lessened by identifying stressors, changing focus, relying on a support system, managing time and energy, and establishing priorities.

Action Steps to Holistic Care
Review the information in this chapter. Complete the following activities.
1. With a partner, prepare a poster that shows two challenges people of different generations face.
2. Find pictures in a magazine, in a newspaper, or online that best demonstrate providing holistic care to a resident. Describe each image and explain why it was selected.
3. Research one growth and development model not discussed in this chapter. Write a brief report that summarizes the theory or model.
4. With a partner, prepare a poster or digital presentation that shows how the body, mind, and spirit interact with each other when a person is happy, sad, stressed, fearful, and tired.

Building Math Skill
Kate planned her tasks and meals for her 7 a.m. to 3 p.m. shift at the long-term care center so she would not feel stressed. She planned 3 hours for hygiene care, 50 minutes for lunch, and 10 minutes for one break. She also knew she would need 1 hour to assist in feeding two residents, 2 hours for special procedures, and 1 hour for shift report and charting. What percent of the shift did she assign to each task and meals?

Preparing for the Certification Competency Examination

To prepare for the nursing assistant certification competency examination, you will need to know content found in this chapter. This content may be tested in the knowledge (written or oral) and skills (hands-on demonstration) portions of the exam. The following areas will be emphasized:
- basic human needs across the life span
- human growth and development
- supportive communication
- behavior that is positive and nonthreatening
- the nursing assistant's role in accommodating spiritual differences
- sources of stress
- appropriate stress-relieving techniques
- signs and symptoms of stress
- time-management skills

These sample test questions are similar to ones you will find on the certification competency exam. See how well you can answer them. Be sure to select the best answer.

1. Which of the following is not an intrinsic motivational factor?
   A. a desire to help others
   B. a desire for recognition
   C. an award
   D. a challenge
2. What qualities are needed to develop a positive relationship?
   A. being in control
   B. knowing all the answers
   C. being caring and professional
   D. showing sympathy
3. A resident sometimes gets mad and yells at the nursing staff. He is very proud and does not want to be in the facility. What would be the best approach to use when you first meet him?
   A. go inside and introduce yourself, and then sit down for a moment and listen to him
   B. tell the resident that no one wants to take care of him
   C. observe the resident in a nonjudgmental way and slowly start taking care of him
   D. go into the room smiling and begin to prepare him for his morning meal

4. As you approach Mrs. S's room, you hear her crying. What should you do?
   A. don't go in; ask someone else to go in and check on her
   B. take a breath, knock, go in, approach Mrs. S, gently touch her shoulder, and ask if you can help
   C. go away, wait for an hour, and then come back to see Mrs. S
   D. go in and tell Mrs. S to stop crying, reminding her that things could be worse
5. Mr. C shares with you that no one cares about him anymore. You've noticed that he has not had visitors this past month. What need is Mr. C expressing?
   A. self-esteem
   B. self-actualization
   C. basic and physiological
   D. love and belonging
6. Mrs. M recently had a hip fracture (break) that required surgery. When you encourage Mrs. M to get up and use her walker to go to the restroom, she refuses. What question should you be asking yourself?
   A. Is Mrs. M having pain or discomfort?
   B. Is Mrs. M angry about her hip surgery?
   C. Is Mrs. M giving you trouble because she doesn't like you?
   D. Is Mrs. M just being difficult because she wants sympathy?
7. Which of the following is one way to create a healing environment that is aware of the body, mind, and spirit?
   A. use behaviors that communicate that residents will get better soon
   B. be present and listen to residents whenever it is appropriate and helpful
   C. talk about ways residents will be able to take care of themselves when they get home
   D. keep busy in residents' rooms and get as much done as you possibly can
8. Which of the following generations is most likely to work very hard?
   A. the baby boomers
   B. millennials
   C. the silent generation
   D. generation Z
9. Mr. E is a 73-year-old man who recently had one leg amputated (surgically removed). He appears very nervous. Which of the following would be the best way to approach him?
   A. feel sorry for Mr. E
   B. encourage Mr. E to try taking deep calming breaths, if he agrees
   C. tell Mr. E to try to think about happy things in his life
   D. reassure Mr. E that there are people who have it worse

10. A nursing assistant wants to help a resident having difficulty with his physical therapy. Which of the following should she do?
    A. observe the resident and talk about what his job was in the service
    B. tell the resident he does not have a good self-image and needs to focus
    C. ask the resident if there is an exercise he used to do that could be changed
    D. get upset and tell the resident he needs to exercise to feel better
11. Which need is fulfilled when a person feels satisfied with his or her state of health, property, and home?
    A. basic needs
    B. love and belonging
    C. self-esteem
    D. safety and security
12. Which part of the nervous system sets off the fight-or-flight response?
    A. central
    B. sympathetic
    C. parasympathetic
    D. subconscious
13. Which of the following would help you achieve a positive work-life balance?
    A. achieving harmony in your life by using stress-management tools
    B. letting your work affect your emotions and home life
    C. ignoring your emotions because they won't affect your work
    D. identifying that work is stressful and realizing that is just the way it is
14. Which of the following statements about stress is true?
    A. Everyone reacts to stress in the same way.
    B. Stress management is easy to include in your life.
    C. Stress cannot be managed; instead, it manages you.
    D. Stress is different for everyone.
15. A nursing assistant in an assisted living facility is responsible for 20 residents. He cannot find enough time to care for all of the residents. He is feeling frustrated and doesn't know what to do. Which of the following should you do to help him?
    A. tell him to complain that he has too much work
    B. agree that it is just too much work for the time he has left on the shift
    C. tell him to quit his job since this is just unfair and it is not the right job for him
    D. ask him if he has set the right priorities for his work

Did you have difficulty with any of the questions? If you did, review the chapter to find the correct answer(s).

Guided Tour

Procedures

Throughout *The Nursing Assistant: Essentials of Holistic Care, Brief Edition*, detailed procedures outline the steps you need to follow to pass the certification competency examination in your state and practice in healthcare. Each procedure contains a rationale, preparation instructions, procedure steps, follow-up actions, and information for reporting and documentation of the care provided. Procedures are easy to follow and are richly illustrated with numerous, professional photographs and drawings. **Best Practice** notes advise you about safety precautions and ways to provide holistic care.

Best Practice: It is important to provide privacy during the admission process. If a resident's family members or friends are present, determine whether they will stay during admission.

Best Practice: When washing your hands, keep your hands and forearms below your elbows. Water should flow down off your fingertips, never up your arms.

Best Practice: Do not turn your back on the sterile field or leave the sterile field unattended. Do not cough, sneeze, talk, or laugh during this procedure. Airborne microorganisms can contaminate sterile items or the sterile field.

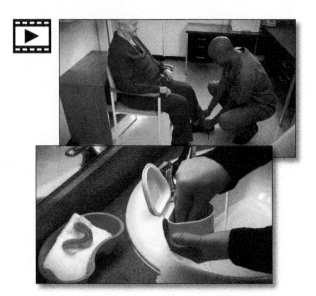

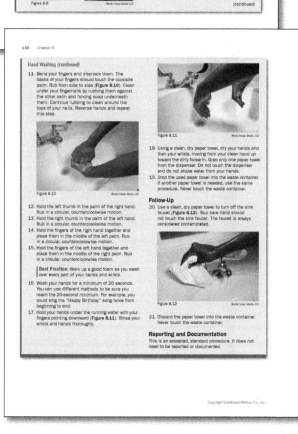

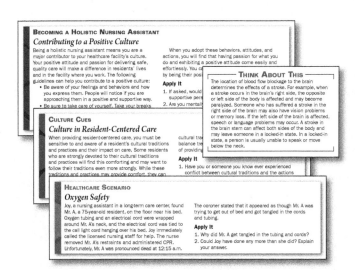

Features

In addition to the *Becoming a Holistic Nursing Assistant* boxes, the text contains other features that address topics of interest in nurse assisting. *Culture Cues* prompt you to examine cultural considerations for improved care. *Healthcare Scenarios* introduce concepts using lifelike situations and ask you to analyze and apply knowledge to dilemmas. *Think About This* features throughout each chapter provide additional information about healthcare topics of interest.

Numerous colorful photographs demonstrate important care guidelines. These images will help you visually understand the concepts being presented. **Detailed illustrations** bring anatomical concepts to life, helping you comprehend body positions and the complex structure of the human body.

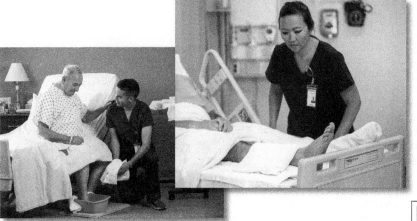

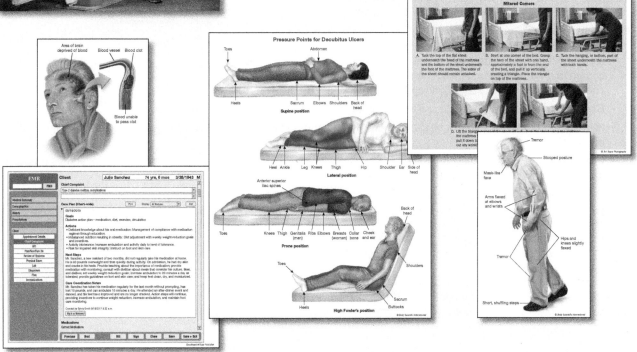

TOOLS FOR STUDENT AND INSTRUCTOR SUCCESS

Student Tools

Student Text

The Nursing Assistant: Essentials of Holistic Care, Brief Edition introduces the field of nurse assisting and outlines the procedures needed to deliver safe, quality care that meets residents' needs. This text focuses on the holistic care of residents—that is, care that attends to all of a resident's needs. The topics covered prepare students for certification and include nursing assistant responsibilities, legal and ethical standards, healthcare teamwork, cultural humility, ways to promote mobility, and ways to assist with hydration and elimination. Infection control, anatomy and disease, personal hygiene procedures, and care for people with disabilities are also covered in this text. At the end of each chapter, practice questions for the certification competency examination assess knowledge and skills gained.

Study Guide

The Study Guide that accompanies *The Nursing Assistant: Essentials of Holistic Care, Brief Edition* includes instructor-created activities to help students recall, review, and apply concepts introduced in the book. The Study Guide also includes procedural checklists and two full practice tests for the certification competency examination.

Instructor Tools

LMS Integration

Integrate Goodheart-Willcox content within your Learning Management System for a seamless user experience for both you and your students. LMS-ready content in Common Cartridge® format facilitates single sign-on integration and gives you control of student enrollment and data. With a Common Cartridge integration, you can access the LMS features and tools you are accustomed to using and G-W course resources in one convenient location—your LMS.

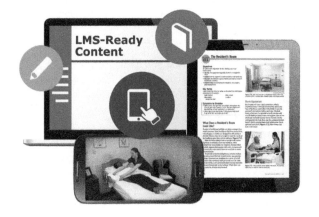

G-W Common Cartridge provides a complete learning package for you and your students. The included digital resources help your students remain engaged and learn effectively:

- **eBook content.** The eBook Reflowable is an enriched digital textbook that works well on all devices and is compatible with screen readers. The eBook also offers complimentary access to digital drill and practice activities.
- **Study Guide content.** Students can have access to a digital version of the Study Guide.
- **Narrated animations.** Ideal for visual learners, these short animations effectively illustrate key concepts from the book.
- **Procedural videos.** These step-by-step videos help students see the tasks required to complete procedures required to pass the certification competency examination.
- **Drill and Practice.** Learning new vocabulary is critical to student success. These vocabulary activities, which are provided for all key terms in each chapter, provide an active, engaging, and effective way for students to learn the required terminology.

When you incorporate G-W content into your courses via Common Cartridge, you have the flexibility to customize and structure the content to meet the educational needs of your students. You may also choose to add your own content to the course.

For instructors, the Common Cartridge includes the Online Instructor Resources. QTI® question banks are available within the Online Instructor Resources for import into your LMS. These prebuilt assessments help you measure student knowledge and track results in your LMS gradebook. Questions and tests can be customized to meet your assessment needs.

Instructor Resources

Online Instructor Resources provide all the support needed to make preparation and classroom instruction easier than ever. Available in one accessible location, the OIR includes Instructor Resources, Instructor's Presentations for PowerPoint®, and Assessment Software with Question Banks. The OIR is available as a subscription and can be accessed at school, at home, or on the go.

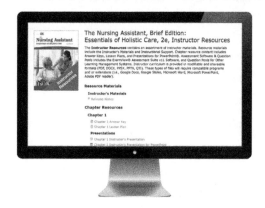

Instructor Resources One resource provides instructors with time-saving preparation tools such as answer keys, editable lesson plans, a quick-reference guide, and other teaching aids.

Instructor's Presentations for PowerPoint® These fully customizable, richly illustrated slides help you teach and visually reinforce the key concepts from each chapter.

Assessment Software with Question Banks Administer and manage assessments to meet your classroom needs. The question banks that accompany this textbook include hundreds of matching, completion, multiple choice, and short answer questions to assess student knowledge of the content in each chapter. Using the assessment software simplifies the process of creating, managing, administering, and grading tests. You can have the software generate a test for you with randomly selected questions. You may also choose specific questions from the question banks and, if you wish, add your own questions to create customized tests to meet your classroom needs.

G-W Integrated Learning Solution

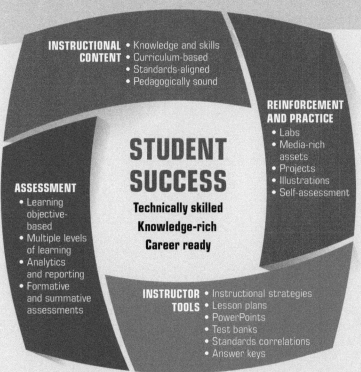

INSTRUCTIONAL CONTENT
- Knowledge and skills
- Curriculum-based
- Standards-aligned
- Pedagogically sound

REINFORCEMENT AND PRACTICE
- Labs
- Media-rich assets
- Projects
- Illustrations
- Self-assessment

STUDENT SUCCESS
Technically skilled
Knowledge-rich
Career ready

ASSESSMENT
- Learning objective-based
- Multiple levels of learning
- Analytics and reporting
- Formative and summative assessments

INSTRUCTOR TOOLS
- Instructional strategies
- Lesson plans
- PowerPoints
- Test banks
- Standards correlations
- Answer keys

The G-W Integrated Learning Solution offers easy-to-use resources that help students and instructors achieve success.

▶ EXPERT AUTHORS
▶ TRUSTED REVIEWERS
▶ 100 YEARS OF EXPERIENCE

EMPLOYABILITY SKILLS · TECHNICAL SKILLS · ACADEMIC KNOWLEDGE · INDUSTRY RECOGNIZED STANDARDS

Brief Contents

Contents

Feature Contents

Culture Cues

Healthcare Scenario

Becoming a Holistic Nursing Assistant

Procedures

Introduction

How exciting to think about becoming a nursing assistant and starting a career in nursing! Maybe you have been thinking about this career choice for as long as you can remember because you have always wanted to help others. Maybe you know someone who is a nurse and would like to be like him or her. Or, maybe you had a nurse take care of you when you were ill, and you knew that was the kind of work you wanted to do someday. Whatever your reason for taking this career path, this textbook will provide you with the knowledge and skills you need to be successful.

In this textbook, you will learn fundamental and important content and procedures to help you deliver safe, quality care. You will also learn about the importance of holistic care; or how understanding the interactions among the body, mind, and spirit can have an effect on the way people maintain wellness and respond to illness. These interactions among the body, mind, and spirit create a connection and harmony that can help people live their lives fully and independently.

As a holistic nursing assistant, you will make a difference in the lives of others by:

- being sensitive to and respectful of yourself and fully understanding your own body, mind, and spirit so you can do the same for others
- being strong, gentle, and caring
- focusing on the unique needs and desires of others to help them be as independent as possible
- being positive and using supportive communication
- paying close attention to the way you walk into a room, the tone of your voice, and the way you communicate with others
- being aware of when others are stressed and helping them understand the importance of maintaining their health and wellness
- creating trust, paying attention and being focused, and showing appropriate concern and respect

The goal of this textbook is to assist you in becoming an effective and successful nursing assistant. As you study the information and detailed procedures in this text, you will learn how to provide holistic care that is appreciated and valued by residents and their families. Be aware that the procedures in this book describe the best general practices. The exact guidelines for procedures in your state may vary, and new knowledge is always shaping the field of nursing, so always check your state's or facility's regulations and policies. Remember:

> *When you touch a body, you touch the whole person, the intellect, the spirit, and the emotions.*
>
> Jane Harrington, American author

I wish you the best as you begin this life-changing journey.

Sue Roe

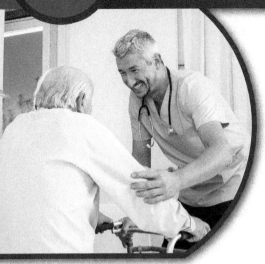

Tyler Olson/Shutterstock.com

Chapter Outline

Section 1.1
Role and Responsibilities

Section 1.2
Professionalism
and Boundaries

Welcome to the Chapter

This chapter provides information you will need to understand your role and demonstrate your responsibilities as a holistic nursing assistant. You will learn about the qualities, behaviors, and professionalism expected of a successful holistic nursing assistant. Further, you will explore the personal and professional boundaries within which a nursing assistant must work. These boundaries are important, because they define what a nursing assistant can and cannot do as a caregiver.

When you become a holistic nursing assistant, you will care for many different people. You may deliver care to **patients**. Patients are people who receive care in a healthcare facility, such as a hospital. Patients need immediate care due to illness or disease and often can expect recovery. A patient's stay in a hospital is usually short. You may also deliver care to **residents**. Residents are people who need ongoing care over a longer period of time. Residents are older and live in long-term care facilities due to age, illness, or inability to care for themselves at home. During your career as a nursing assistant, you may work in many different healthcare facilities and, therefore, may care for both patients and residents. Because this text focuses on long-term care, emphasis will be placed on caring for residents.

Role and Responsibilities

Objectives

To achieve the objectives for this section, you must successfully:

- **describe** the role of a holistic nursing assistant.
- **explain** the requirements for nursing assistants to become certified.
- **discuss** the typical responsibilities of a holistic nursing assistant.
- **list** major duties performed by nursing assistants.

Key Terms

Learn these key terms to better understand the information presented in the section.

activities of daily
   living (ADLs)
ambulating
certification
certified nursing
   assistant (CNA)
compassion
contaminated
empower
holistic care
hospice

infection control
job description
licensed nursing staff
licensed practical/
   vocational nurse
   (LPN/LVN)
patients
registered nurse (RN)
residents
scope of practice
vital signs

Questions to Consider

- Have you ever taken care of someone? Maybe you took care of your mother, friend, younger brother or sister, or even your pet. How did you feel about the responsibility of providing care? What did you do to make sure that the person or pet was cared for properly?
- How would you describe the caregiving role you took or what you had to do? What daily responsibilities, abilities, and attitudes helped you do the best job possible?

What Is a Nursing Assistant's Role?

Becoming a nursing assistant gives you a special opportunity to make a difference in someone else's life. It is also an excellent way to grow personally by gaining knowledge and skills as you journey into an exciting nursing career path.

A *certified nursing assistant (CNA)* is a person who has successfully completed the education and training needed to take and pass a state certification competency examination. The certified nursing assistant helps deliver care and is supervised by

licensed practical/vocational nurses (LPNs/LVNs) and registered nurses (RNs). In some states, a CNA is known as a *nurse aide, registered nursing assistant,* or *licensed nursing assistant.*

Becoming a CNA may be your first step toward becoming a *licensed practical/vocational nurse (LPN/LVN)* or a *registered nurse (RN).* An LPN/LVN is a member of the *licensed nursing staff* who is supervised by an RN. The duties of LPNs/LVNs vary by state, but typically include monitoring and reporting, preparing and giving medications, and inserting catheters. An RN is a licensed nursing staff member who delivers nursing care that includes assessment; providing nursing diagnoses; and planning, implementing, and evaluating care.

A nursing assistant is an important member of the healthcare team and provides care to residents (**Figure 1.1**). Healthcare facilities such as hospitals, community clinics, skilled nursing facilities, residential care or long-term care facilities, *hospices* (healthcare facilities that care for people who are terminally ill), and home healthcare services hire nursing assistants.

Working as a nursing assistant requires much more than just meeting the basic needs of those in your care. Nursing assistants are often the first to communicate with residents and their families. This is because nursing assistants spend more time with residents than LPNs/LVNs or RNs, who may be involved in other work (procedures and tasks).

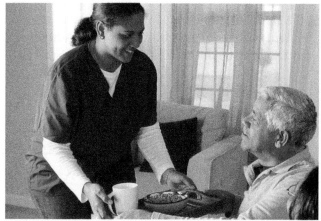

Rob Marmion/Shutterstock.com

Figure 1.1 Nursing assistants work in a variety of settings, including long-term care facilities.

As a result, nursing assistants may be the first ones who observe changes in resident behavior and function or who become aware of residents' specific needs. This information is then reported to the licensed nursing staff for follow-up. The role of the nursing assistant is important and includes many responsibilities.

How Do You Become a Nursing Assistant?

Becoming a nursing assistant requires specialized education and training. The knowledge and skills you learn will help you deliver safe, quality care.

Education and Training

In 1987, the US Congress passed the *Omnibus Budget Reconciliation Act (OBRA)*, which standardized the minimum requirements for certified nursing assistant training programs and evaluation. OBRA is specific to nursing assistants working in nursing homes that receive federal funding. Today, nursing assistant education and training courses that lead to *certification* (a credential that shows a person has completed required education and training) must meet OBRA standards. Since OBRA was passed, states have taken the responsibility of making sure nursing assistant education and training programs meet these standards. States also determine how nursing assistant certification is given, which certification competency examination will be used, and when and where the exam will occur.

The minimum age required to enter a nursing assistant education and training program differs from state to state. Programs range from a minimum of 75 hours to more than 150 hours. Requirements for supervised clinical training include 24 hours or more in long-term care facilities. Some programs also include hospital and other related clinical experiences.

THINK ABOUT THIS

According to the US Bureau of Labor Statistics, employment for nursing assistants is expected to grow 11 percent in the next six years. This growth is faster than the average for all occupations.

The Certification Competency Examination

On completion of a state-approved nursing assistant education and training program, graduates are expected to take the state's certification competency examination. The examination tests knowledge (in a written or oral exam) and skills (as part of a hands-on demonstration). To become certified, a graduate must pass both parts of the examination with a state-determined score. Many resources, including this textbook, provide practice questions similar to those found on the examination.

When a nursing assistant becomes certified, he or she may use the legal title *certified nursing assistant (CNA)*. In some states, a different legal title may be used. Using this title means you have met the requirements to practice as a nursing assistant within the regulations, or *rules*, determined by your state.

Registration as a Nursing Assistant

Federal law requires every state to maintain a *registry*, or list, of nursing assistants. Individuals who successfully complete an approved nursing assistant education and training program and pass the certification competency exam are listed on the registry. The registry also has information about nursing assistants who have been charged with abuse, neglect, and theft.

To work as a nursing assistant, a person must keep an *active status* on the registry. This means that a person's information is up-to-date and that he or she has no charges of abuse, neglect, or the theft or misuse of resident property. Nursing assistants must renew their registration every two years.

Requirements for education or training and the certification competency exam may vary from state to state, and so do regulations for nursing assistants. Be sure to check the specific requirements in your state.

What Do You Need to Know to Become a Holistic Nursing Assistant?

Learning how to be a holistic nursing assistant emphasizes the caring aspect of the nursing assistant's role and strengthens the knowledge and skills needed to provide *holistic care* (care that integrates the body, mind, and spirit). Understanding and using the *Providing Holistic Care Framework*, shown in **Figure 1.2**, will be a helpful guide in this learning process.

The Providing Holistic Care Framework includes the key knowledge and skills you will need to know as a holistic nursing assistant. These knowledge and skills include being professional, using critical thinking, caring and effectively communicating, having cultural humility, and building skills competence. The framework also includes the healthcare environment in which you will work. Holistic nursing assistants must be knowledgeable about different healthcare delivery systems and workplaces, familiar with facility policies and procedures, and capable of working effectively as team members.

The framework show the important interactions between residents; families, friends, and significant others; the holistic nursing assistant; and the healthcare facility. The arrows in the framework represent the support each individual or entity gives to the others. For example, family members support a resident, but may also work closely with a holistic nursing assistant to help make sure the resident's needs are met. Similarly, understanding facility policies and effectively demonstrating procedures help holistic nursing assistants provide safe, quality care.

An effective holistic nursing assistant is aware of a resident's disease process and knows how to respond or take action (for example, by providing assistance with activities of daily living, or ADLs). Holistic nursing assistants are also responsible for responding to residents' needs, emotions, and feelings.

Of great importance in caregiving is sensitivity to the holistic dimensions of the body, mind, and spirit. To provide care that integrates the body, mind, and spirit, holistic nursing assistants must not only respond to physical needs (body), but must also focus on the mind, which includes the resident's needs, wants, feelings, and emotions. Understanding the spirit is also important. The spirit is a person's *higher self*, which includes perceptions, sensations, values, culture, and religion.

By using this holistic approach, caregivers establish an environment that supports the *whole person* and does not just focus on, respond to, and care for a disease. The holistic approach promotes healing and helps residents achieve overall well-being.

As you build your holistic knowledge and skills as a nursing assistant, you will also become aware of how you, as a person, must become sensitive to

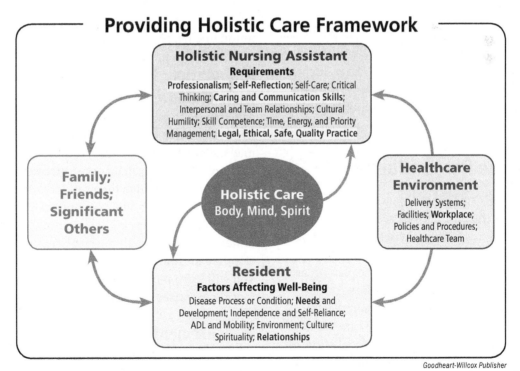

Goodheart-Willcox Publisher

Figure 1.2 The Providing Holistic Care Framework shows the important interactions and support between each entity. The topics covered in Chapter 1 are highlighted in this framework.

your *own* body, mind, and spirit. Holistic caregiving should always include this awareness and sensitivity because it is hard to holistically care for others if you are not aware of your whole self.

This textbook will guide you through the essentials of holistic caregiving. Each chapter will point out a different area of the Providing Holistic Care Framework. This information will be identified at the beginning of each chapter and will be your guide to reading the chapter and becoming a holistic nursing assistant. The topics covered in this chapter are highlighted in Figure 1.2.

In addition, you are encouraged to reflect and journal about what you have learned in each chapter of your textbook. Creating a reflective journal will give you the chance to write and think about both the knowledge and skills you learned and ways you can use them when you begin working as a holistic nursing assistant. It is only through this self-examination and reflection that you can build the confidence and ability to

- be sensitive to special needs and culture;
- understand diseases, conditions, and disabilities;
- use your knowledge and skills competently and safely;
- develop positive and helpful interactions with others; and
- help *empower* (give power to) those in your care.

All of these factors will impact the way you approach, care for, and communicate with residents. Gaining knowledge and developing your skills will allow you to help them achieve the highest levels of well-being possible.

What Are the Responsibilities of a Nursing Assistant?

Providing care is the number-one responsibility of nursing assistants, no matter where they work. The amount of work and type of care required depend on the specific needs of each resident, the plan of care, and the nursing assistant's *job description* (duties, responsibilities, and qualifications). A sample job description is shown in **Figure 1.3**. The care provided also depends on the nursing assistant's legal *scope of practice*, or specific responsibilities, procedures, and actions. Legal scope of practice is determined by each state. While duties may differ depending on the type of healthcare facility in which you work, all nursing

assistants have the same basic responsibilities and requirements.

It is important to be aware of how care is provided. Care should be holistic so that the physical, mental, and spiritual needs of residents and their families are met. This type of care provides assistance with ADLs, pays attention to any changes in condition, responds to needs and requests, offers appropriate emotional support as needed, shows **compassion** (the desire to help another person), and demonstrates *cultural humility* (awareness and sensitivity), among other responsibilities.

Activities of Daily Living (ADLs)

Activities of daily living (ADLs) are actions that people take during a typical day, such as bathing, grooming (combing one's hair), dressing, eating, toileting (urinary and bowel elimination), and *ambulating* (moving about or walking). Nursing assistants are responsible for helping residents complete their ADLs. In some cases, nursing assistants provide all of the care, or they may assist more independent residents as needed. Setting up meals, feeding residents, documenting what and how much residents eat, and assisting with toileting are other important responsibilities. Specific information and procedures to assist in performing ADLs can be found in Chapter 18 and Chapter 20.

Ambulation, Movement, and Exercise

Older residents and those who have illnesses that cause them to be weak or have to stay in bed may need assistance with ambulation. This assistance may include lifting, moving, or transferring residents. Some residents may need assistance with *range-of-motion exercises*, which help residents maintain or improve their flexibility. Nursing assistants also work with residents who need help gaining body strength or need assistance with physical exercise to maintain effective muscular function and general well-being. You will learn more about ambulation and range-of-motion exercises in Chapter 14.

Measurement and Observation

Among the most important responsibilities of a nursing assistant are measuring, documenting, and reporting information about a resident. Information

Certified Nursing Assistant (CNA) Job Description

Job Summary: Assists licensed nursing staff in the provision of basic care for residents and provides necessary unit tasks and functions in compliance with facility policies, procedures, and applicable healthcare standards.

Duties and Responsibilities: Other duties may be assigned.
- Assist residents to meet daily needs while providing a safe environment and ensuring the dignity and well-being of residents.
- Bathe, dress, and undress residents who need help. Assist with other tasks, including but not limited to shaving, nails, and hair.
- Change linens and towels regularly, straighten room, remove soiled linens, and make residents' beds, ensuring that all residents' rooms look neat and clean.
- Ensure that all call lights are in reach of residents and answer call lights within five minutes.
- Serve meals. Assist with eating, if needed.
- Assist with new resident admission.
- Maintain safety and security at all times.
- Report pertinent resident information to licensed nursing staff.
- Complete all forms according to policies and procedures.
- Participate in facility activities, including in-service education and disaster drills.
- Consistently display professional behavior and attitudes and represent the goals and values of the facility.

Qualifications:
- Must have a current and valid Nursing Assistant Certification.
- Must be at least 18 years of age.
- Must be compassionate, mature, sympathetic, and professional at all times.
- Must have good organization and communication skills.
- Must have the ability to read, write, understand, and carry out instructions.
- Must successfully complete all preemployment requirements.
- Must have the physical ability to perform job-related duties, which may require lifting, standing, bending, transferring, stooping, stretching, walking, pushing, and pulling.

Acknowledgment:

I have read this job description and fully understand the requirements for employment. I hereby accept the position of Certified Nursing Assistant (CNA) and will perform all said duties to the best of my ability.

Printed Employee Name: _____

Date: _____

Employee Signature: _____

Figure 1.3 This is an example of a job description for a nursing assistant position.

that nursing assistants measure, document, and report are

- *vital signs*, which include the rates or values of a person's temperature, pulse, respiration, and blood pressure (**Figure 1.4**);
- height and weight;
- fluid intake and output; and
- changes in condition.

Nursing assistants are often the first to know how well a resident is responding to a medicine or treatment. This is because nursing assistants spend more time at the bedside. Any changes in a resident's condition should be immediately reported to the licensed nursing staff. See Chapter 13, Chapter 15, and Chapter 20 to learn more about these observations and measurements.

Procedures

Nursing assistants perform numerous procedures when giving care. These procedures may include providing skin and oral care and admitting, transferring, and discharging residents.

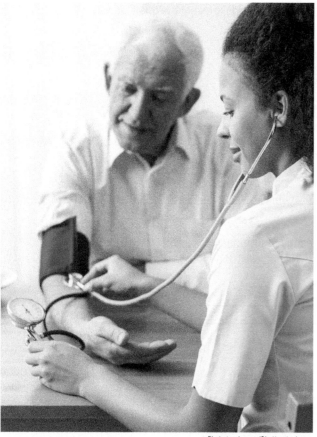

Photographee.eu/Shutterstock.com

Figure 1.4 Nursing assistants measure and document residents' vital signs. This nursing assistant is measuring a resident's blood pressure.

Procedures performed are standardized (made the same) and are found in a healthcare facility policy and procedure manual. Nursing assistants must always perform procedures as directed by the duties and responsibilities of their position and by the healthcare facility. Unless assistance is needed, nursing assistants perform these procedures on their own. However, they are always under the supervision of licensed nursing staff.

Infection Control

Practicing **infection control** lessens the risk of infection. For example, consistently washing hands or rubbing hands with sanitizer (*hand hygiene*) helps prevent the spread of infection. Additionally, the appropriate care and handling of **contaminated** (dirty) objects is important for controlling infection in a healthcare facility. Wearing *personal protective equipment (PPE)*, such as a mask, gloves, protective eyewear, and a gown, is required for specific situations such as the presence of a virulent infection or a resident in isolation (**Figure 1.5**). Infection control also includes observing and reporting environmental situations that might cause the spread of infection. In Chapter 8, you will learn how to follow procedures for hand hygiene and how to properly put on masks, gowns, and gloves.

Communication

Nursing assistants are constantly communicating with residents and their families, other visitors, and healthcare team members. Nursing assistants are also responsible for documenting necessary information in electronic or paper charts and forms, answering the telephone, and taking messages. Communicating electronically has become an important part of healthcare delivery. Electronic communication may include documenting resident information in an *electronic medical record (EMR)*, using mobile devices, or using social media to inform others. Information about communication, documentation, and the use of electronic communication are described in Chapter 11 and Chapter 13.

Environmental Care and Safety

Nursing assistants must keep rooms clean and neat so residents are comfortable and safe. This includes making beds; changing the room temperature and lighting; emptying trash; and removing possible

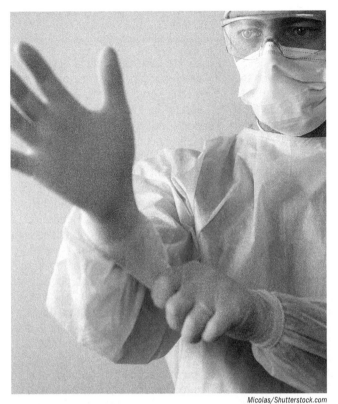

Figure 1.5 To maintain infection control, nursing assistants sometimes wear personal protective equipment (PPE).

Micolas/Shutterstock.com

safety hazards or sources of personal injury, such as spills or objects left on the floor. Practicing environmental safety might also include performing appropriate emergency procedures. You may perform emergency procedures, such as responding to fainting or a seizure, or evacuating residents in case of fires and other environmental emergencies. See Chapter 4, Chapter 5, and Chapter 17 for more information.

Specimen Collection

When directed, nursing assistants collect specimens from residents. Specimens may include *sputum* (mucus from the respiratory system), urine, or *feces* (stool). These specimens help in diagnosing illnesses, preparing for a procedure, or evaluating progress. After collection, specimens are labeled and taken to a clinical laboratory for analyses. Information about collecting specimens can be found in Chapter 16.

What Is a Typical Day for a Nursing Assistant?

When you work as a holistic nursing assistant, you will find that no two days are exactly the same. While there is no "typical" day for a nursing assistant, there are several major duties nursing assistants perform while giving care to residents:

- answering *call lights*, which let staff know that a resident is in need
- assisting with daily needs while promoting independence
- measuring and documenting vital signs
- serving meals and feeding residents when necessary (**Figure 1.6**)
- transporting residents
- lifting or turning residents
- making beds and helping change soiled linens or gowns
- helping maintain personal hygiene
- assisting with toileting
- recording food intake
- measuring and documenting fluid intake and output
- collecting required specimens
- observing and reporting health issues, behaviors, and responses to the licensed nursing staff
- assisting staff with any required tasks involving care
- keeping all lines of communication open
- protecting residents' rights, privacy, confidentiality, and dignity
- being sensitive to and respectful of diversity
- promoting safety and well-being
- making sure all care provided is of the highest quality

When you work as a nursing assistant, you will often perform the same duties daily. Remember that these duties are very important. They will make a difference in the health and well-being of those in your care.

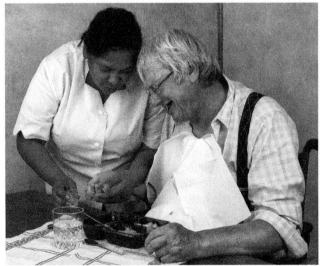

Anneka/Shutterstock.com

Figure 1.6 In a typical day, a nursing assistant might serve meals and feed residents, if necessary.

SECTION 1.1 **Review and Assessment**

Key Terms Mini Glossary

activities of daily living (ADLs) actions that residents take during a typical day; includes bathing, walking, eating, dressing, and toileting.

ambulating moving about or walking.

certification a credential earned when a person has completed the designated education, training, and testing that prepares him or her for a specific field, discipline, or professional advancement.

certified nursing assistant (CNA) a person who has successfully completed the education and training needed to take and pass the CNA state certification competency examination; scope of practice is regulated by the state, and CNAs are supervised by registered nurses (RNs) or licensed practical/vocational nurses (LPNs/LVNs); in some states, CNAs are called *nurse aides, licensed nursing assistants,* or *registered nursing assistants.*

compassion the desire to help another person who is suffering or in pain.

contaminated soiled or dirty as a result of contact or mixture with something that is not clean.

empower to give a person the power to control his or her own destiny and decision making.

holistic care care that is sensitive to a person's values and desires and that integrates a person's physical (body), emotional (mind), and spiritual (spirit) needs to help achieve the highest level of well-being possible.

hospice a healthcare facility or service that provides supportive care for those who are terminally ill and their families; is available on-site at healthcare facilities or in private homes.

infection control policies and procedures used to lessen the risk of spreading diseases and infections.

job description a written document that describes the duties, responsibilities, and qualifications required for a particular position.

licensed nursing staff nursing staff members who have passed state licensing examinations that allow them to perform healthcare tasks within their scope of practice; RNs and LPNs/LVNs.

licensed practical/vocational nurse (LPN/LVN) a person who has successfully completed the education and training needed to take and pass an LPN/LVN state licensing examination; scope of practice is regulated by the state, and LPNs/LVNs provide care under the supervision of

an RN; care can include monitoring and reporting, preparing and giving medications, inserting catheters, and performing wound care.

patients people who visit a healthcare facility, such as a hospital, for a physical examination or for the treatment of an illness or disease.

registered nurse (RN) a person who has successfully completed the education and training needed to take and pass an RN state licensing examination; delivers nursing care, assesses residents, and provides nursing diagnoses; also plans, implements, and evaluates care.

residents people staying in a long-term care facility due to age, illness, or inability to care for themselves at home.

scope of practice the specific responsibilities, procedures, and actions of a healthcare provider, as permitted by state regulations; actions within the scope of practice are allowed only when special educational requirements have been met and when knowledge and skill competency are demonstrated.

vital signs the rates or values of a person's body temperature, pulse, respirations, and blood pressure.

Apply the Key Terms

Write a sentence using each key term properly.

1. ambulating
2. infection control
3. compassion
4. vital signs
5. activities of daily living

Know and Understand the Facts

1. Discuss the role a holistic nursing assistant has when delivering care.
2. Describe four duties a holistic nursing assistant may perform during a "typical day."
3. List three measurements or observations a nursing assistant may be responsible for performing.

Analyze and Apply Concepts

1. Explain how OBRA affects the role and responsibilities of a nursing assistant.

2. Describe three actions a person must take to become a certified nursing assistant.
3. List five responsibilities you will have as a nursing assistant.

Think Critically

Read the following care situation. Then answer the questions that follow.

Jenny is thinking about becoming a nursing assistant. She recently found out she will need to successfully complete a program and then pass an examination to become a nursing assistant. She is concerned about how well she will do in the program, but she is also afraid to take the certification competency examination.

1. What advice would you give Jenny to help her achieve her dream of becoming a nursing assistant?
2. How might Jenny decrease her fears about the nursing assistant program and examination?

Professionalism and Boundaries

Objectives

To achieve the objectives for this section, you must successfully:

- **identify** the qualities and professional behaviors needed to deliver safe, quality care.
- **describe** the personal and professional boundaries of a nursing assistant.

Key Terms

Learn these key terms to better understand the information presented in the section.

attitudes
boundaries
Centers for
   Disease Control and
   Prevention (CDC)
competence
culture

integrity
positive regard
professional
resilience
unethical
values
work ethic

Questions to Consider

- Being *professional* means having knowledge and skills that show others you are competent to do a particular job. Being professional also means demonstrating behaviors and attitudes that are positive and supportive of others. Have you ever been in a position where you were asked to be professional? Maybe this happened at a job or at a special meeting you attended.
- What was the experience of being professional like? Did you have to act and dress differently?
- How comfortable are you acting professional? Is acting in a professional manner something you can do every day, even if it feels uncomfortable?

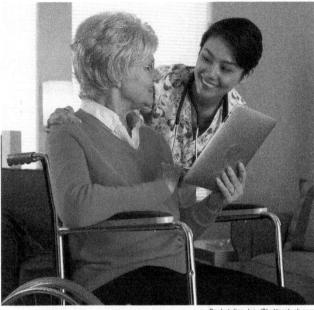

Rocketclips, Inc./Shutterstock.com

Figure 1.7 Being a nursing assistant gives you the opportunity to make a difference in someone's life. You can provide the best care possible by acting professionally.

What Professional Qualities, Attitudes, and Behaviors Are Expected from a Nursing Assistant?

Being *professional* requires the constant, daily demonstration of specific qualities, *attitudes* (ways of thinking or feeling), and behaviors. These are important when delivering safe, quality care. Because working as a nursing assistant can be challenging, being professional is very important. You may work long hours to provide care for ill residents, but the satisfaction of making a difference in someone else's life can make up for feeling tired and frustrated. To know that your professionalism and work are appreciated and valued is priceless (**Figure 1.7**).

Professional qualities, attitudes, and behaviors that make a difference in providing holistic care are those that show you are a thoughtful, caring person. These qualities, attitudes, and behaviors demonstrate your respect for the healthcare facility where you work and for the staff with whom you work. They also help you support and promote the independence and well-being of residents.

Having the qualities, attitudes, and behaviors discussed in this section will help you deliver safe, quality care; keep your skills up-to-date; and make sure the needs of those in your care are met. The healthcare facility's employee handbook may also include specific expectations and guidelines.

Competence

Competent nursing assistants are able to do their jobs well. When you have *competence*, you have learned everything you need to know to feel comfortable completing required procedures safely and appropriately. You also work on keeping your knowledge and skills up-to-date.

Thoughtful, Caring Approach

Thoughtful, caring holistic nursing assistants are often the most successful. It is important to be aware of your approach, be upbeat, and see the positives in what you do. Having an easygoing attitude and a friendly face sends a message to others that you are open and approachable. It lets others know you can be trusted and may help residents feel more comfortable with you. This approach often decreases resident stress. Remember not to spread rumors, share gossip, or act disrespectfully at work. Those in your care need a healing environment.

Professional Appearance

Wearing ironed, clean, wrinkle-free scrubs will help you achieve a professional appearance (**Figure 1.8**).

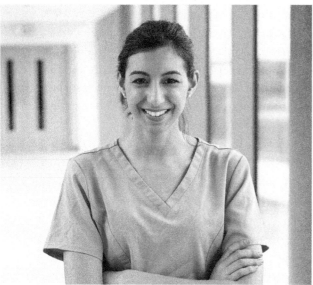

Monkey Business Images/Shutterstock.com

Figure 1.8 Nursing assistants who act professionally look clean and neat. This builds trust with residents and promotes a safe environment.

Underclothing should not be visible. You can wear a neutral-colored, long-sleeve shirt or sweater under the scrubs if cold.

Hair must be clean. If you have long hair, it must be pulled off your collar and away from your face using an elastic band or clip. If makeup is worn, it should be limited to a simple, neutral application of cosmetics. Fingernails should be clean and trimmed short. If nail polish is worn, healthcare facilities usually require that it be clear. Healthcare staff members should not wear artificial nails. The *Centers for Disease Control and Prevention (CDC)*, a US federal agency that helps prevent and control health threats, has guidelines stating that harmful bacteria may grow under artificial nails. These bacteria may be transferred to residents during care. Therefore, having short, clean nails is not a matter of looks, but rather is a matter of safety.

Body art, such as tattoos, must be covered by clothing. Jewelry should be kept to a minimum—for example, small or stud earrings, a watch, and a simple ring such as a wedding band. Body jewelry, including jewelry in the tongue or eyebrow piercings, must be removed.

Physical Stamina

Being an effective nursing assistant requires that you take care of your own health so you have the *physical stamina*, or strength, to perform the duties of your job. Make sure you eat correctly, exercise, and are mindful (aware) of your own well-being.

Respect and Compassion

Holistic nursing assistants understand the importance of treating others with respect and compassion. There are many ways you can show respect for your coworkers and those in your care.

A respectful attitude will help you succeed in your position. Having **positive regard**, or an attitude that is supportive and accepting of others, is another way of demonstrating respect.

As a nursing assistant, you may come across difficult situations that require dignity and compassion. Nursing assistants see residents who are injured, ill, irritable, anxious, lonely, impatient, and depressed. Nursing assistants may also work with residents who are dying. Being compassionate when caring for residents who are dealing with these difficult life situations can ease their pain (**Figure 1.9**). Heartfelt kindness can go a long way.

Work Ethic, Reliability, and Dependability

It is important to arrive to work on time. This demonstrates a positive **work ethic**, or a belief that your work is important. You are responsible to your coworkers and those in your care to be ready for work when you are scheduled. Be thorough, follow policies, immediately let licensed nursing staff know when you observe any changes in a resident's condition, and be accurate and timely in your reporting and documentation.

Trustworthiness

Both your coworkers and those in your care will appreciate working with someone they can trust. Be trustworthy by keeping information confidential and documenting it in the proper place. You must take this part of your role and responsibilities very seriously. It is your legal and ethical responsibility to protect personal and medical information.

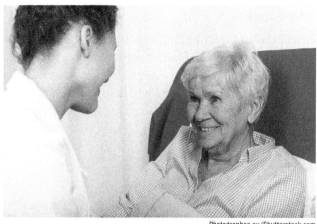

Photographee.eu/Shutterstock.com

Figure 1.9 Nursing assistants promote a healing environment by showing respect and compassion to residents.

Honesty and Integrity

Honesty and **integrity** (strong moral principles) are very important to resident safety. If you make a mistake, you must always tell the truth about what happened. Do not try to cover up the mistake. Residents' health and well-being depend on your honesty. No matter how busy you are or how unimportant you think information is, never leave out details or information about a resident's condition or about care given when reporting or documenting.

Flexibility

Being able to complete a wide range of duties and being able to work independently, when appropriate, are important qualities for any holistic nursing assistant. You may see different residents every day, so become familiar with adjusting to change and to working with new people. You should also be flexible about your schedule, as you may have to work different hours every week, long shifts, or unusual hours.

HEALTHCARE SCENARIO

Employee of the Year

The adult center in your city recently announced that Loretta Sanchez was named employee of the year. Loretta has been employed by the center for the past 15 years as a nursing assistant. The executive director of the center was pleased to share that Loretta was nominated and received the award due to her dedication and loyalty to the center. Loretta's caring and compassionate approach with residents, staff, and families also influenced the selection. In particular, the report noted that Loretta has a very positive attitude,

has a smile on her face, and always has a good word to share. She works well with her team and is ready and willing to take on extra projects and assignments. The executive director of the center stated that Loretta is "an inspiration and a great role model for her peers."

Apply It

1. List Loretta's professional qualities and behaviors.
2. Why do you think the executive director of the center feels Loretta is an "inspiration and a great role model" for her coworkers?

Teamwork

Always work toward being a productive, helpful, and supportive member of the healthcare team. Be aware of and sensitive to ways you can assist other staff. Supporting your coworkers will help increase the quality of your care. This also pays off when other staff members give in return and help you when you need assistance.

Positive Relationships

When you provide care, you will often have close contact with residents' family members, friends, and significant others. Establishing positive relationships with these people will help you provide quality care and create a positive, healing environment. Be calm, kind, supportive, and ready to help when needed. Remember to enjoy what you are doing. A positive attitude will improve the quality of care you provide.

Communication Skills

As a holistic nursing assistant, it is important to understand the differences and diversity of those in your care. Be courteous and communicate clearly and directly when interacting with others in person, on the phone, or by e-mail. Also be sure documentation is well written and easily understood. *Nonverbal communication*, such as gestures and body language, must be considered and should be appropriate to the people you are speaking with and to the situation. You will learn more about developing strong communication skills in Chapter 11.

Resilience

Holistic nursing assistants who demonstrate **resilience** have the ability to recover from or easily adjust to difficulties or change. Resilience is based on your thoughts and understanding of events that are taking place, as well as the emotional energy you have at the time you are dealing with challenging situations or change. To be more resilient, you must see difficulties as growth opportunities rather than avoiding them or shutting down. It is also important to express feelings of gratitude and be appreciative of what you have. Remember to be kind to yourself and to others.

Being professional means putting the resident first. No matter the circumstances, never let your personal feelings and needs get in the way of providing quality care. Being professional also means maintaining high standards. Nursing assistants who act in a professional manner will earn reputations as people who seek the best for those in their care. Acting in a professional manner at work will allow you to relax during your free time, knowing you have done a good job.

Residents depend on nursing assistants. When you are a nursing assistant, residents will put their trust in you. Therefore, you must demonstrate the professional qualities, attitudes, and behaviors you would want to see in somebody who was caring for you or your loved one.

What Are Personal and Professional Boundaries?

As a nursing assistant, you will be expected to demonstrate professional behaviors and establish helping and caring relationships with residents. **Boundaries**, or accepted and expected limits on behavior or actions, are a basic part of all relationships. Both personal and professional boundaries exist for everyone, and particularly for nursing assistants, regardless of the healthcare

---

CULTURE CUES

Understanding Culture

Culture includes traditions, beliefs, rituals, customs, and *values* (ideals) that are learned over time and are specific to a group of people. Think about your own culture and its effect on how you understand and demonstrate professional and caring behaviors. Your family culture may also influence the way you treat others. For example, you may find it difficult to talk with older or sick residents if you have never before communicated with older or ill people in your personal life. You may not have experienced a specific resident's culture and may be unsure how to respond to the resident's specific needs.

Apply It

1. How has your family culture influenced your ability to demonstrate caring behaviors?
2. If caregiving does not come naturally to you, how can you become more comfortable when giving care?
3. Ask your instructor for feedback about ways you can become more comfortable helping others.

facility. Therefore, when acting within your role as a nursing assistant, you must recognize and maintain these boundaries. Maintaining personal and professional boundaries will help you establish appropriate relationships with residents and their families (**Figure 1.10**).

Personal Boundaries

Personal boundaries allow you to protect and take care of yourself. Some personal boundaries, such as not allowing personal abuse or violence, are rigid and absolute. Other personal boundaries, such as allowing someone else to use your cell phone, are more flexible and often need to be worked out between the people in a relationship. Setting personal boundaries lets others know what is acceptable and what the consequences may be if boundaries are crossed.

Professional Boundaries

Professional boundaries are specific to delivering care and are part of a nursing assistant's legal scope of practice. Professional boundaries help you determine the difference between helping behaviors and behaviors that are not helpful. Behaviors that are not helpful, such as not respecting a resident's rights or focusing on yourself rather than on a resident, cross or violate professional boundaries. When boundaries are crossed or violated, an unhealthy relationship can develop.

Crossing and Violating Boundaries

There is a difference between crossing a boundary and violating a boundary, although both actions are inappropriate. Brief, unhelpful acts or behaviors *cross* boundaries. An example of crossing a boundary would be doing something thoughtless or saying something inappropriate, such as telling a resident about the details of your date last night. Acts or behaviors that meet your needs, but not the needs of those in your care, *violate* boundaries. Boundary violations are **unethical** (not in line with accepted rules of conduct), harmful, and in some cases, considered criminal behavior.

Following are examples of crossing or violating a boundary:

- You think a lot about a resident when you are not at work.
- You choose sides with a resident against his or her family or other staff members.

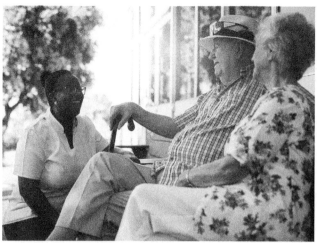

Jacob Lund/Shutterstock.com

Figure 1.10 As a nursing assistant, you will want to establish relationships with both the resident and his or her family.

- You trade assignments with other staff members so you can provide care for a specific resident.
- You share inappropriate personal information.
- You flirt or make sexual comments.
- You share secrets.
- You receive personal gifts after the resident has left the healthcare facility.
- You act in a verbally or physically abusive way.

It is always the nursing assistant's responsibility to maintain both personal and professional boundaries. To do this, use the following guidelines:

- Act and communicate professionally at all times.
- Respect residents' rights.
- Do not visit or spend extra time with a resident who is not part of your work assignment.
- Do not use offensive language.
- Do not make sexual comments or jokes.
- Use touch appropriately.
- Do not accept gifts, loans, money, or other valuables.
- Do not give gifts, loans, or money.
- Do not share personal or financial information.

Nursing assistants are expected to act in the best interest of those they care for and to always respect the dignity of others. This means that a nursing assistant should never seek personal gain at anyone's expense.

The best way to be sure that your care is within professional boundaries is to be aware of and knowledgeable about appropriate boundaries, to have integrity, and to work as a professional.

SECTION **1.2** **Review and Assessment**

Key Terms Mini Glossary

attitudes ways of thinking or feeling about a person, situation, or object.

boundaries accepted and expected limits on behavior or actions.

Centers for Disease Control and Prevention (CDC) a US federal agency responsible for preventing and controlling the spread of infectious diseases and responding to health threats; also provides information and research to the healthcare community.

competence having the knowledge and skills needed to do something well.

culture a set of traditions, beliefs, rituals, customs, and values that are learned over time and are specific to a group of people.

integrity strong moral principles and professional standards.

positive regard an attitude that is supportive and accepting of others.

professional demonstrating an expected level of excellence and competence.

resilience the ability to recover from or easily adjust to difficulties or change.

unethical not in line with accepted rules of conduct.

values beliefs or ideals; set a standard for what is good or bad and significantly influence attitude and behavior; may be shared by people of the same culture.

work ethic a belief in the importance of work; can strengthen a person's character.

Apply the Key Terms

Fill in the blank with the correct key term.

1. When a holistic nursing assistant has an attitude that is supporting and accepting of residents, he is demonstrating _____.
2. Accepted and expected limits on behavior or actions are called _____.
3. A nursing assistant has _____ when everyone he works with knows he has the knowledge and skills to do something well.
4. When holistic nursing assistants demonstrate an expected level of excellence and competence, they are considered _____.
5. A nursing assistant would be _____ if her work was not in line with accepted rules of conduct.

Know and Understand the Facts

1. Identify three professional qualities, attitudes, or characteristics that demonstrate a nursing assistant's caring.
2. List two professional behaviors nursing assistants can demonstrate to show they are competent in delivering care.
3. Describe two examples of professional boundary violations.

Analyze and Apply Concepts

1. Discuss three challenges or difficulties a holistic nursing assistant may have in demonstrating professional behaviors. Explain how these can be overcome.

2. Identify three of your personal boundaries and explain how you are able to keep them.
3. Explain three guidelines that help nursing assistants maintain professional boundaries.

Think Critically

Read the following care situation. Then answer the questions that follow.

Mrs. F has been ill for a long time. Yesterday she was admitted to a long-term care facility because she had pneumonia. Mrs. F had been living with her daughter, who was widowed last year and is still grieving. Mrs. F found it hard living with her daughter because Mrs. F has always been independent. It was also hard for Mrs. F to handle her daughter's difficult behavior. Mrs. F's daughter liked to tell her what to do.

When you introduce yourself to Mrs. F, she turns her back to you and speaks in a harsh voice, saying she hates being in this facility. You can tell Mrs. F is not breathing well. When you go to help, Mrs. F says she does not want you to give her any care this morning. She would rather sleep, so she asks you not to touch her and to stay away.

1. What professional qualities, attitudes, and behaviors would you need to demonstrate in this situation to be sure Mrs. F is provided quality care?
2. What should you report to licensed nursing staff about Mrs. F's behavior?
3. What personal or professional boundaries should you be aware of when caring for Mrs. F?

Key Points

Reviewing the key points for this chapter will help you practice more safely and competently as a holistic nursing assistant and will help you prepare for the certification competency examination.

- The nursing assistant is a member of a healthcare team and provides nursing care under the supervision of an LPN/LVN or an RN.
- Nursing assistants must complete a specific education or training program and pass a certification competency exam to practice as certified nursing assistants (CNAs).
- Holistic nursing assistants provide holistic care, which integrates the body, mind, and spirit. The Providing Holistic Care Framework outlines the components of holistic care.
- The primary responsibility of a nursing assistant is to provide safe, quality care to residents.
- Nursing assistants must act in a professional, ethical manner at all times.
- Nursing assistants must recognize and maintain boundaries that establish appropriate limits in their relationships with residents and their families. Behaviors that violate these boundaries are typically considered unethical, harmful, and in some cases, illegal.

Action Steps to Holistic Care

Review the information in this chapter. Complete the following activities.

1. Select two responsibilities of holistic nursing assistants. Prepare a short paper or digital presentation that identifies and describes two challenges a nursing assistant may have.
2. With a partner, select one professional boundary. Prepare a poster that shows at least three facts other nursing assistants should know about this boundary.
3. Find two pictures in a magazine, in a newspaper, or online that demonstrate professional behavior. Discuss why you believe these images represent professionalism.
4. Research the requirements and scope of practice for nursing assistants in your state. Write a brief report that includes this information and two facts not discussed in this chapter.
5. With a partner, write a song or poem about holistic care and its impact on residents. Include the reasons why holistic care is important, some of the responsibilities of a holistic nursing assistant, and information about professionalism and maintaining boundaries.

Building Math Skill

Janelle, a CNA new to the facility, was asked to measure Mrs. S.'s urinary output. She measured 250 milliliters (mL) and recorded it that way in Mrs. S's chart. When the licensed nurse asks her what Mrs. S's urinary output was in CCs (cubic centimeters), how should Janelle respond?

Preparing for the Certification Competency Examination

To prepare for the nursing assistant certification competency examination, you will need to know content found in this chapter. This content may be tested in the knowledge (written or oral) and skills (hands-on demonstration) portions of the exam. The following areas will be emphasized:

- the nursing assistant's role
- the functions, roles, and responsibilities of nursing assistants
- characteristics of professional behavior

These sample test questions are similar to ones you will find on the certification competency exam. See how well you can answer them. Be sure to select the *best* answer.

1. A nursing assistant who presents a professional appearance
   A. wears a red, printed shirt under her scrubs
   B. keeps her hair below her collar
   C. wears her engagement ring with her wedding band
   D. has short, clean fingernails and wears clear nail polish

2. Nursing assistants who demonstrate caring skills have
   A. an easy-going attitude
   B. a good exercise plan, which they follow
   C. a habit of reading a great deal
   D. a good diet

(Continued)

3. Which of the following must nursing assistants do to become certified?
   A. work in a long-term care facility for a minimum of two years
   B. be in good physical condition
   C. complete an approved education or training program and pass the certification competency exam
   D. receive two positive professional character recommendations

4. What does the term *residents* mean?
   A. people cared for in hospitals
   B. people cared for in hospices
   C. people cared for at home
   D. people cared for in long-term care facilities

5. Which of the following is an example of a boundary violation by a nursing assistant?
   A. taking too much time at a resident's bedside
   B. accepting gifts after a resident has left the facility
   C. putting residents' personal items in the bedside table
   D. helping a resident's family member contact a community resource

6. When nursing assistants provide holistic care, they integrate
   A. body, mind, and spirit
   B. care with medication
   C. therapy with care
   D. culture, ethnicity, and values

7. A nursing assistant with several years of experience has been difficult to work with the last few days. Which of the following approaches could you use to demonstrate professional behavior?
   A. tell the nursing assistant that she needs to be more cheerful
   B. ask the nursing assistant if you can help her
   C. report the nursing assistant's behavior
   D. stay away from the nursing assistant

8. Which of the following healthcare staff members supervises nursing assistants?
   A. doctor
   B. therapist
   C. counselor
   D. licensed nurse

9. Which of the following is *not* a professional boundary violation?
   A. visiting with a resident in your care during your shift
   B. accepting a gift from a family member after a resident is discharged
   C. sharing pictures and stories about your family with residents
   D. defending a resident's desires to his or her family members

10. A nursing assistant is really angry at a nurse on his team. What is the most professional way for him to deal with his anger?
    A. He should post his angry feelings on his blog as soon as he can.
    B. He should ask his supervisor if she can meet with him.
    C. He should send an e-mail message to his supervisor and express his anger.
    D. He should do nothing and just avoid the nurse whenever he can.

11. Which of the following behaviors would lead staff at a local long-term care facility to consider a new nursing assistant "professional"?
    A. working many shifts
    B. leaving work early
    C. maintaining high standards of care
    D. working as quickly as possible

12. Mr. J has been a resident at the city's rehabilitation facility for nearly four weeks. During the last week, he has appeared lonely and depressed. What might a holistic nursing assistant do to support him?
    A. increase his activities
    B. give him snacks several times a day
    C. let him stay in his room longer
    D. ask him about the change in his behavior

13. Which of the following describes OBRA?
    A. a rare disease
    B. a law that standardizes nursing assistant training and education requirements
    C. a law that protects nursing assistants from working in unsafe conditions
    D. a procedure used to prevent residents from falling

14. For which of the following is a new nursing assistant *not* responsible?
    A. helping residents with ADLs
    B. assisting residents with ambulation
    C. discussing residents' conditions with their families
    D. documenting care given in residents' charts

15. When holistic nursing assistants are supportive and accepting of others, they demonstrate
    A. competence
    B. values
    C. integrity
    D. positive regard

Did you have difficulty with any of the questions? If you did, review the chapter to find the correct answer(s).

Welcome to the Chapter

This chapter provides information about how healthcare is delivered in the United States including the types of facilities available, members of the healthcare team, and how healthcare facilities are organized and staffed. Understanding healthcare delivery is important to your success as a holistic nursing assistant. It also provides you with important information that may help you decide where you might work when you become a nursing assistant.

Regardless of where you work in healthcare, you must be fully engaged in what you do and how you care for others. This means you are respectful of and sensitive to others' needs, mentally present when communicating, and self-aware. It also means you self-examine and reflect on your caregiving skills. Learning how to be fully engaged requires you to be an effective critical thinker and communicate professionally.

What you learn in this chapter will help you develop your knowledge and skills to become a holistic nursing assistant. The topics discussed in the chapter are highlighted on the Providing Holistic Care Framework.

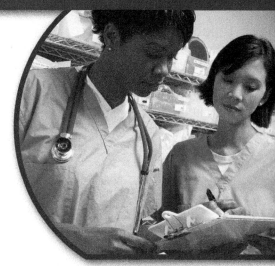

sirtravelalot/Shutterstock.com

Chapter Outline

Section 2.1
Healthcare Facilities
and Teams

Section 2.2
Engagement,
Critical Thinking,
and Communication

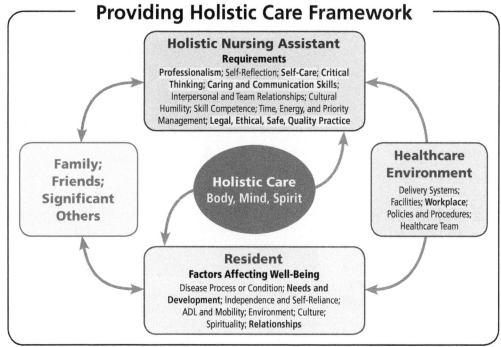

Providing Holistic Care Framework

Holistic Nursing Assistant
Requirements
Professionalism; Self-Reflection; **Self-Care**; Critical Thinking; **Caring and Communication Skills;** Interpersonal and Team Relationships; Cultural Humility; Skill Competence; Time, Energy, and Priority Management; **Legal, Ethical, Safe, Quality Practice**

Family;
Friends;
Significant
Others

Holistic Care
Body, Mind, Spirit

Healthcare
Environment
Delivery Systems; Facilities; **Workplace**; Policies and Procedures; Healthcare Team

Resident
Factors Affecting Well-Being
Disease Process or Condition; **Needs and Development**; Independence and Self-Reliance; ADL and Mobility; Environment; Culture; Spirituality; **Relationships**

Goodheart-Willcox Publisher

Healthcare Facilities and Teams

Objectives

To achieve the objectives for this section, you must successfully:

- **list** important medical discoveries and healthcare leaders who influenced US healthcare delivery.
- **identify** a variety of healthcare facilities.
- **describe** how healthcare is funded.
- **identify** the different levels of a healthcare facility's organizational structure.
- **discuss** how the culture of a healthcare facility influences its effectiveness in delivering care.
- **describe** the healthcare staff you will be working with to provide holistic care.
- **identify** the ways facilities make sure there are enough staff members to provide safe, quality care.

Key Terms

Learn these key terms to better understand the information presented in the section.

acute care	Medicare
census	nursing unit
chain of command	premium
chronic care	primary care
co-payment	provider (PCP)
deductible	private insurance
dementia	ratio
healthcare	Social Security
healthcare services	staffing
immunization	staffing plan
level of care	subacute care
managed care	vaccine
Medicaid	

Questions to Consider

- Have you, a member of your family, or a friend been a patient in a healthcare facility? If so, what type of facility was it? What was the experience like?
- Describe the services the facility offered. Did the services provided help you or others get well?

How Have Healthcare and Medicine Advanced Throughout History?

It was not until the early part of the twentieth century that *healthcare* was delivered as part of an organized system. Previously, healthcare was typically delivered in small communities by family members, some trained doctors, or even the local barber. Over time,

advancements and discoveries allowed the delivery of healthcare to grow into what we know today.

In the mid-1800s, Hungarian doctor Ignaz Semmelweis introduced the practice of doctors washing their hands between patients. This practice significantly reduced death, particularly during childbirth, when infections were often transferred to previously healthy new mothers. The discovery of germs as the cause of disease by Louis Pasteur furthered Semmelweis's mission to improve hygiene practices in healthcare. Florence Nightingale also worked to provide sanitary medical facilities, better hygiene, and proper nutrition, particularly during wartime (**Figure 2.1**). Nightingale is considered the founder of modern nursing because she demonstrated the value of nurses and their positive impact on health outcomes.

After English doctor Edward Jenner successfully administered the first vaccine against smallpox in 1796,

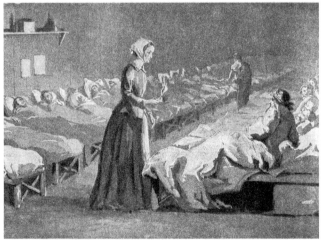

Everett Collection/Shutterstock.com

Figure 2.1 Florence Nightingale served as a nurse during the Crimean War, during which she improved hygiene practices. She also established the first school of nursing and is considered the founder of modern nursing.

the development of other vaccines continued throughout the nineteenth century. *Vaccines* are injections or oral medications that introduce a mild form of a disease so the body builds immunity, or *resistance*, to the disease. The vaccines developed in the 1800s provided *immunization*, or protection, against diseases such as cholera, anthrax, rabies, and typhoid fever. Throughout the 1900s, vaccines were developed for diseases such as diphtheria, whooping cough, tetanus, tuberculosis, measles, mumps, rubella, chicken pox, pneumonia, and meningitis. In the mid-1960s, Dr. Jonas Salk developed a vaccine for polio, a life-threatening disease that had previously left many children paralyzed. Prior to the development of these vaccines, many of these diseases caused epidemics in which a large number of people became very sick or even died.

The twenty-first century brought the wide use of technology to all healthcare facilities. For example, electronic health records (EHRs), rather than paper-and-pen charting, ensure the standardization of policies and procedures and more accurate documentation. Detailed information about the use of EHRs, EMRs, and documentation can be found in Chapter 13. Advancements in robotic surgery, research in stem cells (human cells that can become specific tissues or organs), the Human Genome Project, and the use of evidence-based research (actions based on facts) are all developments influencing healthcare delivery today. These and many other medical discoveries and leaders led the way to establishing what is known today as *modern healthcare.*

What Types of Healthcare Facilities Are Available in the United States?

Medical advances have not only influenced *how* healthcare is delivered, but also *where* it is delivered. Starting in the early 1920s, increasing numbers of healthcare facilities were established. Hospitals replaced homes, for example, as places to treat the ill. Today, there are many different types of *healthcare services* available to those who need care; these services are provided by healthcare facilities. Healthcare facilities fall into three levels, or categories, of care:

1. **Primary care:** the initial medical care a person receives at a doctor's office or a medical clinic. Primary care is used to treat an illness or disease.

2. **Secondary care:** care that focuses only on the prevention of disease or the promotion of health and wellness (well-being). This includes immunization, health education, and health screening. This care might occur in a community or public health clinic or even in a pharmacy.

3. **Tertiary care:** highly specialized care, such as treating trauma (serious injury or shock), burns, or cancer. This type of care is typically found in hospitals or medical centers.

Healthcare delivery may also be described as acute, subacute, or chronic. *Acute care* refers to serious, critical, or surgical care. Acute care is typically given in hospitals. *Subacute care* is provided to a person who has a moderate-to-severe illness, injury, or recurrence of a disease, but who does not require the level of care delivered at a hospital. Often subacute care is given in a specialty facility, or in a long-term care or skilled nursing facility, to people who have a serious episode of a chronic illness or who need intense rehabilitation due to a surgery.

Chronic care applies to those who have a long-term disease or illness that may never go away. Examples of chronic diseases include diabetes; heart or respiratory diseases; conditions that occur at birth, such as cerebral palsy; and diseases of older adults, such as *dementia* (severe loss of mental capacity). Chronic care is often provided in doctors' offices, outpatient clinics, rehabilitation centers, long-term care facilities, or even in people's homes.

A variety of healthcare facilities can be found across the United States:

- **Hospitals:** also called *medical centers*, primarily provide acute or tertiary care for people who have a severe illness or who have experienced trauma that requires surgery or emergency care. Hospitals vary in size and location and can be not-for-profit (do not have to pay taxes), for-profit (owned by investors), or public (funded by the government).

- **Doctors' offices:** staffed with *primary care providers (PCPs)* who may include family practice doctors, internal medicine doctors, nurse practitioners, and physician assistants.

- **Outpatient or community clinics:** provide preventive and wellness care; services offered include annual specialized exams for women (called *well-woman exams*); dental care; and care for the chronically ill. Some outpatient or community clinics have a specific purpose, such as providing only health screenings or immunizations, physical or occupational therapy, or pain management.
- **Urgent-care centers:** sometimes known as *convenient-* or *immediate-care centers*, these facilities treat people with short-term, acute-care needs such as colds, viruses, fractures, sprains, or other minor injuries. Some of these centers are open 24 hours a day, seven days a week.
- **Surgical centers:** also called *surgicenters*, offer a limited range of surgical and diagnostic procedures. These services may include cosmetic surgeries, cataract removals, biopsies (surgical removal of body tissue samples for diagnosis), hernia repairs, or colonoscopies (diagnostic examinations of the large intestine).
- **Skilled nursing facilities:** provide care for people who need short term, around-the-clock care and rehabilitation for conditions such as a stroke, fractured hip, or knee-replacement surgery. The goal is to help patients become well enough to return to their homes and function effectively.
- **Residential care facilities:** there are a variety of levels of residential care facilities that provide services 24 hours per day, seven days a week. These may include independent living, assisted living, continuing care, residential care, or long-term care. Long-term care facilities, or *nursing homes*, are designed to care for residents who can no longer take care of themselves. These residents need medical and licensed nursing care and varying assistance with ADLs, ambulation, feeding, and elimination (**Figure 2.2**).
- **Hospices:** provide care for terminally ill people who have a life expectancy of six months or less. Care may be provided at a residential hospice center, in the home, or in a long-term care facility. In addition to general care services, hospices provide pain relief, grief counseling, family caregiver support, and assistance during the grieving process.
- **Home healthcare services:** employ RNs, LPNs/LVNs, CNAs, caregivers, and home health aides, as well as nonskilled workers to offer services in the home. Home healthcare services may offer companion care, which includes reminding patients to take their medications; cooking meals and feeding; performing light housekeeping; running errands; taking them to appointments; assisting with pet care; and providing conversation or entertainment, such as reading or playing games. Respite care is also offered, which gives family members a break or time off from caring for those who are confined to their beds or dying. Skilled nursing services, such as monitoring blood pressure or providing wound care, may occur daily, weekly, or monthly.
- **Pharmacies:** responsible for filling, dispensing, and refilling prescriptions (**Figure 2.3**). Licensed pharmacy staff members also provide information about medications, including any side effects and interaction between different medications. In some states, pharmacists may give adult immunizations such as flu shots.
- **Laboratories and medical imaging facilities:** provide procedures (checking blood or taking an X-ray) to help with the diagnosis of a disease or condition. These tests also help doctors determine if a patient is getting better.

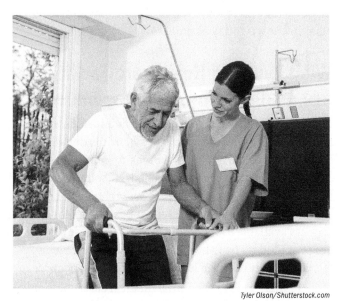
Tyler Olson/Shutterstock.com

Figure 2.2 In long-term care facilities, nursing assistants help residents with ADLs. This nursing assistant is helping with ambulation.

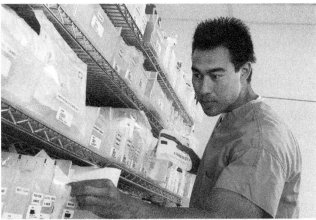

Figure 2.3 Pharmacy staff have different responsibilities in preparing and explaining medications.

How Is Healthcare Funded?

Early in the history of US healthcare, people typically paid cash or bartered (traded goods and services) for their healthcare services. As formal healthcare facilities were developed, how people would pay for healthcare came into question. It was at this time that both public funding and private insurance emerged as options for paying healthcare costs.

Public Funding

Public programs, including Medicare, Medicaid, Children's Health Insurance Program (CHIP), and the Affordable Care Act (ACA), are funded and administered by the federal and state government. They are always influenced by changing healthcare needs, the availability of financial resources, and congressional and executive office directions. As a result, the structure of public programs and the healthcare benefits they offer often change over time. The Centers for Medicare & Medicaid Services (CMS) is the federal agency that oversees Medicare and CHIP. CMS also works with states to provide administration and support for Medicaid. In addition, CMS develops and sets standards for quality care, provides guidance and education, and tracks and shares information about the usage and effectiveness of its programs.

Medicare

Medicare is a health insurance program for people 65 years and older. The funding for Medicare comes from taxes paid to the federal government. Part of every employee's pay is deducted from his or her paycheck to help fund Medicare. Medicare

is considered a prospective payment system (PPS) because payment to providers for healthcare services is based on a predetermined, fixed amount. The removal of a gallbladder, for example, is priced at a certain amount, and that amount is all that is paid to the hospital by Medicare, even if the hospital charges more than that amount for that service.

The federal government also makes automatic paycheck deductions to fund *Social Security*, a program that provides retirement benefits, disability coverage, dependent coverage, and survivor benefits. Employee contributions to Medicare and Social Security are mandatory (required), and employers are also required to pay into these programs. Any US citizen who works a minimum of 10 years qualifies for Social Security and Medicare benefits as soon as he or she turns 65 (**Figure 2.4**).

Medicare is divided into different parts. Part A covers care given in a hospital, skilled nursing facility, nursing home, or hospice, as well as home healthcare services. Part B is medical insurance that covers medically necessary services performed by doctors in their offices or in an outpatient setting. Part B also covers preventive services such as flu shots. Medicare also has a Part C, which is called Medicare Advantage Plans. Part C is a contracted plan between Medicare and a private company; the private company provides both Parts A and B of Medicare and may also offer prescription drug services. Additionally, Medicare has a Part D, which adds prescription drug coverage offered by insurance or private companies approved by Medicare.

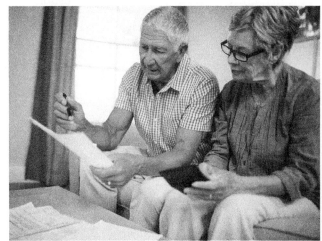

Figure 2.4 After the age of 65, a person who has worked 10 or more years is eligible for Social Security and Medicare.

Medicaid

Unlike Medicare, which is run by the federal government, *Medicaid* funds healthcare at the state level. Medicaid is a program that provides health insurance to people with low incomes, children, pregnant women, seniors, and individuals with disabilities. Each state has its own requirements for those who qualify for Medicaid. Medicaid also offers long-term care insurance, which covers the cost of medically necessary services in long-term care facilities for people with limited financial resources.

The Patient Protection and Affordable Care Act (ACA)

The Patient Protection and Affordable Care Act (ACA) was passed into law in 2010. The purpose of this law is to increase the quality of care and healthcare accessibility, while also decreasing healthcare spending and making healthcare affordable for many who do not have adequate coverage. ACA offers protections for people with preexisting conditions, bans lifetime limits on insurance benefits, offers coverage for individuals under the age of 26 under a parent's healthcare plan, and provides free preventive services, among other benefits. Large employers are required to insure employees, and an insurance marketplace called an *exchange* exists to provide people with a place to shop for free or low-cost private health insurance.

Private Insurance

Private insurance is another way to pay for healthcare. People may have private insurance as a benefit through their work or they may pay for it on their own. Employers typically only pay for a portion of the insurance cost, and the employee is responsible for paying the remainder a *premium*. The premium pays for the specified coverage for the employee and, if elected, his or her family.

Over the years, the cost of these plans has increased, causing some employers to ask their employees to pay for more of these costs. The amount of money a person is required to pay out of pocket to cover healthcare costs is called a *deductible*. Many private insurance plans have *co-payments*, which are fixed amounts that a person pays for specific medical services, such as for a doctor's visit. In these situations, the insurance company pays part of the total fee, but not all of it.

The employer determines the insurance company and coverage offered. Employee benefits may include coverage for a managed care plan or another type of plan that offers a variety of different healthcare services, such as hospitalization, doctor visits, and specialists. Vision or dental plans may also be included in an employee's benefits, as well as prescription drug coverage. These benefits usually change each year, depending on what is available from the private insurance company and how much it will cost the employer.

Long-term care insurance has become more common with increasing life expectancies. This type of insurance generally covers home care, assisted living, adult day care, respite care, hospice, and nursing homes.

Managed Care

During the 1970s, health maintenance organizations (HMOs) were developed in the United States. HMO healthcare facilities were the first to offer *managed care*. Managed care is a form of insurance in which there are contracts with specific healthcare providers who will deliver care at a reduced cost. This group of

---

HEALTHCARE SCENARIO

The Impact of Medicaid

Today, the governor in a neighboring state is proposing to cut $130 million from her state's Medicaid budget. The governor says she will do everything possible so the state's one million Medicaid recipients will notice little change in their healthcare services. However, an interview with Mrs. Pearl Carlson, who lives in the state, shows the concerns of those who use Medicaid. Mrs. Carlson stated, "I worry that, if this happens, I won't be able to afford my husband's care at the long-term care facility he must stay in." The governor is planning a press conference to discuss this change tomorrow at noon at the capitol building.

Apply It

1. From what you have learned about the different financing programs, what effect do you think these cuts could have on the Medicaid program?
2. If this change happens, what might Mrs. Carlson need to do so that her husband has the care he needs? How will this affect their lives?

providers is called the plan's *network*. Each insured person receives most, or all, care from one in-network primary care provider (PCP). The PCP manages and coordinates care and provides a referral if a specialist is necessary. In an HMO, there are also deductibles and co-payments for visits. People who receive care outside the network have to pay for all, or most, of their care.

Managed care can also be offered as a preferred provider organization (PPO). In this approach, the health plan contracts with a broad network of preferred providers from which a person can choose. A primary care provider is not needed, nor are referrals. There are annual deductibles and co-payments for a doctor's visit, which may be higher than in an HMO. People who decide to choose a provider not in the PPO may have to pay a higher amount, pay the provider directly, and then request reimbursement by filing a claim.

While it is important to understand how individuals might pay for their healthcare, it should not matter what insurance arrangements people have. Healthcare staff should treat all residents with the same dignity and respect. Always remember that residents are paying your salary as a nursing assistant, whether it is through federal or state programs, private insurance, or their own out-of-pocket payment.

Which Healthcare Staff Members Work with Nursing Assistants?

One exciting part of working in healthcare is that you will become a member of a healthcare team. Teamwork is of the utmost importance in healthcare because it helps ensure that residents are receiving safe, quality holistic care. To find your place on the healthcare team, you will need to know and understand the different roles and responsibilities of healthcare staff. Several team members are directly involved in the care of residents and work closely with nursing assistants:

- **Doctor (MD or DO):** often called a *physician, primary care provider (PCP), medical doctor (MD),* or *doctor of osteopathic medicine (DO)*; responsibilities include diagnosing illness; evaluating progress; prescribing medications; ordering treatments, laboratory tests, or X-rays; and ordering admissions, transfers, and discharges in and out of healthcare facilities.

- **Registered nurse (RN):** leads the nursing team and is accountable for the coordination of healthcare services; for nursing care; and for the assessment and evaluation of treatments, medications, and progress.
- **Licensed practical/vocational nurse (LPN/LVN):** a licensed caregiver who can administer medications, perform treatments (such as applying sterile dressings), and assist with ADLs.
- **Caregiver:** typically works in assisted living facilities or in people's homes, provides assistance with ADLs as needed, and other support services.
- **Health unit coordinator (HUC):** also known as a *unit secretary* or *unit clerk*, is trained to coordinate the administrative and support responsibilities of a nursing unit or healthcare facility (**Figure 2.5**).
- **Laboratory, medical imaging, and respiratory therapy staff:** responsible for procedures such as drawing blood, collecting specimens, taking X-rays, and providing breathing treatments.
- **Care support staff:** trained on the job, these individuals may work as housekeeping staff, who keep the facility clean and maintain infection control, or transport aides, who assist nursing assistants during transfer or discharge.
- **Case manager:** provides special resources and support for residents, such as planning and implementing assistance for a resident who is going home or aiding in the process of moving a patient from a hospital to a long-term care facility.

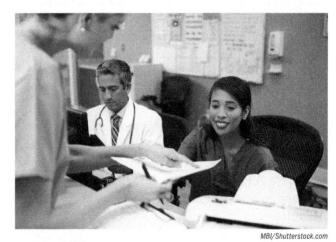

MBI/Shutterstock.com

Figure 2.5 The HUC performs administrative and support functions for healthcare staff.

- **Social worker:** similar to case managers, but social workers have specialized education that emphasizes the psychological, social, and economic aspects of healthcare. Social workers may also assist residents with financial, emotional, or other aspects of their care.
- **Physical therapist (PT):** oversees rehabilitation and restoration under the guidance of a plan of care and with the help of an assistant—either a physical therapy assistant (PTA) or a rehabilitation or restoration aide. Physical therapists may work with residents during recovery to help them achieve the highest levels of function possible (**Figure 2.6**).
- **Speech therapist:** helps residents return to their pre-illness states and restore as much function as possible. For example, a speech therapist might help a resident learn how to swallow and speak again after a stroke.
- **Occupational therapist (OT):** works with residents who have trouble performing daily tasks due to injury or illness to restore their ability to perform ADLs.
- **Dietitian:** helps residents with their nutritional needs by creating special diets, helps residents adjust to new diets, and educates them about these diets.

How Are Healthcare Facilities and Nursing Units Structured?

A healthcare facility's organizational structure includes the staff members who work at the facility, the levels at which staff members work, and each person's decision-making authority. This structure is needed to effectively accomplish the facility's mission and goals. The organizational structure outlines the delivery of care and the communication networks that function based on the facility's *chain of command* (levels of authority).

Most healthcare facilities use a similar organizational structure, although no two organizations are exactly the same. A facility's unique mission, vision, values, leadership, and staff all impact how the organization functions.

Every healthcare facility has a chart illustrating its organizational structure and chain of command (**Figure 2.7**). This chart typically includes four levels that show the facility's organization, positions within the facility, and the names of staff who hold

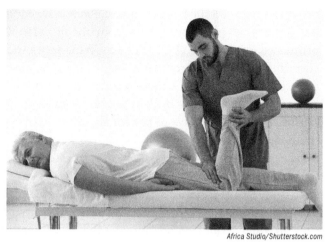

Africa Studio/Shutterstock.com

Figure 2.6 Physical therapists help residents regain flexibility and mobility.

each position. The four different levels shown on the chart will help you understand the facility and who is responsible for different departments.

1. **First level:** as a nursing assistant, you will work at the first level of a facility's organizational structure. You will deliver care on a *nursing unit*, which is an area within a healthcare facility that serves a group of residents. RNs and LPNs/LVNs also work on this level and supervise nursing assistants. A member of the licensed nursing staff is usually assigned as the nurse in charge. This person delegates, or transfers, specific duties you need to perform and will provide guidance (**Figure 2.8**). You should communicate any concerns or resident issues to the nurse in charge.
2. **Second level:** licensed nursing staff members at this level are usually called *nurse managers*. The nurse manager is responsible for supervising and monitoring staff, creating schedules, conducting orientation for new employees, and creating the budget for the nursing unit.
3. **Third level:** staff oversees the entire facility and are considered the top level of the chain of command for nursing. This level includes a chief nursing officer (CNO) or a director of nursing (DON). This nurse has the highest authority over the nursing staff members who work on the nursing unit and is totally responsible for the resident's care, safety, the nursing budget, nursing unit staffing, and the quality of nursing care delivery. The CNO or DON is ultimately responsible for the facility's nursing *reputation*, or how others view the facility.

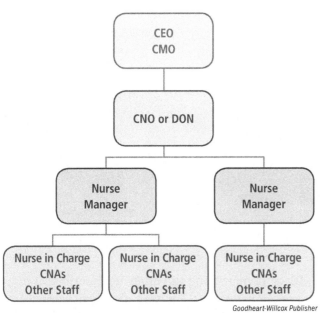

Goodheart-Willcox Publisher

Figure 2.7 An organizational chart like this one outlines the chain of command within a healthcare facility and important communication channels.

4. **Fourth level:** consists of a chief executive officer (CEO) or administrator, who has full authority and responsibility for all staff in the healthcare facility. In many healthcare facilities, there is also a chief medical officer (CMO). The CMO has the same authority as the CEO, but is responsible only for doctors and the care they provide in the facility.

How Does the Culture of a Healthcare Facility Affect Care?

Along with its structure, a healthcare facility also has a culture. *Culture* includes its mission, vision, values, traditions, languages, and customs. Culture also includes the way a facility's staff members feel, think, and behave. Rules and procedures, both official and unofficial, shape the culture of a healthcare facility. For example, in some nursing units, staff birthdays are celebrated at the end of the month and not when they actually occur, laboratory personnel cannot sit in certain areas when they come to draw blood, or wheelchairs can be stored only according to written policy and procedures.

Culture is developed over time, often by the leadership of the facility or nursing unit and by other staff. Different nursing units within the same healthcare facility may have unique cultures. The culture of a facility or nursing unit might be

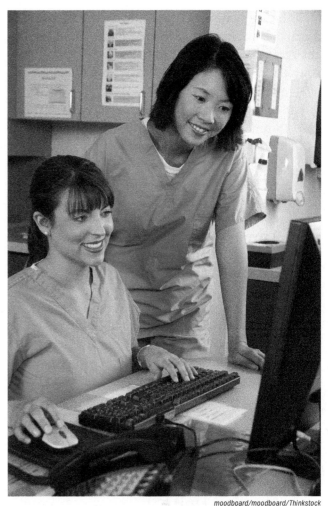

moodboard/moodboard/Thinkstock

Figure 2.8 A member of the licensed nursing staff will be the nurse in charge, supervising and providing help for nursing assistants to perform required tasks.

described as positive or negative. The perception of a particular unit's culture often depends on the personal experiences of staff. The nurse in charge or nurse manager greatly influences the overall culture.

Culture affects the entire healthcare facility and can greatly impact delivery of care. When you begin a new job, it is helpful to determine if you fit within the specific culture of the healthcare facility. To do this, ask yourself if your beliefs and values match well with those of the facility and with the way care is being delivered. Work can become stressful if you find you do not fit well with the facility's culture. Over time, trying to work in a culture that fits poorly with your personality and work style can cause physical and mental fatigue. Since it is unlikely that a facility's culture will change, you will need to make changes in your approach and style if you want to remain working at the facility.

There are some signs that will help you determine if a facility's culture is a good fit for you. If the answers to any of the following questions are not to your liking, then the fit may not be a good one.

- Are staff members recognized for doing a good job?
- Is communication between shifts open, and does it promote a good working environment?
- Do staff members get along well and generally like each other (**Figure 2.9**)?
- Are staff members on a first-name basis with each other?
- Are staff members encouraged to ask questions and give input into how a nursing unit is run?
- Do leaders communicate with staff verbally or use written communications?
- Are there any special rules or policies that can never be broken? Are certain subjects or ideas forbidden from being discussed?
- Is the workplace environment attractive? Is it clean and tidy?
- Are the nursing units noisy or quiet?
- Are there quiet areas or places for the staff to take breaks?
- Are there seating areas for families and visitors?

What Is It Like Working on a Nursing Unit?

Many healthcare facilities operate 24 hours a day, 365 days a year. Each nursing unit in a given facility has an organizational structure similar to the one described earlier.

Healthcare facilities divide the 24 hours in a day into shifts, or periods of time at work. Shifts may be

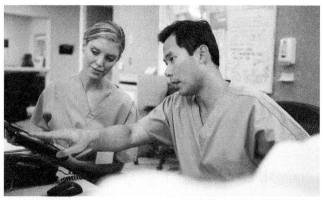
Monkey Business Images/Shutterstock.com

Figure 2.9 Each healthcare facility has a culture. How you fit in with this culture will make a difference in your job satisfaction.

8, 10, or 12 hours long and often are described as *day, evening,* or *night shifts*. For example, if you worked an eight-hour day shift, you might start work at 7:00 a.m. and work until 3:00 p.m. If you worked a 12-hour day shift, you might start work at 7:00 a.m. and work until 7:00 p.m. The lengths and structures of shifts are determined by facility policy, services provided, and sometimes the types of residents. Healthcare facilities may also have overlapping shifts, where staff members are asked to work shifts that cover the busier parts of the day. An example of an overlapping shift would be a shift that lasted from 11:00 a.m. to 7:00 p.m.

Healthcare delivery is usually a 24-hour responsibility in long-term care facilities and hospitals, so a traditional Monday-through-Friday, 40-hour workweek may not apply (**Figure 2.10**). For example, you may be assigned to work a 12-hour shift three days a week or for six days in a two-week period. If you work eight-hour shifts, you will probably work five days a week or for 10 days in a two-week period. There are usually requirements

---

BECOMING A HOLISTIC NURSING ASSISTANT
Contributing to a Positive Culture

Being a holistic nursing assistant means you are a major contributor to your healthcare facility's culture. Your positive attitude and passion for delivering safe, quality care will make a difference in residents' lives and in the facility where you work. The following guidelines can help you contribute to a positive culture:

- Be aware of your feelings and behaviors and how you express them. People will notice if you are approaching them in a positive and supportive way.
- Be sure to take care of yourself. Take your breaks to give yourself the energy you need during a shift and eat healthy snacks.
- Be *mindful*, or mentally present and aware.

When you adopt these behaviors, attitudes, and actions, you will find that having passion for what you do and exhibiting a positive attitude come easily and effortlessly. You can even encourage others to follow by being their positive role model.

Apply It

1. If asked, would people say you are a positive and supportive person? Explain your answer.
2. Are you mentally present when you work with others? If not, what can you do to be more present?
3. What healthy habits do you have? What can you do to become even healthier?

for how many weekends and holidays staff must work. For example, often staff are required to work every other weekend and some holidays. Other policies related to scheduling are typically specific to the healthcare facility, the nursing unit, and sometimes the type of care being given.

How Are Healthcare Facilities Staffed?

Staffing is the process of determining the numbers and types of healthcare staff needed to care for a group of residents on a nursing unit. Staffing a nursing unit can be complicated because the need for staff and the financial objectives of the healthcare facility must be balanced. The nurse manager of the nursing unit is usually responsible for its staffing. In a healthcare facility, the mix of staff should include those with skills that match the nursing unit's *census* (number of residents) and required *levels of care* (types of care). During one shift, staffing needs might change due to changes in:

- the number of residents who are admitted, transferred to another facility, or discharged
- the levels of care needed due to changes in condition

The *ratio* (the number of residents per each healthcare staff member) is also considered when developing the *staffing plan* for a nursing unit. The staffing plan is a formal document that shows the mix and types of staff members who will work on each shift in the nursing unit. In a typical nursing unit, there are usually 10 residents for each nursing assistant. In units where residents have more serious conditions, the ratio may change so there are fewer residents for each nursing assistant.

The actual mix of the types and levels of staff is determined by the healthcare facility. Some hospitals, for example, do not hire nursing assistants; instead, they hire only RNs, LPNs/LVNs, and other healthcare

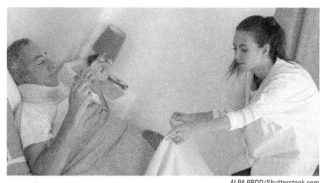

ALPA PROD/Shutterstock.com

Figure 2.10 Healthcare is a 24-hour responsibility. As a nursing assistant, you may have to work unusual shifts, such as night shifts or shifts during the holidays.

providers. Other facilities may not use LPNs/LVNs. In long-term care facilities, there are usually many nursing assistants and LPNs/LVNs and a smaller number of RNs.

If a census falls below a set level, corrections must be made. They might include sending staff home or transferring staff to another nursing unit. If the census increases and there are not enough staff members, staff members may be transferred from another unit or called in from home. Internal or external staffing agencies may also be temporarily used to meet the need. Sufficient staffing has a direct impact on providing safe, quality care. If there are not enough staff members, for example, certain important procedures might not be performed, and this can affect safety and resident well-being.

Staffing can be a challenge because it is always difficult to know in advance what the census will be on a particular shift or over time. Even with this lack of consistency, staffing must always be as accurate as possible. Maintaining the necessary numbers and types of staff needed in each nursing unit is very important to providing safe, quality care.

SECTION 2.1 Review and Assessment

Key Terms Mini Glossary

acute care serious, critical, or surgical care; typically delivered in hospitals.

census the number of residents on a nursing unit.

chain of command the levels of staff in a facility with regard to authority; from top to bottom, staff members at each level have direct authority over staff members below them.

chronic care care given to those who have long-term diseases or illnesses.

co-payment a fixed fee, paid by the patient, for specific medical services covered partially by health insurance.

deductible the amount of money that a health insurer, program, or employer requires people to pay out of pocket as their share of the cost for health insurance coverage.

dementia a progressive, permanent, severe loss of mental capacity that interferes with a person's ability to lead a normal life.

healthcare the prevention, diagnosis, and treatment of diseases; the management of acute and chronic illnesses; and the promotion of wellness.

healthcare services screening, diagnostic, and evaluation activities that assist and support the restoration, maintenance, or improvement of health.

immunization a method of providing protection against diseases causing the body to respond to the specific antigens.

level of care the type of care needed for a particular resident.

managed care a form of insurance in which there are contracts with specific healthcare providers who will deliver care at a reduced cost.

Medicaid a US law in 1965 that provides a combination of federal and state financing to offer healthcare at the state level for those with low incomes; participants must meet certain income requirements to qualify.

Medicare a US law passed in 1965 that supplies federal funds to deliver healthcare to people who are 65 years of age or older, who are under 65 years and have disabilities, or who have end-stage renal disease.

nursing unit an area in a healthcare facility in which care is delivered; typically designated by a floor name, area, or type of illness (as in an *Alzheimer's* or *surgical unit*).

premium the amount of money paid, usually on a schedule, to an insurance company for a specific insurance policy.

primary care provider (PCP) a doctor, nurse practitioner, or physician assistant who is responsible for monitoring a person's overall healthcare needs and coordinates care across healthcare services when necessary.

private insurance a plan for the payment of healthcare services; may be purchased by an employer on the employee's behalf or by an individual.

ratio the number of residents in a healthcare facility or unit assigned to each member of the healthcare staff.

Social Security a US law in 1935 that provides retirement benefits, disability coverage, dependent coverage, and survivor benefits; is funded by mandatory payments by employers and employees.

staffing the process of determining the numbers and types of healthcare staff needed to take care of a group of residents on a nursing unit.

staffing plan a formal document that outlines the mix and types of healthcare staff members who will work on each shift in the nursing unit.

subacute care care provided to a person who has a moderate-to-severe illness, injury, or recurrence of a disease, but who does not require acute care in a hospital.

vaccine a mixture given orally or by injection containing a weakened or killed antigen, which causes the body to develop antibodies specific to that antigen to protect a person against a specific disease.

Apply Key Terms

An incorrect key term is used in each of the following statements. Identify the incorrect key term and then replace it with the correct term.

1. Medicaid supplies federal funds to deliver healthcare to people who are 65 years of age or older, who are under 65 years and have disabilities, or who have end-stage renal disease.
2. The process of determining the numbers and types of healthcare staff needed to take care of a group of residents on a nursing unit is called a ratio.
3. A patient has a serious, critical, or surgical problem and is in a hospital because he requires subacute care.
4. A vaccine is a method of providing protection against diseases by introducing a weakened or killed antigen to cause the body to develop antibodies specific to that antigen.
5. The number of residents on a nursing unit is called a co-payment.

Know and Understand the Facts

1. Identify the three levels of care.
2. Describe the roles of three different staff members with whom nursing assistants will work on the healthcare team.

3. Describe what makes up the culture in a healthcare facility.

Analyze and Apply Concepts

1. Define *acute care*, *subacute care*, and *chronic care*. Which types of patients fall into each of these categories?
2. In what two ways do you think you, as a holistic nursing assistant, could contribute to making a facility's culture positive?
3. Discuss four different ways in which healthcare is funded.

Think Critically

Read the following care situation. Then answer the questions that follow.

Marion's mother is no longer able to take care of herself at home. She is forgetful and has not been able to get around like she used to. While Marion would like her mother to stay at home or even move into Marion's home, Marion feels that a healthcare facility offers better care for her mother.

1. What care options are available if Marion's mother stays in her own home?
2. If Marion decides that it will not be possible for her mother to stay at home, what type of healthcare facility might work best, and why?

Engagement, Critical Thinking, and Communication

Objectives

To achieve the objectives for this section, you must successfully:

- **demonstrate** ways to engage residents who receive your care.
- **examine** the characteristics of a critical thinker.
- **explain** how to communicate effectively.
- **describe** the functions of a healthcare team and team member roles.
- **demonstrate** how you can be an effective healthcare team member.

Key Terms

Learn these key terms to better understand the information presented in the section.

anxiety	mindfulness
bias	nonverbal
deduction	communication
engagement	rational
humility	self-reflection
intuitive	stress
journal	systematic
meditation	verbal communication

Questions to Consider

- When was the last time you stopped and took a quiet walk, either by yourself or with a good friend?
- Take a walk today. This time, stop to appreciate what you see. For instance, observe today's sunset, admire its colors, and feel the warmth it brings. Don't think about anything else except the feelings and emotions you have at that very moment. Stay with this experience for at least two minutes. Were you able to focus on the sunset and let all other thoughts and feelings fade away? How did you feel when you looked away?

Why Is Engagement Important?

People enter healthcare facilities because they are ill, are injured, or can no longer care for themselves. When this happens, some people feel *stress*, which is a physical or psychological response to a situation that causes worry or tension. People may also feel *anxiety* (uneasiness and nervousness) or feel lonely or depressed. Some people express these feelings as sadness, hopelessness, withdrawal, or even anger. At this time, attention, support, and care from a holistic nursing assistant can make a huge difference in a person's mental and emotional well-being.

Engagement refers to complete involvement and commitment. In your role as a holistic nursing assistant, being engaged means focusing your attention completely on those in your care. You may engage with residents when you first enter their rooms, while you provide care, or as you prepare to leave their rooms. Engagement can also occur when you are answering a call light. It is also important to engage with your coworkers.

When you are engaged, you take the time to fully address the needs and desires of another. This allows you to give attention that shows others you care about them and provides others with a positive, helpful experience. It has been found that a resident's satisfaction increases when a caregiver takes notice and responds to the resident's needs, answers questions, and acknowledges the resident's presence. Increased satisfaction can decrease a resident's stress and anxiety, which may help the resident heal more rapidly, increase the resident's efforts to follow his or her treatment plan, and improve the resident's cooperation with caregivers.

There are two skills you can learn to achieve engagement—*mindfulness* and *self-reflection*. Having these skills allows you to observe the interactions you have with others and better understand the role you play in them. These skills usually need to be learned and then practiced.

Being Mindful of Others

Have you ever driven somewhere and found that, when you arrived, you did not remember the details of the drive? Have you ever been to dinner with your family and afterwards not remembered a word that was said? These situations—in which you are physically, but not mentally, present—may occur because you are not paying attention. When you pay attention, you are mindful and are present in the moment. You can see situations for what they really are. Being mindful also means being open to your thoughts and feelings, as well as the thoughts and feelings of others, without *bias* (unfair beliefs) or judgment.

Mindfulness can be integrated into daily living in two ways—through informal activities or through a more formal approach called **meditation**. Meditation helps you achieve mindfulness by allowing you to free your mind from thoughts and feelings that may be stressful (**Figure 2.11**). Meditating daily can provide you with time to truly relax and be with yourself.

Informal mindfulness activities can include taking a few minutes out of each day to pay attention to simple activities such as washing your face. This awareness can make you more aware of the physical act of washing and of the emotional response to how washing your face feels. This takes just a few minutes and can help you start your day more mindfully.

Sometimes events during the day are stressful and cause you to feel nervous or anxious. You can regain your sense of being present and mindful by stopping what you are doing for just a few minutes and consciously taking five slow, deep breaths without thinking about anything else. It is helpful if you think

of the word *strong* when you inhale and the word *calm* when you exhale. This simple action can change your focus from feeling anxious and stressed to being present and mindful.

Whether you become more mindful through informal or formal practice, you will soon find that mindfulness spreads to your communications with others. Practicing mindfulness will help you become more fully engaged with your residents, coworkers, friends, and family.

Practicing Self-Reflection

Nursing assistants who practice self-reflection are mindful not only of others, but also of themselves. They examine the work they have done and ways it can be improved. Self-reflection is like giving yourself a work performance review. Self-reflection need not occur at a specified time; you can reflect on your performance when it is convenient. The key is to be honest about your performance. You must regularly reflect on your behavior and actions for self-reflection to become a part of your daily routine. One way to accomplish self-reflection is to be self-aware and to keep a **journal** (written record) of your thoughts and feelings about your work performance and experiences.

Journaling is most effective when you write your thoughts and feelings so they can be saved, read again, and compared with later entries. Journaling is not the same as keeping a diary. When you journal, you list specific actions, resulting thoughts and feelings, and further actions that are meant to improve your skills as a nursing assistant.

How Can You Become a Critical Thinker?

Another important skill that you need to be effectively and appropriately engaged, be self-aware, and to self-reflect is critical thinking. Critical thinking is helpful in many situations, both personal and professional. As a nursing assistant, you will apply critical thinking to work through specific aspects of care delivery.

Critical thinking is a cognitive (mental) process that helps you examine your thinking and the thinking of others. As a critical thinker, you will reflect on what has been done and determine if you are accurate and on target when thinking about specific situations. The best way to understand and learn critical

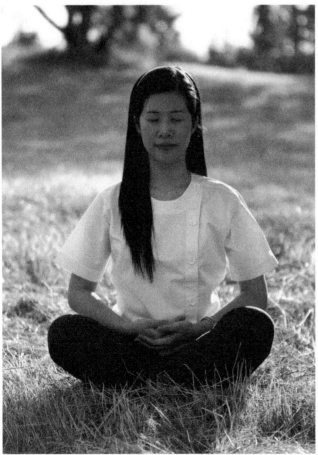

jannoon028/Shutterstock.com

Figure 2.11 Meditation involves emptying your mind of stressors and negative thoughts and instead focusing on the moment.

thinking is to remember its key components. Critical thinking requires the following:

- the ability to be purposeful, *rational* (having clear thinking), and *systematic* (orderly) when examining a situation
- focus and presence
- the ability to form conclusions and make decisions
- an attitude of inquiry
- the ability to reflect on your thinking

Experience and knowledge can help you think critically; however, having little experience or knowledge will not stop you from being a critical thinker. In nursing, critical thinking is an important skill, particularly when you are asked to help solve a problem, observe a resident, or learn something new.

An effective critical thinker has several characteristics. Review the following list and consider which of these characteristics you demonstrate:

- stops and thinks carefully about a situation before acting
- is able to see complex situations and work with them
- can use *deduction*, or use specific information to develop reasonable conclusions
- is able to modify judgments when new information is uncovered
- is objective and reasonable
- is *intuitive* (perceptive) and curious
- is creative
- communicates clearly and logically
- is willing to listen
- can consider multiple viewpoints and shows interest in other people's ideas
- demonstrates confidence and perseverance
- is responsible and accountable
- possesses *humility* (modesty) and integrity
- is truthful and recognizes limitations
- can control feelings rather than letting feelings be in control
- regards problems as exciting challenges

How Can Staff Members Communicate Effectively?

Along with mindfulness and critical thinking, effective communication is an essential part of working in a healthcare facility. It is important that you learn how staff members in your facility communicate so you can interact effectively with residents and their families, visitors, the leadership team, and others. The goal is always for you to communicate in a way that promotes healing and well-being.

As you learned in Chapter 1, nursing assistants are the first line of communication with residents and their families. Nursing assistants spend the most time with residents. Because of this, it is very important that nursing assistants always share relevant information with licensed nursing staff and clearly and effectively provide resident information verbally, nonverbally, and in writing.

The chain of command, which you learned about earlier, plays an important role in a facility's communication practices. Knowing with whom to discuss your concerns, as well as the concerns of your residents, is part of understanding a facility's chain of command. You should always communicate and work out any issues or problems with the nurse in charge first. This maintains the chain of command. If this approach does not work, the next person to communicate with is the nurse manager.

Verbal and Nonverbal Communication

Properly, effectively, and clearly communicating any concerns and issues can help encourage a positive response to and resolution of a potential problem. How you communicate is very important. *Verbal communication*, which includes speaking clearly and using the appropriate words, is important; however, communication is more than the words you say. Nonverbal communication can also make a big difference in how people receive and respond to what you say.

Nonverbal communication includes gestures, facial expressions, body movements, and even your tone of voice. Pay attention to your nonverbal communication to accurately express your thoughts and feelings. If you are feeling angry, this can come across to others through your nonverbal communication. Therefore, avoid angry facial expressions, such as

frowning. If you are happy, express this appropriately. Do not cross your arms when you want people to feel your concern and openness. Older individuals may think actions such as crossing your arms or leaning on furniture express negativity or are disrespectful (**Figure 2.12**).

Written Communication

Another type of communication in healthcare facilities is *written communication*, which includes documentation, letters, memorandums (or *memos*), e-mails, reports, policies, and procedures. Communication, particularly written communication, is used to share information among staff in healthcare facilities. This helps establish mutual understanding about a resident's needs, improves decision making, and helps staff members provide the best holistic care possible. You will learn more about communication in Chapter 11 and Chapter 13.

Professional Communication

In Chapter 1, you learned about professional boundaries and behaviors. Maintaining these boundaries is a requirement for all nursing assistants. Professional communication will help accomplish this. To communicate professionally, you should:

- always speak in a courteous and polite manner
- never use first names when addressing residents and their families, and instead use Mr., Mrs., or Ms. and the person's last name
- use only respectful language and never use names such as *sweetie* or *honey*
- be clear and concise in your directions
- always take the time to respond to residents and their families

---

THINK ABOUT THIS

Research has found that effective communication in healthcare facilities can increase productivity, decrease employee turnover, and establish and maintain a positive work environment.

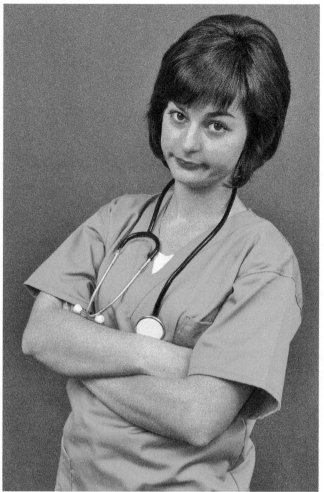

Kristo-Gothard Hunor/Shutterstock.com

Figure 2.12 Some residents may believe crossing one's arms is a sign of disrespect. What do you think this nursing assistant's body language communicates?

- let residents communicate their own thoughts and feelings, and then convey this information as accurately as you can to the licensed nursing staff
- never use offensive or slang language
- never make sexual comments or suggestions
- never share your own personal problems and information with residents or their families
- only share your personal information with those who need this information
- be conscious of your nonverbal communication and how you come across to others
- never post pictures or comments about your workplace on social media
- never send an angry or emotional e-mail or post similar comments on Facebook, Twitter, or other social media websites

What Are the Functions of a Healthcare Team?

Developing strong communication skills is an important part of working successfully with the rest of the healthcare team. The healthcare team, which may consist of a combination of RNs, LPNs/LVNs, HUCs, and nursing assistants, plays a vital role in shaping the facility's culture. No matter where you work as a nursing assistant, you will always be delivering care alongside some of these staff members on the nursing unit. In some cases, respiratory therapists, transport aides, and social workers will also be part of the healthcare team. When these healthcare providers are also included, the healthcare team is usually called an *interdisciplinary healthcare team*. Whatever its composition, the healthcare team is always responsible and accountable for delivering safe, quality care.

Successful Teams

The goal of any team is to work well together, or exhibit *teamwork* to achieve specific outcomes. The healthcare team's primary goal is to deliver safe, appropriate, and effective care to residents so residents achieve their optimal levels of wellness. How well the healthcare team functions can make a difference in this outcome.

For a team to function at its best, its members must trust one another, communicate effectively to establish clear goals, make decisions as a group, and handle conflicts appropriately to ensure a good working relationship.

Team Life Cycle

Successful teamwork does not happen overnight. Teams have a *life cycle*, or a series of developmental stages that influences their ability to achieve their primary outcome. A team's life cycle includes the following stages:

1. **Forming**: the team is established, and team members get to know one another. Team members learn to trust one another and develop positive relationships.
2. **Storming**: effective and ongoing communication becomes increasingly important as conflicts develop between team members. In this stage, learning how to handle conflicts helps make optimal teamwork possible.

3. **Norming**: team members have worked through their differences and determined ways to work together and make effective decisions.
4. **Performing**: team members work well together, resulting in the achievement of the team's intended outcomes.

Establishing a well-functioning and successful team is not always easy. It takes work and practice. Sometimes teams have a hard time moving past the forming stage because of turnover (the number of staff members who leave a healthcare facility) on a unit. Other teams may not move out of the storming stage because team members cannot work through differing opinions and successfully handle conflict. Teams are also affected by the characteristics of their members, such as age, gender, and ethnicity. The leader of the team has a great deal of influence over how well a team will progress through its life cycle (**Figure 2.13**).

How Can I Be an Effective Member of the Healthcare Team?

Working on a healthcare team is a very important part of daily work as a holistic nursing assistant. Each team member has a special role. The following behaviors and actions will help you become an effective team member and a contributor to a successful healthcare team:

- Be dependable. Show up on time and be responsive to the team's efforts.

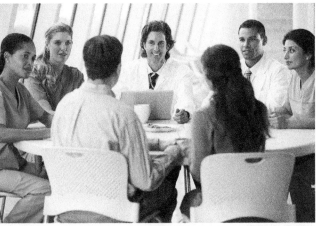
MBI/Shutterstock.com
Figure 2.13 Teams have life cycles. It takes work and practice to become an effective and well-functioning team.

- Participate by sharing your ideas, perspective, and experiences.
- Value the contributions of others.
- Listen and show understanding.
- Speak honestly, but do not blame or judge others.
- Disagree without being rude or argumentative.
- Be positive and open to new ideas.
- Treat everything you hear as an opportunity to learn and grow.
- Show respect and integrity by not sharing confidential information with others.
- Always seek understanding and clarification.

CULTURE CUES

Diversity in the Healthcare Team

On the healthcare team, diversity among team members offers differing viewpoints and perspectives. A diverse team may include people of various ages, people from different countries, and people who practice different religions. Diversity among team members can make a team stronger because everyone brings their special perspectives to the team. These differing perspectives can also create conflict within the team. When team members make an effort to appreciate their team's diversity, learn to trust one another, and communicate effectively

despite their differences, the team will be able to make appropriate and effective decisions and achieve team outcomes.

Apply It

1. What experiences have you had working on a team? What personal strengths do you think you would bring to a team?
2. If you were a member of a diverse team, what special actions could you take to help the team be successful?

SECTION 2.2 **Review and Assessment**

Key Terms Mini Glossary

anxiety a feeling of worry, uneasiness, or nervousness.

bias an unfair belief that some people, objects, or situations are better than others.

deduction the use of specific information to reach a conclusion.

engagement the practice of being fully involved and committed to the task at hand.

humility modesty; the quality of not putting one's self first.

intuitive perceptive about a situation; having insight.

journal a written record of observations and experiences.

meditation the practice of emptying the mind of thoughts, feelings, and emotions to reach a state of relaxation through concentration.

mindfulness the practice of being aware and mentally present in every situation by focusing on what is being said, what is being done, or what is happening in the environment.

nonverbal communication the use of gestures, facial expressions, tone of voice, or body movements to convey a message.

rational having the ability to think clearly and make decisions based on facts.

self-reflection the practice of looking at one's self in an honest and truthful way and being open to any changes that may be needed.

stress a physical or psychological response to a situation that causes worry or tension.

systematic using a specific method; orderly.

verbal communication the use of spoken words to convey a message.

Apply Key Terms

An incorrect key term is used in each of the following statements. Identify the incorrect key term and then replace it with the correct term.

1. The use of gestures, facial expressions, tone of voice, or body movements to convey a message is called verbal communication.
2. When a resident feels worried, uneasy, or nervous, they have stress.
3. A nursing assistant is practicing deduction when she practices looking at herself in an honest and truthful way and being open to any changes that may be needed.
4. When a nursing assistant is fully involved and committed to the task at hand, he has humility.
5. Engagement is being aware and mentally present in every situation by focusing on what is being said, what is being done, or what is happening in the environment.

Know and Understand the Facts

1. Discuss what it means to engage residents.
2. Identify one formal and one informal approach to mindfulness.
3. Identify the key components of critical thinking.
4. List three characteristics of a critical thinker.
5. List five ways you can be an effective healthcare team member.

Analyze and Apply Concepts

1. Describe how mindfulness can contribute to effective caregiving.
2. Describe two informal exercises a person can use to help develop mindfulness.
3. Explain two strategies that can be used to increase engagement.
4. Discuss five ways you can communicate professionally.

Think Critically

Read the following care situation. Then answer the questions that follow.

Lately, it has been difficult to care for Mr. J. Mr. J has not wanted to get up, bathe, or talk with other residents. This behavior is unusual for Mr. J. During the last week, you noticed Mr. J's behavior getting worse. You have been busy and have tried to be helpful and aware, but that does not seem to be working. Each time you walk into Mr. J's room, he turns away.

1. What might be the first action that you, as a holistic nursing assistant, could take the next time you walk into Mr. J's room?
2. What might you say to Mr. J?
3. What engagement strategies could you use to find out what has happened to Mr. J. that is causing this change in behavior?

Summary and Review

Key Points

Reviewing the key points for this chapter will help you practice more safely and competently as a holistic nursing assistant and will help you prepare for the certification competency examination.

- Healthcare services fall into three levels of care: primary, secondary, and tertiary care. Care may also be categorized as acute, subacute, or chronic.
- A variety of healthcare facilities are available in the United States, and each facility specializes in a particular type of care.
- Public funding to pay for healthcare costs includes Medicare, Medicaid, and coverage under the Patient Protection and Affordable Care Act. Private insurance is available to individuals, often through their employer.
- Healthcare facilities are structured to ensure effective communication and decision making through a chain of command. Additionally, facilities have unique cultures that influence the feelings and behaviors of their staff.
- Practicing engagement, mindfulness, and self-reflection will improve the quality of care given.

Action Steps to Holistic Care

Review the information in this chapter. Complete the following activities.

1. Select one way in which healthcare is funded. Prepare a short paper or digital presentation that describes three issues related to healthcare funding not included in this chapter. Discuss one issue that promotes quality and one that ensures a safe environment.
2. With a partner, write a song or poem about the importance of mindfulness.
3. Find two pictures in a magazine, in a newspaper, or online that best demonstrate working as a holistic nursing assistant in a healthcare facility. Describe each image and provide a reason why you selected it.
4. Research a healthcare facility in your community. Write a brief report describing its organizational structure and where nursing assistants work in the facility. Also discuss the mission and values. Explain whether you might like working in this facility.

Building Math Skill

There are 32 residents in the subacute care unit at the Village Skills Center. In the staffing plan, the ratio of residents to each nursing assistant has been set at 8:1 per shift. The ratio is lower in this unit because of the required level of care for each resident. How many nursing assistants will be needed on each shift?

Preparing for the Certification Competency Examination

To prepare for the nursing assistant certification competency examination, you will need to know content found in this chapter. This content may be tested in the knowledge (written or oral) and skills (hands-on demonstration) portions of the exam. The following areas will be emphasized:

- the variety of available healthcare facilities and services provided
- healthcare staff and their roles
- the roles and functions of healthcare teams
- ways of communicating and working with members of healthcare teams
- professional communication

These sample test questions are similar to ones you will find on the certification competency exam. See how well you can answer them. Be sure to select the *best* answer.

1. A nursing assistant is working in a residential care facility. What type of facility is this?
   A. a place where people who have had a stroke can regain their function and abilities
   B. a place where people who have been injured in a car accident can recuperate
   C. a place where people can get cosmetic or other types of surgery
   D. a place where people who need 24-hour supervised care can live and receive care

2. Mrs. G's insurance requires a deductible. What is a deductible?
   A. a type of insurance older adults get
   B. the premium that families pay to cover their children
   C. the cost of private insurance policies
   D. the amount of money paid out-of-pocket for healthcare services

3. What should you do as a holistic nursing assistant to be an effective team member?
   A. share only personal opinions and give advice
   B. disagree without being rude or argumentative
   C. decline when asked to participate
   D. review everything said using your own experience

4. A nursing assistant likes his coworkers and appreciates the praise he gets from the licensed nursing staff. He also enjoys the residents in his care. You could say that the nursing assistant's values fit in well with which of the following?
   A. the facility's structure
   B. the facility's culture
   C. the facility's staffing
   D. the facility's strategy

5. What type of care is given to people who are required to stay in a hospital?
   A. acute care
   B. chronic care
   C. subacute care
   D. subchronic care

6. When communicating, a nursing assistant should show she understands the chain of command by first sharing resident concerns with which staff member?
   A. her coworkers
   B. the DON
   C. the nurse in charge
   D. the nurse manager

7. A nursing assistant who is mindful does which of the following?
   A. makes a resident's bed
   B. is aware of call lights ringing
   C. is present and focused on residents' needs
   D. keeps residents' rooms tidy and clean

8. Mrs. D has just turned 65. She has worked full-time since she was 35 and is planning on retiring soon. For what type of public insurance is she now eligible?
   A. Medicaid
   B. Medicare
   C. CHIP
   D. managed care

9. When nursing assistants engage with residents, they are being which of the following?
   A. compliant
   B. present
   C. happy
   D. noticed

10. Which of the following factors are most important to the staffing of a unit?
    A. census and level of care
    B. level of care and doctor's preferences
    C. census and available resources
    D. staff education and training

11. Which category of care focuses on disease prevention and wellness?
    A. secondary care
    B. tertiary care
    C. acute care
    D. primary care

12. Which of the following is *not* an example of professional communication?
    A. speaking in a courteous and polite manner
    B. speaking clearly and being concise in your directions
    C. using first names when addressing residents and their families
    D. always taking the time to respond to residents and their families

13. Which of the following provides direct services for people who need long-term chronic care?
    A. hospice
    B. hospital
    C. nursing home
    D. pharmacy

14. A nursing assistant is working in a hospice. What type of facility is this?
    A. a place where people who have had a stroke can regain their function and abilities
    B. a place where people who have been injured in a car accident can recuperate
    C. a place where people who are dying can receive care and comfort
    D. a place where people who need 24-hour supervised care can live and receive care

15. Which of the following describes the culture of a healthcare facility?
    A. the structure and organizational chart
    B. the beliefs, customs, and attitudes
    C. the different types of personnel
    D. the communication levels of the facility

Did you have difficulty with any of the questions? If you did, review the chapter to find the correct answer(s).

3 Legal and Ethical Practice

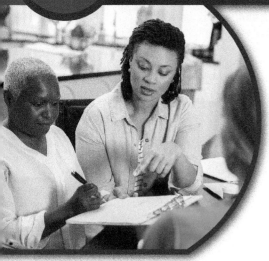

asiseeit/E+/via Getty Images

Welcome to the Chapter

To gain a better understanding of the roles and responsibilities of a nursing assistant, you must know the nursing assistant's scope of practice; regulations that affect healthcare facilities; and the healthcare laws and regulations that you, as a nursing assistant, will need to follow. Legislation and regulations that affect nursing assistants include the Nursing Home Resident Rights and laws related to elder neglect and abuse. In this chapter, you will also learn about why ethical practice is important and how ethical decisions are made.

What you learn in this chapter will help you develop your knowledge and skills to become a holistic nursing assistant. The topics discussed in the chapter are highlighted on the Providing Holistic Care Framework.

Chapter Outline

Section 3.1
Healthcare Laws, Regulations, and Scope of Practice

Section 3.2
Ethics, Problem Solving, and Decision Making

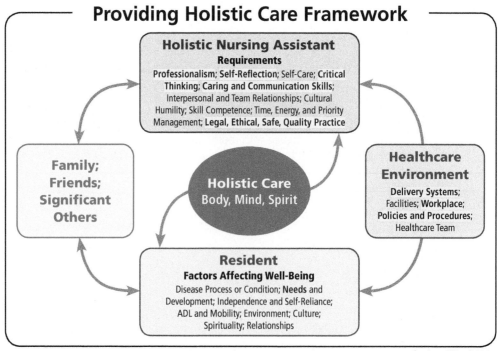

Providing Holistic Care Framework

Holistic Nursing Assistant
Requirements
Professionalism; Self-Reflection; Self-Care; Critical Thinking; Caring and Communication Skills; Interpersonal and Team Relationships; Cultural Humility; Skill Competence; Time, Energy, and Priority Management; **Legal, Ethical, Safe, Quality Practice**

Family; Friends; Significant Others

Holistic Care
Body, Mind, Spirit

Healthcare Environment
Delivery Systems; Facilities; **Workplace; Policies and Procedures;** Healthcare Team

Resident
Factors Affecting Well-Being
Disease Process or Condition; **Needs** and Development; Independence and Self-Reliance; ADL and Mobility; Environment; Culture; Spirituality; Relationships

Goodheart-Willcox Publisher

Healthcare Laws, Regulations, and Scope of Practice

Objectives

To achieve the objectives for this section, you must successfully:

- **describe** the laws that influence healthcare and how organizations are regulated.
- **explain** the key laws and regulations nursing assistants must know.
- **follow** the legal scope of practice for a nursing assistant.
- **abide** by resident rights.
- **respond** to any observed mistreatment, neglect, and elder abuse.
- **identify** ways to avoid negligence and malpractice.

Key Terms

Learn these key terms to better understand the information presented in the section.

abuse	liability
accreditation	libel
assault	licensure
battery	malpractice
civil law	neglect
confidentiality	negligence
criminal law	regulation
defamation of character	rehabilitation
elder abuse	self-determination
false imprisonment	slander
informed consent	The Joint Commission (TJC)

Questions to Consider

- Have you ever watched a television show—perhaps a medical drama—where laws were violated or broken? Maybe the situation had to do with abuse, neglect, or theft.
- What happened to the victim when the law was broken? What feelings or emotions were involved, and how did they affect the victim's life? What happened to the person who violated or broke the law?

What Are Laws and Regulations?

The United States legal system has a long and rich history. *Laws* are formal rules or actions enforced by a legal authority such as the US government, a state, a county, or a city. *Regulations* are rules or requirements that are based on laws and that healthcare facilities and staff must follow. Regulations are usually enforced by an authority, such as the federal or state government.

There are different types of law in the United States. *Constitutional law* is a system of laws that governs a nation, such as those laws found in the US Constitution. *Common law,* or *case law,* is a system of laws established as a result of decisions usually made in a court of law.

Federal laws, such as laws regarding income tax, affect everyone in the United States. States also pass laws that must be obeyed. *State laws,* such as traffic laws, affect only those who live in that state. Within a state, there are also county and city governments that pass their own laws, such as city sales tax.

There are many federal laws that require healthcare facilities to meet specific regulations and standards. State laws also focus on areas of healthcare that include resident rights, safety, and licensure (**Figure 3.1**).

How Do Accreditation and Licensure Affect Healthcare?

Delivering healthcare services means making decisions and providing care that can make a difference in the outcome of a resident's life. Therefore, healthcare facilities must adhere to very high standards and always comply with federal and state laws.

Healthcare facilities must also follow accreditation and licensure rules and regulations. *Accreditation* determines that a healthcare facility meets established

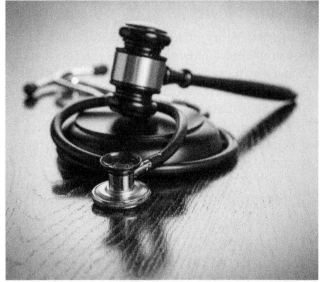

Andy Dean Photography/Shutterstock.com

Figure 3.1 Laws regulate many parts of healthcare delivery, including licensure of healthcare facilities, scope of practice, and the rights of residents.

professional and community standards that promote safety and quality. Seeking accreditation is a voluntary decision made by a healthcare facility. *Licensure* means a healthcare facility meets standards set by law and has the legal permission to deliver care. Unlike accreditation, licensure is mandatory.

Accreditation

Private organizations usually accredit healthcare facilities. For example, ***The Joint Commission (TJC)*** accredits hospitals, ambulatory healthcare services, behavioral healthcare services, home healthcare services, and nursing and ***rehabilitation*** (recovery) centers. The majority of healthcare facilities seek accreditation by at least one major accrediting body, such as TJC. Other organizations accredit rehabilitation centers, trauma centers, chest pain centers, and primary stroke centers.

Licensure

Licensure of healthcare facilities usually occurs at the state level. Specific agencies within a state's health department set the standards for licensure. These agencies also oversee healthcare facilities through routine monitoring, site visits, and consultation. An example of a licensing body would be an agency located in a state's health department that licenses long-term care facilities such as nursing homes.

What Is the Legal Scope of Practice for Nursing Assistants?

The *legal scope of practice* describes, using laws and regulations, what nursing assistants can and cannot do and who supervises them. In all cases, the licensed nursing staff must supervise nursing assistants. Nursing assistants must also have the range of skills and qualifications necessary to perform their responsibilities properly. If using the title *CNA*, they must have a certification.

Understanding Regulations and the Scope of Practice

The legal scope of practice for nursing assistants is defined by regulations. These regulations were established by the Omnibus Budget Reconciliation Act (OBRA), which is a federal law. Since OBRA was passed, each state has determined the legal scope for a nursing assistant's practice in that state.

Regulations regarding scope of practice are usually found in a nurse practice act (NPA) or in other forms of regulation, such as those set by a state's department of health. State regulations outline a nursing assistant's responsibilities in that state, including limits on duties and responsibilities and the definition of competent practice.

Determining Your Scope of Practice

To find out if a responsibility is in your scope of practice, always ask yourself these three questions:

1. Do I have the education and training to perform this responsibility?
2. Is the responsibility allowed by my state's regulations or laws?
3. Is the responsibility allowed by my healthcare facility's policies and regulations?

If the answers to all of these questions are *yes*, it is safe to perform the responsibility. If the answer to any one of these questions is *no*, then it is not safe to perform the responsibility. If you don't know the answers to any of these questions, ask the licensed nursing staff (**Figure 3.2**).

Some states require specific hours of training for a particular competence, such as preventing, recognizing, and reporting resident abuse. In others there may be an addition to the responsibilities of a nursing assistant discussed in Chapter 1. This might include the delivery of some medications as part of a nursing assistant's scope of practice. This added responsibility usually requires additional training and certification. An individual who is responsible

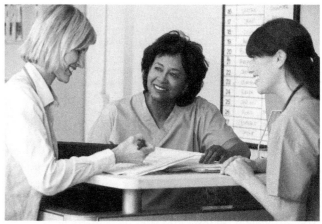

MBI/Shutterstock.com

Figure 3.2 As a nursing assistant, you should always ask the licensed nursing staff if you have a question or are uncertain about your scope of practice.

for specified medications is often called a *certified medication aide, medication assistant,* or *medication technician.* Review the regulations in your state to determine whether this role is included in the nursing assistant's scope of practice and what requirements a nursing assistant must meet to perform these responsibilities.

Working Outside the Scope of Practice

When you work within the legal scope of practice, you know the limitations of your position and are aware of your *liability* (legal responsibility) when practicing as a nursing assistant. Nursing assistants who work outside their legal scope of practice may be disciplined by both their healthcare facilities and by the regulatory bodies that oversee certification in their states. Working outside the scope of practice may affect residents, nursing staff, and doctors. It may also result in disciplinary, criminal, or civil actions.

Disciplinary Actions

The first type of action, *disciplinary action,* is taken when a policy or procedure in a healthcare facility has not been followed appropriately or correctly. Violations that require disciplinary actions can range from being late to work or not following the dress code to not completing a care assignment or not performing a procedure correctly. These violations are usually handled according to a facility's disciplinary policy and procedure. Consequences depend on the frequency or severity of the violation. These may include counseling by a supervisor, suspension from duties for a period of time, or termination. Issues that become formal complaints may be reported to the state board of nursing or state department of health.

Criminal Actions

Criminal actions are taken when someone breaks or violates a *criminal law.* Violations of criminal law may be misdemeanors or felonies. *Misdemeanors* are less serious crimes. Examples of misdemeanors include petty theft, trespassing, or public intoxication. Fines, probation, or community service are often the penalties for a misdemeanor.

Felonies are more serious crimes, such as homicide (murder), arson (setting a fire), or robbery. A person found guilty of a felony beyond a reasonable doubt is often sentenced to time in prison. Felonies committed in a healthcare facility are handled by the state's legal system. When criminal offenses occur, the state board of nursing or department of health may also be involved.

Civil Actions

A *civil action* occurs in response to a violation of a *civil law* (a law that deals with disagreements between individuals and organizations). Negligence and malpractice are two violations of civil law. They are also called *torts* because physical or emotional injury occurs as a result of failing to deliver proper care.

Negligence is the unintentional failure to act or provide care, possibly resulting in injury. An example of negligence might be a busy nursing assistant forgetting to check on a hot compress he or she put on a confused, frail resident's leg. When the nursing assistant returned to the room and removed the compress, the skin on the resident's leg was very red.

Malpractice is more serious, occurs when professional standards are not followed (known as a *breach of duty*), and always results in an injury. An example of malpractice might be the continued failure to properly and regularly turn a frail, immobile resident in bed as ordered. This would cause the resident to spend long periods of time in the same position, resulting in skin breakdown and the formation of decubitus ulcers.

When there is a civil action due to negligence or malpractice, the result is monetary compensation for the extent of injury determined. When civil actions are taken, the state board of nursing or department of health responsible for nursing assistants may also be involved.

To prevent negligence and avoid malpractice:

- give care only within your legal scope of practice
- know and understand all healthcare facility policies and procedures
- always ask for instruction if you are not sure how to do a procedure
- be honest, particularly if you have made a mistake, and inform licensed nursing staff immediately
- document appropriately and effectively (see Chapter 13 for documentation)
- maintain resident privacy and confidentiality of information

Which Laws and Regulations Affect Nursing Assistants?

Overseeing healthcare laws and regulations is primarily the responsibility of doctors, nursing administrators, quality improvement staff, and people working in finance. While a facility's chief executive officer (CEO), chief nursing officer (CNO), or director of nursing (DON) are ultimately accountable for following these laws and regulations, several important regulations are also the responsibility of nursing assistants.

Healthcare facilities, particularly those receiving Medicare and Medicaid funds, must follow specific guidelines and standards. State laws and requirements for licensing long-term care facilities may place additional regulations. These regulations and standards include important requirements, such as maintaining a restraint-free environment. Nursing assistants must learn a facility's specific regulations and understand how these regulations affect the facility's policies; procedures; and delivery of safe, quality care.

Key laws and regulations that nursing assistants must know and follow include the Health Insurance Portability and Accountability Act (HIPAA) and Nursing Home Resident Rights.

Health Insurance Portability and Accountability Act (HIPAA)

In 1996, the US federal government enacted the *Health Insurance Portability and Accountability Act (HIPAA)* to ensure that personal medical information is stored and shared securely, thus maintaining confidentiality. Two parts of HIPAA—the Privacy Rule (2003) and Security Rule (2005)—affect the daily work of nursing assistants. These rules define and protect resident rights and their personal health information.

HIPAA states that *health information* is considered any paper, oral, or electronic record shared with a healthcare provider, insurer, or similar body that can be used to identify a resident. This includes details concerning a resident's past, present, or future physical or mental health; any healthcare received; and payment information related to healthcare. Any information collected that identifies (or could potentially be used to identify) a resident must be protected. This type of information is called *individually identifiable health information* or *protected health information (PHI)*. The HIPAA Privacy Rule covers protected health information collected by any means,

and the HIPAA Security Rule covers any electronic protected health information.

HIPAA is very specific about what types of information can and cannot be shared. For example, a resident may provide a doctor's office a written release that dictates what information can be given to other healthcare providers. This shared information may be needed to provide follow-up care or for insurance purposes. Penalties for disclosing confidential information without a resident's permission range from civil suits to discipline, the loss of a job, and fines.

Confidentiality

In addition to following HIPAA requirements, maintaining the *confidentiality* of resident information is an important part of any healthcare provider's responsibility. To maintain confidentiality, healthcare providers must consider any information communicated by a resident private. They must also know the limits on and procedures for sharing this information. If healthcare providers share information inappropriately, it can be considered an *invasion of privacy*.

Nursing assistants should always remember the following *never* statements about confidentiality:

- *Never* discuss any resident information, including progress, with anyone who is not directly involved in care.
- *Never* read the chart of a resident who is not in your care.
- *Never* remove any resident information from where it is stored.
- *Never* discuss a resident with another staff member in a public place (for example, a cafeteria or parking lot) where information may be overheard.
- *Never* talk about a resident in a way that would allow other people, such as your friends, family, or even acquaintances, to identify the resident.

You must never use electronic mail (e-mail) or social media to communicate anything that might violate confidentiality or to disclose any information about the healthcare facility, residents and their families, or other staff. While residents may discuss their own information on electronic media or publish it on social media, you cannot. If you do, it is considered a violation of ethics, professional standards, policies, and the law.

It is important to remember that content once posted or sent on electronic or social media can be circulated to unintended others. Once posted, the content usually cannot be deleted from an electronic or social media site. Also be aware that it is still a violation of confidentiality if a resident's personal information is communicated to intended recipients even if it is only read by them. It is also not acceptable to discuss or refer to residents on electronic or social media using initials, a nickname, room number, diagnosis, or condition.

Proper and ethical behavior and actions are essential when using electronic and social media. Follow these guidelines to maintain confidentiality:

- Never discuss on electronic media or post or publish on social media sites (closed, open, or secret) comments or messages that contain information, details, or identifying information about residents, including photographs, images, memorials, and tributes.
- Never post or publish information that may lead to the identification of residents. Using privacy settings is not enough to guarantee privacy.
- Never take photos or videos of residents on personal devices, including cell phones.
- Use caution with out-of-facility online social contact with residents or former residents and their families. Direct contact from a resident does not give you permission to respond and become involved in a personal relationship.
- Never post content or otherwise speak for your employer unless you have been given permission.
- Promptly report any identified violation of confidentiality or privacy to the licensed nursing staff.
- Always follow your facility's electronic and social media policies and procedures.

Nursing Home Resident Bill of Rights

In addition to maintaining confidentiality, nursing assistants are responsible for supporting and promoting a safe environment and good quality of life for residents. The Nursing Home Resident Rights used in long-term care contain standards that must be displayed and shared with residents. This document outlines legal and ethical responsibilities for all healthcare providers and facilities. Typically, a bill of rights guarantees privacy of information, a safe environment, fair treatment, and the ability to make one's own medical decisions, among other rights.

In 1987, Nursing Home Resident Rights were established under OBRA and the Nursing Home Reform Act. Nursing homes must meet these federal resident rights requirements if they receive Medicare or Medicaid funds. OBRA and the Nursing Home Reform Act require that resident rights be protected and promoted and place a strong emphasis on individual dignity and *self-determination* (the ability to make choices based on one's own preferences). Some states also have additional laws or regulations that determine resident rights for long-term care facilities and other residential care centers. Residents must be informed of their rights in a language they understand. These rights must be provided in writing and signed by residents upon admission and during their stays. As a nursing assistant, you must abide by and respect the following resident rights:

- freedom from abuse (verbal, physical, mental, or sexual), mistreatment, and neglect
- freedom from physical restraints
- privacy
- have personal items in one's room, manage one's own money, live with a spouse, and privately send and receive personal mail and e-mail
- receive accommodation for medical, physical, psychological, and social needs and full disclosure about medical conditions and treatments
- make one's own schedule and visit with family and friends

CULTURE CUES

Culture and Care

There are times when culture and its related values may impact ways in which nursing assistants act. This may lead nursing assistants to behave inappropriately. For example, if a nursing assistant comes from a culture that believes healthcare providers are authority figures, she may tend to be bossy with residents and expect them do things according to her way and her schedule.

Apply It

1. Is it acceptable for nursing assistants to be bossy if they come from a culture where this is customary behavior? Explain your answer.
2. Certain behaviors can sometimes be viewed as a violation of resident rights. Which rights could a bossy nursing assistant's behavior be seen as violating?

- be treated with respect and dignity
- exercise self-determination, which includes leaving a healthcare facility temporarily or permanently, with or without a doctor's permission (if this right is not upheld, the resident's stay can be seen as *false imprisonment*)
- communicate freely
- participate in the review of one's plan of care, access one's health information, and be fully informed in advance about any changes in care, treatment, or status in the facility (**Figure 3.3**)
- have an advocate or representative
- be told in writing about all nursing home services and fees
- make complaints without discrimination or reprisal

Many facilities have *resident councils*. A resident council is provided with a meeting space and a facility representative who listens and responds to grievances and recommendations of the council.

Informed Consent

When certain medical or surgical procedures are needed, residents must sign an **informed consent** prior to the procedures being performed. These procedures are determined by a doctor and guided by a doctor's order. Residents must understand their treatment choices and the related risks. Either the resident or the resident's legal guardian must be given a detailed explanation of each procedure, including the benefits and risks. Doctors may delegate the responsibility of providing this explanation and getting the resident's signature to licensed nursing

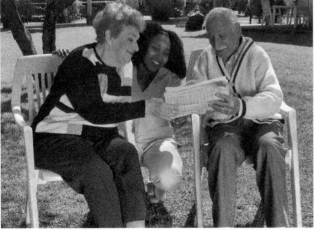

GagliardiPhotography/Shutterstock.com

Figure 3.3 Residents have the right to involve their family members in care.

staff. When informed consent documents are signed, the resident accepts the risks and grants permission for the specific procedure to be performed.

Healthcare providers must always have a resident's verbal permission to give care. Remember that it is not acceptable to force someone to do something he or she does not want to do. Using threats or force to make someone do something is considered *coercion* and an invasion of privacy. To gain verbal consent, you must follow these steps:

1. Carefully explain what you plan to do.
2. Make sure the resident understands.
3. Provide the resident with opportunities to ask questions.
4. *Never* give care against the resident's wishes. Report any refusals of care to the licensed nursing staff.

Neglect and Mistreatment

One important right of residents is the right to freedom from neglect or mistreatment. Holistic nursing assistants must prevent neglect or mistreatment, be able to recognize it if it does happen, and know how to report it. While it is important to be aware of neglect and mistreatment in any care delivery environment, it is particularly significant when caring for older adults, who are one of the most at-risk populations.

Neglect is the failure to provide necessary care that meets a resident's daily needs, such as treatments, medication, food, clothing, hygiene, or shelter. Neglect can be accidental. For example, a healthcare provider may forget to perform treatments or deliver medications. Neglect may also be deliberate. Neglect can cause injury to the resident and may result in sores on the skin, weight loss, dehydration, complaints of hunger or thirst, a body that is not clean, and soiled clothes and bed linens. If you observe any of these signs of neglect, you must immediately report them to the licensed nursing staff.

Defamation of character, which consists of false statements made about a person that damage his or her reputation, is a form of mistreatment. Defamation of character is called **libel** when the statements are written, or **slander** when the statements are spoken. Both libel and slander can result in a legal action.

Assault, Battery, and Abuse

While doing harm of any kind to another person is unacceptable, assault and battery are the most serious types of harm and are considered criminal acts.

Assault refers to any words or actions that a person finds threatening, causing the person to fear harm. *Battery* is the act of touching a person without his or her permission. If you perform a procedure without a resident's consent, it *may* be considered battery. This is why you must always ask for permission from residents prior to performing a procedure, even if they do not understand.

Abuse is a deliberate action, such as assault or battery, that causes harm. There is never an excuse for abusing another person. Abuse can happen to anyone. *Elder abuse*, or deliberate actions that harm seniors, is particularly concerning because seniors may be defenseless due to illness and the loss of cognition (understanding) and mobility. Seniors' dependence on caregivers and family can make them very vulnerable to the frustrations and anger of others, which can lead to abuse.

Elder abuse may be physical, verbal, financial, or sexual:

- **Physical abuse**: the use of force that causes injury and pain. It includes grabbing, hitting, slapping, pulling hair, shaking, or using a restraint inappropriately.
- **Verbal, mental, or emotional abuse**: the use of words or actions that cause emotional pain or injury. It includes threatening physical harm or abandonment, laughing at or teasing a person, insulting or harassing (annoying or pestering) a person, isolating a person, or keeping a person alone in a room over a long period of time with the door closed.
- **Financial abuse**: the theft or misuse of another person's money or property.
- **Sexual abuse**: the touching of a person's body parts in inappropriate ways, suggestive comments or gestures, inappropriate photography, or rape.

Signs and symptoms of abuse include:

- unexplained bruises or injuries, such as broken bones
- burns with unusual shapes
- bite marks
- dry, cracked, or bleeding skin or red marks
- severely poor personal hygiene, such as matted or missing hair, broken and un-brushed teeth, body odor, or decubitus ulcers
- changes in personality or fear when being touched
- attempts to cover abused areas with clothing
- statements by a resident that suggest neglect or abuse

If abuse or neglect is suspected, the licensed nursing staff must be told. Nursing assistants are not responsible for determining if a resident is being abused, but *are* responsible for observing and reporting any signs or symptoms of abuse. If signs of abuse are not reported, the nursing assistant can be legally liable, as reporting this information is required by federal and state laws.

If nursing assistants are accused of abuse, they are usually suspended until a full investigation is performed. Typically, the healthcare facility conducts an investigation; however, state agencies such as adult protective services and the state board of nursing or state department of health may also be involved.

SECTION 3.1 **Review and Assessment**

Key Terms Mini Glossary

abuse a deliberate action (physical, verbal, financial, or sexual) that causes harm.

accreditation an official determination that a healthcare facility meets professional and community standards that promote safety and quality.

assault any words or actions that a person finds threatening or that cause a person to fear harm.

battery the act of touching a person without his or her permission.

civil law a type of law that deals with disagreements between individuals and organizations; money is awarded to the victim for injuries or damages.

confidentiality the act of keeping personal information that has been shared with the healthcare staff private.

criminal law a type of law that punishes criminal offenses; includes imposing a fine or a prison sentence to keep offenders and others from acting unlawfully again.

defamation of character false statements made about a person that damage his or her reputation.

elder abuse a deliberate action (physical, verbal, financial, or sexual) that causes harm to an older adult.

false imprisonment illegal confinement in which a person is held against his or her will by another, resulting in restraint of movement; the person can be confined using force or threats.

informed consent the legal process of getting written permission prior to giving care or conducting procedures.

liability legal responsibility.

libel false written statements made about a person that damage his or her reputation; a type of defamation of character.

licensure official permission given to a person or facility to deliver care; based on meeting standards set by law.

malpractice a form of negligence in which a caregiver does not comply with the standards expected and set by his or her discipline's regulatory body, resulting in resident injury.

neglect the failure to provide necessary care that meets a resident's daily needs.

negligence the unintentional failure to act or provide care that a sensible person would; can result in injury.

regulation in healthcare, a rule or requirement that healthcare facilities and staff members must follow; usually enforced by an authority, such as the federal or state government.

rehabilitation a period of recovery in which healthcare staff members help residents regain their strength and mobility with the goal of learning to function independently.

self-determination the process of making choices and decisions based on a person's own preferences and interests.

slander false spoken statements made about a person that damage his or her reputation; a type of defamation of character.

The Joint Commission (TJC) a private regulatory agency that accredits various healthcare facilities, such as hospitals, behavioral health agencies, home healthcare services, and nursing and rehabilitation centers; facilities that pursue accreditation by TJC must meet specific guidelines and standards for safety and quality.

Apply the Key Terms

Describe the differences between each pair of key terms.

1. accreditation and licensure
2. civil and criminal laws
3. assault and battery
4. libel and slander
5. negligence and malpractice

Know and Understand the Facts

1. List the three questions holistic nursing assistants should ask themselves to determine if they are working within their scope of practice.
2. What is informed consent?
3. What are five signs of elder abuse?

Analyze and Apply Concepts

1. Describe how Nursing Home Resident Rights affect the kinds of care you will provide as a nursing assistant.
2. What are three ways a nursing assistant can maintain confidentiality? Include electronic communications and social media.
3. List the steps you would take if you suspected that elder abuse was taking place in your healthcare facility.

Think Critically

Read the following care situation. Then answer the questions that follow.

Dominick, a new nursing assistant, has been taking care of Mr. C for the past week. He has become quite friendly with Mr. C and likes Mr. C's family very much. Mr. C and his family also like Dominick. Dominick feels he should do extra for Mr. C, but he sometimes forgets to ask the RN whether what he wants to do is acceptable. For example, Dominick makes sure Mr. C's family brings in vitamins and food supplements so Mr. C can get stronger. He also tries to get Mr. C to ambulate even when Mr. C does not want to. Dominick has started walking out with Mr. C's family when they leave the healthcare facility; he lets them know how Mr. C is doing and what more they can do to help him. Dominick has been invited to dinner with Mr. C's family next week, and he is thinking he will go.

1. In what ways is Dominick acting within his legal scope of practice as a nursing assistant?
2. In what ways is Dominick practicing outside his legal scope of practice?
3. Is Dominick violating confidentiality? Explain your answer.
4. Which resident rights is Dominick supporting, and which may he be violating?
5. Is Dominick doing anything in his care that might be considered abuse?

Objectives

To achieve the objectives for this section, you must successfully:

- **identify** ethical principles and their impact on care.
- **explain** the importance of a code of ethics.
- **discuss** the importance of ethical practice.
- **explain** the relationship between problem solving and decision making.
- **describe** the process that is used for ethical decision making.

Key Terms

Learn these key terms to better understand the information presented in the section.

beneficence	nonmaleficence
dilemma	prognosis
ethics	veracity
fidelity	

Questions to Consider

- Have you ever been in a situation in which someone told you to act in a way that made you feel uncomfortable? Perhaps you were told to take something that, while a small item, was not yours to take. You did it because the person who told you to was your friend and said it would be all right.
- Have you been in a situation where you knew you should have helped someone who was struggling, but you chose not to, telling yourself you were too busy when you were not?
- How did you feel about your decisions and actions in these situations? Looking back, should you have made a different decision? Why?

What Does It Mean to Act Ethically?

You must act ethically to be a professional. *Ethics* are principles that guide conduct; they help us determine what is the right or wrong thing to do. A person's ethics and values are influenced by his or her parents, significant others, teachers, friends, and experiences. Each person has his or her own set of values. Some people might value education or happiness, while others value earning a lot of money or enjoying leisure time. Values influence a person's attitudes and behavior and are the basis of ethics and a person's ethical practice. It is important for you to know and understand your values so you can determine how they might affect your ability to practice ethical caregiving.

Principles of Ethical Caregiving

There are several important ethical principles in caregiving. These principles specify how residents should be seen and approached and how healthcare staff should practice ethically:

- **Autonomy**: residents should maintain their own values and uniqueness.
- **Freedom**: residents should function independently and make their own decisions (**Figure 3.4**).
- **Confidentiality**: residents have the right to privacy and to the expectation that information will not be shared in an unethical or illegal manner.
- *Beneficence*: healthcare staff have a moral obligation to do good.
- *Nonmaleficence*: healthcare staff have the moral obligation to avoid doing harm.
- *Veracity*: healthcare staff must be honest, represent themselves truthfully, and admit if they work outside their legal scope of practice. This honesty will help residents make informed decisions.
- *Fidelity*: healthcare staff are faithful and do not abandon those in their care.
- **Justice**: healthcare staff treat all residents fairly.

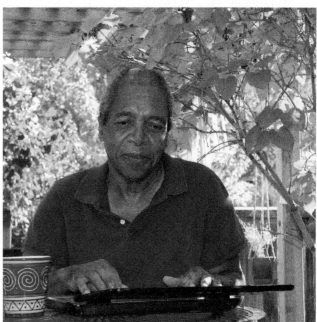

Oscar C. Williams/Shutterstock.com

Figure 3.4 Ethical caregiving respects the resident's right to freedom, which includes functioning independently.

Codes of Conduct and Ethics

All professions or disciplines have a code for conduct and ethics, called a *code of conduct* or a *code of ethics*. These guidelines set standards for care delivery and practice and direct actions and behaviors (**Figure 3.5**). Some codes of conduct or ethics are outlined in a state's nurse practice act (NPA) or in other regulations. You can check to see if your state's regulations for nursing assistants have a code of conduct or ethics. If a code of conduct or ethics is set out in regulations, this means it is enforced by law. Codes of conduct or ethics can also be set by a discipline's professional association, and the members of that discipline or profession are expected to follow the code's guidelines.

Why Are Ethical Problem Solving and Decision Making Important?

Life is full of problems, which can be big or small and simple or complex. In healthcare, problems are an everyday occurrence. Successful holistic nursing assistants are comfortable with this reality and find ways to identify problems and solve those they are able to. Your skills in problem solving will be especially important when there are situations that violate principles of ethical caregiving or codes of conduct. Having an awareness and understanding of the problem-solving and decision-making process will help you provide helpful information when resolving ethical issues and dilemmas.

Sample Code of Ethics for Nursing Assistants

For my residents, I will...	For my fellow healthcare staff, I will...	For the healthcare facility, I will...	For myself, I will...
• provide competent, high-quality care • be dependable • treat you with respect and dignity • ensure a safe environment • recognize and follow your bill of rights • recognize and appreciate your beliefs and values • protect your privacy and property • keep personal information confidential, including on social media and in electronic communication • care for you in a positive, approachable manner • be supportive and encouraging when communicating with your family	• be sensitive to your needs, values, and beliefs • listen to your opinions and recommendations • work as a cooperative, trustworthy team member • help you, whenever I am able, to ensure quality care • be patient and supportive in all my communications with you	• follow all policies and procedures • perform only those duties that are within my legal scope of practice • follow directions given by licensed nursing staff within my scope of practice • attend all facility and educational meetings requested • fully and accurately document care • report errors and incidents immediately and truthfully	• know the limits of my role and responsibilities • perform only those skills that I have the competence and preparation to do • carry out directions and instructions to the best of my ability • come to work with a positive attitude • be conscientious about my work • when caring for residents, I will not use my cell phone to make personal calls • be respectful in all of my relationships • be accountable for my actions • always ask the licensed nursing staff if I have any questions about care, procedures, and guidelines for use of social media and electronic communication

Goodheart-Willcox Publisher

Figure 3.5 A Code of Ethics sets the standards for the way you practice and deliver care.

The strategy used to respond to problems is called the *problem-solving and decision-making process* (**Figure 3.6**). The best way to start is to look at a problem as a question or issue that requires a solution. Use the following six-step process:

1. **Identify the problem:** you cannot solve a problem unless you recognize it as a problem. Once you are aware of a problem, the identification step lets you to focus on the difference between what *is* happening and what *is supposed to be* happening.
2. **Examine the problem:** look at the factors that influence the problem, ask others what they see, and search for factual evidence to help you understand what is happening. If a problem is not examined carefully and fully, the alternatives that are identified will likely be faulty, and the decision made will not solve the problem.

3. **Determine alternatives:** examining the problem can show you possible courses of action. Alternatives must be realistic and should respond to the problem as it was identified.
4. **Select an alternative:** identify the alternative that best solves the problem. Sometimes a specific alternative is selected based on the resources available, such as time or money. If this is the case, be sure you are not sacrificing the best solution for a quick fix.
5. **Implement:** all aspects of the alternative should be put in place.
6. **Evaluate:** the process of evaluation determines whether the alternative selected solved the problem. If the problem continues, then the problem-solving and decision-making process starts again.

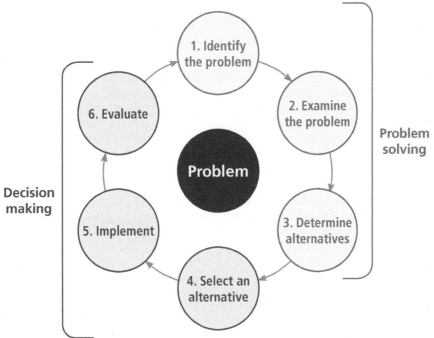

Goodheart-Willcox Publisher

Figure 3.6 The problem-solving and decision-making process helps healthcare professionals make decisions.

How Are Ethical Dilemmas Solved?

There are many ethical **dilemmas** in healthcare that come from situations in which there is not a clear right or wrong decision. These are examples of ethical dilemmas that occur in healthcare. You may see some of them in the facility in which you work:

- a resident who refuses care and treatment
- a family that requests that the ventilator for a comatose resident be turned off, because there is no hope of recovery
- the performance of procedures that are not medically necessary
- the covering up of mistakes
- a situation in which there are too few donor organs for those who need them
- a family that requests that a resident not be told he or she is dying

Ethics Committees

To deal with ethical dilemmas, healthcare facilities usually refer specific ethical issues to an *ethics committee*. The ethics committee uses ethical decision making to help assess and resolve ethical problems involving care. The size of the committee is usually consistent with the needs of the facility. Committee members are selected based on their interest in the welfare of others, experience, integrity, and respect for others. Most members of the committee are doctors, licensed nursing staff, and other healthcare providers. The committee also includes members of the clergy, social workers, and community members (**Figure 3.7**).

The work of an ethics committee is confidential and deals only with ethical matters. The facility's code of ethics; other guidelines, such as facility policy and current standard practice; and deep consideration of the facts and issues at hand are used to help make decisions. Recommendations are made with the purpose of educating and providing guidance for the facility and family members.

The Nursing Assistant's Role in Ethical Practice

As a holistic nursing assistant, you will not typically be part of an ethics committee, although you may be asked by the licensed nursing staff to provide information

---

HEALTHCARE SCENARIO

An Ethical Dilemma

Recently, a medical journal reported that an ethics committee was asked to meet about a resident who had a massive stroke and was transferred to a local hospital. After hospitalization, the resident was returned to the skilled nursing and rehabilitation unit in the long-term care facility in which he had been living. He was on a ventilator, and was maintained with intravenous and tube feedings. He had total right-side paralysis and was not able to communicate with his family. He was also recently diagnosed with early-stage dementia. The family asked the committee to meet because there was conflict about how to continue care. The man's grown children wanted to see if he would recover, but his wife believed he would want to die and was requesting that he be taken off the ventilator. There was no documentation to determine what the resident would prefer.

To address this ethical dilemma, the committee followed its typical procedure:

- clarifying and assessing the facts, issues, and goals to determine if there was enough information to make a decision
- identifying what steps to take, what the consequences were for each potential action, and if actions violated core ethical values or principles
- making a recommendation and implementing it
- monitoring and evaluating to see if changes were needed

Apply It

1. Which ethical principles would the committee be considering in this situation?
2. According to the sample code of ethics in this section, how should a nursing assistant practice ethically while caring for this resident and communicating with his wife and children?

you learned when caring for residents. You will be responsible for providing this information, and you are also always responsible for practicing ethically every day. Be aware that residents or family members may ask you questions about care delivery, treatments, and the *prognosis* (likely outcome) of a resident's condition. You may even be asked what you would do. It is very important that you always practice ethically and follow the code of conduct. If you are unsure how to practice ethically, you must always ask the licensed nursing staff.

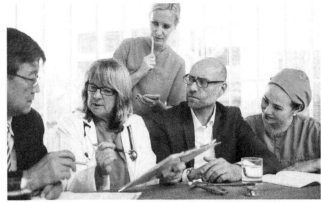

Rawpixel.com/Shutterstock.com

Figure 3.7 Ethics committees meet concerning specific ethical dilemmas. They help advise healthcare staff and families.

SECTION 3.2 Review and Assessment

Key Terms Mini Glossary

beneficence the moral obligation to do good.
dilemma a choice between two difficult options; options may be desirable or undesirable.

ethics principles that guide behavior with respect to what is right and wrong.
fidelity the quality of being faithful and not abandoning those who need care.
nonmaleficence the moral obligation to avoid harm.

prognosis a projection of the likely course and outcome of a disease and the potential for recovery.
veracity honesty; the act of providing full disclosure to enable residents to make informed decisions.

Apply the Key Terms

Write a sentence using each key term properly.

1. beneficence
2. fidelity
3. nonmaleficence
4. prognosis
5. veracity

Know and Understand the Facts

1. What are ethics?
2. Identify four principles of ethical caregiving.
3. What is a code of ethics?
4. How is an ethics committee used in healthcare?
5. Identify the six steps of the problem-solving and decision-making process. Give an example of each.

Analyze and Apply Concepts

1. List two ways in which ethics committees help with ethical dilemmas and decision making.
2. Describe how problem solving and decision making influence each other.
3. Identify a recent problem you solved. Describe how you could have applied the six-step problem-solving and decision-making process. Would the outcome have been different?

Think Critically

Read the following care situation. Then answer the questions that follow.

Mr. D, a new resident in the assisted living facility where you work, was hospitalized recently with abdominal pain. He had a series of tests, which revealed he has cancer of the stomach. Mr. D's daughter does not want her father to know that he has cancer. She is very upset and thinks it's better if he knows less. The doctor is concerned, as a treatment plan needs to be made to determine the best way to care for Mr. D. He thinks Mr. D should be making these decisions. Mr. D's daughter thinks she should. While you care for Mr. D, he asks if you have his test results because he really feels that there is something wrong with him.

1. What should you say to Mr. D?
2. Do you believe that you would be practicing ethically if you checked to find out what was wrong with Mr. D? Explain your answer.
3. What should you do next to show you are practicing ethically?

3 Summary and Review

Key Points

Reviewing the key points for this chapter will help you practice more safely and competently as a holistic nursing assistant and will help you prepare for the certification competency examination.

- Regulations are enforced by state and federal laws. Healthcare facilities follow accreditation and licensure rules and regulations that guarantee safety and quality standards.
- The legal scope of practice determines what nursing assistants can and cannot do and who supervises them.
- Confidentiality is an important responsibility.
- All communications by and about a resident must be kept private.
- The Nursing Home Resident Rights state how residents must be treated. These rights include privacy of information, a safe environment, fair treatment, and the ability to make their own medical decisions.
- Principles of ethical caregiving include autonomy, freedom, beneficence, nonmaleficence, veracity, fidelity, justice, and confidentiality.
- A code of conduct or ethics outlines standards for practice. If ethical problems occur, an ethics committee uses ethical decision making to help assess and resolve the issue.

Action Steps to Holistic Care

Review the information in this chapter. Complete the following activities.

1. Select one ethical principle discussed in the chapter. Prepare a short paper or digital presentation that describes three issues related to this principle.
2. With a partner, select one type of elder abuse. Prepare a poster that shows at least three facts about this type of abuse and ways to prevent and report it.
3. Research current scientific information about an ethical dilemma. Write a brief report that describes three current facts about the dilemma.
4. Find two pictures online that represent a nursing assistant's code of ethics. Describe the behaviors and attitudes shown in the images.

Building Math Skill

Judith has 10 patients to care for today. Six of her residents need a shower, but only three need her assistance; two require a complete bed bath, but one of these residents has a private nurse who takes care of her. The last two residents had bowel movements in bed on the previous shift and have already been bathed. How many of her residents need her assistance with bathing?

Preparing for the Certification Competency Examination

To prepare for the nursing assistant certification competency examination, you will need to know content found in this chapter. This content may be tested in the knowledge (written or oral) and skills (hands-on demonstration) portions of the exam. The following areas will be emphasized:

- the nursing assistant's role as outlined in regulatory and professional guidelines
- the legal limits of nursing assistant practice
- healthcare laws and regulations
- the Nursing Home Resident Rights
- ways of protecting residents from neglect, mistreatment, and abuse
- types of elder abuse
- ways of reporting neglect, mistreatment, and abuse
- nursing assistant ethics
- the nursing assistant standards of conduct

These sample test questions are similar to ones you will find on the certification competency exam. See how well you can answer them. Be sure to select the *best* answer.

1. During morning care, a nursing assistant notices bruises and teeth marks on a resident's body. She tells the licensed nursing staff that she suspects which of the following?
   A. malpractice
   B. libel
   C. abuse
   D. slander

2. Which of the following describes the legal scope of practice for nursing assistants?
   A. the boundaries that define what a nursing assistant can and cannot do
   B. standards of care defined by regulation
   C. the type of holistic care given to residents
   D. how well a nursing assistant does his or her work when practicing

3. If a nursing assistant unintentionally fails to act or provide care, resulting in harm to a resident, this is called which of the following?
   A. liability
   B. malpractice
   C. negligence
   D. libel

4. Which of the following is a document that sets and guides nursing practice?
   A. code of behavior
   B. code of discipline
   C. code of practice
   D. code of ethics

5. A nursing assistant has been praised for demonstrating ethical behavior. Which behavior may have helped him earn that reputation?
   A. He asks other staff to do some of his work.
   B. He maintains confidentiality.
   C. He spends a lot of time talking with the family.
   D. He likes residents to think he is a friend.

6. A person commits a serious criminal offense and goes to jail. What type of criminal offense did the person commit?
   A. felony
   B. certification
   C. misdemeanor
   D. due process

7. A nursing assistant wants to determine if a specific responsibility he has been given is part of his scope of practice. Which of the following should he do to make that determination?
   A. He should ask his friend Joe, who is also a nursing assistant.
   B. He should ask his mother, who is an RN.
   C. He should review the regulations for nursing assistants.
   D. He should look at his healthcare facility's procedure manual.

8. When a nursing assistant came to work on Monday, the RN asked her to do a procedure she did not have the training or education to perform as a nursing assistant. If the nursing assistant did the procedure, which of the following would she be violating?
   A. accreditation
   B. boundaries
   C. confidentiality
   D. scope of practice

9. A nursing assistant needs to perform care for her residents quickly. Mr. A does not want his morning care, but because the nursing assistant is so busy, she performs it anyway. Which resident right was violated?
   A. freedom from coercion and invasion of privacy
   B. freedom from mistreatment and neglect
   C. freedom from verbal abuse and coercion
   D. freedom from physical abuse

10. As Mrs. K is being prepared for a special procedure, the doctor asks her to sign a written permission form that explains the procedure and its risks. What is the name of this document?
    A. informed consent
    B. bill of rights
    C. code of conduct
    D. protected health information

11. What is the major difference between certification and licensure?
    A. Certification is voluntary, and licensure is mandatory.
    B. Certification costs more than licensure.
    C. Licensure takes longer to get than certification.
    D. Unlike certification, licensure does not require the meeting of standards.

12. A nursing assistant wrote a false statement about another nursing assistant. Which of the following did she commit?
    A. slander
    B. abuse
    C. mistreatment
    D. libel

13. A new nursing assistant is learning about Nursing Home Resident Rights. He knows very little about what is included. Which of the following sentences would best describe it to him?
    A. Nursing Home Resident Rights are a set of requirements that protect residents in nursing homes from harm and empowers residents to make their own healthcare decisions.
    B. Nursing Home Resident Rights are a set of requirements that ensure that older people have proper insurance over their lifetimes.
    C. Nursing Home Resident Rights are a set of requirements that protect older people from spending too much money.
    D. Nursing Home Resident Rights are a set of requirements that ensure that healthcare staff have good employee benefits.

14. Why is HIPAA an important law in healthcare?
    A. It protects healthcare staff from retaliation.
    B. It protects the families of residents.
    C. It protects the environment in healthcare facilities.
    D. It protects the privacy of healthcare information.

15. What should a nursing assistant do if she suspects that a resident is being abused?
    A. She should ask the family about the abuse.
    B. She should ask the resident about the abuse.
    C. She should tell the licensed nursing staff.
    D. She should call the police.

Did you have difficulty with any of the questions? If you did, review the chapter to find the correct answer(s).

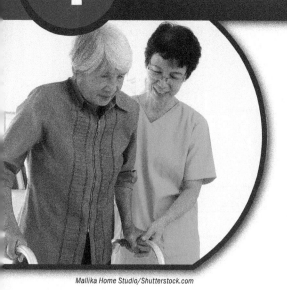

Mallika Home Studio/Shutterstock.com

Welcome to the Chapter

This chapter provides information you will need to maintain a safe culture and environment for yourself and those in your care. It focuses on identifying potential hazards, the importance of proper body mechanics, preventing common accidents and injuries, properly reporting safety issues, and keeping residents free from harm. The chapter also explains best practice and quality measures to promote and maintain a safe culture, the need for safety plans, safety awareness, and the importance of safety checks.

What you learn in this chapter will help you develop your knowledge and skills to become a holistic nursing assistant. The topics discussed in the chapter are highlighted on the Providing Holistic Care Framework.

Chapter Outline

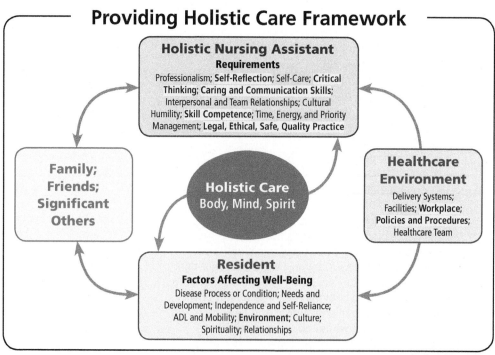

Providing Holistic Care Framework

Holistic Nursing Assistant
Requirements
Professionalism; **Self-Reflection**; Self-Care; **Critical Thinking**; **Caring and Communication Skills**; Interpersonal and Team Relationships; Cultural Humility; **Skill Competence**; Time, Energy, and Priority Management; **Legal, Ethical, Safe, Quality Practice**

Family; Friends; Significant Others

Holistic Care
Body, Mind, Spirit

Healthcare Environment
Delivery Systems; Facilities; **Workplace**; **Policies and Procedures**; Healthcare Team

Resident
Factors Affecting Well-Being
Disease Process or Condition; Needs and Development; Independence and Self-Reliance; ADL and Mobility; **Environment**; Culture; Spirituality; Relationships

Goodheart-Willcox Publisher

A Culture and Environment of Safety

Objectives

To achieve the objectives for this section, you must successfully:

- **describe** the importance of a culture of safety, safety checks, and compliance with the healthcare facility's safety plans.
- **identify** potential hazards, common accidents and injuries, and ways to prevent and properly report these issues.
- **include** safety awareness and risk prevention as important parts of daily nursing assistant practice.
- **explain** the four main principles of body mechanics.
- **demonstrate** proper body mechanics when working with residents.

Key Terms

Learn these key terms to better understand the information presented in the section.

always events	minimum data set (MDS)
bloodborne pathogens	near misses
body mechanics	needlesticks
clinically adverse events	never events
connective tissue	pathogens
culture of safety	plan of care
decubitus ulcer	posture
entrapment	sharps
harm	transparency
joints	

Questions to Consider

- Safety is an important need that all people share. How would you define *safety*?
- How can you make sure that you and people important in your life remain safe?
- When you become a nursing assistant, what safety practices do you think will become most important?

Safety has always been an important and desired outcome in healthcare, and it is more important today than ever. Both government and private agencies work to make sure quality and safety standards are achieved. Hospitals and long-term care facilities are expected to regularly monitor and report specific measures of quality and safety. As a result, the performance of healthcare facilities in reporting and meeting set standards is tied to financial reimbursement (the money a facility receives). If care given in a facility does not meet safety and quality standards, Medicare and some insurance companies may not pay the facility for the cost of care.

The Centers for Medicare & Medicaid Services (CMS) monitors quality measures such as clinical care, patient outcomes, and recent hospital experiences. Quality measures also exist for other types of facilities. CMS requires long-term care facilities to perform initial assessments of residents on admission, conduct periodic assessments, and develop *minimum data sets (MDSs)*. An MDS is a complete assessment by licensed nursing staff of a resident's mobility, transfer skills, and ADLs, and is used to identify health problems. The MDSs establish a foundation for the assessment of all residents. Assessment information is used to help develop, review, and revise the resident's *plan of care* (a document that guides the delivery of care to each resident). The goal is to coordinate care and services so the highest possible physical, mental, and psychosocial well-being is achieved. A *resident assessment instrument (RAI)* must be used to gather specific information and be sure residents are provided a level of care that promotes quality of life.

What Does Safety Mean in Healthcare?

Quality of care and safety are connected. A healthcare facility must use safe practices to achieve required quality standards and measures. For example, both the environment and the equipment used must be safe. Healthcare staff members must maintain safety standards and follow facility safety plans (**Figure 4.1**).

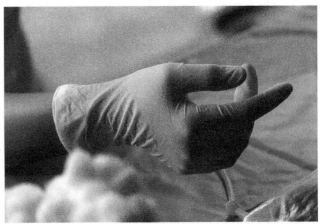

Pornprasit/Shutterstock.com

Figure 4.1 Safety standards, such as the use of PPE, keep healthcare staff and residents safe.

Being safe and promoting safety are daily responsibilities of nursing assistants. Definitions of safety should guide your practice as a holistic nursing assistant. Organizations such as the World Health Organization (WHO), Agency for Healthcare Research and Quality (AHRQ), Institute of Medicine (IOM), and National Quality Forum (NQF) offer definitions of safety that are commonly used in healthcare. The following are important guidelines drawn from the safety definitions and standards of these organizations:

- Be aware and mindful of safety at all times.
- Always work to prevent errors or *harm* (unintended injury).
- Learn from errors that do occur.
- Demonstrate *transparency* (honesty) in reporting safety issues.
- Work to be sure there is a culture of safety that includes all healthcare staff members, facilities, and residents.

How Can You Recognize a Culture of Safety?

The Centers for Disease Control and Prevention (CDC) defines a *culture of safety* as the shared commitment of a healthcare facility's leadership and staff to ensure a safe work environment. A healthcare facility with a culture of safety has the needed systems, procedures, and teamwork to achieve safe, high-quality performance from the nursing and healthcare staff. Healthcare facilities that have a culture of safety promote *always events*. Always events are routine activities and processes that are so important they must *always* be performed consistently and without error. For example, always events result in effective admissions into and out of facilities.

Unfortunately, it is impossible to eliminate all errors in a healthcare facility. When errors do occur in a culture of safety, the focus is on *what happened*, not on *who did it*. The goal of this approach is to bring failures and issues out into the open immediately and deal with them in a blame-free, nonjudgmental, and nonthreatening way. As a result, in a culture of safety, *clinically adverse events* (medical errors) and *near misses* (unplanned health outcomes that do not cause harm) can be reported without fear of punishment. A culture of safety is always willing to respond to and resolve all safety concerns.

THINK ABOUT THIS

Cultures use colors differently to signal warnings or danger. In the United States, the color red is often used as a warning of danger. Healthcare facilities use red or sometimes orange to identify hazards. Other cultures may use different colors to communicate warnings. Chinese culture, for example, uses the color yellow for this purpose.

Sometimes nursing and healthcare staff members may fail to think or act safely due to lack of time, inexperience, or shortcuts. This type of behavior does not support a culture of safety. To create a culture of safety, nursing assistants must:

- follow all safety principles, policies, and procedures
- be aware of safety issues
- be sure that all equipment is working properly
- pay attention to how personal, cultural, and ethnic differences impact safety
- voice opinions and concerns about safety to the licensed nursing staff
- suggest solutions to problems
- report errors both informally to the licensed nursing staff and formally through documentation
- report errors in a timely and specific way using the facility's policy, procedure, and forms

Using a safety-oriented approach demonstrates that you value and are committed to your own personal safety and the safety of others.

How Do Nursing Assistants Ensure Safety?

Hazards and accident risks for residents in long-term care facilities include falls; burns; *decubitus ulcers* (sores on the skin caused by pressure); blood clots; medication errors; *entrapment* (a harmful event in which the resident falls between the bed and side rails); and healthcare-associated infections (HAIs), such as *Staphylococcus* (staph) or urinary tract infections and pneumonia. The majority of these complications are temporary and treatable; however, some of them may cause life-threatening injuries or even contribute to death. Nursing assistants are responsible for making sure residents are safe by avoiding never events, preventing accidents, conducting safety checks, preventing injuries related to *sharps* (objects that can penetrate the skin), wearing PPE when appropriate, and following facility safety plans.

Avoiding Never Events

Never events are actions or errors that lead to serious resident harm, disability, or death. Never events are serious, reportable events and are grouped into seven categories: surgical events, product or device events, resident protection events, care management events, environmental events, radiologic events, and criminal events. Some examples of never events are:

- a fall while a resident is receiving care
- an infection or decubitus ulcer due to improper or lack of care
- a burn (from any source) from a procedure

As a holistic nursing assistant, you must avoid never events by always following facility policy and practicing safely.

Preventing Accidents

Preventing accidents requires personal awareness of safety hazards, safety promotion, following safety policies and the facility's safety plan, understanding risks, using safety equipment, and infection prevention and control. For example, as a nursing assistant, you can prevent the risk of providing care to the wrong resident by always checking the resident's identification. To properly check resident identification, use two identifiers. These might include the resident's name, a facility-assigned identification number or bar code, date of birth, phone number, Social Security number, address, or photo. In most instances, you can say the resident's name, ask the resident to give you his or her name, and compare the name with the identification bracelet (**Figure 4.2**). In some healthcare facilities,

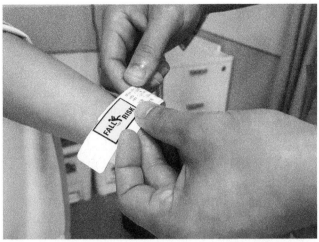

Monet_3k/Shutterstock.com

Figure 4.2 Checking the identification bracelet makes certain you are delivering care to the correct resident.

such as in assisted living, residents may not want to wear identification bracelets. In this case, you can use at least one identifier verification and their photo, which can be found in the EMR (**Figure 4.3**). You may also need to verify the identification of residents who are unable to communicate. Follow facility policy for this identification verification.

Following these general guidelines will also help keep residents safe by reducing the risk of an accident:

- Make sure there is adequate lighting when you work around and with residents.
- When transferring residents between beds, stretchers, or wheelchairs, always lock the equipment wheels before moving the resident.
- Make sure all equipment is in good repair and functions properly.

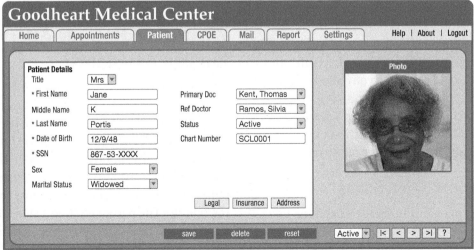

Goodheart-Willcox Publisher, Brian Eichhorn/Shutterstock.com

Figure 4.3 Upon admission, a resident's photograph is normally taken and saved in the EMR to be used for identification purposes.

Conducting a Safety Check

Safety checks play an important role in reducing risks and preventing accidents. You should perform a safety check as you give care in a resident's room and always before you leave the resident's room. During a safety check, make sure the resident is safe and comfortable in bed, in a chair, or in a wheelchair. The bed or wheelchair must be in the locked position so that it does not roll when the resident moves into or out of the bed or wheelchair. If side rails are used on the bed, the resident must be situated to prevent entrapment. Entrapment can cause injury or death. If side rails are not used, the bed must be placed in its lowest position so the resident does not fall.

After positioning a resident properly, check that any tubing (for example, from an intravenous catheter, or *IV*, used to administer fluids) is attached properly and is not kinked. Place the call light in an easy-to-find place for the resident. Pick up any used items or clean up any spills that may be on the floor. Position any furniture or obstacles so they will not get in the way if the resident moves around the room.

Preventing Sharps-Related Injuries and Needlesticks

Sharps-related injuries are caused by sharp objects that break the skin. **Needlesticks** are punctures of the skin by needles (for example, from an IV). These pose another safety risk, as puncture wounds from used needles can transmit **pathogens** (disease-causing microorganisms). When handling exposed sharps or needles, pay attention to the safety of the resident and other staff. Visually check trays and other surfaces (including the bed) that may contain waste materials from a procedure. Make sure no sharps or needles are left behind after procedures.

Sharps and needles must be disposed of in designated *sharps containers* (**Figure 4.4**). When disposing of sharps and needles, do not bring your hands close to the opening of the sharps container, and never place your hands or fingers into the container. Visually check the sharps container for hazards, such as overfilling, which can cause injuries from exposed sharps.

Following Facility Safety Plans

The *facility safety plan* outlines policies and procedures that need to be followed by all healthcare staff. These plans comply with federal, state, and local laws and regulations related to health and

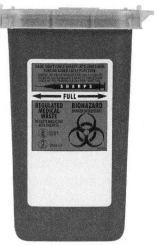

Thom Hanssen Images/Shutterstock.com

Figure 4.4 Used sharps and needles should be disposed of in sharps containers.

safety. They also comply with facility-specific requirements. Facilities often have departments or staff responsible for maintaining and updating the plan, investigating and reducing or removing hazards or risks, and conducting research to achieve compliance. Facility safety plans usually include regulations and guidelines related to the following workplace safety concerns:

- fire safety
- biosafety (related to the treatment of human blood, body fluids, body tissues, or pathogenic organisms)
- radiation and chemical safety
- hazardous waste and materials (HAZMAT) management and emergency response
- accident investigation, mitigation (to reduce or remove accident risks), and reports such as incident reports

What Work Hazards Affect Nursing Assistants?

The Occupational Safety and Health Administration (OSHA) estimates that 5.6 million nursing and healthcare staff members are at risk for occupational exposure to **bloodborne pathogens** (infectious micro-organisms in the blood) such as HIV, the hepatitis B virus (HBV), and the hepatitis C virus (HCV). To reduce these risks, nursing assistants should follow the bloodborne pathogen precautions outlined in Chapter 8. Other safety hazards include needlesticks, other sharps-related injuries, and musculoskeletal disorders (MSDs).

Nursing staff members have reported high rates of MSDs, such as back and shoulder injuries. The most common cause of MSDs is moving and repositioning residents. Other risk factors for developing MSDs include:

- overexerting
- performing multiple lifts
- lifting a resident alone
- lifting uncooperative or confused residents
- lifting residents who cannot support their weight or who are heavy
- performing work beyond your physical capabilities
- moving an object or resident improperly
- moving a resident in a confined space or awkward position
- not being adequately trained in body mechanics

What Are Body Mechanics?

Most musculoskeletal disorders can be prevented by using proper body mechanics. *Body mechanics* are actions that promote safe, efficient movement by using the correct muscles and movements to avoid straining muscles or joints. Proper body mechanics allow nursing assistants to safely and efficiently complete tasks such as positioning residents.

Mobility, or the ability to move, enables you to walk, climb stairs, or drive a car. Mobility is essential for your well-being and the well-being of residents. It occurs only through the contraction of muscles. When muscles contract, they move bones with the help of *connective tissue* (which joins muscles and bones together). For example, two muscle groups contract to move your upper arm: the biceps located on the front of your upper arm and the triceps located on the back of your upper arm. The contraction of these muscles is aided by connective tissue.

Principles of Body Mechanics

Proper body mechanics prevent muscle and joint strain and promote good posture. *Posture* refers to the way in which a person holds his or her body.

Four main principles characterize proper body mechanics:

1. **A stable center of gravity** is established when you keep your back straight and bend only at the knees and hips.

2. **A line of gravity** is established when you keep your back straight and lift objects close to your body.
3. **A wide base of support** is established when you keep your feet shoulder-width apart (about 12 inches), place one foot slightly in front of the other, slightly bend your knees to absorb any impact, and turn with your feet first. These practices provide maximum stability while lifting.
4. **Proper body alignment when standing** occurs when you tuck in your buttocks, pull your abdomen in and up, keep your back flat, hold your chest up and slightly forward, stretch your waist, center your shoulders above your hips, hold your head up, and tuck your chin in. Your weight should lean forward and should be supported by the outsides of your feet.

Benefits of Proper Body Mechanics

Proper body mechanics help ensure resident safety by preventing nursing and healthcare staff injuries during care. Using proper body mechanics (for example, by properly picking up and lifting items during everyday life) also leads to good posture (**Figure 4.5**). Good posture:

- aligns bones and *joints* (locations where two or more bones meet) and reduces any stress between them
- reduces wear and tear on joints
- strengthens the spine and muscles
- conserves energy

Think about your own posture. On a scale of 1–10, with 10 being the best, how would you rate your posture? Do you stand up straight or do you hunch your back? If you gave yourself a low rating, what do you think causes you to have poor posture? What might you do to improve your posture?

How Are Proper Body Mechanics Used?

As you complete daily activities, be mindful of your body mechanics. The following guidelines can help you remember to use proper body mechanics while performing your everyday duties:

- Move in a smooth and coordinated way, not in a jerky way.

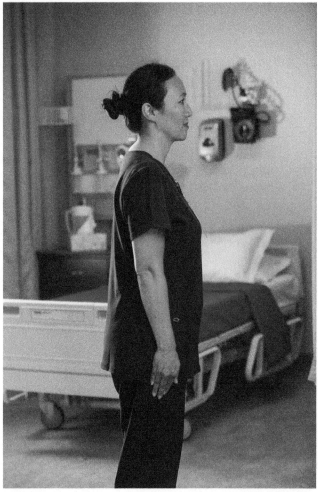

© Tori Soper Photography

Figure 4.5 Proper body mechanics result in good posture. Good posture can reduce the chance of injury and saves energy.

- Because lifting an object can be difficult, pull, push, or roll the object instead.
- When possible, lift, move, or carry objects with both hands.
- Whenever possible, use your strongest muscles—shoulders, upper arms, hips, and thigh muscles—instead of your back muscles.
- When caring for a resident in bed, keep your work close to your body. Place equipment and supplies on the bedside table and move the bedside table close to you when you are performing a procedure. This approach puts less strain on your back, legs, and arms.
- Keep your work at a comfortable height and raise the resident's bed (after locking the wheels) or stand at a counter, when appropriate, to avoid bending at the waist.
- Most importantly, maintain good physical health to reduce your chance of injury on the job.

Proper body mechanics also apply to the movements involved in standing, sitting, lifting, and reaching. The following describes the proper body mechanics associated with various body positions. As you read, try to copy the body positions described. Use a mirror to see how well you are doing or ask a friend to watch you and give you feedback.

Standing

Using proper body mechanics when standing results in proper alignment and correct posture. When you are standing, your shoulder blades should be back, your chest should be forward, and the top of your head should align with the ceiling. Keep your knees straight and avoid tilting your pelvis in any direction. Wear comfortable shoes that support the arches of your feet.

Sitting in a Chair

When you are sitting in a chair, proper body mechanics result in proper posture and alignment and reduce the risk of strain (**Figure 4.6**). When you are sitting, your buttocks should lie at the very back of the chair. Keep your back straight and your shoulders back. Your knees should be bent at right (90°) angles at the same height or higher than your hips. Your feet should lie flat on the floor.

Lifting an Object

Lifting objects without using proper body mechanics can cause strain and injury. When lifting, use your strong leg muscles. Bend your knees and hips and keep your back straight. Lower your body down using your legs until you are level with the object you are trying to lift. Use your arms to support objects and keep your elbows close to your side. Never bend at the waist with your legs straight (called *stooping*). Using your leg muscles, lift straight up in one smooth motion to return to an upright position (**Figure 4.7**).

Reaching for an Object

When reaching for objects, use proper body mechanics to reduce strain and prevent possible falls and injury. Before reaching for an object, make sure it is not too heavy or large for you to move safely. Stand directly in front of the object and make sure you are

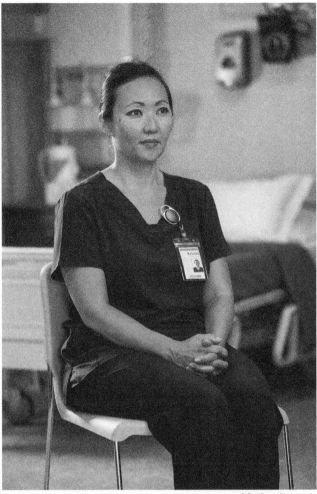

© *Tori Soper Photography*

Figure 4.6 In correct body alignment while sitting, the buttocks should lie at the very back of the chair, and the knees should be bent at a right angle.

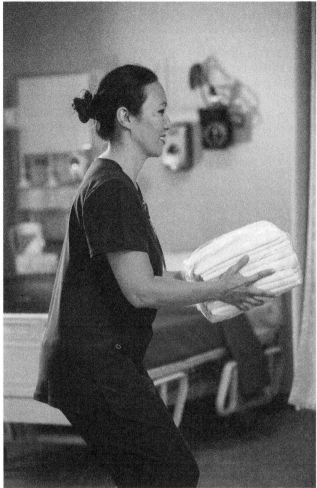

© *Tori Soper Photography*

Figure 4.7 Keep your back straight when lifting objects. Bend only at the knees and hips.

close to it. As you reach for the object, avoid twisting or stretching your body. Stand on a stool or ladder to reach high objects. Before using the stool or ladder, make sure it is stable and will support you.

Why Do Some Healthcare Staff Members Wear Back Belts?

Some healthcare facilities ask that healthcare staff members wear specially designed *back belts* to protect against back injuries during care. Unless it is required, wearing a back belt is usually a matter of choice, because research has not shown that back belts actually prevent back injuries. If a back belt is used, it should be worn properly. Wearing a back belt should never be a substitute for proper body mechanics and good lifting skills.

There are several types of back belts. Back belts typically worn in healthcare facilities are lightweight, elastic, and worn around the lower back. Some back belts have suspenders that hold them in place.

As a holistic nursing assistant, you will be responsible for following safety principles and practices at all times and for using good body mechanics, both during work and in your everyday life. Being aware and taking extra steps to prevent hazards and harm can make a difference in your life and in the lives of others.

SECTION 4.1 **Review and Assessment**

Key Terms Mini Glossary

always events routine activities and processes that are so important they must be performed consistently and without error.

bloodborne pathogens infectious microorganisms in the blood; can cause disease.

body mechanics actions that promote safe, efficient movement without straining any muscles or joints.

clinically adverse events medical errors.

connective tissue a type of body tissue that connects or supports other body tissues, structures, and organs; composed of collagen fibers that provide strength and elastic fibers that enable flexibility.

culture of safety the shared commitment of a healthcare facility's leadership and staff to ensure a safe work environment.

decubitus ulcer a skin condition caused when continuous pressure on the skin and on bony areas restricts blood flow and creates a sore; also called a *bedsore* or *pressure ulcer*.

entrapment a harmful event in which a resident falls between the bed and side rails.

harm unintended physical injury that requires additional monitoring, treatment, or hospitalization; may result in death.

joints locations where two or more bones connect.

minimum data set (MDS) complete assessment by licensed nursing staff of residents' mobility, transfer skills, and ADLs to identify health problems.

near misses unplanned health outcomes that do not cause harm, even though they have the potential to; considered *close calls*.

needlesticks puncture wounds caused by needles.

never events actions or errors that result in harm, death, or significant disability; usually preventable.

pathogens disease-causing microorganisms.

plan of care a written plan that provides directions and serves as a guide to delivering individualized, holistic care; also called a *service plan*.

posture the way in which a person holds his or her body; the manner in which the body remains upright against gravity when sitting down, lying down, or standing up.

sharps objects such as needles, razors, broken glass, and scalpels that can penetrate the skin.

transparency lack of secretive or hidden information; honesty.

Apply the Key Terms

Two key terms are used in each of the following sentences. Identify the key terms.

1. Entrapment occurs when a resident falls between the bed and side rails; this can cause an unintended injury called harm.
2. In a culture of safety—a shared commitment of a healthcare facility's leadership and staff to ensure a safe work environment—the goal is to prevent never events, actions or errors that result in harm, death, or significant disability.
3. Body mechanics are actions, such as having a good posture, that promote safe, efficient movement without straining any muscles or joints.
4. A near miss is an unplanned health outcome that does not cause harm, even though it may be a close call, such as a needlestick, which is a puncture wound caused by needles.
5. To prevent clinically adverse events, or medical errors, holistic nursing assistants should provide a level of care that aims for always events or performing consistently and without error.

Know and Understand the Facts

1. List three common hazards or risks for residents in healthcare facilities.
2. Why are safety checks important?
3. What is a safety plan, and what does it usually include?
4. Identify the four main principles of body mechanics.
5. What are three benefits of using proper body mechanics?

Analyze and Apply Concepts

1. What are the characteristics of a culture of safety?
2. How can a nursing assistant help maintain a culture of safety?
3. List three actions a holistic nursing assistant should perform when conducting a safety check.
4. Describe proper body mechanics for sitting in a chair.
5. List two guidelines for incorporating proper body mechanics into your daily life.

Think Critically

Read the following care scenario. Then answer the questions that follow.

Veronica has cared for older adults at her facility for the past five years and prides herself in the care she provides. She feels that all healthcare staff members should have the same level of commitment. Yesterday, Veronica saw Daniel, another nursing assistant, taking care of Mrs. G, who is 85 years old and has Alzheimer's disease. Mrs. G had a cold, and Daniel did not wash his hands when he entered the room. Daniel also did not make sure Mrs. G was safe in her bed when he briefly left the room. When lifting an object from the floor, Daniel did not use body mechanics. This is not the first time Veronica has noticed Daniel's lack of safety awareness.

1. What risks or safety hazards did Veronica observe?
2. Should Veronica mind her own business or should she report Daniel's actions? Explain your answer.
3. If Veronica does report Daniel's actions, what should she say, and whom should she tell?

Fall Prevention

Objectives

To achieve the objectives for this section, you must successfully:

- **identify** the causes of falls and those who are at risk for falling.
- **describe** ways to prevent falls.
- **explain** what a nursing assistant should do if a resident falls.

Key Terms

Learn these key terms to better understand the information presented in the section.

commode	hypothermia
gait	incident report
gait belt	osteoporosis

Questions to Consider

- Falls are more common among older adults; however, OSHA reports that slips, trips, and falls cause 15 percent of all accidental deaths, second only to traffic fatalities. Have you ever fallen? What was the cause of your fall?
- Could the fall have been prevented? If so, explain what you could have done.

Falls can cause serious injury, especially for older adults. One out of every three adults age 65 or older falls each year. More falls occur as a person ages. Those who fall once are likely to fall again.

Falls cause 25 percent of all hospital admissions and 40 percent of admissions to long-term care facilities. Most falls happen in a resident's room between 10:00 p.m. and 6:30 a.m. This period of time causes more risks because there are usually fewer staff members and less activity in a resident's room at night. Residents are more likely to leave their beds to go to the bathroom without asking for help and may fall.

Twenty to thirty percent of people who fall suffer moderate-to-severe injuries such as dislocations, bruising, cuts to the skin, muscle tears, hip fractures, or head traumas. Injuries are more likely to affect residents who have **osteoporosis** (a condition of porous bones). Bones weakened by osteoporosis increase a person's risk of falling, and if a person with osteoporosis does fall, the injury is usually more severe.

What Causes Falls?

Falls happen for a variety of reasons. Not enough handrails, a slippery tub, an icy sidewalk, or even a pet can cause a person to fall. Falls can also occur because of poor or unstable footwear and poor lighting. Health issues may also increase a person's risk of falling. For example, low blood pressure, sensory loss (poor eyesight), stroke, dementia, medications, and nervous system disorders such as Parkinson's disease can cause a person to fall. A person's ability to get up after a fall can also affect the outcome. Immobility after a fall can cause complications such as dehydration, decubitus ulcers, **hypothermia** (a condition of low body temperature), and pneumonia.

Older adults need to be particularly careful about falls, as age alone is a high risk factor. Many older adults rely on assistive devices such as walkers and canes. However, these devices can increase the risk of falling if they fit poorly or are defective. An older adult is also more likely to fall if he or she has difficulty with balance, strength, perception, vision, range of motion, or coordination.

When caring for a resident who may be at risk for falling, you should always pay attention to the resident's:

- balance and strength
- potential loss of sensation or sensory impairment
- level of vision and hearing
- joint range of motion and **gait** (manner of walking)

Balance, gait, muscle, or range-of-motion exercises can be very helpful for preventing falls in some residents. Building strength and balance also promotes self-confidence, which decreases a resident's likelihood of falling.

How Can Falls Be Prevented?

Nursing assistants play a vital role in preventing residents from falling. The first step in preventing falls is identifying residents who are at risk for falls. Usually, a doctor, licensed nursing staff member, or physical therapist will assess a resident. This assessment will review a resident's medications, any fall risk factors, and strategies to overcome risks. The assessment provides information for a *fall risk program*, which is developed as part of a resident's plan of care.

Identification of Residents with Increased Fall Risk

Healthcare facilities often use a visual alert, such as a sign, picture, or wristband, to show that a resident has an increased risk for falling. Fall risk images are located either within a resident's room or in the hall near the doorway (**Figure 4.8**). Some facilities may use resident seat monitors, bed and chair exit alarms, and wrist or room motion monitors to alert nursing staff that an at-risk resident is mobile without assistance. A resident's independence must always be balanced with safety needs.

Observation and Prevention Strategies

Nursing assistants use a variety of fall-prevention strategies to prevent resident harm. First, work slowly and steadily when you provide assistance with ADLs and ambulation. Do not rush residents. Follow the acronym *ACT*:

- be **A**ware.
- **C**orrect risks.
- **T**ake precautions.

Strong observation skills can help prevent resident falls. Holistic nursing assistants should frequently monitor and observe residents and listen for calls for help, banging, or falling objects. In facilities that use bed and chair alarms, nursing assistants can listen for alarms that tell them a resident may have gotten out of bed or a chair. The following guidelines will also help holistic nursing assistants practice safely and prevent falls:

- Be sure there is a working call light always within each resident's reach. Instruct residents to call for assistance instead of trying to get up themselves. Answer call lights promptly.

- Keep the resident's bed at the lowest possible level and place mats around the bed, if necessary. If side rails are used, keep them in the down position for mobile residents.
- Make sure the resident's room is well lit and does not have glare (especially important for residents with poor eyesight).
- Keep the room clean, dry, and uncluttered. Place the resident's personal items within his or her reach. Clean up small, nonhazardous spills immediately or block off the area if you must wait for someone to clean up the spill.
- Check to be sure there are no wires, cords, or other tripping hazards in the room.
- Encourage residents to use handrails and grab bars, especially in bathrooms and ambulating areas (for example, hallways). Provide shower chairs, if needed.
- Be sure chairs are stable and well-built, are at a good height, and have armrests to assist residents who want to stand.
- Be aware of any changes in a resident's medications and understand how changes may affect the resident. Observe for dizziness, sleepiness, and blood pressure changes.
- Keep a bedside *commode* (chair containing a place to go to the bathroom) nearby, so it can be used safely (**Figure 4.9**). If needed, install high toilet seats so residents do not have to bend down too far when using the toilet.
- Check with the licensed nursing staff before applying creams, bath oils, or powders to a resident's skin, because these substances can make the skin slippery.
- If a resident wears eyeglasses, be sure the eyeglasses fit properly and are nearby so the resident can reach them easily.
- Discourage residents from wearing long gowns or robes.
- Be sure ambulatory residents have sturdy, nonskid shoes or footwear. Also check canes, walkers, and chair legs for nonskid tips. Lock the wheels on beds and wheelchairs whenever a resident is moving into or out of the bed or wheelchair.
- Provide assistive devices, such as a *gait belt* (a safety device that fits around the waist), when a resident ambulates (**Figure 4.10**).
- If a resident begins to fall while ambulating, ease him or her down using guidelines provided in Chapter 14.

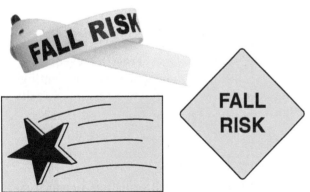

Ilze_Lucero/Shutterstock.com, Goodheart-Willcox Publisher

Figure 4.8 Fall risk bracelets, signs, and falling stars signal that a resident has an increased risk for falling.

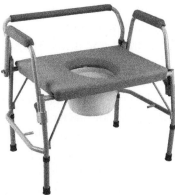

Figure 4.9 A bedside commode allows residents to eliminate without walking to the bathroom.
focal point/Shutterstock.com

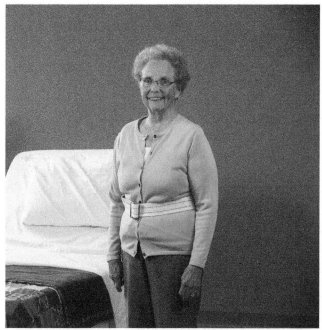

Figure 4.10 When worn around the resident's waist, a gait belt allows the nursing assistant to assist the resident in standing, transferring, and ambulating.
© Tori Soper Photography

Always remember to report resident falls immediately and to report any changes in a resident's condition. Document and report your observations and any actions taken. Resident safety and fall prevention should be top priorities for all nursing assistants.

What Should Be Done if a Resident Falls?

If a resident falls, you must act quickly. Stay with the resident and do not move him or her. The fall may have caused an injury, and moving the resident can make injuries worse. Tell a member of the licensed nursing staff immediately and then stay as he or she checks the resident. The nurse's assessment will determine the next action. Once the assessment is completed, the resident's vital signs may need to be taken frequently. You will need to observe the resident for unusual changes, such as headache, fever, drowsiness, dizziness, vomiting, or double vision. Be sure to notify the licensed nursing staff if these occur.

A resident's recovery from a fall depends on the extent of injury and the resident's medical condition prior to the fall. Regaining mobility is always the goal, especially for older adults, who can rapidly lose strength and function if immobile.

BECOMING A HOLISTIC NURSING ASSISTANT
Precautions for Preventing Falls

Holistic nursing assistants must always be aware of fall risks and be sure appropriate precautions are in place. The following are actions you can take to help prevent falls:

- As you walk down a hall in the facility, look around you. Observe all of the residents and their rooms and identify any possible safety hazards.
- Using proper body mechanics, pick up anything on the floor that should not be there and clean up any spills on the floor.
- Move potential obstacles in common areas. For example, move tables, chairs, or carts in the dining room or hallways so residents can ambulate safely.

- Make sure that residents' rooms do not have any furniture, lamps, rugs, or other items that might become a fall risk.
- Pay attention to resident footwear. Be sure residents' shoes provide good support, have closed backs, and securely tied shoelaces.
- Always think ahead about the needs of residents, particularly if you think residents may try to ambulate without assistance.
- Remind residents and family members about the facility's safety measures for preventing falls.

Apply It

1. What actions could a nursing assistant take to anticipate resident needs and prevent falls?
2. Name two other ways to prevent residents from falling.

An *incident report*, or *occurrence* or *accident report*, will likely be required if a resident falls. Incident reports record information about unusual events, such as resident injuries. The purpose of an incident report is to document the exact details of an incident and provide factual information for reviewing and responding to the event. Incident reports document the details of any injuries, such as falls, needlesticks, or burns; errors in care; resident complaints; faulty equipment; and incidents that put residents or staff members at risk.

An incident report must be written as soon as possible after the event. This ensures that details are not forgotten or remembered incorrectly. Incident reports are completed according to facility policy and procedure, and the appropriate facility form is used. Details should be recorded in sequence, be accurate and complete, and include objective (factual) information. If subjective information (the resident's viewpoint) is recorded, it should have exactly what the resident said. Write only what was observed. Do not make assumptions or place blame. Usually, the following information is requested:

- where and when the incident occurred
- the events surrounding the incident
- whether injury was a direct result of the incident

Reporting incidents is critical to maintaining a safe environment. Never try to cover up or hide an injury or mistake.

SECTION 4.2 **Review and Assessment**

Key Terms Mini Glossary

commode a chair that contains a place to go to the bathroom; can be used as a toilet by residents with mobility challenges.

gait a manner of walking.

gait belt a belt worn around a resident's waist that serves as a safety device when a resident stands and ambulates; also called a *transfer belt* when used for moving a resident.

hypothermia a condition of abnormally low body temperature.

incident report a document that records information about an unusual event, such as a resident injury; also called an *accident report* or *occurrence report*.

osteoporosis a condition of porous bones; characterized by low bone density.

Apply the Key Terms

Complete the following sentences using key terms in this section.

1. The specific manner in which a person walks is called a(n) _____.
2. A resident fell while getting out of bed. The holistic nursing assistant should complete a(n) _____ to document information about the fall.
3. A resident is mobile but too weak to walk to the bathroom. The nursing assistant should put a(n) _____ by the bedside for him to use.
4. A person who has abnormally low body temperature is said to have _____.
5. The nursing assistant is helping a weak resident out of bed. He uses a safety device called a(n) _____ to help the resident stand.

Know and Understand the Facts

1. What are three common causes of falls among older adults?
2. List four actions that can help prevent resident falls.
3. Describe the purpose of an incident report.
4. List three ways in which facilities can let staff know that a resident is a fall risk?

Analyze and Apply Concepts

1. What does *ACT* stand for?
2. Describe the first two actions a nursing assistant should take when a resident falls.
3. Identify three important guidelines to follow when completing an incident report.
4. What might a nursing assistant be asked to observe after a resident has fallen?

Think Critically

Read the following care situation. Then answer the questions that follow.

Mr. T has been at a skilled nursing facility for only one week, and Luis, a new nursing assistant, has been assigned to take care of him. Mr. T is 73 years old and is very thin. He was admitted to the facility after falling several times at home and has some bruises on his arms and legs. Mr. T is very independent and does not like to use his walker. Luis has been assigned to help Mr. T with his morning shower and to make sure he ambulates several times a day.

1. What are two reasons why Mr. T may be considered a fall risk?
2. What actions should Luis take to prevent Mr. T from falling?
3. What should Luis do if Mr. T does fall?

Restraint-Free Care

Objectives

To achieve the objectives for this section, you must successfully:

- **identify** different types of restraints.
- **discuss** alternative strategies to restraints.
- **identify** situations in which a restraint may be ordered.
- **explain** how to observe, monitor, and care for residents in restraints.

Key Terms

Learn these key terms to better understand the information presented in the section.

Alzheimer's disease (AD)　　　restraint
range of motion (ROM)

Questions to Consider

- Have you ever been held somewhere without your permission or kept back physically from doing something?
- If so, what was it like to be restrained? How did you feel?

As a holistic nursing assistant, you will care for some residents whose physical activity requires monitoring (checking) due to disease or medications. For example, residents with dementia or ***Alzheimer's disease (AD)*** may be disoriented, confused, aggressive, or may tend to wander. AD is a degenerative brain disease that leads to memory loss, confusion, disorientation, and changes in personality and mood. When residents exhibit these behaviors, doctors may order restraints to keep residents from falling or harming themselves or others.

The decision to use a ***restraint*** (a device or substance that restricts movement) is very difficult, and healthcare facility policies and federal and state regulations regarding the use of restraints must be followed. Preventive or alternative measures must be tried before restraints can be applied. If restraints are used, they must be ordered by a doctor and usually applied by licensed nursing staff. Some states allow nursing assistants to apply restraints with a doctor's order and under the direction and supervision of the licensed nursing staff. There should be training on their use, careful observation, monitoring, and special care of residents who have restraints applied.

What Is a Restraint?

A restraint is anything that prevents a resident from moving freely. Restraints can be physical or chemical. A *physical restraint* is a device, material, or equipment that is placed on or near a resident and restricts his or her freedom of movement. A *chemical restraint* is a medication that makes a resident drowsy or sleepy and unable to move freely. Restraints can be used only to treat medical conditions or prevent residents from causing physical harm to themselves or others.

If restraints are necessary, they must be used in ways that do not cause injury or emotional harm. Observation and monitoring of a restrained resident's physical and psychological status (condition) are important and required.

Types of Physical Restraints

Only the least restrictive restraints may be applied in healthcare facilities. The type of restraint is determined by the doctor, who will choose a restraint that keeps the resident safe and also provides the greatest amount of freedom.

Physical restraints used in healthcare facilities should never be makeshift (such as a bedsheet, for example). Restraints should always be designed and purchased for a specified use and should be the correct size. Examples of physical restraints include:

- a vest or trunk restraint (**Figure 4.11**)
- a belt
- soft-padded wrist or ankle restraints (**Figure 4.12**)

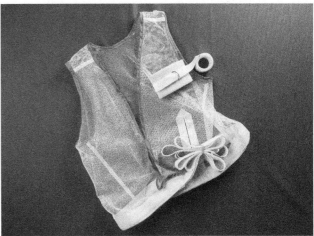

© Tori Soper Photography

Figure 4.11 A vest restraint secures a resident's trunk to a bed or chair.

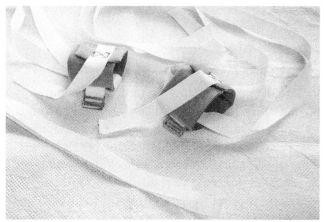
Kim M Smith/Shutterstock.com

Figure 4.12 Wrist restraints secure a resident's arms and hands to a bed or chair.

- a lap tray to keep a resident from falling forward or out of a chair
- a mitten used to stop a resident from pulling on a urinary catheter

Tucking a resident into bed too tightly is considered a restraint. The side rails on a resident's bed are also considered restraints. Side rails are often used to assist with and enhance the mobility of residents, enabling residents to move in bed and get in and out of bed. When side rails prevent residents from leaving their beds or become dangerous they are considered physical restraints.

Risks Associated with Restraint Use

Several risks are related to the use of restraints. Bruises, choking, loss of muscle tone, decubitus ulcers, falls, and loss of dignity are just a few examples. Residents can become depressed, withdrawn, or agitated (restless) when their movements are restricted. The use of side rails as restraints has also led to severe injury and death, as struggling residents become trapped between the side rails and the bed mattress while trying to leave the bed. This is called *entrapment*. There are seven entrapment zones (**Figure 4.13**). Each entrapment zone has great potential for causing injury or death.

As a result of possible entrapment, many long-term care facilities avoid using side rails. Instead, beds are lowered close to the floor, and bed wheels are locked for safety. If a resident is at risk for falling out of bed, mats are placed next to the lowered bed. Some beds that do have rails have *mobility rails*, which are smaller than side rails and provide handholds for residents who need help getting in and out of bed.

In long-term care centers that use side rails, licensed nursing staff members must perform ongoing

assessments of the resident's physical and mental status to allow side rail use. If used, side rails must be in proper working order. The bed used should have a proper-sized mattress or a mattress with raised foam edges. There should never be a gap wide enough to entrap a resident's head or body between the mattress and the bed or side rail. Close monitoring is required to ensure safety and to determine if a resident's status has changed.

How Is a Restraint-Free Environment Promoted and Maintained?

The use of restraints is regulated by state and federal laws. For example, Medicare- and Medicaid-certified nursing homes cannot use restraints except to treat medical symptoms. Certified nursing homes must provide care that maintains or improves residents' quality of life. As a result, the goal of care is always to keep residents free from harm using restraint alternatives.

One key action that helps avoid the use of restraints is answering call lights immediately. Answering call lights immediately helps prevent residents from wandering, becoming confused, or getting out of bed. Responding quickly to resident needs and offering physical, behavioral, or emotional support can be used as alternatives to restraints. Following are some other guidelines, usually directed by the plan of care, for providing alternatives to restraints:

- Place the call light close to the resident or attach the call light to the resident's gown or clothing (**Figure 4.14**). Remind the resident to use the call light.
- Suggest that the resident be moved to a room or bed more visible to the nursing or healthcare staff.
- Always keep the resident's bed in the lowest position possible. This reduces the risk of injury if the resident falls.
- Check on residents who are at risk for harm more often. Increase the frequency of rounds from every hour to every 15 minutes.
- Use alternative restraint devices, such as door, bed, and chair alarms or recliners that can be adjusted to upright or fully extended, reclined positions.
- Remind family members or special private sitters hired by the family to monitor the resident, particularly during the night hours.

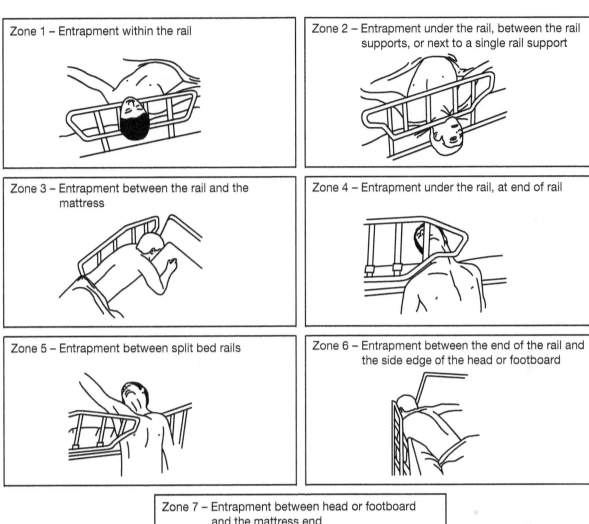

Zone 1 – Entrapment within the rail

Zone 2 – Entrapment under the rail, between the rail supports, or next to a single rail support

Zone 3 – Entrapment between the rail and the mattress

Zone 4 – Entrapment under the rail, at end of rail

Zone 5 – Entrapment between split bed rails

Zone 6 – Entrapment between the end of the rail and the side edge of the head or footboard

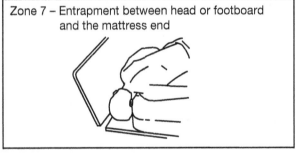

Zone 7 – Entrapment between head or footboard and the mattress end

US Food and Drug Administration

Figure 4.13 The seven entrapment zones describe the seven areas in which a resident can become entrapped.

- Place a dim night-light in the room so the resident can safely walk to the bathroom at night without tripping or falling. For residents who are not a fall risk, you might also place a bedside commode or urinal close to the bed within the resident's reach.
- Remind the resident to use grab rails in the hallways and bathrooms (**Figure 4.15**).
- Redirect the resident from trying to pull on a catheter, tube, or IV. A long-sleeve gown or robe over an IV may prevent a resident from pulling it out.

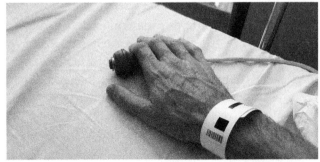

Lloyd Carr/Shutterstock.com

Figure 4.14 Easy access to a call light and a prompt response from nursing staff will reassure residents that their needs will be responded to quickly, discouraging them from trying to get out of bed when it is unsafe to do so.

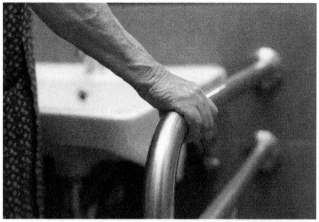

Figure 4.15 Using grab rails in the hallways and bathrooms will help residents ambulate safely.

- Encourage the resident to use his or her eyeglasses, hearing aids, cane, or walker. Explain that these devices will help the resident better respond to the environment and socialize with others.
- Decrease resident confusion by providing links to reality. For example, you could turn on the television or radio or place a calendar and clock in the room.
- Provide distraction for residents by visiting, holding hands, providing enjoyable activities, encouraging residents to hold on to a favorite item, offering a snack or something to drink, and promoting socialization with other residents.
- Be aware of actions that may cause aggressive or combative behaviors and learn what actions may be calming.
- Provide care that allows the resident to live as independently as possible, such as assisting with walking; scheduled toileting; and independent eating, dressing, and bathing programs.
- Tell residents when their behavior is unsafe. Provide safety reminders. Reward residents with praise when they act safely.

The goal of care is to provide as much independence as possible while still keeping the resident safe. Research shows that a safe environment can be provided without physical restraints, which restrict freedom and can create other serious risks. Safe care can often be provided using alternative safety measures that fit individual needs and assure the best possible quality of life.

While all healthcare facilities work toward providing restraint-free care, restraint-free care is not always possible. Sometimes restraints are needed to keep a resident safe and free from harm. Holistic nursing assistants can help prevent any issues or challenges related to restraints by:

- applying restraints in the correct manner, if directed and supervised by the licensed nursing staff, using proper procedure
- providing excellent care
- monitoring and observing residents
- reporting any problems to the licensed nursing staff immediately

When Should Restraints Be Used?

Restraints should only be used to protect residents from harming themselves or others when preventive actions or alternative measures have failed. Restraints should *never* be used for the convenience of the nursing and healthcare staff or to punish the resident.

The use of a restraint requires a doctor's order. In a restraint order, the doctor must give the medical reason for the restraint, the conditions under which the restraint can be used, and the length of use. Before a restraint can be used, a resident's family member or guardian is consulted, and the family member or guardian must sign an informed consent document if the resident is unable. Because residents have the right to make decisions about their care and treatment, restraints cannot be used without the consent of residents, their family members, or guardians. The resident and his or her family member or guardian must be informed about the potential risks of using the restraint.

Restraint use must be monitored, and its effectiveness must be continuously observed and evaluated. Nursing assistants must be aware of healthcare facility policy regarding the use of restraints.

How Are Restraints Safely Applied and Monitored?

Once the doctor has ordered a restraint and the informed consent document has been reviewed and signed, licensed nursing staff members have full responsibility for applying, monitoring, and removing restraints. Licensed nursing staff members assess the resident's condition and then plan for and provide preventive actions for restraint safety. Only in emergencies can licensed nursing staff members apply short-term restraints without a doctor's order.

Nursing assistants provide direct care to residents with restraints; may apply and remove restraints, if directed and supervised by the licensed nursing staff; and observe and report residents' conditions and responses to restraints. Nursing assistants must always follow the healthcare facility's procedure for applying a restraint and must not make any changes to the approved procedure.

Applying a Restraint

The procedure for applying a restraint varies depending on the type of restraint and the facility. The following general guidelines ensure the resident's comfort and the safe, proper application of the restraint:

- Tell the resident (and family members, if present) what you are doing and why. For example, you could say, "Mrs. J, I am going to put this padded, soft restraint on your right wrist because you are trying to pull out the IV on your left arm. You need the IV to receive your medication."
- Check that you have the right restraint type and size. The restraint should not be frayed or torn. Check the fit of the restraint by making sure three fingers will fit between the restraint and the resident's body (**Figure 4.16**).
- Always apply the restraint over clothing, not on bare skin. Padding should be used for any areas where a bone seems to be sticking out (bony projections).

- Be sure the resident is properly positioned in bed while wearing the restraint.
- Never tie a restraint to a movable part of the bed or to a movable chair. For example, a vest restraint should never be tied to a side rail.
- Check that the restraint does not interfere with the resident's breathing or circulation.
- Do not put a restraint on an arm with an IV; on skin that is burned, sore, or injured; or on a broken arm or leg.
- Make sure the resident cannot reach the ties of the restraint.
- Tie the restraint using a slipknot for quick release (**Figure 4.17**).
- Put the call light in a place the resident can easily use it.
- Assure the resident and/or family members that you and other healthcare staff members will regularly observe and check on the resident.
- Report to the licensed nursing staff immediately if the resident or a family member does not want the restraint. If the resident is stable, you can leave the room to give the report. If the resident is not stable, use the call light or ask someone to get a licensed nursing staff member so you can stay in the room.

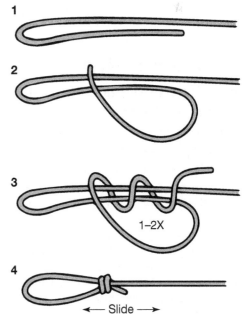

Goodheart-Willcox Publisher

Figure 4.17 To tie a slipknot, follow the four steps in this illustration.

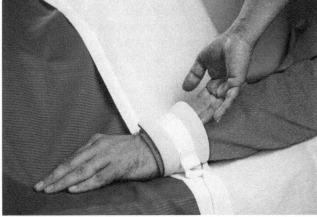

© Tori Soper Photography

Figure 4.16 You should be able to fit three fingers between the resident's body and the restraint used.

Observing a Restrained Resident

Restrained residents must be observed, or checked on, regularly. Observing residents means monitoring their physical and emotional reactions and responses to the restraint. Depending on the resident's condition, you may need to observe the resident every 5, 10, or 15 minutes. Stable and safe residents may be observed hourly, but licensed nursing staff members make this decision. When observing a resident, carefully think about the following:

- **The resident's physical state**: Is the resident safe from injury? Is the resident's skin pink, blue, or gray? Is the skin warm or cool to the touch? What is the color of the resident's lips or nails? Is the restraint comfortable—not too tight or loose? Does the resident feel tingling in any restrained body part? Does the resident have a decreased or absent pulse? Is the resident breathing normally? Does he or she appear weaker than usual? Is the resident complaining about pain on or near the restraint? Are nutrition, elimination, and hygiene needs being met?
- **The resident's emotional state**: Is the resident afraid or nervous? What is the resident saying about the restraint? Does the resident appear confused? Is he or she upset, angry, or agitated?

- **The resident's response to the restraint**: Is the restraint keeping the resident from harm? Has the resident improved enough that he or she no longer needs the restraint? Have the behaviors that caused the use of the restraint disappeared?

If you notice that something is not normal or correct during observation, report it to the licensed nursing staff immediately. Fix any problems you are qualified and able to fix (for example, readjusting the restraint). If you cannot fix the problem, call for help, but do not leave the resident alone.

Residents in restraints need more frequent care than residents without restraints. Care for residents with restraints should be given at least every two hours and more often when needed. Restraints should be released for at least 10 minutes during care. Care for residents with restraints should include a plan for:

- sufficient movement and toileting
- *range of motion (ROM)*, or the amount of voluntary motion, for the restrained body parts (unless the resident is sleeping)
- turning and positioning, if the resident is not able to turn and position himself or herself
- skin care, as needed
- cleaning, bathing, and drying
- food and fluids

BECOMING A HOLISTIC NURSING ASSISTANT
Caring for Residents with Restraints

When caring for residents with restraints, you should be aware of and sensitive to the influence restraints have on the body, mind, and spirit. Be respectful by paying attention to and including the following guidelines in your care:

- Know residents and their routines and preferences. Give the type and level of care that meets their needs.
- When residents know you, they feel more relaxed and comfortable. Ask if it is possible to have the same resident assignment regularly.
- Involve residents in their care. Explain what you're doing in ways residents can understand. This can lower fear and anxiety.

- Be involved with residents and listen carefully to their feelings, concerns, and fears. Share any important information you learn with the licensed nursing staff, so that the information can be included in the plan of care.
- Give residents time to rest and participate in social and physical activities, as appropriate.
- Promote relaxation. Provide warm baths, warm drinks (tea or warm milk), a gentle back massage, or other integrative modalities (alternatives to conventional medicines), if available and appropriate.

Apply It

1. Think about the experience of being in a restraint. How would you feel?
2. Which holistic care approaches do you think you could use when giving care? Which strategies might present a greater challenge? Explain your answers.

Observations about restraints should always be documented. Be sure you are familiar with the documentation procedures and forms required by your healthcare facility. Some facilities use *restraint flow sheets*, which track the care given (such as monitoring every two hours, turning, or positioning). Other facilities require progress notes that include the same information and also comment on how well residents are adjusting to restraints. It is important to know which form is required by your healthcare facility.

How Is Restraint Use Discontinued?

The use of restraints can be discontinued only when there is a doctor's order. The discontinuation of a restraint is ordered when a resident's behavior has improved to the point that the restraint is no longer needed. Restraints are usually removed gradually according to a plan that includes the use of alternative safety measures. Restraints should never suddenly be removed, as they can bruise and damage the skin and strain joints. Licensed nursing staff members may ask nursing assistants to continue closely observing a resident for a short period of time after a restraint has been discontinued. This helps keep the resident safe and free from harm.

SECTION 4.3 Review and Assessment

Key Terms Mini Glossary

Alzheimer's disease (AD) a degenerative brain disease and the most common form of dementia; results in progressive memory loss, confusion, disorientation, and changes in personality and mood; advanced cases lead to decline in cognitive and physical functioning.

range of motion (ROM) the amount that a person can move a joint voluntarily.

restraint any physical equipment or chemical substance that prevents a resident from moving freely.

Apply the Key Terms

Identify the key term used in each sentence.

1. The resident has a bruised joint and has limited range of motion.
2. A nursing assistant is caring for a resident with memory loss, who is confused and disoriented. He was recently diagnosed with Alzheimer's disease (AD).
3. A nursing assistant reported to the licensed nursing staff that the resident she is caring for is becoming very restless, agitated, confused, and seems to be unsafe. The licensed nurse calls the doctor to see if a restraint might be needed.

Know and Understand the Facts

1. What are physical restraints?
2. What are three types of physical restraints?
3. What are chemical restraints?
4. What is entrapment, and how can it be prevented?
5. Identify two risks associated with the use of restraints.

Analyze and Apply Concepts

1. What are four alternative safety measures to using restraints?
2. What is one reason the use of restraints might be ordered by a doctor?

3. Describe three observations that nursing assistants must make when residents are in restraints.
4. Name three actions nursing assistants should take when caring for a resident in a restraint.

Think Critically

Read the following care situation. Then answer the questions that follow.

Tom is a nursing assistant at a long-term care facility. Today, he is providing care for a newly admitted resident—Mr. C, a 65-year-old Hispanic gentleman. Mr. C was transferred from the hospital about two hours ago and was admitted after a serious car accident. Mr. C is very agitated and does not speak English well. He seems to be trying to remove his IV and get out of bed. He is moaning and appears to be in a lot of pain. Tom has been asked by a member of the licensed nursing staff to check on Mr. C to see how he is doing.

1. What should Tom immediately do to make sure Mr. C is safe?
2. What should Tom say to the licensed nurse about his observations regarding Mr. C's present condition?
3. Do you think Mr. C should be put in restraints? If not, how should the situation be handled? If you think he should be in restraints, what would be the next steps?

Fire, Chemical, Electrical, and Oxygen Safety

Objectives

To achieve the objectives for this section, you must successfully:

- **describe** ways to prevent fires and eliminate chemical and electrical risks.
- **identify** what to do in case of a fire.
- **explain** the actions required to safely care for residents using oxygen.

Key Terms

Learn these key terms to better understand the information presented in the section.

fire triangle
flow meter
nasal cannula

personal protective equipment (PPE)
RACE
safety data sheet (SDS)

Questions to Consider

- Have you ever experienced a fire—either small or large?
- If you have experienced a fire, what was your immediate reaction? Were you unable to move, or did you get a burst of energy and immediately take action?
- Did you use some form of fire suppression, such as a fire extinguisher? If so, what was that experience like?

Healthcare facilities face high risks because of their large populations of non-ambulatory residents and the difficulty of evacuation (removal). As a result, nursing and healthcare staff members must know how fires can start and how to prevent them. They must be knowledgeable about fire safety rules, plans, and procedures. They must also know how to prevent fires and what to do if a fire starts.

How Do Fires Start?

For a fire to start, three elements must be present—fuel, oxygen, and heat. These three elements form the *fire triangle*. Fuel is any flammable solid, liquid, or gas. If any one part of the fire triangle is missing, a fire will not start.

You can help prevent fires by keeping heat away from flammable items. For example, you should keep resident clothes away from potentially hot items, such as a frayed electrical wire.

How Should a Nursing Assistant Respond to a Fire?

When you begin working as a nursing assistant, you may hear a facility fire alarm or an overhead announcement, even if you do not see a fire. If the facility fire alarm sounds or if you are alerted by an overhead announcement, follow the facility guidelines and:

- listen for the facility code announcement to identify the location of the fire
- close the nearest resident, office, laboratory, and utility room doors
- clear the corridors and elevator lobbies on the floor of the fire alarm and on other floors, if instructed
- remain alert and await further instructions on the announcement system
- do not evacuate unless specifically instructed to do so
- resume normal activities when the facility code indicates all is clear

If a fire starts in your facility, you must act very fast. The first few minutes can be a matter of life and death. Use the **RACE** system and always follow your healthcare facility's specific fire plan (**Figure 4.18**).

You should try to extinguish a fire using a fire extinguisher *only* after the rescue, activate the alarm, and confine the fire steps are completed and the fire department is on the way. Do *not* use fire extinguishers unless you are trained and confident about using them.

Classes of Fire and Types of Fire Extinguishers

There are several types of fire extinguishers. Each is designed to extinguish a particular class of fire:

- **Class A fire**: ordinary, solid materials such as wood, paper, cloth, or trash; a water or multipurpose dry chemical extinguisher is used.
- **Class B fire**: gasoline, oil, paint, or other flammable liquids; a carbon dioxide or multipurpose dry chemical extinguisher is used.
- **Class C fire**: wiring, fuse boxes, computers, or other electrical sources; a dry chemical or multipurpose dry chemical extinguisher is used.

Understanding the RACE Acronym

Acronym	Actions to Be Taken
R—Rescue	Remove residents from danger by helping them to a safe place (usually designated by the facility fire plan). Move residents outdoors only if there is no safe indoor option. Unlock bed wheels to move residents quickly. All personal items should be left behind.
A—Activate alarm	Follow the facility fire plan procedure and tell a fellow staff member, call the fire department, activate a manual pull station, or send out the prescribed code over the announcement system.
C—Confine the fire	Close fire doors behind the last person leaving an area. Confining the fire limits the spread of heat and smoke as residents are moved elsewhere on the floor or out of the building.
E—Extinguish	Extinguish the fire if you can do so safely without causing danger to anyone. Only a staff member who is competent using a fire extinguisher and who has a clear, unobstructed exit should use the extinguisher. In all other cases, qualified, professional firefighters should extinguish the fire.

Goodheart-Willcox Publisher

Figure 4.18 The RACE system consists of four steps: rescue, activate the alarm, confine the fire, and extinguish.

- **Class D fire**: powders, flakes, or shavings from metals; a class D extinguisher is used.
- **Class K fire**: combustible fluids, such as oils and fats; a dry or wet chemical extinguisher is used.

Fire extinguisher checks should be performed on a regular basis by a designated person, who should make sure extinguishers are fully charged and ready for use in case of an emergency. The facility fire plan should show when fire extinguishers must be checked.

Using a Fire Extinguisher

Once you have obtained the proper fire extinguisher for the type of fire present, you must use the extinguisher as you were trained. When using a fire extinguisher, remember the acronym *PASS* (**Figure 4.19**):

- **P—Pull** the lock pin.
- **A—Aim** the nozzle low at the base or bottom of the fire or flames.

┌─── **THINK ABOUT THIS** ───┐

Seventy-seven percent of all estimated deaths from fires occur in people's homes. Burns from the fire and smoke inhalation are primary symptoms leading to death. Bedrooms are the leading specific location where these deaths occurred (US Fire Administration). Older adults are most at risk for fire-related injuries because they may have difficulty escaping from a fire.

- **S—Squeeze** the handles together while holding the extinguisher straight.
- **S—Sweep** the nozzle from side to side at the base of the flames until the fire is extinguished.

A slight kickback may accompany the activation of the extinguisher. Carbon dioxide extinguishers may make a noise as the extinguishing agent rushes out of the extinguisher. Before using an extinguisher, identify an exit behind you in case the fire extinguisher fails to operate properly or you cannot completely extinguish the fire.

How Can a Fire Be Prevented?

Preventing fires is a very important part of a nursing assistant's responsibilities. Taking specific actions to prevent fires will help keep residents free from harm:

- Know the locations of smoke detectors and fire alarms in your facility. Smoke detectors should never be disabled. A periodic beep or chirp from a smoke detector means the battery is low and must be changed immediately. If you hear this, report it to the licensed nursing staff.
- Know the facility fire plan, the locations of fire extinguishers, and the proper methods of using fire extinguishers. Become familiar with the facility's escape routes and actively participate in facility fire drills.

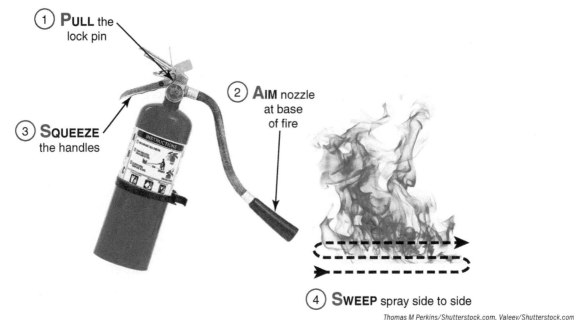

① **PULL** the lock pin

② **AIM** nozzle at base of fire

③ **SQUEEZE** the handles

④ **SWEEP** spray side to side

Thomas M Perkins/Shutterstock.com, Valeev/Shutterstock.com

Figure 4.19 The four steps in extinguishing a fire are pulling the lock pin, aiming the nozzle, squeezing the handles, and sweeping the nozzle from side to side.

- Check that sprinklers are in working order and are not obstructed by any objects. Do not store items near sprinkler heads, as items may prevent water from spraying on the fire.
- Keep hallways and exit doors clear.
- Store flammable materials properly.
- Enforce no-smoking rules.
- Teach mobile residents about fire safety. Educating residents about responding in the event of a fire is an important method for ensuring safety.
- Show residents the proper escape routes from their rooms. Remind mobile residents to use the stairs and not the elevator if there is a fire. Let those who use wheelchairs, canes, or walkers know that assistance will be provided.
- Tell residents to shut the door if a fire is blocking the doorway, as this will help keep the fire out. Residents or nursing assistants should also put towels or blankets along the bottom of the door to keep smoke out of the room (**Figure 4.20**). If they are able, residents should yell for help or call 9-1-1 from their room phone, if they have one.
- Instruct residents to feel the door before opening it if they hear a fire alarm. The door should not be opened if it feels hot. If the door is hot, a fire is just on the other side. Opening the door will spread the flames and smoke into the room. If the door is hot, the resident should put a towel or blanket along the bottom of the door to keep the smoke out and signal or call for help.

What Are Electrical and Chemical Hazards?

Nursing assistants must also be aware of electrical and chemical hazards. Understanding these hazards helps nursing assistants maintain the safety of residents, family members, and facility staff.

Electrical Safety

Electrical hazards can result in electrical shock, electrical fires, and explosions. There are four main types of electrical injuries: electrocution, electrical shock, burns, and falls caused by contact with electricity.

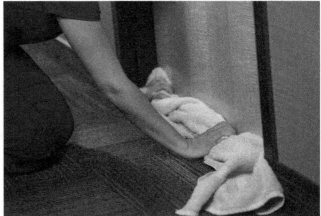

© Tori Soper Photography

Figure 4.20 A towel or blanket will help prevent smoke from entering the room.

Hazards include electrical cords that are damaged or aging, faulty electrical equipment, and damaged electrical wall outlets. The facility safety plan should provide directions regarding electrical safety. OSHA standards must also be met. General guidelines must also be observed to maintain electrical safety:

- Never overload electrical outlets or use an item with a damaged electrical cord. Do not use extension cords, and do not turn on an electrical razor while oxygen is in use.
- Check that all equipment used for residents has been inspected and is safe. Many facilities use stickers or tags to identify electrical equipment as safe.
- Be sure there is sufficient working space around all electrical equipment to permit the safe operation and maintenance of equipment.
- Check that all outlets near sources of water are properly grounded with a three-pronged outlet to prevent shocks or electrocution.
- Do not plug in or unplug electrical equipment when your hands are wet.
- Keep all electrical appliances at least 3–4 feet from any sink, tub, shower, or stove.
- If you are concerned about an electrical outlet or piece of equipment, do not use it. Report it to the licensed nursing staff.

Chemical Safety

Many hazardous chemicals are present in healthcare facilities, causing the threat of toxic exposure for residents and healthcare staff. Toxic exposure to hazardous chemicals can result from topical and spray medications; anesthetic gases; and chemicals used to clean, disinfect, and sterilize work surfaces and equipment.

OSHA hazard standards and facility-specific guidelines for chemical safety are often outlined in the facility safety plan. Know the information provided in the facility's **safety data sheet (SDS)**, or *material safety data sheet (MSDS)*, for each hazardous chemical. The SDS contains information about potential hazards; the safe use, storage, and handling of chemical products; and emergency procedures. Check that all hazardous chemicals are clearly labeled and wear appropriate **personal protective equipment (PPE)**, such as gloves, goggles, and gowns, when handling hazardous detergents and chemicals. If the eyes or body are exposed to hazardous chemicals, quickly flush the body or eyes using facility equipment according to procedure (**Figure 4.21**).

What Is Oxygen Therapy?

Oxygen therapy is a lifeline for many people. Without oxygen therapy, some people might not survive a respiratory illness or might not be able to perform simple ADLs. Oxygen is safe to use under the right conditions and can be used at home or in healthcare facilities. Oxygen will not explode or burn, but can cause things that are already burning to burn hotter and faster.

The need for oxygen therapy is determined by a doctor. The doctor also identifies the *rate*, or amount, of oxygen to be delivered per minute based on what the resident needs. In healthcare facilities, licensed nursing staff members are responsible for setting up oxygen equipment and tubing and adjusting the rate of oxygen given to a resident. The nursing assistant observes that the amount of oxygen delivered is accurate and that equipment and tubing are properly placed. Any changes or problems are reported by the nursing assistant to the licensed nursing staff.

The following supplies are typically used for administering oxygen:

- **Flow meter**: also called a *regulator*; ensures that a resident gets the prescribed amount of oxygen (1–6 liters per minute, if delivered through a nasal cannula)

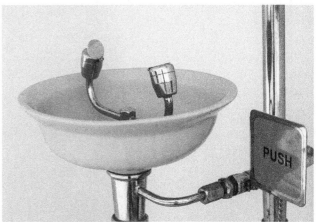

Figure 4.21 Healthcare facilities may have emergency showers and eyewash stations to flush the body and eyes if they are exposed to hazardous chemicals.

- **Pressure gauge**: shows the amount of oxygen being delivered
- **Oxygen tubing**: used to move oxygen from the tank, cylinder, or wall unit to the resident (**Figure 4.22**)
- *Nasal cannula*: most commonly used to deliver oxygen; has two small prongs that deliver oxygen into the nose; prongs are placed about 1/2 inch into the nostrils (**Figure 4.23**)
- **Masks**: used if a resident has difficulty breathing through the nose or needs a large amount of oxygen; covers the nose and mouth
- **Humidifier**: adds moisture to oxygen and prevents the resident's nasal passages from drying

Oxygen tanks and cylinders are labeled with a United States Pharmacopeia (USP) code and are marked with a colored diamond that reads *Oxygen*. The USP code indicates that the oxygen is being used for medical purposes. Oxygen tanks and cylinders

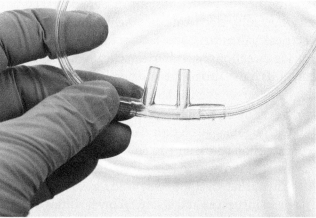

MedstockPhotos/Shutterstock.com

Figure 4.23 A nasal cannula is most often used when a low to medium flow of oxygen is required.

contain gas under high pressure. If they are not handled correctly, their high pressure can cause serious damage, injury, or death.

All supplies and equipment involved in oxygen therapy must be kept clean and in good, working order. Any connections should be in good condition. As a holistic nursing assistant, report any needed repairs to the licensed nursing staff. Keep equipment clean and safe by wiping down the outsides of the equipment with a damp, soapy cloth on a regular basis. If the resident is using a humidifier, empty the water from the reservoir and wash the reservoir in hot, soapy water every day. Nasal cannulas and masks are usually changed at least every two to four weeks. The tubing should be changed at least once a month. Change the tubing and mask often if the resident has a cold or the flu; however, always check facility policy regarding changing equipment, nasal cannulas, tubing, and masks.

Promoting Oxygen Safety

Oxygen must always be used safely. Follow these important safety rules both in healthcare facilities and at home:

- Make sure precautions for oxygen safety are posted outside any room or building in which oxygen is used or stored.
- When oxygen is in use, prevent static electricity (for example, from skin rubbing on sheets or blankets and the use of hand sanitizer).
- Prevent fires by never using oil-based face creams, hair dryers, or electrical razors while oxygen is in use. Instead, use water-based cosmetics or creams.

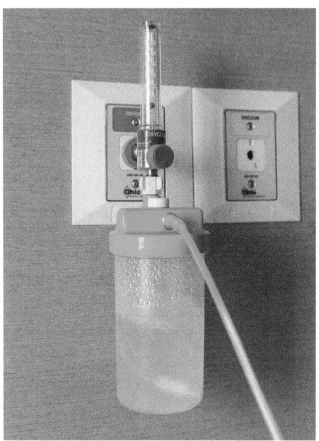

Jsnow my wolrd/Shutterstock.com

Figure 4.22 Oxygen tubing connects the oxygen mask or nasal cannula to the source of oxygen (in this case, an oxygen wall unit).

Oxygen Safety

Joy, a nursing assistant in a long-term care center, found Mr. A, a 75-year-old resident, on the floor near his bed. Oxygen tubing and an electrical cord were wrapped around Mr. A's neck, and the electrical cord was tied to the call light cord hanging over his bed. Joy immediately called the licensed nursing staff for help. The nurse removed Mr. A's restraints and administered CPR. Unfortunately, Mr. A was pronounced dead at 12:15 a.m.

The coroner stated that it appeared as though Mr. A was trying to get out of bed and got tangled in the cords and tubing.

Apply It

1. Why did Mr. A get tangled in the tubing and cords?
2. Could Joy have done any more than she did? Explain your answer.

- Maintain oxygen therapy precautions (such as keeping a resident away from flammable items or static electricity) and follow facility procedures when transporting residents receiving oxygen.
- Place no-smoking signs throughout the facility and the room in which oxygen is being used.
- Keep tanks and cylinders, if used, at least 10 feet from open flames, space heaters, large windows, or any other source of heat. Make sure that stored oxygen tanks and cylinders will not tip over or fall. Keep liquid oxygen upright so that it does not spill. Liquid oxygen may cause skin damage.
- Do not use cleaning solutions, paint thinners, or aerosol spray cans near oxygen, as these can ignite a fire.
- Never use grease or oil near oxygen, as these are flammable materials. Grease and oil can be found in hand lotions, hair lubricants, and petroleum jelly. Aerosol sprays, such as hairsprays, are also flammable and should not be used near oxygen equipment.
- If the person receiving oxygen therapy is cooking, ensure that the cannula is secured over the ears and behind the head, not under the chin.
- Secure tubing to the side of clothing with a large safety pin (though be sure not to puncture the tubing). This will keep the tubing away from any heat source.

Caring for Residents on Oxygen Therapy

Residents receiving oxygen therapy need safe, quality care. As a holistic nursing assistant, you should observe and report skin irritation, changes in breathing, changes in vital signs, or changes in

the operation of equipment to the licensed nursing staff. You should also do the following:

- Make sure an *Oxygen in Use* sign is posted on the door to the room and on the wall over the bed.
- Regularly check oxygen flow, as directed by the licensed nursing staff, and remove possible tubing kinks that can minimize or prevent the flow of oxygen.
- Keep any tubing off the floor.
- Be sure the cannula or mask and tubing are placed correctly, as they can easily be disturbed when a resident moves or sleeps.
- Observe the skin around the nasal cannula or mask for irritation. Give frequent skin care to the face or nose. Use water-soluble lubricants on these sensitive skin areas and do not use any oil-based products.
- Tuck some gauze under the nasal cannula and oxygen tubing to prevent the skin under the nose and behind the ears from becoming sore (**Figure 4.24**).

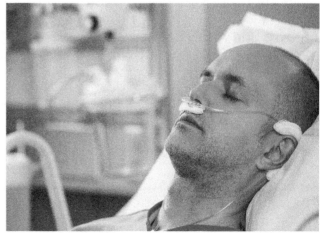

© Tori Soper Photography

Figure 4.24 Placing gauze beneath the nasal cannula and its tubing can reduce soreness around the nose and ears.

- Promote breathing comfort for residents in bed by keeping the head of the bed raised. Use pillows to support residents who are seated.
- Observe changes in skin color. Gray or blue skin could indicate that the resident is not getting sufficient oxygen. Immediately let the licensed nursing staff know if this occurs.

- Remove items that may cause a fire (for example, electrical equipment that may cause sparks or flammable fluids).

SECTION 4.4 **Review and Assessment**

Key Terms Mini Glossary

fire triangle the three elements—fuel, oxygen, and heat—needed to start a fire.

flow meter a medical device used to make sure a resident receives the prescribed amount of oxygen.

nasal cannula a narrow, flexible plastic tube used to deliver oxygen through the nostrils.

personal protective equipment (PPE) specialized clothing and accessories, such as gloves, gowns, masks, goggles, and other pieces of equipment, that are worn to protect against infection or injury.

RACE an acronym for the process of responding to a fire; stands for *rescue, activate alarm, confine the fire,* and *extinguish.*

safety data sheet (SDS) a document found in the facility safety plan; contains information about the potential hazards of a chemical product and use, storage, handling, and emergency procedures.

Apply the Key Terms

Think about the definitions of the following key terms. Describe one difference between each pair of key terms.

1. flow meter and nasal cannula
2. fire triangle and RACE
3. personal protective equipment (PPE) and safety data sheet (SDS)

Know and Understand the Facts

1. What are the three elements needed to start a fire?
2. What does *RACE* stand for?
3. What does *PASS* stand for?
4. Identify two pieces of equipment used in oxygen therapy. Explain how each piece is used.

Analyze and Apply Concepts

1. What should a nursing assistant do if a fire alarm is activated in the facility?
2. Describe five guidelines a nursing assistant should follow to prevent a fire.
3. Explain two actions a nursing assistant can take to maintain electrical safety.
4. Identify five oxygen safety guidelines that must be followed.

Think Critically

Read the following care situation. Then answer the questions that follow.

Mary is a nursing assistant at a skilled nursing facility and is caring for Ms. J, who was transferred from the hospital with moderate respiratory distress caused by serious pneumonia. Ms. J is 75 years old and very independent. She is mobile, but will need oxygen therapy while she recovers. Ms. J is not happy about being in the skilled nursing facility and complains about the nasal cannula. Her nose is sore, and she does not like the sign that shows she is on oxygen.

1. What can Mary do to help Ms. J with her nasal cannula and sore nose?
2. If you were Mary, how would you explain the importance of the sign to Ms. J?
3. Identify three oxygen safety guidelines Mary should follow when caring for Ms. J.

Key Points

Reviewing the key points for this chapter will help you practice more safely and competently as a holistic nursing assistant and will help you prepare for the certification competency examination.

- Preventing risks and accidents requires personal awareness about safety hazards, safety promotion, safety policies, infection control, risk management, and the use of safety equipment.
- Proper body mechanics allow you to complete tasks safely and efficiently without straining your muscles or joints.
- To prevent falls, always work slowly and steadily and *ACT* (be aware, correct risks, and take precautions).
- A restraint-free environment must be promoted and maintained whenever possible. A doctor's order is required to use a restraint and all federal, state, and facility policies must be followed to ensure that residents have a good quality of life.
- Nursing assistants should always use fire-prevention skills and be familiar with the facility's fire safety plan.
- When caring for residents on oxygen therapy, observe and report signs of skin irritation, changes in breathing and vital signs, or changes in the operation of equipment to the licensed nursing staff.

Action Steps to Holistic Care

Review the information in this chapter. Complete the following activities.

1. Prepare a short paper or digital presentation that describes how nursing assistants contribute to a culture of safety. Discuss how a culture of safety supports quality and ensures a safe environment.
2. With a partner, write a song or a poem about fire safety. Include how fires can start and how to prevent them.
3. Research current scientific information about electrical and chemical safety in healthcare facilities. Write a brief report describing three current facts not covered in this chapter.
4. Find two pictures in a magazine, in a newspaper, or online that best represent correct body mechanics. Explain why you selected these images.

Building Math Skill

Oxygen therapy was ordered for Mrs. M because she was having difficulty breathing. Prior to placing the nasal cannula, she was breathing slowly and with difficulty at a rate of 12 breaths per minute. One hour later when you checked her respirations, they were very fast and shallow at 26 breaths per minute. When you report this change to the licensed nursing staff, what will you say the increase is in breaths per minute?

Preparing for the Certification Competency Examination

To prepare for the nursing assistant certification competency examination, you will need to know content found in this chapter. This content may be tested in the knowledge (written or oral) and skills (hands-on demonstration) portions of the exam. The following areas will be emphasized:

- general resident safety
- safety hazards
- accident prevention and reporting
- body mechanics
- fall prevention
- use of restraints
- fire prevention and oxygen safety

These sample test questions are similar to ones you will find on the certification competency exam. See how well you can answer them. Be sure to select the *best* answer.

1. A doctor has ordered restraints for Mr. S. Which of the following is true?
   A. Mr. S will be at a lower risk for developing respiratory problems.
   B. Mr. S will be at a greater risk for developing decubitus ulcers.
   C. Mr. S will become more hungry and thirsty.
   D. Mr. S will be at a greater risk for falling out of bed.

2. A fire starts in Mr. G's room. The first thing a nursing assistant should do is
   A. try to put out the fire
   B. get Mr. G out of the room safely
   C. pull the fire alarm
   D. inform a member of the licensed nursing staff

(Continued)

3. Mr. D has been identified as a fall risk. The first thing a nursing assistant should do is
   A. put a restraint on Mr. D
   B. tell Mr. D to be careful getting out of bed
   C. advise Mr. D's family that he is a fall risk
   D. put a fall risk sign on Mr. D's bed or outside his door

4. A nursing assistant sees that Mrs. C, who is in restraints, is half out of bed. What should the nursing assistant do?
   A. put the restraint back on tightly so Mrs. C cannot move
   B. leave the restraint off and report to the licensed nursing staff
   C. call for help to get Mrs. C back to bed and reapply the restraints
   D. put a different type of restraint on Mrs. C

5. A nursing assistant sees that Mr. J is not getting enough oxygen through his tubing. What should the nursing assistant do?
   A. turn up the oxygen
   B. turn off the oxygen
   C. check the oxygen tubing for kinks
   D. ask Mr. J to take deeper breaths

6. To prevent back strains and injuries, nursing assistants should
   A. wear sturdy shoes
   B. not try to lift very heavy residents without help
   C. ask for help on all of their activities
   D. use correct-size bed sheets when making beds

7. To make sure electrical safety is achieved, a nursing assistant should do all of the following *except*
   A. use extension cords to keep equipment away from a water source
   B. not unplug equipment with wet hands
   C. not switch on an electrical razor while oxygen is in use
   D. leave sufficient working space around all electrical equipment to permit safe operation

8. Which of the following is *not* a principle of proper body mechanics?
   A. narrow base of support
   B. line of gravity
   C. stable center of gravity
   D. proper alignment when standing

9. Which of the following is *not* an important safety guideline?
   A. be aware and mindful of safety at all times
   B. always work to prevent errors or harm
   C. learn from errors if they occur
   D. never report an error because you can get in trouble

10. A nursing assistant has been asked to lift a resident. Which of the following actions should she take to use proper body mechanics?
    A. She should bend over the resident.
    B. She should push and not pull.
    C. She should stay close to the resident.
    D. She should take small breaks.

11. During a safety check, a nursing assistant should
    A. turn off the television
    B. make sure the call light is accessible
    C. close the bathroom door
    D. straighten the bed linens

12. A nursing assistant must complete an incident report about a fall. What should be included in the incident report?
    A. the person the nursing assistant thinks is to blame
    B. detailed facts about what the nursing assistant witnessed
    C. the resident's actions prior to the fall
    D. the resident's attire during the fall

13. A nursing assistant's left eye was exposed to a chemical spray during cleaning. What should the nursing assistant do?
    A. quickly report the exposure to the licensed nursing staff
    B. see the doctor after getting home
    C. quickly flush the eye per facility procedure
    D. wipe the eye with a clean, wet dressing

14. To prevent falls, a nursing assistant should
    A. provide comfortable chairs for residents
    B. move possible obstacles in common areas and resident rooms
    C. place extra blankets on the resident in bed
    D. assist residents in dressing and wearing loose-fitting clothing

15. When an error occurs in a culture of safety, the focus is on
    A. what happened, not who did it
    B. who made the error and the result
    C. how many times the error was made
    D. what will happen to the person who made the error

Did you have difficulty with any of the questions? If you did, review the chapter to find the correct answer(s).

Welcome to the Chapter

This chapter provides information about the different types of medical emergencies you may come across as a nursing assistant and the best ways to respond to them. Medical emergencies include anaphylaxis, asphyxia, burns, chest pain, choking, fainting, heart attack (*myocardial infarction*), hemorrhage, poisoning, shock, and stroke (*cerebrovascular accident*). You will learn about first aid, first-responder responsibilities, cardiopulmonary resuscitation (CPR), and automated external defibrillators (AEDs). This chapter also includes important local and global issues concerning disasters, disaster preparedness, terrorism, bioterrorism, violent attacks, pandemics, and effects of climate change.

The information and procedures presented in this chapter will help you build the knowledge and skills needed to become a holistic nursing assistant. Check with your instructor to ensure that these procedures are within your state's regulations for nursing assistant practice. The topics discussed in the chapter are highlighted on the Providing Holistic Care Framework.

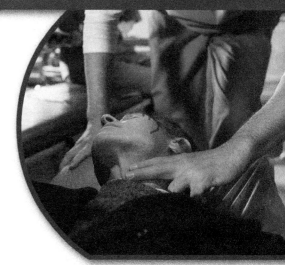

LightField Studios/Shutterstock.com

Chapter Outline

Section 5.1
Medical Emergencies

Section 5.2
Disasters, Pandemics, and Terrorism

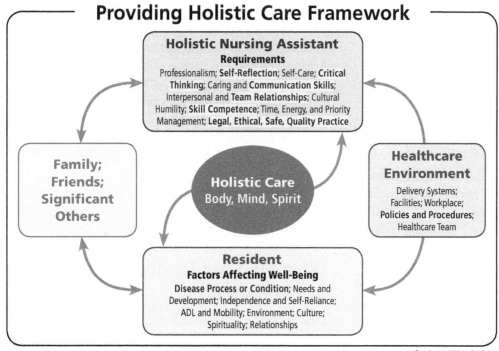

Providing Holistic Care Framework

Holistic Nursing Assistant
Requirements
Professionalism; **Self-Reflection**; Self-Care; **Critical Thinking**; Caring and **Communication Skills**; Interpersonal and **Team Relationships**; Cultural Humility; **Skill Competence**; Time, Energy, and Priority Management; **Legal, Ethical, Safe, Quality Practice**

Family; Friends; Significant Others

Holistic Care
Body, Mind, Spirit

Healthcare Environment
Delivery Systems; Facilities; Workplace; **Policies and Procedures**; Healthcare Team

Resident
Factors Affecting Well-Being
Disease Process or Condition; Needs and Development; Independence and Self-Reliance; ADL and Mobility; Environment; Culture; Spirituality; Relationships

Goodheart-Willcox Publisher

Medical Emergencies

Objectives

To achieve the objectives for this section, you must successfully:

- **describe** the nursing assistant's responsibilities during medical emergencies.
- **recognize** when it is appropriate to act as a first responder.
- **explain** guidelines for giving first aid, performing CPR, and applying an AED.
- **demonstrate** procedures for responding to choking, fainting, seizures, and hemorrhage.

Key Terms

Learn these key terms to better understand the information presented in the section.

abdominal thrusts
allergen
anaphylaxis
angina
asphyxia
automated external
   defibrillator (AED)
basic life support (BLS)
cardiopulmonary
   resuscitation (CPR)
diabetes mellitus

fibrillation
grand mal seizure
Hands-Only™ CPR
hemorrhage
myocardial infarction
petit mal seizure
pulse
rule of nines
seizures
shock
stroke

Questions to Consider

- Have you ever experienced a medical emergency such as a broken leg, a severe burn, or a cut that bled a lot? What did you do? How did you feel? Were you scared?
- Did someone help you during or after the emergency? If so, what did the person do? Did the person's actions help make you feel better?
- Has someone you know experienced a medical emergency? If so, what did you do to help? If you did not know what to do, how did you feel?

What Is a Medical Emergency?

A *medical emergency* is a sudden, acute, and serious illness or injury. Many medical emergencies have long-lasting effects. Medical emergencies can result from trauma (such as severe cuts, burns, and broken bones) or medical conditions (such as strokes and heart attacks). No matter where or how a medical emergency occurs, response and care must be immediate. Many areas in the United States have *emergency medical services (EMS)*, which can be reached by calling 9-1-1.

First responders are people who arrive first at an emergency. The immediate actions of first responders depend on the location of the emergency. Within a healthcare facility, nursing assistants must respond to all medical emergencies by:

- immediately turning on the emergency call light to alert staff that there is an emergency
- always following facility policy and considering safety and comfort during and after procedures

Outside a healthcare facility, your first actions as a first responder should be to call 9-1-1 and give your name and location to the 9-1-1 operator. Then provide basic first aid according to your understanding of first aid and help to the best of your ability. Do not try to perform a procedure if you do not feel prepared. First responders may only do more if they have special education and training (certification or licensure). Examples of first responders who have specialized training include emergency medical technicians, paramedics, licensed nursing staff members, and doctors.

What Are Good Samaritan Laws?

Good Samaritan laws protect people who voluntarily help during a medical emergency outside a healthcare facility. In many states, laws define the scope of what can be done by a Good Samaritan. In some states, a person who witnesses a medical emergency must, at the very least, call for help. In other states, a person does not need to provide care unless it is part of his or her job description. People who respond to medical emergencies must be very careful when giving care. Many Good Samaritan laws protect a person against charges of negligence, unless reckless actions were taken that resulted in injury or worsened a situation. As a nursing assistant, you need to know the emergency care laws in your state.

Good Samaritan laws do not apply to emergency services in a healthcare facility. In a healthcare facility, it is your duty and responsibility to help in an emergency.

What First Aid Guidelines Are Important?

First aid is the process of observing and responding to a medical emergency, such as an injury, poisoning, burn, or medical issue (for example, a heart attack or stroke). First aid is performed at the beginning of and during an emergency. It begins with determining the level of the emergency. Then, action should be taken based on accepted standards of care.

Every emergency is different, but in all instances, timing is very important. Try to find trained healthcare providers immediately. Until this trained help arrives, follow general first aid guidelines. By doing this, you can make the difference between a person's life and death.

If you are witness to an emergency, do not panic. Call for help (9-1-1) immediately (**Figure 5.1**). When speaking with a 9-1-1 operator, remember the following first aid guidelines:

1. Provide as many facts as possible.
2. Give the operator the person's name (if you know it), gender (male or female), and approximate age.
3. Describe the symptoms, but only the symptoms you see or are told. Symptoms might include bleeding and its location, the site of burns, or complaints of chest pain.
4. Describe your exact location and how trained healthcare providers can get there.
5. Answer any questions you are asked to the best of your ability.

Pay attention to your own safety. Notice your surroundings and evaluate the situation. For example, never jump into a pool to save a drowning person if you are not a strong swimmer.

Always consider infection control. If you suspect a person may have a communicable (contagious) disease, wear gloves and a mask, if possible. Avoid direct contact with the person's blood. If contact does occur, clean the blood off as soon as possible.

Do not move the person except for safety reasons, such as fire. Moving the person may increase the chance of paralysis or death due to spinal cord damage.

If a person's condition or situation is *not* getting worse, always wait for trained healthcare providers to arrive. Remember to *do no harm*. You can further injure a person who is stable (whose condition is not worsening) by performing a procedure for which you have no training. Be honest with yourself about what you are able to do.

Reassure the person that trained healthcare providers have been called and that you will stay until they arrive (**Figure 5.2**). As much as possible and appropriate,

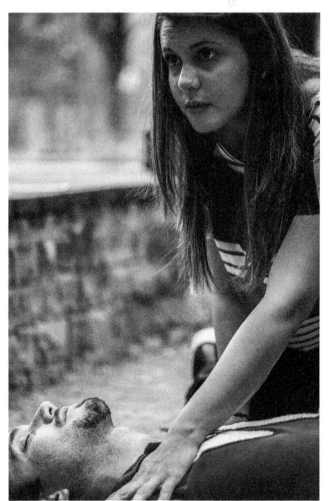

pixelaway/Shutterstock.com

Figure 5.2 After calling for emergency help, stay with the person and perform basic life support depending on your level of training until help arrives.

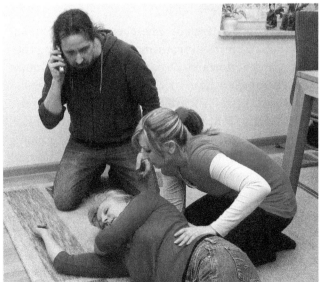

Miriam Doerr Martin Frommherz/Shutterstock.com

Figure 5.1 If you witness an emergency situation, call 9-1-1 immediately.

keep the area free from distractions such as onlookers, noise, or other disturbances. This type of support can help the person remain calm and promote safety.

What Is Basic Life Support?

As a nursing assistant, you must become certified in *basic life support (BLS)* and therefore will be expected to administer CPR, if needed. Certification is earned by satisfactorily completing a course offered by the American Heart Association, the American Red Cross, or other approved agencies or providers. Topics learned in basic life support typically include the *chain of survival* (**Figure 5.3**), CPR techniques, bag-mask techniques, rescue breathing, and choking relief.

Cardiopulmonary Resuscitation (CPR)

In many emergencies, one of the first actions you can take is to perform cardiopulmonary resuscitation (CPR). *Cardiopulmonary resuscitation (CPR)* is an emergency lifesaving procedure for a person whose breathing or heartbeat has stopped. The term *cardiopulmonary* means "pertaining to the heart and lungs," while *resuscitation* means "to revive." CPR supports blood circulation and breathing. It includes manual, external chest compressions (to make the heart pump) and rescue breaths (to restore breathing until trained healthcare providers arrive). CPR may be necessary after a person suffers an electric shock; drowning; or *cardiac arrest*. During cardiac arrest, the heart stops beating suddenly and without warning. Cardiac arrest can be caused by a heart attack.

According to the American Heart Association, more than 350,000 sudden, out-of-hospital cardiac arrests occur in the United States each year. Of those cardiac arrests, 70 percent happen at home. The person becomes unconscious, stops breathing, and has no *pulse* (the beat of the heart as felt through the walls of an artery near the surface of the skin). The skin will be cool, pale, and gray. The person often appears healthy right before cardiac arrest.

Responding quickly to cardiac arrest can help prevent death. A person's chance for survival drops 7 to 10 percent for every minute a normal heartbeat does not begin again. CPR performed immediately can double or triple a person's chance of survival.

The American Heart Association identifies the best approach for CPR based on the amount of training a person has:

- People trained in CPR and confident in their ability should conduct *conventional CPR*. Conventional CPR begins with chest compressions and also includes clearing the airway and performing rescue breathing. The acronym *CAB* will help you remember these steps: Compressions, Airway, and Breathing.
- People *not* trained in CPR should provide *Hands-Only™ CPR*. This involves performing chest compressions at a rate of around 100–120 compressions per minute until trained healthcare providers arrive. Chest compressions force blood through the cardiovascular system.

Hands-Only™ CPR is CPR *without* rescue, or mouth-to-mouth, breathing. Hands-Only™ CPR can be used for teens or adults who suddenly collapse and are not breathing. Conventional CPR with compressions and rescue breathing is recommended for infants and children.

Conventional CPR

Conventional CPR includes chest compressions, airway clearing, and rescue breathing (CAB). Clearing the airway and performing rescue breathing should never be attempted without formal training. The steps of conventional CPR are different for infants and children than for teens and adults. When giving CPR to children, use the same steps as for adults, but only compress the chest 1½ inches. If the child's chest is very small, use only one hand. Following are the steps of conventional CPR:

Chest Compressions—C

1. Check the carotid pulse located on the side of the person's neck. Place your index finger and middle finger on the neck to the side of the windpipe to feel the pulse. Check the pulse for no more than 10 seconds.

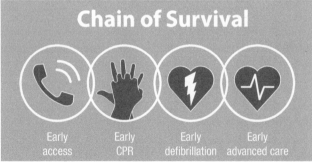

Figure 5.3 The chain of survival includes early access, early CPR, early defibrillation, and early advanced care. All of these links in the chain increase the chance of survival.

Dzm1try/Shutterstock.com

2. If there is no pulse, prepare to start chest compressions. Be sure the person is lying on his or her back (in the supine position), and if possible, on a hard surface. Get on your knees and bend over one side of the person.

3. Using the heels of your hands, place one hand on top of the other. Interlock your fingers. Your dominant hand should touch the person's chest. With your arms straight and your shoulders directly over your hands, use your body weight to push hard and fast in the center of the person's chest on the sternum. Perform 30 chest compressions with no interruptions. For teens and adults, compress the chest to a depth of 2 inches. For children, compress the chest 1½ inches. It is helpful to count out loud each time you allow the chest to move back to its normal position between compressions.

Airway—A

4. After 30 chest compressions, clear the airway by tilting the head and lifting the chin. Put your palm on the person's forehead and gently tilt the head back. With your other hand, gently lift the person's chin forward to open the airway (**Figure 5.4**).

Rescue Breathing—B

5. After clearing the airway, quickly check for normal breathing for no more than 10 seconds. Check for breathing by looking for chest motion, listening for normal breath sounds, and feeling the person's breath on your cheek and ear. Gasping is not normal breathing. If the person is not breathing or is gasping, then begin rescue breathing.

6. Give mouth-to-mouth breathing or mouth-to-nose breathing if the mouth is injured or cannot be opened. If possible, use a barrier device to prevent contact with the person's mouth, secretions, and other body fluids (**Figure 5.5**). After clearing the airway and covering the mouth to form a seal, give two rescue breaths, each lasting one second. After the first breath, watch to see if the chest rises. Then give the second breath and resume chest compressions. Follow a cycle of 30 chest compressions, followed by two rescue breaths.

7. Perform five cycles of CPR (lasting a total of two minutes) before using an available ***automated external defibrillator (AED)***, which is a medical device that delivers an electrical shock through the chest to the heart. An AED is used if a person is not responding to CPR. It can be used twice between a set of five CPR cycles. If an AED is not available, continue CPR until the person starts to move, an AED becomes available, trained healthcare providers arrive, or you become physically exhausted and cannot continue.

Hands-Only™ CPR

The following steps should be used when performing Hands-Only™ CPR. Begin by calling 9-1-1 (or send someone to do so) and following the first aid guidelines discussed earlier in this section. Check to see if the person is conscious. You can tap or shake the person's shoulder and ask, "Are you okay?" (**Figure 5.6**). Also look at the person's chest to see if he or she is breathing (if the chest is rising and falling). If the person is unconscious and is not breathing or is gasping, proceed. You can also check the carotid pulse.

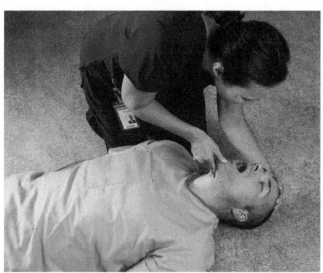

© Tori Soper Photography

Figure 5.4 Clear the airway by tilting the person's head back and lifting the chin.

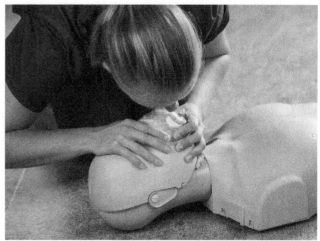

© Tori Soper Photography

Figure 5.5 Sometimes barrier devices are used to help ensure infection control.

An automated external defibrillator (AED) shocks the heart to stop *fibrillation* (irregular heart rhythm) and allow a normal heart rhythm to begin again (**Figure 5.7**). Using an AED is an important part of responding to a medical emergency.

AEDs can be found in a variety of places, such as ambulances, police cars, and public and private locations (doctors' offices, airports, and sports arenas). AEDs are lightweight, battery-operated, and easy to use. Some use video, on-screen text, or verbal directions to guide the user. The AED tells the user if and when a shock should be given to the heart. The AED also provides step-by-step instructions based on the person's heart rhythm.

To use an AED, follow these guidelines:

1. Provide two minutes of CPR at your level of training. After the two minutes of CPR, use an AED.
2. Always practice safety when using an AED. An AED gives an electrical shock, so check for any water nearby. Water conducts (transmits) electricity, so using an AED in or near water may cause shock. If there is water nearby, carefully move the person to a dry area.
3. Turn on the AED's power.
4. Uncover the person's chest, if it is not already uncovered. Remove any metal necklaces or underwire bras and check for body piercings that may get in the way. Metal can conduct electricity and cause burns. To remove a bra, you can cut the center and pull the bra away from the skin. If the person has a lot of chest hair, use the tools provided with the AED to trim or shave it quickly.

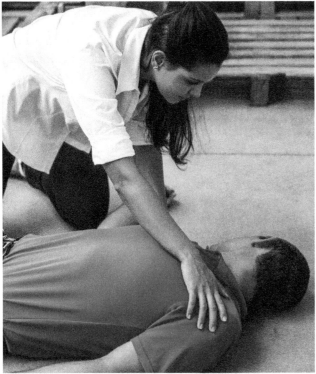

pixelaway/Shutterstock.com

Figure 5.6 Always check level of consciousness and breathing before beginning CPR.

If there is no pulse, begin chest compressions following the guidelines listed for conventional CPR. But, instead of the 30 chest compressions per minute used with conventional CPR, give 100–120 compressions per minute, with no interruptions. You can time your compressions to the beat of the disco song "Stayin' Alive" or use some other familiar method. The chest should be compressed to a depth of two inches and then released. Do not remove your hands from the sternum. It is helpful to count out loud each time you allow the chest to move back to its normal position between compressions. Continue chest compressions until the person starts to breathe, an AED becomes available, trained healthcare providers arrive or you become physically exhausted and cannot continue.

Hands-Only™ CPR improves a person's chance of survival. Performing it is simple enough that it should not be feared.

Automated External Defibrillator (AED)

The rate and rhythm of a person's heartbeat is controlled by an internal electrical system in the heart. Some people have problems with heart rhythm. The heart may beat too fast or too slow, beat irregularly, or stop due to cardiac arrest.

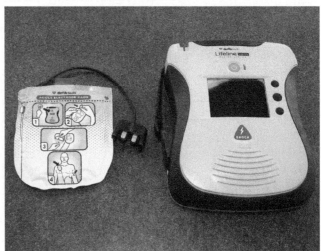

Goodheart-Willcox Publisher

Figure 5.7 An AED is an emergency medical device that shocks the heart to bring it back to normal rhythm.

5. AEDs have sticky pads with sensors called *electrodes*. Apply the pads to the person's chest (**Figure 5.8**). The AED should also have extra pads available. Be sure the person's chest is dry. Lean over the person and place one pad on the right center of the person's chest above the nipple. Place the other pad slightly below the other nipple and to the left of the rib cage. Make sure the sticky pads make a good connection with the skin. If the connection is not good, a *Check electrodes* message will appear on the AED's screen.

6. Check for a medical alert bracelet to see if the person has any implanted devices, such as a pacemaker. Implanted devices are also visible under the skin of the chest or abdomen. Move the defibrillator pads at least one inch away from any implanted devices or piercings so the electrical current can flow freely between the pads. Also remove any medication patches on the chest and wipe the skin.

7. Check that the wires of the electrodes are connected to the AED. Make sure no one is touching the person and then press the AED's *Analyze* button. Stay clear while the machine checks the person's heart rhythm. The AED will determine if a shock can help restore normal heart rhythm. If a shock is needed, the AED will let you know. The shock may be delivered automatically by the AED, or you may be prompted to press the *Shock* button.

8. Stand clear of the person and make sure others are clear before you push the AED's *Shock* button.

9. After the shock, begin CPR again.

10. The AED will automatically reanalyze the person's heart rhythm to determine if another shock is needed.

11. If a shockable heart rhythm is not detected, the AED will prompt you to check the person's pulse and continue performing CPR.

12. If the person is still not responding, continue CPR until the person moves or until trained healthcare providers arrive. Stay with the person until help arrives. Report all the information you know.

How Should Chest Pain, Heart Attacks, and Strokes Be Handled?

Chest pain (angina), heart attacks, and strokes are medical emergencies and require quick response. There are actions you can take to respond to these medical emergencies outside a healthcare facility. If these medical emergencies occur within a healthcare facility, follow the facility's policy.

Chest Pain

Angina, or chest pain, is any major discomfort around the chest. Angina is a common complaint that may or may not be caused by heart disease. While chest pain may be located in the chest area, it can easily spread to the back, neck, lungs, esophagus (the tube that carries food and liquids from the mouth to the stomach), or abdomen (stomach).

Stable angina is caused by physical activity that makes the heart work harder and that demands more blood than what is available due to narrowed arteries. Stable angina usually lasts for a few minutes and disappears with rest or prescribed medications. *Unstable angina*, which is more serious, can occur even at rest and is unexpected. Unstable angina may occur due to a rupture of plaque (a build-up of fat and other substances), causing blockage in the artery. Unstable angina lasts longer and may not disappear with prescribed medications. Unstable angina is a medical emergency.

Until the cause of angina has been determined, angina should be considered a sign of a heart-related problem. Get immediate help by either calling 9-1-1 or taking the person to an emergency department. If angina is caused by a heart attack, trained healthcare providers can determine how to continue to increase the person's chance of survival.

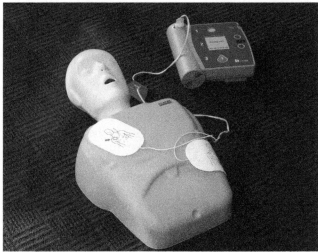

Goodheart-Willcox Publisher

Figure 5.8 One pad should lie on the right center of the person's chest over the nipple. The other pad should lie to the left of the rib cage below the other nipple.

Heart Attack

A *myocardial infarction*, or *heart attack*, occurs when blood flow to part of the heart muscle is blocked. Plaque ruptures within the coronary artery, causing a blood clot to form and cause blockage. The heart muscle becomes severely damaged and dies. Heart attacks can cause cardiac arrest.

Many heart attacks begin with hardly noticeable symptoms, such as discomfort or pain that comes and goes. Other initial symptoms may include lightheadedness; cold sweats; or mild, spreading pain (which some people mistakenly think will improve through rest or sleep). Women may experience different symptoms from men. Women are more likely to have generalized chest pain; pain in the arms, back, or jaw; sweating; nausea; or fatigue. Some people have a *silent heart attack* with no symptoms. A silent heart attack is more common among women and people with *diabetes mellitus* (excessive sugar in a person's blood).

In general, a person having a heart attack may have some or all of these signs and symptoms:

- discomfort or pain that is described as a tight ache, pressure, fullness, severe and crushing feeling, or squeezing in the chest
- pain that lasts more than a few minutes in the left, right, or both arms or below the breastbone
- pain, numbness, or tingling down the left arm (**Figure 5.9**)
- discomfort that spreads to the back, jaw, or throat
- fullness, indigestion, or a choking feeling that may feel like heartburn
- sweating, nausea, vomiting, or dizziness
- extreme weakness or shortness of breath during exercise or at rest
- rapid or irregular heartbeats
- anxiety or a feeling of impending doom

If possible, call 9-1-1 within five minutes of the occurrence of these symptoms. The quicker treatment occurs, the better the outcome will be. If a person is not allergic to aspirin, he or she can chew and swallow one non-coated aspirin (325 mg) since chewing works faster than swallowing aspirin whole. Aspirin slows down the growth of a blood clot. This helps blood flow through the coronary artery and keeps heart muscle cells from dying.

Keep the person who is experiencing these symptoms calm and quiet, loosen the person's clothing if it is tight, and have the person sit or lie

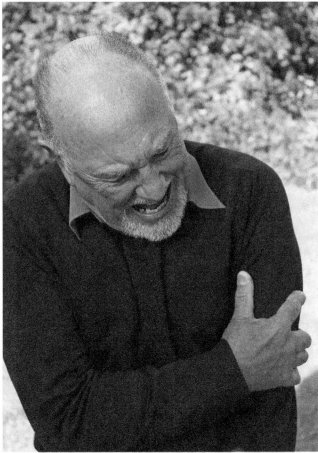

Giideon/Shutterstock.com

Figure 5.9 Pain in the left arm is one sign of a heart attack.

down and raise his or her head to breathe better. Check the person's respirations and pulse often. If the person stops breathing, start CPR based on your level of training.

Stroke

A *stroke*, or *cerebrovascular accident (CVA)*, is the fifth leading cause of death in the United States. It is also a leading cause of disability. A stroke occurs

---

THINK ABOUT THIS

The location of blood flow blockage to the brain determines the effects of a stroke. For example, when a stroke occurs in the brain's right side, the opposite or left side of the body is affected and may become paralyzed. Someone who has suffered a stroke in the right side of the brain may also have vision problems or memory loss. If the left side of the brain is affected, speech or language problems may occur. A stroke in the brain stem can affect both sides of the body and may leave someone in a locked-in state. In a locked-in state, a person is usually unable to speak or move below the neck.

Risk Factors for Heart Disease and Stroke

Members of particular ethnic groups are at higher risk for heart disease than others. Individuals from these groups may be more likely to have a medical emergency. Heart disease is the leading cause of death for African-Americans and Hispanics. Native Americans, Alaska natives, Asians, and Pacific Islanders face heart disease as the second leading cause of death.

According to the American Stroke Association, compared to Caucasians, African-Americans are nearly twice as likely to suffer a stroke, and Hispanics also have an increased risk. African-Americans and Hispanics are more likely to die following a stroke than Caucasians.

Apply It

1. For what medical emergencies does your culture have increased risk?
2. How can you be respectful of a person's culture when responding to a medical emergency?

---

when a blood vessel carrying oxygen and nutrients (substances that provide nourishment needed to maintain life) to the brain becomes blocked by a clot or ruptures. When this happens, a part of the brain cannot get the blood and oxygen it needs.

Some signs of a stroke include:

- a severe headache
- weakness and tingling in the arms, legs, or face
- paralysis on one side
- difficulty waking
- sudden confusion
- slurred speech and drooping eyelids
- facial drooping
- drooling
- change in vision
- difficulty with speech
- change in vital signs

If a person shows signs of a stroke, get immediate help by calling 9-1-1 or take the person to the emergency department. Keep the person warm, do not offer food or fluids, and provide CPR at your level of training, if needed.

What Is Anaphylaxis?

Many people have allergies to medications (such as aspirin or antibiotics), foods (such as nuts, fish, and shellfish), and insect stings. Some people respond with mild to moderate allergic reactions, and others experience anaphylaxis. *Anaphylaxis* is a severe allergic reaction that can affect the whole body. An allergic reaction usually occurs within minutes of exposure to an *allergen*, or substance that causes an allergic reaction (**Figure 5.10**). Anaphylaxis, however, can occur 30 or more minutes after exposure to an allergen.

Not everyone has the same allergic reactions. Symptoms of an allergic reaction may include:

- skin reactions such as hives, itching, and flushed or pale skin
- swelling of the face, eyes, lips, or throat
- a feeling of warmth throughout the body
- the sensation of a lump in the throat
- constriction (tightening) of airways, which can cause wheezing and troubled breathing
- a weak, rapid pulse
- nausea, vomiting, or diarrhea
- dizziness, fainting, or unconsciousness

If someone is experiencing moderate-to-severe symptoms of an allergic reaction or anaphylaxis, do not wait to see if the person gets better. Symptoms of anaphylaxis must be acted on immediately, and

Common Allergens

Type	Examples
Skin contact	• Poisonous plants • Pollen • Animal scratches • Latex
Inhalation	• Mold and mildew • Animal dander • Dust • Pollen
Ingestion	• Medications • Nuts and shellfish
Injection	• Bee stings

Goodheart-Willcox Publisher

Figure 5.10 There are many types of allergens that can be inhaled, swallowed, injected, or touched.

emergency treatment is needed even if symptoms start to improve. Get emergency treatment right away. Untreated anaphylaxis can lead to death within 30 minutes.

Take the following actions to help someone having an allergic reaction:

1. Call 9-1-1 immediately and follow the first aid guidelines discussed earlier in this section.
2. Determine whether the person has an epinephrine auto-injector to treat the allergic reaction. If the person does, ask if the person needs help with the injection. If help is needed, press the auto-injector against the middle of the person's outer thigh. Inject into the skin or muscle. In an emergency, the injection can be given through clothing (**Figure 5.11**).
3. Have the person lie still on his or her back and loosen tight clothing. Cover the person with a blanket, if available.
4. Do not give the person anything to drink. If the person is vomiting or bleeding from the mouth, turn the person to the side to prevent choking.
5. If there are no signs of breathing, coughing, or movement, begin CPR depending on your level of training until the person starts moving or until trained healthcare providers arrive.

What Is the Best Method for Responding to Burns?

Burns are a serious threat to a person's health. The skin is the body's first line of defense against infection. A *burn* is a break in the skin. A burn increases the risk of infection at the burn site and possibly throughout the body.

The amount of damage a burn causes depends on its location, depth, and the body surface it covers. The ***rule of nines***, usually used for adults, provides you with a guide to determine the percentage of the body burned (**Figure 5.12**). It applies only to second- and third-degree burns. It estimates the body surface area (BSA) burned using multiples of nine. For example, a burn affecting the head and neck would be reported as nine percent. The rule of nines can also help determine what treatment is needed (for example, if fluid replacement is necessary).

Burns are also classified by depth. There are three depth classifications: first degree, second degree, and third degree. The degree of a burn can change

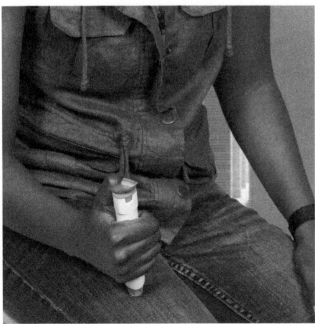

Rob Byron/Shutterstock.com

Figure 5.11 The epinephrine auto-injector should be placed against the middle of the outer thigh.

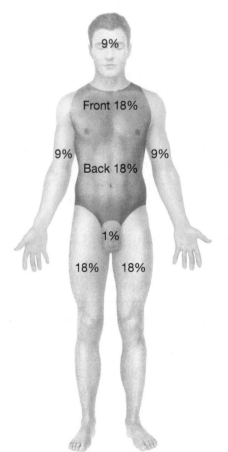

© Body Scientific International

Figure 5.12 The rule of nines estimates the percentage of body surfaces burned using multiples of nine.

over time. For example, a sunburn that was originally considered a first-degree burn can blister and become a second-degree burn over a few hours.

- **First-degree burns:** the least severe burns, affecting only the surface or outer layer of the skin. These burns may cause redness, mild swelling, skin that is tender to the touch, and pain. Most first-degree burns are easily treated by quickly and gently removing jewelry or tight clothing, holding the burned area under cool water for 10–15 minutes or applying a clean towel dampened with cool water, using aloe vera lotion on the affected area, or using over-the-counter pain medications.

- **Second-degree burns:** deeper than first-degree burns, these may cause red, white, or splotchy skin; swelling; pain; and blistering of the skin. Do not attempt to break blisters. Get medical help if large blisters develop or if signs of infection occur, such as oozing from the burned area, increased pain, redness, and swelling. If blisters break on their own, gently clean the area with mild soap and water, apply an antibiotic ointment, and cover the area with a nonstick gauze bandage.

- **Third-degree burns:** the most severe of burns, third-degree burns affect all layers of the skin and underlying fat. Nerves, blood vessels, muscle, and bone can also be affected. Burned areas may be charred black or white and become leathery. The person may have difficulty breathing, and if smoke inhalation has occurred, may suffer other serious effects. Call 9-1-1 immediately and be sure the person is safe. Check for signs of breathing, coughing, or movement. If the person is unconscious, perform CPR depending on your level of training until trained healthcare providers arrive. Do *not* remove burned clothing that is stuck to the skin. Elevate burned areas above the heart, if possible. Do not use cold water for large, severe burns. This may cause a serious loss of body heat (known as *hypothermia*) or a drop in blood pressure and decreased blood flow (shock). Rather, cover the burned area with a cool, moist bandage or clean cloth.

What Should Be Done if Someone May Be Poisoned?

People are injured or die as a result of poisoning every day. Poisoning can be either *accidental* (such as a child swallowing a cleaning product) or *intentional* (poisoning yourself on purpose). Most poisons, such as cyanide, paint thinners, or household cleaning products, are swallowed, but poisons can also enter the body through the skin, by inhalation (breathing it in), intravenously (by injection), through radiation exposure, or by eating spoiled food. Residents with dementia and Alzheimer's disease are at increased risk for poisoning.

A person can be poisoned and not show symptoms for hours, days, or even months. For example, a person may take a large dose of aspirin for extreme pain, which seems harmless. Over a long period of time, however, the long-term effects of the aspirin can slowly poison the person and cause an overdose. The delay in seeking medical help can result in lasting or permanent damage.

When a person has been poisoned, it can be difficult to determine what type of poisoning has occurred. Some signs and symptoms of poisoning are similar to those of common illnesses such as strokes, seizures, and head injuries. Typical signs and symptoms of poisoning include:

- abnormal skin color
- burns or redness around the mouth and lips

HEALTHCARE SCENARIO

Degrees of Burns

Yesterday's news covered a fire that partially burned a home next to yours. You know family members who were involved in the fire. It was reported that two little girls had blistering burns on both of their hands. They were trying to save their cat. The father was coughing severely, was lying on the ground, and had very burned pants. The mother was rubbing her face, which was very red, as she cried.

Apply It

1. If you were a first responder in this situation, what would you do first?
2. Given the information in the news report, what level of burn do you think each family member has?
3. Based on the levels of the burns you identified, what actions should you take?

- breath that smells like chemicals such as gasoline or paint thinner
- nausea and vomiting
- difficulty breathing
- restlessness and irritability
- seizure
- confusion or disorientation

If you suspect that someone has been poisoned, look for clues, such as empty pill bottles; scattered pills; and burns, stains, or odors on the person or nearby objects. Children may have applied medicated patches to their skin or swallowed small batteries. Call the US National Poison Control Center at 1-800-222-1222 or the Regional Poison Control Center to ask questions about possible poisoning. Have the pill bottle, medication, cleaning product, or other suspected container or material available so you can talk about it.

Call 9-1-1 or go to a local emergency department if a person shows active signs of poisoning, if an infant or toddler has been poisoned, or if the poisoning was intentional (even if the substance itself is not harmful). After calling 9-1-1, do the following until trained healthcare providers arrive:

- If a person has swallowed poison, check the person's mouth and remove any poison that remains. If the person swallowed household cleaner or another chemical, read the container's label and follow instructions for accidental poisoning.
- If poison is on a person's skin, remove any contaminated clothing with gloves. Rinse the skin for 15 to 20 minutes in a shower or with a hose.

- If poison is in a person's eye, gently flush the eye with cool or lukewarm water for 20 minutes or until help arrives. Use an eyewash station, if available.
- If a person has inhaled poison, move the person into fresh air as soon as possible.
- If the poisoned person is vomiting, and lying on the floor, turn his or her head to the side to prevent choking.
- If the poisoned person is not breathing or has no pulse, begin and continue CPR depending on your level of training until trained healthcare providers arrive.

Before trained healthcare providers arrive, gather any pill or vitamin bottles, packages or containers with labels, plants, or other information about the suspected poison. Be ready to describe the person's symptoms, the age and weight of the person, any medications being taken, and any information about the suspected poisoning (for example, the amount swallowed and the time since the poisoning occurred).

What Should Be Done if Someone Is Choking?

Choking is a medical emergency that blocks the flow of oxygen to the lungs and the rest of the body. Lack of oxygen causes *asphyxia*, a condition in which the body is deprived of oxygen, leading to the loss of consciousness or death. If you witness someone choking, you must act quickly. For adults, breathing in foreign objects, such as a piece of food, usually causes choking. For children, swallowing a small

---

BECOMING A HOLISTIC NURSING ASSISTANT

Responding to Medical Emergencies

Medical emergencies are frightening for everyone involved. Your first action when responding to a medical emergency should always be to get help. Whether the emergency is happening to you or someone else, always remain calm. If you are aiding another, focus on that person. Listen carefully and use your observation skills. Only do what you know how to do. Never try to be a hero. Instead, be helpful, supportive, and comforting. Remember that, when you are calm and reassuring, the person will be able to sense your emotional state. A fast response and calmness during an emergency can make a positive difference in recovery.

Apply It

1. Think about an emergency you witnessed in the past. What did you do first? Did you effectively help yourself or another person?
2. Were you able to stay calm in the situation? If so, how did you do that? If you were not calm, what might you have done differently to become calm?

object usually causes choking. Older adults whose swallowing is difficult or weak are more at risk of choking.

Blockages that cause choking can be partial or complete:

- **Partial blockage**: the person is coughing a lot, but can speak, and can breathe. Encourage the person to continue coughing. Stay with the person and call 9-1-1 for help. Do not strike the person on the back or perform abdominal thrusts. If the person is coughing, his or her body is doing its job of trying to get rid of the object.
- **Complete blockage**: the person cannot speak and makes high-pitched sounds or grabs at the throat with his or her hands (**Figure 5.13**). These are universal signs of distress. Take quick action by performing quick inward and upward **abdominal thrusts** (formerly known as the *Heimlich maneuver*) using your fist.

The abdominal thrusts may be combined with a series of back blows to help the choking person. When giving a back blow, lean the choking person forward and strike his or her back between the shoulder blades five times using the heel of your hand (**Figure 5.14**). The American Red Cross suggests using the *five-and-five method*, in which five

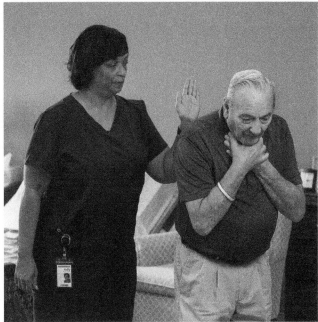

© Tori Soper Photography

Figure 5.14 Back blows should be given between the shoulder blades of the choking person using the heel of your hand.

back blows are followed by five abdominal thrusts. The American Heart Association's recommendation does *not* recommend using back blows. Instead, they say to use only abdominal thrusts.

In this section of the chapter, you will learn several procedures for responding to emergencies. As you review and learn these procedures, remember to:

- always ask for help if you need it
- always follow your facility's policies
- consider the safety and comfort of the resident before, during, and after each procedure

Each procedure is organized so you can clearly understand how to perform it effectively when delivering care. *Best Practice* reminders are included to point out important strategies and actions that help ensure safety and quality care. In each procedure, you will find:

- the reason for performing the procedure (*Rationale*)
- important steps to take before starting the procedure (*Preparation*)
- the procedure itself (*The Procedure*)
- important steps to take after the procedure is completed (*Follow-Up*)
- directions for reporting and documenting the procedure (*Reporting and Documentation*)

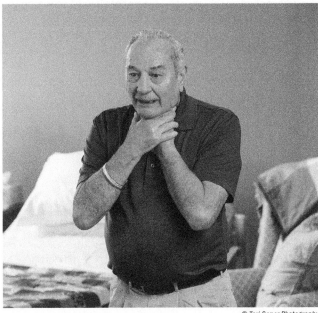

© Tori Soper Photography

Figure 5.13 Grasping the throat with the hands is a universal sign of distress.

Procedure

Responding to Choking Using Abdominal Thrusts

Rationale

Foreign objects can block a person's airway and cause choking. Relieving choking can prevent injury or death. The following procedure should be used with adults and children over one year of age. It should not be used with children under one year of age.

Preparation

1. Follow first aid guidelines and remain calm.
2. Call for help or have someone else call for help. If you are in a healthcare facility, press the emergency call light. Otherwise, call 9-1-1.

The Procedure: Choking—Conscious Adult or Child (Over One Year of Age)

3. Reassure the choking person that you are there to help. Check the person's ability to breathe.
4. If the person is coughing, wait to see if coughing dislodges, or removes, the object.
5. If coughing does not dislodge the object, stand or kneel behind the person. Wrap your arms around the person's waist.

   > **Best Practice:** If possible, let the person's arms hang free. Many people will continue to grasp their throat.

6. Make a fist with one hand.
7. Place the thumb side of your fist against the person's abdomen, slightly above the navel (belly button), and well below the sternum.
8. Grasp your closed fist with your other hand. Do not tuck your thumb inside your fist. Avoid pressing on the person's ribs with your forearms.
9. Press forcefully into the abdomen with the thumb side of your fist. Use quick, inward and upward thrusts to dislodge the object (**Figure 5.15**).
10. Perform five abdominal thrusts and then check to see if the object is visible or has been expelled (forced out).
11. Remove the object only if you see it. To open the person's airway, tilt the person's head back and lift the chin. Look into the person's mouth for the object. Grasp and remove the object if it is within reach.

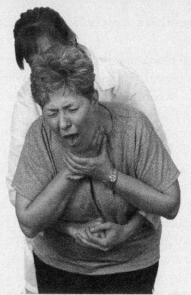

Figure 5.15   aceshot1/Shutterstock.com

> **Best Practice:** Do not sweep your fingers in the person's mouth or try to remove an object you cannot see. Make sure you can reach the object. Trying to remove an object you cannot see or reach may push the object farther into the throat and cause more difficulty.

12. If the object is not visible or has not been expelled, keep performing abdominal thrusts until the object is expelled or the person loses consciousness (stops responding). If the person loses consciousness, follow the steps for an unconscious, choking adult or child (over one year of age).

The Procedure: Choking—Unconscious Adult or Child (Over One Year of Age)

13. Put on disposable gloves, if available, following the procedure in Chapter 8.
14. Turn the person so he or she is lying on his or her back.
15. Check for a pulse (locate the carotid pulse on the person's neck or follow the procedure in Chapter 15). If there is a pulse, open the airway by tilting the head back and lifting the chin. Deliver one breath and watch to see if the chest rises. If the chest does not rise, try one more time.
16. If rescue breaths do not cause the chest to rise, begin conventional or Hands-Only™ CPR depending on your level of training.
17. Every 30 compressions, open the person's airway and look for the foreign object in his or her mouth.
18. If you can see the object, remove it, but do not push it farther down into the throat.

19. Continue performing CPR and checking for the object until the object is expelled or until trained healthcare providers arrive.

Follow-Up

20. If you are not in a healthcare facility, report your observations and actions to the trained healthcare providers when they arrive.
21. If you are in a healthcare facility, take the person's vital signs once the object has been expelled and let the licensed nursing staff know what happened.
22. Remove and discard (appropriately throw away) your gloves, if used.
23. Wash your hands to ensure infection control (see Chapter 8 for the appropriate procedure).
24. If you are in a healthcare facility, make sure the person is comfortable once the object has been expelled. Place the call light and personal items within reach.

25. Conduct a safety check (for example, checking that the bed wheels are locked and person's positioning in is appropriate) before leaving the room. The room should be clean and free from clutter or spills.
26. Remove, clean, and store equipment in the proper location. Remove soiled linens and discard disposable equipment.
27. Wash your hands or use hand sanitizer before leaving the room.

Reporting and Documentation

28. Update a licensed nursing staff member with the person's vital signs. (Measuring and recording vital signs will be discussed in Chapter 15.)
29. If you are in a healthcare facility, report any specific observations, complications, or unusual responses to the licensed nursing staff. Document this information, along with the care provided, in the chart or EMR.

What Happens When a Person Faints?

Fainting is a brief loss of consciousness (awareness) and is considered a medical emergency. Fainting is also called *syncope* or *passing out*. It is caused by a drop in blood flow to the brain.

Reasons for fainting include fatigue (exhaustion), hunger, certain medications, dehydration, heart conditions, age, or the temperature or airflow in a room. Signs that a person may faint include:

- a pale face
- skin that feels cold and clammy (moist)
- perspiration
- a weak pulse
- shallow breathing
- trembling and shaking
- complaints of dizziness or blurred vision

To help prevent fainting when a resident gets out of bed, allow the resident to sit on the side of the bed for a few minutes, dangle the legs to increase blood flow, and breathe deeply to promote the spread of oxygen throughout the body. If a resident is dizzy or faint, do not let him or her stand. Have the resident lie back down until a member of the licensed nursing staff arrives. Consider any signs of fainting a medical emergency even if the person only says he or she feels faint. This prevents possible injury.

Procedure

Responding to Fainting

Rationale

Fainting is a sudden loss of consciousness due to a lack of blood supply to the brain. When consciousness is lost, a person is likely to fall, and injuries can occur.

Preparation

1. Follow first aid guidelines and remain calm.

2. Call for help or have someone else call for help. If you are in a healthcare facility, press the emergency call light. Otherwise, call 9-1-1.

The Procedure

3. Reassure the person that you are there to help.
4. If you have observed signs that the person is about to faint, assist her to a safe position using proper body mechanics. Help her sit or lie down before fainting occurs. Do not leave the person alone.

(continued)

Responding to Fainting *(continued)*

5. If the person is sitting and feels like she is about to faint, have her bend forward and place her head in front of her knees for at least five minutes (**Figure 5.16**). If the person is lying down and there are no related risks, place her on her back and raise her legs approximately 12 inches so they are above the heart. This increases blood flow to her brain.

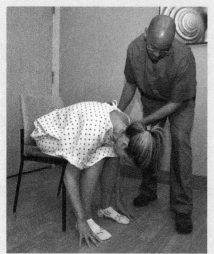

Figure 5.16   *Wards Forest Media, LLC*

6. Check the clothing around the person's neck, chest, and abdomen. Loosen any tight clothing that may restrict breathing.
7. If fainting occurs when the person is standing, slowly lower the person to the floor using your body to support the weight.

8. When on the floor, turn the person's head to the side in case of vomiting. Check breathing and pulse. Call for help. Do not leave the person.
9. Do not let the person get up for at least five minutes after the fainting.
10. Do not give the person anything to eat or drink, unless directed by a trained healthcare provider.
11. Do not leave the person alone as you wait for trained healthcare providers to arrive.

Follow-Up

12. If you are not in a healthcare facility, report your observations and actions to the trained healthcare providers when they arrive.
13. Wash your hands to ensure infection control.
14. If you are in a healthcare facility, let the licensed nursing staff know. Make sure the person is comfortable and place the call light and personal items within reach.
15. Conduct a safety check before leaving the room. The room should be clean and free from clutter or spills.
16. Remove, clean, and store equipment in the proper location. Remove soiled linens and discard disposable equipment.
17. Wash your hands or use hand sanitizer before leaving the room.

Reporting and Documentation

18. If you are in a healthcare facility, report any specific observations, complications, or unusual responses to the licensed nursing staff. Document this information, along with the care provided, in the chart or EMR.

What Is the Appropriate Way to Respond to a Seizure?

Seizures are sudden changes in the brain's normal electrical activity that cause changed or loss of consciousness. A seizure may be the result of a disease such as epilepsy, tumors, or nervous system disorders. Seizures can also be the result of a head injury, so you should act quickly if you witness someone having a seizure. Seizures can occur at any age and generally last from a few seconds to several minutes.

There are two different types of seizures: partial seizures and generalized seizures. *Partial seizures* include motor seizures, sensory seizures, and autonomic seizures. *Motor seizures* occur in the muscles and cause the hands and fingers to jerk. *Sensory seizures* are tingling sensations. *Autonomic seizures* cause changes in breathing rate, sweating, and heart rate.

Generalized seizures can be one of two types: petit mal seizures and grand mal seizures. A person having a ***petit mal seizure*** will have less or no awareness of his or her surroundings and will not be able to respond to you. He or she may stare and may have facial or body twitches.

A person having a ***grand mal seizure*** will have tonic and clonic phases. In the *tonic phase,* muscles stiffen, and air is forced out of the lungs. A person usually groans and then loses consciousness. The person may also fall to the floor, turn blue, and bite his or her tongue. In the *clonic phase,* muscles contract and relax, which causes jerking and rhythmic movements of the arms and legs. Bowel and bladder control may be lost. Consciousness returns slowly and gradually after a grand mal seizure. This type of seizure may last a few seconds or as long as 10 minutes.

Procedure

Responding to a Seizure

Rationale
Preventing injury and maintaining an open airway are primary goals when responding to a seizure.

Preparation
1. Follow first aid guidelines and remain calm.
2. Call for help or have someone else call for help. If you are in a healthcare facility, press the emergency call light. Otherwise, call 9-1-1.

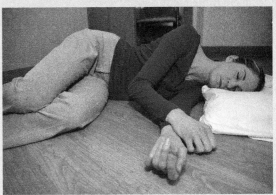

Figure 5.17   *Wards Forest Media, LLC*

The Procedure
3. Reassure the person that you are there to help.
4. Never try to stop a seizure.
5. Note the time the seizure started.
6. Lower the person to the floor if the person is standing using your body to support her weight. This will protect her from falling.
7. Maintain an open airway. Turn the person onto her side and make sure her head is also turned to promote the drainage of any saliva or vomit.
8. Protect the person's head by placing something soft under her head. This will help prevent the head from striking the floor during a seizure. Use a pillow, chair cushion, folded jacket, blanket, or towel. You may also hold the person's head in your lap.
9. Loosen tight clothing and jewelry around the person's neck. Clear the area of equipment or sharp objects. The person may strike these objects during the seizure.
10. Do not force the mouth open. Do not put any objects or your fingers between the teeth. Do not try to limit or control movements.
11. Note the time the seizure ends and place the person in a recovery position (lying on her side). The head should be turned to the side to allow saliva to drain from the mouth (**Figure 5.17**).

Follow-Up
12. If you are not in a healthcare facility, report your observations and actions to the trained healthcare providers when they arrive.
13. Wash your hands to ensure infection control.
14. If you are in a healthcare facility, let the licensed nursing staff know. Make sure the person is comfortable and place the call light and personal items within reach.
15. Conduct a safety check before leaving the room. The room should be clean and free from clutter or spills.
16. Remove, clean, and store equipment in the proper location. Remove soiled linens and discard disposable equipment.
17. Wash your hands or use hand sanitizer before leaving the room.

Reporting and Documentation
18. If you are in a healthcare facility, report any specific observations, complications, or unusual responses to the licensed nursing staff. Document this information, along with the care provided, in the chart or EMR.

What Is a Hemorrhage, and How Can It Be Controlled?

A *hemorrhage*, which is the loss of a large amount of blood over a short period, is a medical emergency. You must act quickly if a hemorrhage occurs.

There are two types of hemorrhages: internal hemorrhages and external hemorrhages. *Internal hemorrhages* occur inside the body. Signs of an internal hemorrhage are pain, shock, vomiting, coughing up blood, and loss of consciousness. In *external hemorrhage*, blood may spurt or flow steadily out from an opening in the body, such as from the nose or mouth, or from a wound or injury that may happen anywhere on the body.

When a person loses a large amount of blood, he or she may go into *shock*. In shock, there is not enough oxygen available to the organs and tissues of the body. When a person is in shock, blood pressure drops; the pulse is rapid and weak; the skin is cool, clammy, and pale; and the person may lose consciousness. Trained medical providers must treat a hemorrhage immediately to prevent death.

The signs and symptoms of a hemorrhage include:
- a pale or cyanotic (blue and discolored) face
- low blood pressure
- increased, but weak, heart rate
- rapid, shallow respirations
- feelings of weakness and helplessness
- restlessness
- complaints of thirst
- coldness, shaking, or trembling

To control the bleeding of an external hemorrhage, you can use direct or indirect pressure. Direct pressure is applied to the bleeding wound. Indirect pressure is applied to a pressure point near or on top of the wound. Pressure points exist where blood vessels are located close to the surface of the skin (**Figure 5.18**). When these points are pressed, blood flow to the wound slows. Combined with direct pressure, this will help stop bleeding. Pressure can be applied using the fingers, thumb, or heel of the hand.

Pressure points, especially the carotid artery, should be used with extreme caution. Sometimes indirect pressure can cause tissue damage.

Pressure Points

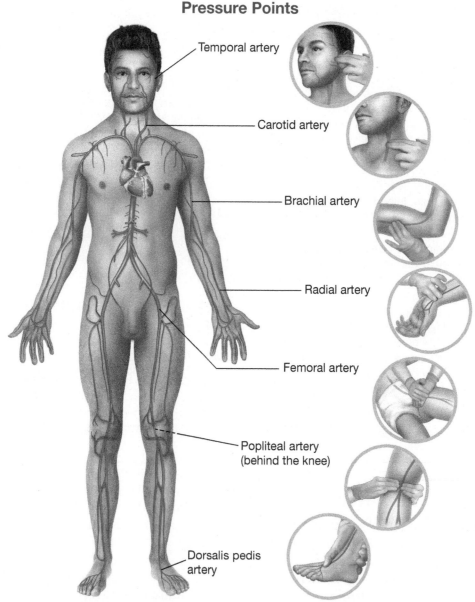

- Temporal artery
- Carotid artery
- Brachial artery
- Radial artery
- Femoral artery
- Popliteal artery (behind the knee)
- Dorsalis pedis artery

© Body Scientific International

Figure 5.18 Applying pressure to these points near the wound will help slow bleeding.

Procedure

Responding to and Controlling Bleeding

Rationale
A hemorrhage can be life threatening if not stopped. Hemorrhages can occur internally or externally, and they are often caused by an injury.

Preparation
1. Follow the first aid guidelines and remain calm.
2. Call for help or have someone else call for help. If you are in a healthcare facility, press the emergency call light. Otherwise, call 9-1-1.

The Procedure: Internal Hemorrhage
3. Reassure the person experiencing a hemorrhage that you are there to help.
4. Keep the person flat, warm, and quiet.
5. Do not give the person any fluids.
6. Do not remove any objects that may have caused the hemorrhage.
7. Wait calmly with the person for trained healthcare providers to arrive.

The Procedure: External Hemorrhage
8. Reassure the person experiencing the hemorrhage that you are there to help.
9. Put on disposable gloves, if available.
10. Apply firm, steady, direct pressure to the bleeding site (**Figure 5.19**). Do not stop applying pressure until the bleeding stops.

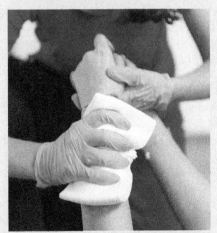

Figure 5.19   *Microgen/Shutterstock.com*

11. Use a sterile (free of germs) dressing, if available. If a sterile dressing is not available, apply a clean material, such as a towel or cloth, and keep it in place with a bandage or tape.
12. If possible, raise the affected area of the body (hand, arm, foot, or leg). This will help slow down blood flow to the area. Wrap the wound when the bleeding stops.
13. Watch for bleeding through the bandage. If you have the knowledge to do so, apply indirect pressure on a pressure point to try to slow the bleeding.
14. Keep the person warm by covering him with a blanket.
15. Do not give the person anything to eat or drink.
16. Wait calmly with the person for trained healthcare providers to arrive.

Follow-Up
17. If you are not in a healthcare facility, report your observations and actions to the trained healthcare providers when they arrive.
18. Remove and discard your gloves, if used.
19. Wash your hands to ensure infection control.
20. If you are in a healthcare facility, let the licensed nursing staff know. Make sure the person is comfortable and place the call light and personal items within reach.
21. Conduct a safety check before leaving the room. The room should be clean and free from clutter or spills.
22. Remove, clean, and store equipment in the proper location. Remove soiled linens and discard disposable equipment.
23. Wash your hands or use hand sanitizer before leaving the room.

Reporting and Documentation
24. If you are in a healthcare facility, report any specific observations, complications, or unusual responses to the licensed nursing staff. Document this information, along with the care provided, in the chart or EMR.

SECTION **5.1** **Review and Assessment**

Key Terms Mini Glossary

abdominal thrusts an emergency procedure in which a person places his or her fist just above the navel of a choking person, covers his or her fist with the other hand, and performs quick inward and upward thrusts.

allergen any substance that the body perceives as a threat, causing an allergic reaction.

anaphylaxis a severe allergic reaction that can affect the whole body; may cause skin reactions, swelling, trouble breathing, rapid pulse, nausea, and dizziness.

angina chest pain or discomfort; there may be a sensation of squeezing, pressure, heaviness, or tightness in the center of the chest.

asphyxia a lack of oxygen in the body; may be caused when breathing stops due to a blockage or swelling in the trachea.

automated external defibrillator (AED) a medical device that gives an electric shock to the heart to stop irregular heart rhythm and allow normal heart rhythm to begin.

basic life support (BLS) care given to a person experiencing respiratory arrest, cardiac arrest, or airway blockage;

includes giving cardiopulmonary resuscitation (CPR), using an automated external defibrillator (AED), and relieving a blocked airway.

cardiopulmonary resuscitation (CPR) an emergency procedure in which air is breathed into a person's mouth or nose to provide ventilation; external chest compressions help oxygenated blood flow to the brain and heart.

diabetes mellitus a disorder in which there are excessive amounts of glucose (sugar) in a person's blood due to insufficient production of insulin (the hormone that regulates glucose) or insulin resistance; commonly referred to as *diabetes*.

fibrillation an irregular heart rhythm.

grand mal seizure a generalized seizure in which a person may experience loss of consciousness and violent muscle contractions; caused by abnormal electrical activity in the brain.

Hands-Only™ CPR an emergency procedure in which uninterrupted chest compressions restore heartbeat and promote blood circulation; is a procedure for those not trained in conventional CPR.

hemorrhage the excessive loss of blood over a short period of time due to internal or external injury.

myocardial infarction a sudden medical emergency that occurs when blood flow to part of the heart muscle is blocked, causing the heart muscle to become severely damaged and die; can cause loss of heart function, or cardiac arrest; also known as a *heart attack*.

petit mal seizure a generalized seizure in which a person has no or lessened awareness and responsiveness and may lose consciousness; caused by abnormal electrical activity in the brain.

pulse the beat of the heart measured through the walls of a peripheral artery.

rule of nines a method of determining the surface area of the body affected by burns.

seizures sudden changes in the brain's normal electrical activity; cause a change in or loss of consciousness.

shock a condition in which the organs and tissues of the body do not have sufficient oxygen.

stroke a sudden blockage or rupture of a blood vessel in the brain; can cause a loss of consciousness, partial loss of movement, and speech impairment; also called a *cerebrovascular accident (CVA)*.

Apply the Key Terms

Write a sentence using each key term properly.

1. anaphylaxis
2. angina
3. hemorrhage
4. seizure
5. shock

Know and Understand the Facts

1. What are three responsibilities nursing assistants have during medical emergencies?
2. Describe the role of the first responder.
3. What specific actions should you take to help someone who is in anaphylaxis?
4. How can you tell if someone has been poisoned?
5. What should you do if a person has a second-degree burn?

Analyze and Apply Concepts

1. Explain the importance of following Hands-Only™ CPR guidelines.
2. List the steps required to effectively use an AED.

3. Explain the procedures for responding to choking in adults and children over one year of age.
4. Describe the actions a nursing assistant should take if a resident has a seizure.

Think Critically

Read the following care situation. Then answer the questions that follow.

Jean, your best friend's grandmother, became very pale, clutched her chest, and started to collapse like she was fainting while she was making you and your friend lunch. You know that Jean had been sick last month and that she takes medication. She had been fine just a few minutes before and had been laughing and telling a great story. You are sitting closest to Jean.

1. What signs should you look for to tell if Jean might be having a heart attack?
2. What is the first action you should take?
3. What should you do to keep Jean safe?

Disasters, Pandemics, and Terrorism

Objectives

To achieve the objectives for this section, you must successfully:

- **describe** types of disasters, pandemics, and terrorism.
- **explain** how a nursing assistant can respond to a disaster, pandemics, and terrorism appropriately.

Key Terms

Learn these key terms to better understand the information presented in the chapter.

bioterrorism
cyberattacks
evacuation
pandemics

Questions to Consider

- Have you ever experienced a disaster, such as a hurricane or tornado? If you have, what was it like? Did you know about the disaster ahead of time? If you did, what precautions did you take?
- If you have not experienced a disaster, have you watched or read the news about one? During the disaster, what actions were taken by emergency response personnel? What happened after the disaster? How did watching the disaster feel?

Medical emergencies have a small impact. For example, only one person suffers from a heart attack. The impact of a disaster is much bigger, affecting many people, and potentially causing large-scale destruction of life and property and affecting local and global health. Both medical emergencies and disasters require quick action and preparation to save lives and improve recovery.

What Are Disasters, Pandemics, and Terrorism?

According to the World Health Organization (WHO), a *disaster* causes human, material, economic, and environmental loss and limits a community's ability to function. Disasters can range from natural disasters (such as earthquakes, hurricanes, avalanches, wildfires, and tornados) to aircraft crashes, *arson* (fires set intentionally to cause damage), explosions, and epidemics (outbreaks of a disease that affects a large number of people).

> **THINK ABOUT THIS**
>
> The United States ranks second in the world for its number of natural disasters. Natural disasters tend to be related to the weather. For example, tornados are more common in the United States than in any other country. Other natural disasters include heat waves, cyclones, earthquakes, and floods. Wildfires also destroy property and threaten lives.

Disasters can also be caused by changes in climate. *Climate change* is an unusual pattern of weather related to changes in oceans, land surfaces, and ice sheets, which happen over time—usually decades or longer. For example, changes in ocean temperatures can lead to increased wind speeds in tropical storms.

Pandemics occur when there is a worldwide spread of a disease and most of the populations affected do not have immunity (body's ability to prevent the disease) against the disease. In a pandemic, the disease may affect people of all ages, with some being more severely affected than others. Pandemics differ from epidemics. An epidemic occurs when there is a sudden increase in the number of people in one area or country who have a specific disease. When that same disease spreads across several countries, affecting large numbers of people, it becomes a pandemic. An example of a pandemic is COVID-19.

Terrorism is violence that is politically motivated. Examples of terrorism include the September 11, 2001, attacks in New York and the Boston Marathon bombing. Terrorist attacks can also include biological and chemical threats, the use of nuclear weapons, *cyberattacks* (illegal attempts to gain access to a digital device or network to cause harm), and bombings. Violent attacks that are not politically motivated (for example, mass shootings) can also have devastating consequences. Terrorism and violent attacks are disasters and often cause a large number of casualties (deaths or injuries), damage to buildings, the need for heavy law enforcement, widespread media coverage, work and school closures, travel restrictions, and possibly evacuation.

Bioterrorism is the intentional use of pathogens such as viruses and bacteria to cause illness or death in people, animals, or plants. Bioterrorism agents can be spread by air, through water, or in food. They are categorized based on their ability to spread and the severity of illness or number of deaths they cause.

What Is the Best Way to Respond to a Disaster?

If a disaster or terrorist attack occurs while you are working as a nursing assistant, follow the healthcare facility's policies, procedures, and disaster plans (**Figure 5.20**). If the disaster is a pandemic, there will also be specific policies and procedures to be followed. Disaster plans are typically discussed with staff members during orientation, and specific training and practice are given to be sure staff members are ready. As a nursing assistant, you must be prepared.

It is also helpful to be prepared for disasters that may occur outside a healthcare facility. Consider creating a supply kit and disaster and communication plan. Disaster and communication plans should include responsibilities, emergency contacts, pet safety guidelines, procedures, safe spots for different types of emergencies, *evacuation* routes (routes for the removal of people or objects from a dangerous area), and a shelter location. Practicing these plans twice a year will improve your ability to make them happen. It is also important to familiarize yourself with emergency plans for the places where you and your family spend time (for example, schools, faith organizations, and sporting events). Further preparation includes:

- teaching children how and when to call 9-1-1 for help
- learning your community's warning signal
- showing family members how and when to turn off the water, gas, and electricity (**Figure 5.20**)

- teaching family members how to use and where to find fire extinguishers
- checking your emergency supplies throughout the year to replace batteries, food, and water as needed

If a disaster occurs in your community, follow these steps to respond:

1. Remain calm.
2. Follow the advice of local emergency officials.
3. Listen to your radio or television for news and instructions.
4. If the event occurs near you, check for injuries. Give first aid and get help for seriously injured people.
5. Check and shut off damaged utilities.
6. Check on your neighbors, especially older adults or people with disabilities.

Agencies and organizations in the United States typically work together and coordinate their efforts to prepare for and respond to disasters. The primary organizations include the following:

- **American Red Cross**: a nonprofit, volunteer organization that responds to disasters regardless of size or scope (**Figure 5.21**). The American Red Cross is responsible for mass care, including food, shelter, distribution of disaster relief supplies, first aid, and disaster welfare information.

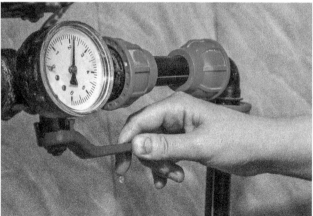

Figure 5.20 Knowing the location of a water shutoff valve like this one can help prepare you for an emergency situation.

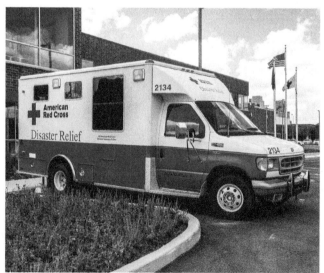

Figure 5.21 The American Red Cross responds to disasters of any scale.

- **Centers for Disease Control and Prevention (CDC)**: a federal agency that focuses on preparedness to support the US Department of Homeland Security. The CDC protects the public from health threats and assists with public health and medical preparedness.
- **Federal Emergency Management Agency (FEMA)**: a federal agency that helps in disasters recognized by the US president. Some of FEMA's work involves community recovery tasks such as rebuilding bridges, roads, and public buildings.

- **US Department of Homeland Security**: a federal agency responsible for the National Response Framework and Plan. This agency supports citizen and community preparedness and ensures that first responders have the resources needed to respond to a violent attack or natural disaster.

The Food and Drug Administration (FDA) and the Environmental Protection Agency (EPA) also provide protection against bioterrorism and ensure water security.

SECTION 5.2 Review and Assessment

Key Terms Mini Glossary

bioterrorism the use of harmful agents and products with biological origins (including pathogens or toxins) as weapons.

cyberattacks illegal attempts to gain access to a digital device or network to cause harm.

evacuation the intentional removal of people or objects from a dangerous area.

pandemic worldwide spread of a disease among people who have no immunity against the disease.

Apply the Key Terms

An incorrect key term is used in each of the following statements. Identify the incorrect key term and then replace it with the correct term.

1. A cyberattack occurs when harmful agents and products with biological origins are used as weapons.
2. When an illegal attempt is made to gain access to a digital device or network to cause harm, it is called an evacuation.
3. Bioterrorism is the intentional removal of people or objects from a dangerous area.

Know and Understand the Facts

1. List three different types of disasters.
2. Explain why bioterrorism and terrorist attacks are considered disasters.
3. Describe the roles and responsibilities of three different agencies or organizations in preparing for and responding to disasters.

Analyze and Apply Concepts

1. Why are disaster plans so important?
2. What is the most important thing a nursing assistant can do to be prepared for a disaster?
3. Identify three important actions a person can take to be prepared for a disaster.

Think Critically

Read the following care situation. Then answer the questions that follow.

Bianca works in a long-term care facility. She is a new nursing assistant and recently moved from a city in which tornados were common. While she lived there, she had to evacuate her home three times due to a tornado, and her home was heavily damaged once. She is very frightened of tornados and wants to be prepared to help residents if one strikes.

1. What is the most important thing Bianca can do to be sure she is ready if a disaster occurs?
2. How can Bianca decrease her fears about disasters?
3. If Bianca prepares a personal disaster plan, what should she include?

Summary and Review

Key Points

Reviewing the key points for this chapter will help you practice more safely and competently as a holistic nursing assistant and will help you prepare for the certification competency examination.

- First aid is the initial process of evaluating and responding to a medical emergency. First responders arrive first at an emergency, and their immediate actions are to call 9-1-1 and provide basic first aid. When responding to an emergency in a healthcare facility, turn on the emergency call light immediately.
- Nursing assistants need to be certified in conventional CPR, which includes chest compressions and rescue breaths. A person who is not certified in conventional CPR should use Hands-Only™ CPR. Using an AED can stop an irregular heart rhythm so normal rhythm returns.
- If you witness a person choking, fainting, having a seizure, or hemorrhaging, remain calm and respond appropriately.
- Natural disasters, pandemics, and terrorism can cause the loss of life and property damage.
- As a nursing assistant, one of the best ways to respond to a disaster is to become familiar with your healthcare facility's policies, procedures, and disaster plans. Being prepared is your most important responsibility.

Action Steps to Holistic Care

Review the information in this chapter. Complete the following activities.

1. Select one medical emergency discussed in this chapter. Prepare a short paper or digital presentation that identifies and describes the three most important actions to take when responding to the emergency.
2. Create a poster or digital presentation explaining how to use an automated external defibrillator (AED). For each step, include both a visual (photograph, image, or illustration) and written description.
3. With a partner, prepare a poster that lists at least four facts about emergency care for strokes and heart attacks. Include how these actions can slow down or reduce injuries and complications.
4. Create a supply kit and disaster and communication plan for your family in the event of a possible natural disaster in your area. Discuss your preparations with your family, making sure each person knows their role, identify evacuation routes, and practice your plans. Then write a brief report.

Building Math Skill

Krishna, an experienced nursing assistant, is taking a walk outside at lunchtime when he sees a man fall to the ground. He immediately uses his cell phone to call 9-1-1 and follows first aid guidelines. It is clear that CPR is needed. He starts conventional CPR, in which he is certified. He has to do four cycles of CPR before trained professionals arrive. How many chest compressions did he give and how many rescue breaths?

Preparing for the Certification Competency Examination

To prepare for the nursing assistant certification competency examination, you will need to know content found in this chapter. This content may be tested in the knowledge (written or oral) and skills (hands-on demonstration) portions of the exam. The following areas will be emphasized:

- principles and goals of basic emergency care
- basic first aid principles
- signs of medical emergencies such as anaphylaxis, asphyxia, burns, choking, fainting, hemorrhage, poisoning, shock, and stroke
- CPR and abdominal thrusts
- responses to and documentation of emergency situations according to standards of care

These sample test questions are similar to ones you will find on the certification competency exam. See how well you can answer them. Be sure to select the *best* answer.

1. An AED is used to help during
   - A. the control of bleeding
   - B. CPR
   - C. abdominal thrusts
   - D. a seizure

2. A nursing assistant knows that a second-degree burn has
   - A. slight redness
   - B. white, leathery skin
   - C. blistering
   - D. charred white skin

3. What is the most important responsibility of the US Department of Homeland Security?
   A. evacuating people from their homes
   B. maintaining the National Response Framework and Plan
   C. rebuilding towns and highways
   D. making sure the water is safe during a disaster

4. What is a first responder?
   A. the first person who knows the victim
   B. the first person who hears about an emergency
   C. the first person who knows what to do in an emergency
   D. the first person to arrive at an emergency

5. When giving Hands-Only™ CPR, you should
   A. perform chest compressions with your hands
   B. perform rescue breaths, but not chest compressions
   C. perform rescue breaths and chest compressions
   D. do nothing, but call for help

6. Mrs. G is grabbing her throat with her hands. She is most likely
   A. having a seizure
   B. having a stroke
   C. choking
   D. having a heart attack

7. How is CPR performed?
   A. using rhythmic breathing
   B. using chest compressions
   C. using abdominal thrusts
   D. using a firm back slap

8. On which type of burn should you *not* use cool water?
   A. first-degree burn
   B. fourth-degree burn
   C. second-degree burn
   D. third-degree burn

9. What is the difference between a disaster and a medical emergency?
   A. A disaster requires fewer resources than a medical emergency.
   B. A disaster does not require the help of organizations and agencies.
   C. A disaster affects larger groups of people than a medical emergency.
   D. A disaster is not as serious as a medical emergency.

10. Mr. D was recently admitted to a long-term care facility. When you give him morning care, you notice that his right eyelid is drooping and that he is having trouble speaking. These are symptoms of a
    A. stroke
    B. heart attack
    C. seizure
    D. anaphylaxis

11. After arriving at a medical emergency, what is the first thing a nursing assistant should do?
    A. check for consciousness
    B. take vital signs
    C. reassure the person
    D. call for help

12. When responding to a medical emergency in a healthcare facility, nursing assistants should always
    A. use basic first aid principles
    B. consult with a supervisor first
    C. follow facility policy
    D. wait until a licensed nursing staff member arrives

13. Ms. C is eating lunch in the dining room and is showing signs of fainting. What should you do after calling for help?
    A. continue to talk with Ms. C to redirect her attention
    B. have Ms. C bend forward and place her head in front of her knees
    C. offer Ms. C a glass of water and some crackers
    D. move Ms. C to her bed so she is lying flat

14. Jody has a severe allergic reaction that affects her whole body when she eats nuts. This is called
    A. anaphylaxis
    B. aphagia
    C. asphyxia
    D. angina

15. Which of the following is an important principle in giving first aid?
    A. stand back and let others help
    B. take control and tell others what to do
    C. push yourself to perform challenging tasks
    D. know your limits when helping

Did you have difficulty with any of the questions? If you did, review the chapter to find the correct answer(s).

6 Holistic Care

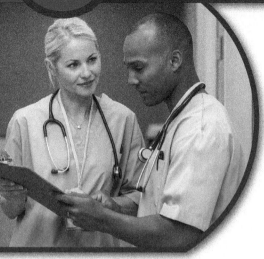

Rido/Shutterstock.com

Chapter Outline

Welcome to the Chapter

This chapter provides information about the different levels and types of nursing care delivered in healthcare facilities. You will also learn about the role holistic nursing assistants play in the nursing process and about the importance of policies and procedures for safe and competent practice. Members of the licensed nursing staff will delegate (transfer) work to nursing assistants. It is important that delegated tasks be completed in an accurate and timely manner. Nursing assistants may also be asked to perform procedures for residents entering a facility (admission), moving within or to another facility (transfer), and leaving a facility (discharge).

The information and procedures presented in this chapter will help you build the knowledge and skills needed to become a holistic nursing assistant. Check with your instructor to ensure that these procedures are within your state's regulations for nursing assistant practice. The topics discussed in the chapter are highlighted on the Providing Holistic Care Framework.

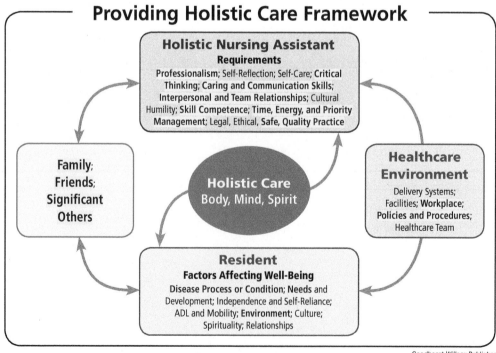

Providing Holistic Care Framework

Holistic Nursing Assistant
Requirements
Professionalism; Self-Reflection; Self-Care; Critical Thinking; Caring and Communication Skills; Interpersonal and Team Relationships; Cultural Humility; Skill Competence; Time, Energy, and Priority Management; Legal, Ethical, Safe, Quality Practice

**Family;
Friends;
Significant
Others**

Holistic Care
Body, Mind, Spirit

**Healthcare
Environment**
Delivery Systems;
Facilities; Workplace;
Policies and Procedures;
Healthcare Team

Resident
Factors Affecting Well-Being
Disease Process or Condition; Needs and Development; Independence and Self-Reliance; ADL and Mobility; Environment; Culture; Spirituality; Relationships

Goodheart-Willcox Publisher

Levels and Types of Nursing Care

Objectives

To achieve the objectives for this section, you must successfully:

- **describe** the different levels and types of nursing care delivery.
- **recognize** the process of delegation and its impact on delivering care.

Key Terms

Learn these key terms to better understand the information presented in the section.

accountable
cognitive status
continuity

delegate
tracheostomy

Questions to Consider

- Have you ever been asked to do something by a friend or coworker? Maybe you were asked to do a job or task that was part of your friend's responsibilities or to attend a meeting in your coworker's place.
- When your friend or coworker requested your help, did he or she give you the information you needed to decide if you were able to help him or her? If he or she did not, what would have helped in your decision making?
- If you did what was asked of you, did your friend or coworker follow up to see how it went?

What Are Levels of Care?

Every healthcare facility provides varying levels of care to meet the special needs of each resident. As you learned in Chapter 2, *levels of care* describe the types and amounts of care that residents need to achieve the best result or outcome. Providing the right level of care helps a resident in a long-term care facility remain as independent as possible. For example, the level of care an older adult needs helps determine whether a healthcare facility has the staff and resources to meet the older adult's needs. Knowing the level of care a resident requires also helps healthcare staff evaluate the resident's insurance to determine what care will be covered.

Determining Levels of Care

Levels of care are usually evaluated before a resident selects a long-term care facility. This helps

to make sure the facility will offer the care needed. For example, someone with dementia might need special memory care and should choose a facility that offers this care.

Level of care is evaluated again once a resident has entered and spent some time in the healthcare facility. After the information provided by doctors and nurses is reviewed, medical needs are considered, including the level of nursing staff needed for specific care. The nursing staff needed may range from a nursing assistant to an RN. Personal care needs are also important in evaluating level of care. This might include the amount of help needed to complete ADLs. A resident's *cognitive status* (ability to think clearly, make decisions, and remember) is also considered. Self-care abilities, such as a resident's ability to swallow medications, also influence the level of care. Once these factors are considered by the doctor and licensed nursing staff, a *level-of-care assignment* is made.

Assigning Levels of Care

As a resident's needs or conditions change over time, so do the level of care assignments. Typically, an initial evaluation places residents in facilities that will best meet their care needs. When people seek long-term care, it is often helpful for them to consider both current and future needs and choose a facility that meets both. This way, when residents have more advanced needs, they do not need to move to a new facility. Levels of care in a long-term care facility include skilled, intermediate, and supportive care.

Skilled Care

Skilled care requires 24-hour, hands-on care in a healthcare facility. This level of care may also include physical therapy, rehabilitation therapy, speech therapy, or wound care. Skilled care is typically needed for only a short period of time. Depending on the services needed, Medicare limits the number of days it will pay for care in a skilled care facility. The goal of skilled care is to improve a resident's medical condition so the level of care can be changed to intermediate.

Intermediate Care

Intermediate care is provided for those who require assistance with ADLs, such as bathing or hygiene. Care is usually provided by nursing assistants, caregivers, home health aides, or even family members. Licensed nursing staff and doctors must continually monitor progress and assess healthcare needs. Intermediate care can occur in a person's home or in a healthcare facility such as *assisted living*.

Supportive Care

Individuals who need *supportive care* may require special rehabilitation. These services could include **tracheostomy** care (care for a surgical opening in the trachea), care for multiple medical problems (called *comorbidities*) that require blood pressure or medications to be monitored, or respiratory therapy (**Figure 6.1**). This care may be given in a person's home by an RN or LPN/LVN. This level of care also includes *end-of-life care*, which provides for a person's physical, emotional, and spiritual needs.

What Are Different Types of Nursing Care Delivery?

Nursing care is delivered in different ways in healthcare facilities. A facility's belief about providing resident care usually determines how nursing care

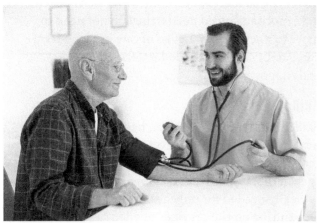

Africa Studio/Shutterstock.com

Figure 6.1 Supportive healthcare services include monitoring blood pressure.

is delivered. The medical conditions of residents are also considered, as are the numbers and types of nursing staff available. The goal is to match needs with the best, most cost-effective care possible.

When you start to work at a healthcare facility as a holistic nursing assistant, it is important to identify the type of nursing care delivery used at the facility. Identifying the way care is delivered will give you a better understanding about your role. Nursing care may be delivered in six ways:

- **Total patient care:** one licensed nursing staff member provides all the care required for each assigned resident during his or her shift. Because this type of care requires a large number of licensed nursing staff, it is not often used today.
- **Functional nursing:** available nursing staff members complete all required care tasks needed for an assigned group of patients or residents. Medications may be given by an RN, an LPN/LVN might do all treatments, and a nursing assistant might measure vital signs and help residents meet their hygiene needs.
- **Team nursing:** led by an RN who coordinates a small team of staff to provide care for a group of residents. Team member cooperation is needed so the team leader can plan, assign, assist with, teach, coordinate, and delegate care assignments to the staff on the unit.
- **Primary nursing:** one licensed nursing staff member (usually an RN) coordinates and also provides all individualized care during the full length of a resident's medical condition or illness. The goal is to achieve **continuity** (an uninterrupted sequence of events) by having a licensed nursing staff member coordinate and provide direct care. Popular in the 1970s, primary nursing is considered too expensive to use today.
- **Progressive care:** the delivery of care is determined by the degree of an illness and the level of care needs. For example, a patient in a hospital receiving progressive care who is well enough to leave a critical care unit may move to a *step-down unit* if he or she is still too sick to be cared for on a general medical unit.

CULTURE CUES

Culture in Resident-Centered Care

When providing resident-centered care, you must be sensitive to and aware of a resident's cultural traditions and practices and their impact on care. Some residents who are strongly devoted to their cultural traditions and practices will find this comforting and may want to follow their traditions even more strongly. While these traditions and practices may provide comfort, they can also be barriers to effective treatment. For example, dietary limitations due to a particular disease or condition may be a challenge to a resident's long-standing cultural traditions and practices. Finding ways to balance treatment with culture is an important part of providing care.

Apply It

1. Have you or someone you know ever experienced conflict between cultural traditions and the actions needed to maintain life and well-being?
2. How was the conflict handled? If it wasn't settled, what was the outcome?

• **Resident-centered care:** residents are the focus of care and the primary sources of information about how care is best delivered. Care delivery is holistic and also specific to each resident. Residents are encouraged to express needs and preferences, and to learn about their own diseases or conditions. The goal of resident-centered care is to deliver care that meets each resident's needs while promoting self-reliance and independence. For example, in resident-centered care, a resident who requires insulin (the hormone that regulates blood sugar) due to a new diagnosis of diabetes will learn how to balance nutrition, exercise, rest, and relaxation.

How Does Delegation Influence Delivery of Care?

One responsibility of the licensed nursing staff is to *delegate* tasks to a nursing assistant. By delegating the task, the licensed nursing staff is asking a nursing assistant to take the responsibility of performing the task. Sometimes the delegated tasks are routine, and other times they may require special knowledge or skill. No matter what the delegated task is, it must always be a part of your scope of practice as a nursing assistant. You must be able to do the task safely and accurately.

An example of delegation would be an RN asking that, during the care you provide Mrs. R today, you monitor her blood pressure, taking it every two hours because it was unusually high this morning. The RN also asked that you report back and document the results each time you take Mrs. R's blood pressure.

When a licensed nursing staff member delegates a task to a nursing assistant, he or she also transfers the responsibility for performing that task. If the nursing assistant accepts the task, he or she becomes responsible for performing it correctly. Trust is an important part of delegation. How much licensed nursing staff members trust a nursing assistant's ability determines what will be delegated.

Delegation and the Licensed Nursing Staff

Delegation is a legal act within a licensed nursing staff member's scope of practice. Nursing assistants cannot delegate a task. Licensed nursing staff members are always *accountable* (responsible) for the completion of delegated tasks, even if a nursing assistant is giving the care. When delegating tasks, licensed nursing staff members must be aware of the nursing assistant's scope of practice, skill level, and performance. The written policies and procedures of the healthcare facility must also be considered.

When delegating, licensed nursing staff members must observe the five rights of delegation, which are provided in a guide by the National Council of State Boards of Nursing. According to these guidelines, licensed nursing staff members must be sure:

1. the **right task** is delegated
2. the delegation occurs under the **right circumstance**
3. the task is delegated to the **right person**
4. the **right direction and communication** are given
5. the **right supervision and evaluation** are provided

Acceptance of a Delegated Task

When you begin working as a nursing assistant, it is your responsibility to let the licensed nursing staff know if you believe you do *not* have the skill to accomplish a delegated task. Sharing such concerns will help you be sure residents receive safe and accurate holistic care. When you recognize your limitations as a nursing assistant, you act in a professional manner. You are also giving licensed nursing staff members information they need to help you develop your skills and abilities. Doing this strengthens collaboration and will improve your ability to work as a team.

SECTION 6.1 Review and Assessment

Key Terms Mini Glossary

accountable responsible; able to explain any actions taken.

cognitive status the ability to understand, think clearly, and remember.

continuity an uninterrupted connection or sequence of events.

delegate to transfer duties to another competent person; the person who delegates the responsibility is still accountable for the proper completion of the tasks involved.

tracheostomy a surgical opening in the trachea; a tube is inserted into the opening to help people who have difficulty breathing.

Apply the Key Terms

Fill in the blank with the correct key term.

1. When an RN transfers duties to a nursing assistant, she _____ the task.
2. When a resident has difficulty with his breathing, a doctor may perform a(n) _____, which is a surgical opening in the trachea.
3. Nursing assistants who are responsible and able to explain the actions they take are _____.
4. A resident's _____ is considered when his ability to understand, think clearly, and remember is evaluated.
5. _____ is an uninterrupted connection or sequence of events.

Know and Understand the Facts

1. Describe three levels of resident care.
2. Identify two types of nursing care delivery.
3. Explain the five rights of delegation.

Analyze and Apply Concepts

1. Describe the level of care a resident might receive if he or she were provided skilled nursing care.

2. Explain how care would be delivered if team nursing is used.
3. Discuss what you should do if you are delegated a task you do not know how to do.

Think Critically

Read the following care situation. Then answer the questions that follow.

Tasia is assigned to Ms. O, a 78-year-old resident who badly broke her leg. Ms. O was in the hospital for one week before being transferred to an assisted living facility. The doctor has ordered physical therapy as well as daily dressing changes. Ms. O will likely need three weeks of care before she is allowed to go home. Today, a member of the licensed nursing staff delegated Ms. O's dressing change to Tasia. Tasia learned how to change a dressing, but she is worried that she may not do the procedure well.

1. What level of care is Ms. O receiving?
2. What type of nursing care delivery do you think is being provided in this facility?
3. How would you suggest Tasia deal with her worries about being delegated the dressing change?

SECTION 6.2 The Nursing Process, Policies, and Procedures

Objectives

To achieve the objectives for this section, you must successfully:

- **explain** the nursing process and the role of the nursing assistant.
- **discuss** the importance of understanding and obeying healthcare policies.
- **recognize** the differences between policies and procedures.
- **describe** how following written healthcare procedures maintains safe, quality practice.

Key Terms

Learn these key terms to better understand the information presented in the section.

assessing
evidence-based practice
nursing diagnosis
nursing process

plan of care
priorities
standards of care

Questions to Consider

- What policies and procedures do you have to follow in your life? Have you found any of your school's policies and procedures helpful? If so, how and in what ways have they helped?
- Have you had to follow policies and procedures that are not helpful or are frustrating? What could you do to handle these issues?

1. **Assessing:** information about the physiological, psychological, emotional, sociological, economic, lifestyle-related, and spiritual aspects of a resident is collected through observation, a physical examination, medical history, or an interview with the resident. Assessment by licensed staff is ongoing during care.
2. **Making a nursing diagnosis:** a health problem or the cause of a health problem is identified, such as sleep deprivation (a lack of sleep), that can be helped through nursing care. A resident's risk for developing further problems is also determined during this step. The nursing diagnosis is used by licensed nursing staff to develop a plan of care.
3. **Planning:** a written document, called a *plan of care* (or *service plan*) is developed to guide the delivery of individualized, holistic care. The licensed nursing staff and resident identify measurable and achievable goals and *priorities* (actions of high importance) for each identified health problem. The resident's family members and other healthcare team members may also be involved.

What Is the Nursing Process?

One important part of delivering care is following a set of guidelines called *standards of care*. Created by the nursing profession, standards of care are methods, processes, and actions. In nursing, one standard of care is called the *nursing process*.

The nursing process is led by an RN, who uses critical thinking, analytical skills, and *evidence-based practice* (the use of research findings to guide decisions) to plan and deliver safe, quality care. The nursing process begins on admission to a healthcare facility and continues for as long as a resident needs care. There are five steps in the nursing process: *assessing*, making a *nursing diagnosis*, planning, implementing, and evaluating (**Figure 6.2**).

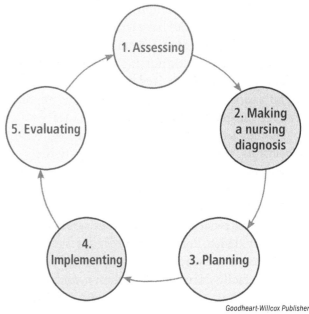

Goodheart-Willcox Publisher

Figure 6.2 The nursing process consists of five steps.

4. **Implementing:** care is carried out based on the plan of care. This may include direct care, education and instruction of residents, or referrals (recommendations) for follow-up therapies to achieve the highest level of wellness. Care and any actions taken are always documented in a resident's chart or EMR.

5. **Evaluating:** this step is ongoing throughout care. As nursing actions are completed and licensed nursing staff evaluate the achievement of goals, changes may be needed. As a result, new goals may be identified.

Why Is the Nursing Process Important?

As a holistic nursing assistant, when asked, you will participate in the nursing process by providing your observations of a resident's status and information about your interactions with residents. Licensed nursing staff will use this information during the planning, implementing, and evaluating steps. Your observations must be accurate and timely (at the right time). You should also report any changes to the licensed nursing staff.

What Are Policies and Procedures?

In addition to plans of care, healthcare policies and procedures are written by facilities to provide a consistent way of accomplishing your work. All healthcare facilities have written policies and procedures that set required guidelines for the care you deliver as a holistic nursing assistant. Policies and procedures are required by several regulatory organizations and agencies, such as Medicare, that oversee the quality and safety of healthcare.

Policies and procedures set boundaries, directions, and guidelines that make sure the actions taken by healthcare staff are based on good evidence and best practice. Policies and procedures are usually specific to a healthcare facility, but are based on external rules and standards, research, and factual evidence. Policies and procedures also take into account the way a healthcare facility delivers care, the facility's resident population, and doctors' approaches in caring for residents with specific diseases and conditions.

Policies and procedures are always located in a place that is easily found by all healthcare staff. Policies and procedures concerning resident care are usually found in a facility's policy and procedure manual or, in some facilities, may be found online. Policies and procedures related to administrative tasks and employee behavior are found in a facility's employee handbook.

The goal is to make sure all staff members are guided by policies and are performing tasks according to set procedures. This helps guarantee accuracy, safety, and consistency to avoid errors.

Policies

Policies are rules or guidelines developed by a healthcare facility and its staff. Healthcare facilities may have policies on proper dress, behavior, or benefits (for example, how many vacation days staff members may have). Facilities may also have care-related policies, such as a policy about hand hygiene.

Procedures

Procedures are specific and consistent actions or steps taken to deliver care. Procedures are always based on policies. Procedures are very detailed and tell you exactly how to perform a task. In Section 6.3, you will learn the procedures for admitting, transferring, and discharging residents from facilities.

How Do Policies and Procedures Ensure Safe, Quality Care?

Policies and procedures are developed to guide and assist healthcare staff. All healthcare staff members are responsible for obeying policies and following procedures. Policies and procedures are meant to help deliver care, not to make it difficult. They are written to be followed. Without policies and procedures in place, errors can be made, and care can be inconsistent, creating anxiety and feelings of being unsafe for both staff and residents. In some cases, ignoring a policy or procedure can lead to harm and a legal or ethical problem for healthcare staff and the healthcare facility. Therefore, when you work as a nursing assistant, it is not appropriate to take shortcuts or decide there is a better or easier way to complete a task.

If you change the way a policy is interpreted or do not follow a procedure, this can lead to disciplinary action. A better way of dealing with a challenging or difficult policy or procedure is to bring this information to a member of the licensed nursing staff. When doing this, always identify the specific policy or procedure that needs to be reviewed. Also explain which part of the policy or procedure is not working and include a recommendation for how it can be improved. Recommended changes should always relate to improving care. The licensed nursing staff can bring this information to members of the facility administration, who have the authority to review and rewrite policies and procedures, if needed.

SECTION 6.2 **Review and Assessment**

Key Terms Mini Glossary

assessing examining a situation so it can be evaluated.

evidence-based practice the process of locating and using research findings to guide decisions made about care delivery.

nursing diagnosis the identification of a health problem or the cause of a health problem; does not identify a specific disease.

nursing process assessing, identifying problems, planning, implementing, and evaluating to deliver safe, quality care.

plan of care a written plan that provides directions and guides delivery of individualized, holistic care; also called a *service plan*.

priorities items or actions of high importance.

standards of care methods, processes, and actions healthcare providers follow.

Apply the Key Terms

Identify the key term used in each sentence.

1. Assessing; making a nursing diagnosis; and planning, implementing, and evaluating care is called the nursing process.
2. The facility you work for expects that evidence-based practice will be used to guide decisions made about care delivery.
3. Every day, the written plan of care provides directions and guides your delivery of individualized, holistic care as a nursing assistant.
4. RNs in your facility use a nursing diagnosis to identify a health problem or the cause of a health problem.
5. It is very important to follow the methods, processes, and actions, or the standards of care, to be sure you provide consistent, safe, quality care.

Know and Understand the Facts

1. What is a standard of care and why is it important?
2. Identify the five steps in the nursing process.
3. Explain the difference between a policy and a procedure. Give an example of each.
4. Describe the importance of a resident plan of care.

Analyze and Apply Concepts

1. Identify two ways in which nursing assistants participate in the nursing process.
2. What might happen if a policy or procedure is not followed?

3. What should a nursing assistant do if he or she thinks a policy or procedure is not helpful?
4. What influences the development of a facility policy?
5. Identify two ways policies and procedures help make sure safe, quality care is provided.

Think Critically

Read the following care situation. Then answer the questions that follow.

Over the past year, the facility in which Louis works has twice changed the procedure for putting on gloves for protection before entering a room where a resident has been isolated due to a contagious disease. A member of the nursing administration decided to change the procedure for a second time after reading a newly published article on the subject. Louis is frustrated because he had just learned the procedure well when it changed. Louis decides to continue following the old procedure since that is what he knows. After all, he is an experienced nursing assistant, and the procedure has worked in the past. Louis wonders, *Why should I change how I put on gloves?*

1. Is Louis doing the right thing by continuing to use the old procedure? Explain your answer.
2. Why do you think the nursing administration chose to change the procedure?
3. What actions should the licensed nursing staff take to ensure that Louis and other staff members follow the new procedure?

Admission, Transfer, and Discharge

Objectives

To achieve the objectives for this section, you must successfully:

- **describe** the procedure for admission to a healthcare facility and the nursing assistant's role.
- **list** the steps that are taken to be sure there is a safe transfer within a facility or to another facility.
- **explain** the procedure for discharge from a facility.

Key Terms

Learn these key terms to better understand the information presented in the section.

discharge plan sphygmomanometer
pulse oximeter

Questions to Consider

- Have you ever had to pack up and leave quickly after a vacation? What actions did you take to make sure you took all your personal belongings? If someone helped you, how did you make sure they took all your belongings?
- When you packed up quickly, did you or your family leave something behind? How did that experience feel? What did you do to get back or replace the lost items?

In this section of the chapter, you will learn about procedures you may need to know as part of your role and responsibilities as a nursing assistant working in some facilities. These procedures include admission to a healthcare facility, transfer within or to another healthcare facility, and discharge from a healthcare facility.

What Is the Procedure for Admission to a Healthcare Facility?

Admission to a healthcare facility occurs when people can no longer take care of themselves or have serious illnesses or conditions. People are usually *admitted to*, or enter, a hospital (and become a patient) or long-term care facility (and become a resident). In hospitals,

---

THINK ABOUT THIS

A recent estimate by the Centers for Disease Control and Prevention (CDC) states that there are 1.3 million residents in long-term care facilities in the United States. According to the American Hospital Association (AHA), an estimated 36 million admissions occur each year in US-registered hospitals.

---

there are two major types of admission: emergency admission and elective admission. *Emergency admission* occurs when someone goes to the emergency department. From there, the person may be admitted to a hospital. *Elective admission* usually occurs if a person has a scheduled procedure or surgery. Sometimes people are admitted to a hospital because they need to be observed for a short period of time until decisions can be made about their conditions or illnesses (**Figure 6.3**).

Admissions to long-term care facilities are almost always elective. The decision to enter a long-term care facility is made when a person is no longer able to independently live at home. Usually, the person needs some assistance with ambulation, eating, or hygiene and may need special treatments or the administration and monitoring of medications.

Specific policies and procedures are used to collect needed information and prepare people for admission. Sometimes healthcare staff members complete the paperwork for admission in the admitting office of the facility. Other times, the paperwork is completed in a patient's or resident's room by a person from the admitting office, a HUC, a member of the licensed nursing staff, or a nursing assistant. Room preparation and the admission process may be the responsibility of the nursing assistant or another assigned healthcare staff member, depending on directions from the licensed nursing staff.

The information needed for admission usually includes a person's personal information, employment information, closest relatives, insurance carriers, reasons

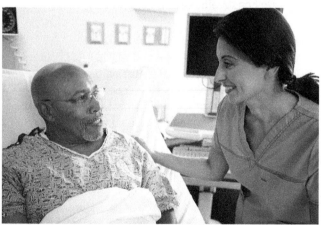

MBI/Shutterstock.com

Figure 6.3 Not all patients in a hospital are admitted because of medical emergencies. Some require observation until a condition is diagnosed or treatment begins.

for admission, and medications. Admission documents are used to help collect necessary information. A clothing and personal belongings list is also completed as part of the admission process to document all items that remain in the facility. Other forms that require a signature include privacy practices and treatment agreements.

Hospitals usually provide an admission kit that includes a water pitcher, a cup, a basin, toothpaste, a toothbrush, soap, lotion, and other hygiene items.

In long-term care facilities, the admission kit might not include hygiene items such as a toothbrush or toothpaste, because residents often bring their own.

The admission procedure focuses on making sure people are oriented to and made comfortable in the facility and their rooms, are aware of their rights, and have rooms that are prepared with needed supplies and equipment. Once residents are settled into their rooms, treatments ordered by their doctors are started.

Procedure

Admission to a Healthcare Facility

Rationale

When nursing assistants help during admission, they prepare the room, assist with gathering necessary information, and help with orientation to the healthcare facility and room.

Preparation

1. Wash your hands or use hand sanitizer before entering the room.
2. Bring the necessary equipment into the room. Place the following items in an easy-to-reach place:
   - instruments for measuring vital signs, such as a thermometer, *sphygmomanometer* for measuring blood pressure (**Figure 6.4**), stethoscope, and *pulse oximeter* for measuring oxygen in the blood (**Figure 6.5**)

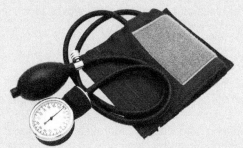

Figure 6.4   *Sergej Razvodovskij/Shutterstock.com*

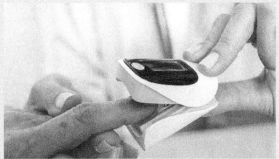

Figure 6.5   *Click and Photo/Shutterstock.com*

   - an intravenous (IV) pole, if needed
   - a specimen container for collection of a urine sample, if ordered by the doctor
   - any other items requested by the licensed nursing staff

   Place the following items on or inside of the bedside stand:
   - an admission kit
   - a bed pan and urinal (for men)
   - towels and washcloths
3. Prepare the bed by pulling back the bed covers and placing the bed in a low position (if not already there) so the resident can easily enter the bed. Lock the bed wheels so the bed does not roll or move (**Figure 6.6**).

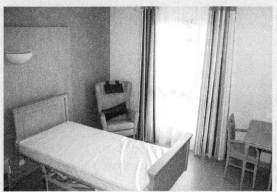

Figure 6.6   *sylv1rob1/Shutterstock.com*

4. Ensure that the call light is easily accessible and within the resident's reach.

The Procedure

5. When the resident arrives at the room, a licensed nursing staff member will check the resident's name with any admission forms.
6. Introduce yourself using your first or preferred name and title. Explain that you work with the licensed nursing staff and will be assisting with the admission.

(continued)

Admission to a Healthcare Facility *(continued)*

7. If instructed by the licensed nursing staff, place an identification bracelet on the resident's wrist if he or she is not already wearing one.

> **Best Practice:** Some facilities may use alternative methods of identification, such as identifying residents using a photo in the EMR. Check your facility's guidelines for verifying a resident's identify.

8. Use Mr., Mrs., or Ms. and the last name when conversing.

9. Explain the part of the admission procedure you will be doing in simple terms, even if the resident is not able to communicate or is disoriented (confused).

10. Provide privacy by closing the curtains, using a screen, or closing the door to the room.

> **Best Practice:** It is important to provide privacy during the admission process. If a resident's family members or friends are present, determine whether they will stay during admission.

11. Get the approved admission forms for the resident. You may have to ask the licensed nursing staff for these forms. Admission forms are usually filled out electronically using a tablet, laptop, or computer on wheels.

12. As directed by the licensed nursing staff, ask the resident the questions on the admission forms, assuming the admission forms have not already been completed. If the resident is disoriented or unable to answer questions, you may have to ask family members the questions, if they are with the resident.

13. A member of the licensed nursing staff or a social worker may explain to the resident what his or her rights are and provide a booklet on the topic. The resident's photo may also be taken for identification purposes.

14. If the resident has a roommate, make introductions.

15. Let the resident stay dressed, if approved, or help the resident change into a gown or pajamas.

16. Help the resident into bed or into a chair, as directed by the licensed nursing staff.

17. An RN will usually conduct a resident assessment. Assist with the assessment by measuring vital signs, height, and weight.

18. Complete the resident's clothing and personal belongings list (per facility policy). Along with the licensed nursing staff, sign the list to verify which belongings have been left in the room and if any valuables have been put in the facility's

safe. You may be asked to label the resident's belongings.

19. Unless a family member or friend wishes to assist, put away the resident's clothes and personal items.

20. Provide the resident with an orientation to the room by doing the following:
    - Identify and explain the purposes of items in the bedside stand.
    - Explain how to use the overbed table.
    - Show the resident how to use the call light, bed controls, TV, and light control.
    - If there is a telephone in the room, explain how to make a telephone call and place the telephone within reach.
    - Show the resident where the bathroom is and how to use the bathroom's emergency call light.

21. Explain the facility's visiting hours and policies, as well as where to find the nurses' station, chapel, dining room or cafeteria, and any other areas specific to the facility. Also explain how to identify different staff. Some facilities have different colored uniforms or different types of identification badges for staff members.

22. Explain any ordered activity limits, such as bed rest or ambulation restrictions.

23. Explain when meals are served and how to request snacks.

24. If fluids are allowed per the doctor's orders, fill the water pitcher and cup in the resident's room.

25. Provide a denture cup, if needed, and label it with the resident's name, room number, and bed number.

> **Best Practice:** If handling dentures, use disposable gloves. Wash your hands before and after discarding the disposable gloves to ensure infection control.

Follow-Up

26. Wash your hands to ensure infection control.

27. Make sure the resident is comfortable and place the call light and personal items within reach.

28. Conduct a safety check before leaving the room. The room should be clean and free from clutter or spills.

29. Wash your hands or use hand sanitizer before leaving the room.

Reporting and Documentation

30. Report the completion of admission. Report any specific observations, complications, or unusual responses to the licensed nursing staff. Document this information, along with the care provided, in the chart or EMR.

BECOMING A HOLISTIC NURSING ASSISTANT

Admission and Anxiety

Admission to any healthcare facility is often hard on residents and their families. Residents have fears and are nervous about no longer being able to care for themselves at home. Unfortunately, many residents never return home. When residents enter a long-term care facility, they leave behind friends, family, and even pets to live in a new, strange place with people they do not know. Many times, the decision was not the resident's, but was made by the resident's family. Once residents enter a long-term care facility, they are being taken care of rather than taking care of themselves. This is even more frightening for residents who are no longer mobile or who have dementia. Needing someone to assist you with every move, when you were once independent, can be a hard reality to accept.

There are several ways holistic nursing assistants can ease fear and nervousness to make a resident more comfortable. These might include:

- making eye contact when communicating
- asking questions or giving instructions slowly and clearly
- being patient and waiting for an answer to a question before asking another
- using a pleasant and even tone of voice
- expressing body language, gestures, or movements that are open, relaxed, and accepting
- smiling and showing concern, when appropriate

Apply It

1. Which approaches do you already take when interacting with people who are fearful or nervous? Are there any approaches that are new and that you need to learn? How will you go about doing that?
2. What other approaches can you think of that might also help decrease fear or nervousness for a resident?

What Are the Steps for Transfer?

Sometimes residents are transferred to a different location in the same healthcare facility or to another facility entirely. Sometimes it is due to a change in condition; for example, if a resident's cognitive status has changed, the resident may need to be moved to memory care, which may be in the current facility or in a new facility. A resident may have a stroke and need to be hospitalized. Or, a resident's needs may have changed so that they require a different type of care facility, such as a hospice.

Like admission, a transfer requires a written doctor's order. Licensed nursing staff members may delegate transfer responsibilities to nursing assistants or HUCs. A staff member from social services often assists residents and their families in locating a facility that will meet treatment needs and is covered by insurance.

Forms are used for the transfer procedure. Transfer forms usually request information about the destination, diagnosis, medications, treatments, allergies, physical and mental assessments, the level of independence, safety concerns, and personal belongings.

Some residents become frightened during the transfer procedure. This is especially common among older adults, who may not understand the reasons for the transfer. In these situations, it is important that you stay calm and reassure and reorient the resident as necessary (**Figure 6.7**). Make sure the transfer is safe. Seek assistance from another staff member to help with the transfer, if needed.

HEALTHCARE SCENARIO

Admission Concerns

Today, at 9 p.m., the news shared that a local healthcare facility reported higher-than-expected numbers of admissions. This had an impact on the resident care and on staffing. A reporter interviewed the facility administration, doctors, nurses, and several residents. During the interviews, it was clear that the healthcare staff and residents were concerned about whether the high numbers of residents entering the facility would affect safety and the delivery of quality care.

Apply It

1. What can nursing assistants do during admission to ensure safety?
2. Identify steps in the admission procedures where quality of care might be at risk. Discuss how this can be prevented.

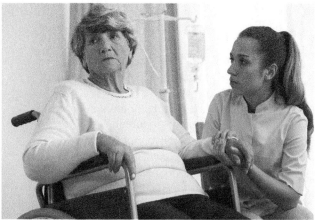

Figure 6.7 There may be some fear and nervousness during transfer. You can help by reassuring these residents during the process.

If the transfer occurs between units in a facility, the destination unit is notified about the transfer, and a nursing assistant or other assigned healthcare staff member usually accompanies the resident. The nursing assistant or other assigned healthcare staff member checks in with the licensed nursing staff on the new unit and transfers the paper chart, assuming the information has not already been shared electronically.

If the transfer is to another facility, a licensed nursing staff member will contact the destination facility about the time of the arrival. A nursing assistant or other assigned healthcare staff member will accompany the resident to the transport vehicle. At the transport vehicle, those responsible for transport will take responsibility for the resident, his or her documents, and any belongings and valuables not taken by the family.

What Is the Procedure for Discharge from a Healthcare Facility?

While the procedure for discharge is more likely for patients leaving hospitals, residents may also leave a long-term care facility to go home. Discharge from a facility can only occur when there is a written doctor's order.

Sometimes patients or even residents decide to terminate treatments or care prescribed by a doctor while in a healthcare facility. Patients may also decide to leave a healthcare facility earlier than when a doctor believes is best. If patients leave a healthcare facility such as a hospital, against a doctor's wishes,

they are making these decisions *against medical advice (AMA)*. If this situation occurs, the patient or resident is asked to sign a release indicating that the healthcare facility and those providing care are not liable (responsible) for any harm resulting from ending care or early discharge.

A nursing assistant or HUC may assist with discharge by following doctors' orders and completing tasks delegated by the licensed nursing staff. Sometimes a transport aide or volunteer will take the patient or resident to a waiting vehicle once discharge is completed (**Figure 6.8**).

A discharge form must be completed before the resident leaves a healthcare facility. Discharge forms include all of the necessary information gathered, such as personal information, medical diagnoses, insurance carriers, and a clothing and personal belongings list.

In addition to discharge forms, discharge also requires a **discharge plan**. The discharge plan provides instructions listing medications, activity levels, treatments to continue at home, and follow-up appointments with the doctor. These instructions are provided by the licensed nursing staff.

Be sure to practice safety during discharge. Make sure that there are no opportunities for the patient or resident to trip or fall when getting ready to leave. Safety is also important during the transfer from wheelchair to the transport vehicle. Get assistance from another staff member, if needed.

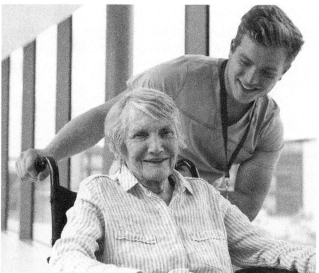

Figure 6.8 Nursing assistants and other healthcare staff members provide an escort to transport vehicles upon discharge.

Procedure

Discharge from a Healthcare Facility

Rationale

During the discharge process, the nursing assistant may assist the licensed nursing staff as directed with completing paperwork, packing personal belongings, and helping with safe transport.

Preparation

1. Ask the licensed nursing staff if there are doctor's orders for the procedure and if there are any specific instructions listed in the plan of care.
2. Obtain the discharge forms ordered by the doctor. You may have to ask the licensed nursing staff for these forms.
3. Wash your hands or use hand sanitizer before entering the room.
4. Knock before entering the room.
5. Introduce yourself using your first or preferred name and title. Explain that you work with the licensed nursing staff and will be assisting with discharge.
6. Greet the resident and ask the resident to state his or her full name, if able. Then check the resident's identification bracelet.
7. Use Mr., Mrs., or Ms. and the resident's last name when conversing.
8. Explain the part of the discharge procedure you will be doing in simple terms.

The Procedure

9. Provide privacy by closing the curtains, using a screen, or closing the door to the room.
10. Help the resident get dressed. Then help collect and pack the resident's belongings and any needed equipment.
11. Return any valuables that have been kept in the facility's safe to the resident. Check the belongings against the list created during admission.

> **Best Practice:** Family members may want to assist with the discharge. Include the family members, as directed by the licensed nursing staff and as appropriate. Take care that the family's involvement does not interfere with safe discharge.

12. During discharge, observe and report any issues regarding the resident's ability to complete ADLs, as well as any of his or her concerns or fears, to the licensed nursing staff.

> **Best Practice:** Practice safety during the discharge process. Get assistance from another staff member, if needed.

13. Notify the licensed nursing staff when the resident is ready for final discharge instructions. At this time, an RN will usually:
    - provide the resident with prescriptions ordered by the doctor
    - communicate discharge instructions
    - have the resident sign clothing and personal belongings forms
14. Help escort the resident in a wheelchair from the unit to the transport vehicle.
15. Lock the resident's wheelchair and assist the resident into the transport vehicle.
16. Help move the resident's belongings into the transport vehicle.

Follow-Up

17. Return the wheelchair and cart (if used) to the storage area for cleaning.
18. Put on disposable gloves and practice infection control to prevent transmission of any possible pathogens (bacteria or viruses).
19. Clean the room and prepare it for a new occupant. The housekeeping staff may share some of the following duties:
    - stripping the bed and cleaning the room
    - disposing of dirty linen
    - making the bed using clean linen
20. Remove and discard your gloves.
21. Wash your hands to ensure infection control.

Reporting and Documentation

22. Report the completion and time of discharge, the staff who assisted with the discharge, the way in which the resident was transported, the people who accompanied the discharged resident, the resident's destination, and any observations and responses to the licensed nursing staff. Also document this information in the chart or EMR.

SECTION 6.3 **Review and Assessment**

Key Terms Mini Glossary

discharge plan a set of instructions given at the time of discharge; may include the doctor's instructions about activity level, medications, continued treatment, important changes in condition, and follow-up appointments with the doctor.

pulse oximeter a medical device, usually applied to the end of a finger, that indirectly measures the amount of oxygen in the blood; oxygen content is recorded as a percentage.

sphygmomanometer a medical device used to measure blood pressure; includes a cuff that wraps around a person's upper arm and a measuring device.

Apply the Key Terms

Complete the following sentences using the key terms in this section.

1. A set of instructions given at the time of discharge, which may include the doctor's instructions about activity level, medications, continued treatment, important changes in condition, and follow-up appointments with the doctor, is called a(n) _____.
2. A(n) _____ is a medical device, usually applied to the end of a finger, that indirectly measures the amount of oxygen in the blood.
3. The medical device that measures blood pressure and has a cuff that wraps around a person's upper arm and a measuring device is called a(n) _____.

Know and Understand the Facts

1. Identify two types of admission to a healthcare facility.
2. Describe the processes of admission, transfer, and discharge.
3. Identify two examples of needed information that is collected during admission.
4. What is a discharge plan, and how is it used?

Analyze and Apply Concepts

1. Explain how to prepare a room for admission.
2. Using what you have learned so far, identify two actions you could take to help a resident better adjust to admission to a healthcare facility.

3. Identify three steps a nursing assistant performs to be sure there is a safe and effective transfer.
4. What information is needed for a safe and effective discharge?

Think Critically

Read the following care situation. Then answer the questions that follow.

You have just admitted a new resident, Mrs. H. Once she settles into her bed, you check her vital signs and weight. Mrs. H seems very upset and agitated. Her blood pressure is above normal. She seems to have trouble understanding what you are saying. You think she may not understand English very well. You are concerned that she may not remember everything you told her during admission. In particular, you are concerned that she does not understand how to call for help using the call light.

1. What can you do to be sure Mrs. H understands what you are saying?
2. What actions can you take to help Mrs. H become more calm?
3. How can you help Mrs. H remember what you have told her?
4. Would you need to inform a member of the licensed nursing staff about Mrs. H's blood pressure reading? Explain your answer.
5. What steps can you take to help Mrs. H learn how to use the call light?

Summary and Review

Key Points

Reviewing the key points for this chapter will help you practice more safely and competently as a holistic nursing assistant and will help you prepare for the certification competency examination.

- Levels of care are the types and amounts of care that residents require. The three levels of care are skilled care, intermediate care, and supportive care.
- The types of nursing care delivery typically seen today are functional nursing, team nursing, progressive care, and resident-centered care.
- Delegation occurs when a licensed nursing staff member asks a nursing assistant to perform specific tasks. These tasks must always be within a nursing assistant's scope of practice.
- The nursing process is a method in which licensed nursing staff members use critical thinking, analytical skills, and supporting evidence to plan for and deliver care. This process has five steps: assessing, making a nursing diagnosis, planning, implementing, and evaluating.
- Policies and procedures set boundaries, directions, and guidelines so that actions taken by healthcare staff are based on good evidence and best practice.
- The three procedures involved in moving residents into, between, and out of healthcare facilities are admission, transfer, and discharge.

Action Steps to Holistic Care

Review the information in this chapter. Complete the following activities.

1. Select one type of nursing care delivery. Prepare a short paper or digital presentation that discusses the nursing assistant's role and responsibilities within this type of care delivery.
2. Write a short poem or limerick that expresses what nursing assistants should do when accepting a delegated task.
3. With a partner, prepare a poster that identifies and describes the top three most important practices that should be included in one of the procedures discussed in this chapter.
4. Admission to, transfer within, or discharge from a healthcare facility can leave a resident feeling nervous or uncertain. List possible reasons for the nervousness. Then come up with ways you, as a holistic nursing assistant, can help the resident be more comfortable.

Building Math Skill

Today will be a very busy day for Mariana. The charge nurse has designated the following tasks: preparing a room for each of two admissions that will occur this morning, getting Mr. Q ready for transfer to a rehabilitation hospital in the afternoon, and cleaning the room of a resident who will be discharged right after lunch. How many admissions, transfers, and discharges will Mariana be taking care of in the morning, and how many in the afternoon?

Preparing for the Certification Competency Examination

To prepare for the nursing assistant certification competency examination, you will need to know content found in this chapter. This content may be tested in the knowledge (written or oral) and skills (hands-on demonstration) portions of the exam. The following areas will be emphasized:

- professional work habits
- the importance of the delegation process
- facility policies and procedures
- admission, transfer, and discharge skills

These sample test questions are similar to ones you will find on the certification competency exam. See how well you can answer them. Be sure to select the *best* answer.

1. During which step in the nursing process might a nursing assistant provide information?
   A. making a nursing diagnosis
   B. appraising
   C. evaluating
   D. activating

2. If a resident receives 24-hour direct care in a healthcare facility, what level of care would be assigned?
   A. intermediate care
   B. skilled care
   C. long-term care
   D. supportive care

(Continued)

3. Which of the following *best* describes a policy?
   A. a set of steps
   B. a process
   C. an action
   D. a rule or guideline

4. A new nursing assistant is giving care assigned by a member of the licensed nursing staff. What type of nursing care delivery is being practiced on his unit?
   A. total resident care
   B. team nursing
   C. resident-focused care
   D. supplemental care

5. Which of the following is one of the five rights of delegation?
   A. right action
   B. right process
   C. right person
   D. right environment

6. Mr. L, an older gentleman, is being transferred to a long-term care facility after suffering a mild stroke. What is the first thing that must be done after the doctor's order is received and before the transfer can occur?
   A. Mr. L's permission must be obtained.
   B. Transport must be arranged.
   C. The RN must call Mr. L's destination facility.
   D. Mr. L's belongings must be packed.

7. A nursing assistant has been asked to discharge Mr. S from a rehabilitation facility. Mr. S plans to go home with his wife. Which of the following actions should the nursing assistant *not* take?
   A. help Mr. S gather all of his belongings
   B. make sure there is a doctor's order for Mr. S's discharge
   C. let the licensed nursing staff know Mr. S is ready for his discharge orders
   D. let Mr. S's wife help him to their car

8. A member of the licensed nursing staff has delegated a task to a nursing assistant who works on the day shift. The task is part of the nursing assistant's scope of practice, but she does not remember how to do it correctly. Which of the following should the nursing assistant do?
   A. take more time to do the task
   B. ask another nursing assistant to help her
   C. tell the licensed nursing staff she needs some training before she can do the task
   D. tell the licensed nursing staff that she doesn't think she will have time today to do the task

9. What is the first action a nursing assistant should take when admitting a resident?
   A. make sure the bed and bedside stand are ready
   B. get the admission kit and ensure that it contains all necessary components
   C. check with the licensed nursing staff and consult the admission forms
   D. tell the resident's roommate about the arrival

10. Why is a discharge plan important?
    A. It provides information about the patient's history.
    B. It provides a set of instructions for the patient.
    C. It provides data on the patient's family.
    D. It provides information about the patient's pain.

11. Which of the following explains why nursing assistants should always follow facility procedures?
    A. Procedures provide helpful information needed to provide care.
    B. Procedures are written at a level at which they can be understood.
    C. Procedures ensure that all healthcare providers give consistent care.
    D. Procedures are simple and provide just a few steps to follow.

12. A new nursing assistant received a delegated assignment to prepare a room for resident admission. Which healthcare staff member on her unit delegated this assignment?
    A. the RN
    B. the HUC
    C. the doctor
    D. the social worker

13. Which of the following is a level of care that provides physical and rehabilitation therapy?
    A. progressive
    B. supportive
    C. skilled
    D. intermediate

14. How are level-of-care assignments used?
    A. to decide on the best facility based on a person's needs
    B. to determine how to share a resident's progress with his or her family
    C. to help design facilities so they provide the best services
    D. to put standards in place so that the environment is safe

15. Before a patient or resident can be admitted, transferred, or discharged, which of the following must occur?
    A. The family must agree to the decision.
    B. The patient must be provided information.
    C. The RN must provide an assessment.
    D. There must be a doctor's order.

Did you have difficulty with any of the questions? If you did, review the chapter to find the correct answer(s).

Welcome to the Chapter

This chapter will help you understand what motivates people, how to recognize human needs, and how people grow. This will help you feel empathy for others, which can help you build understanding and openness. You will also learn how behavioral and generational differences can make it difficult to develop positive, productive communication and relationships. As a holistic nursing assistant, you can learn to respond to and overcome differences using the skills and knowledge in this chapter.

You will also learn how your *body*, *mind*, and *spirit* affect how you feel and behave. You will find out that each is important to understanding yourself, achieving a healthy lifestyle, and helping others do the same. With this understanding, you will be able to grow and strengthen your relationships. Developing holistic relationships will directly influence the way you communicate with others and the quality of care you deliver.

In this chapter you will also learn about the power of stress and ways to manage stressful situations. You will identify ways to set personal and professional priorities. Setting these priorities will help you to better manage your time and energy and establish a positive work-life balance.

What you learn in this chapter will help you develop your knowledge and skills to become a holistic nursing assistant. The topics discussed in the chapter are highlighted on the Providing Holistic Care Framework.

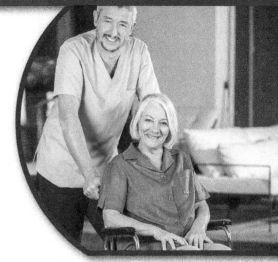

Tyler Olson/Shutterstock.com

Chapter Outline

Section 7.1
Human Needs, Growth and Development, and Behavior

Section 7.2
Body, Mind, and Spirit

Section 7.3
Work-Life Balance

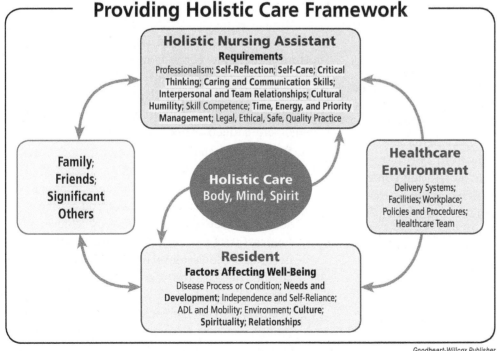

Providing Holistic Care Framework

Holistic Nursing Assistant
Requirements
Professionalism; Self-Reflection; Self-Care; Critical Thinking; Caring and Communication Skills; Interpersonal and Team Relationships; Cultural Humility; Skill Competence; Time, Energy, and Priority Management; Legal, Ethical, Safe, Quality Practice

Family;
Friends;
Significant
Others

Holistic Care
Body, Mind, Spirit

Healthcare
Environment
Delivery Systems; Facilities; Workplace; Policies and Procedures; Healthcare Team

Resident
Factors Affecting Well-Being
Disease Process or Condition; **Needs and Development**; Independence and Self-Reliance; ADL and Mobility; Environment; **Culture**; **Spirituality**; Relationships

Goodheart-Willcox Publisher

Human Needs, Growth and Development, and Behavior

Objectives

To achieve the objectives for this section, you must successfully:

- **discuss** the types, components, and theories of motivation.
- **list** the human needs that impact the attitudes, feelings, and behaviors of others.
- **explain** why human needs must be satisfied to achieve well-being.
- **describe** the stages of human growth and development.

Key Terms

Learn these key terms to better understand the information presented in the section.

behavior	overt
covert	rapport
empathy	respect
generation	self-actualization
generation gap	self-esteem
genuine	self-respect
homeostasis	stereotypes
motivation	

Questions to Consider

- What needs do you have in your life? For example, you may need to live in a safe environment, get good grades to reach your career goal, or feel appreciated by your friends.
- How important are your needs? What can you do to better meet your needs? What do you think would happen if your needs were not met? How would you feel?

How Are People Motivated?

When people have **motivation**, they choose to act on something they want. These actions are often related to personal or professional goals. For example, a person may be motivated to go back to school because he or she wants to learn new skills to find a better job.

There are two types of motivation. The first is *extrinsic* (or external). Extrinsic motivation comes from outside influences, such as receiving awards, getting a raise in salary, or avoiding punishment. *Intrinsic* (or internal) motivation comes from within a person. It is often called *self-motivation*. Intrinsic motivations are determined by your values, beliefs, and emotions, or by a desire to complete an important challenge or achieve personal satisfaction. Intrinsic factors that create motivation include curiosity, a challenge, or a need to help others.

The two types of motivation can work together or conflict with each other. For example, a person may be offered a challenging new job (intrinsic motivation) with an increased salary (extrinsic motivation). The same person can, however, turn it down (extrinsic motivation) because it conflicts with being able to spend time with his or her children (intrinsic motivation).

There are several theories (ideas) of motivation. One of these theories suggests that people have strong reasons for performing various actions. This theory is best represented by Maslow's hierarchy of needs, which shows that people have different levels of needs and are motivated by both extrinsic and intrinsic factors.

What Are Human Needs?

All people have needs. A person's needs change throughout his or her life. In the 1940s, psychologist Abraham Maslow developed a hierarchy (method of ordering or ranking) to help people understand human needs. This hierarchy, called *Maslow's hierarchy of needs*, is still used to explain human needs and how these needs affect a person's motivation to act or to behave in certain ways. Maslow believed that human needs are ordered (or ranked) from lowest to highest. The lowest needs are *basic needs* (the need for food, water, sleep, and elimination). The highest level of needs was called *self-actualization*. Self-actualization happens when people believe they have fully developed their creative, educational, or social potential. Maslow's hierarchy of needs is shown as a pyramid, with basic needs at the bottom and high-level needs at the top (**Figure 7.1**). Maslow believed that needs influence a person's actions, behaviors, and feelings. He also believed that people must meet needs at the bottom of the hierarchy (basic needs) before meeting needs at the next level.

1. **Basic needs:** includes the need for food, water, sleep, and elimination (urination and bowel movements). Consuming adequate amounts of water, eating a nutritious diet, and getting sufficient sleep will help your body achieve **homeostasis** (an internal balance). When basic needs at the lowest level of Maslow's hierarchy are met, needs at the next level for security and safety are important.

2. **Security and safety:** includes the need to feel as though you have a safe and secure place to live; enough money; and are happy with your health,

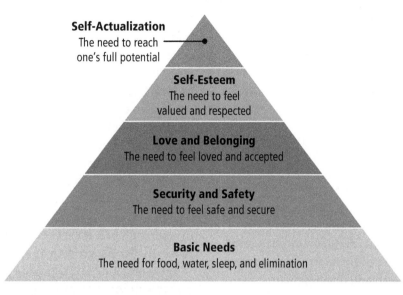

Self-Actualization
The need to reach
one's full potential

Self-Esteem
The need to feel
valued and respected

Love and Belonging
The need to feel loved and accepted

Security and Safety
The need to feel safe and secure

Basic Needs
The need for food, water, sleep, and elimination

Figure 7.1 Maslow's hierarchy of needs contains five levels of needs: basic needs, security and safety, love and belonging, self-esteem, and self-actualization.

property, and home. As a holistic nursing assistant, you will have to listen carefully to what residents are saying to understand their levels of safety or security. Demonstrating *empathy* (understanding for another person's feelings and emotions) can help you form a deeper relationship with residents without violating professional boundaries (**Figure 7.2**).

3. **Love and belonging:** Needs related to love and belonging can only be achieved after safety and security needs have been met. People may express a lack of love or feeling that they belong. Drooping shoulders, crossed arms, or staring off into space may show that someone is lonely. Comments such as "I feel lost" or "I wish I could join those ladies over there" can also help identify loneliness. You may not be able to change residents' feelings of loneliness, but you can empathize and try to find ways to overcome the loneliness such as talking with them or having them participate in activities.

4. **Self-esteem:** a person's confidence and regard (positive opinion) of him or herself describes his or her *self-esteem*. You can show *respect* (admiration and appreciation) and acknowledge residents' feelings, needs, and knowledge. You can help strengthen resident self-esteem by showing interest in what residents have done in their lives and the experiences they have had. For example, you might ask a resident if he or she has a story about helping a family member or doing something special for a friend. Recognizing personal value and self-worth is one way to strengthen resident self-esteem and help fulfill needs at this level.

5. **Self-actualization:** the highest level is achieved when a person becomes everything he or she hoped to be and has fully developed his or her potential. Self-actualization is different for each person and does not stop at a particular age. Meaningful life events can bring new awareness that can potentially lead to greater self-actualization. Respect that residents have the ability to solve their own problems and are special because of their knowledge and experiences. As a holistic nursing assistant, your support should bring out residents' very best qualities. Achieving self-actualization can make the difference between an impersonal, ordinary relationship and one that is *genuine* (honest, open, and sincere).

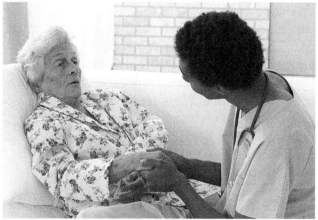

Figure 7.2 With the resident's permission, you can hold her hand while talking to express your empathy. This will help form a deeper relationship.

Your knowledge and awareness of Maslow's hierarchy of needs can affect your relationships with coworkers and residents. Be sure to determine where your residents fall on the hierarchy of needs by observing and communicating with them about their needs so you can provide safe, quality care.

How Do People Grow and Develop?

People grow physically. They become taller and increase their weight, and their appearance and body functions also change. People also develop mentally, emotionally, and socially based on their special characteristics. Change happens throughout life. Genetics (heredity), family history, and the environment in which a person lives can influence growth and development.

Growth can be discussed in several ways. Doctors use *growth charts*, which show average growth patterns (for example, how much an average toddler weighs at two years of age). As people grow physically, they are also developing critical thinking and problem-solving skills, learning language, and building skills to communicate with others.

Growth and development usually happen in steps or stages. For example, children must learn to walk before they can run. Simple skills are developed first and build to skills that are more difficult. Each stage of development has a specific purpose, or task, that must be completed before the next stage can take place. Growth and development are different for every person. They can happen unevenly, or in *spurts*. For example, a person may grow faster physically than he or she develops emotionally.

Physical Development

Physical growth charts track the growth of infants, children, and adolescents by comparing physical growth with specific measurements that are expected at certain ages. These charts are available for both girls and boys. Growth charts might measure body length or height from birth to three years of age or track the weight of a child over time. There are several different age categories for periods of physical growth, including infancy (birth to 1 year), toddlerhood (1–3 years), the preschool years (4–5 years), the school-age years (6–12 years), and adolescence (13–18 years).

Psychosocial Development

Psychosocial development refers to mental, social, and emotional changes. Psychosocial development occurs in a series of stages, sometimes called *life stages*. Jean

Piaget's theory of cognitive (mental) development, published in the early 1900s, states that, as children develop, they become able to perform increasingly more difficult daily functions and activities. For example, children ages 7–11 can pay attention to more than one situation at a time. This is something they were not able to do when they were younger.

Another popular approach to growth and development is Erik Erikson's theory of psychosocial development, which was developed in the 1950s. Erikson believed that certain conflicts (physiological or social issues) occur at different stages of growth in a person's life. If these issues and conflicts are resolved, people grow to be successful human beings.

Erikson's model is thought to be one of the best ways to understand human growth and development. The model includes eight stages of growth: infancy, toddlerhood, preschool years, school-age years, adolescence, early adulthood, adulthood, and aging years. Erikson believed that every person passes through these stages. When each stage is successfully completed and conflicts are resolved, a person reaches the potential for his or her age group.

For example, according to Erikson, when you resolve the central conflict of the adolescent stage, you will achieve **self-respect** (appreciation and acceptance of yourself). This is important because respecting one's self is the basis for respecting others, no matter what age you are. Erikson also believed that during the aging years people reflect or think back on their lives. In this stage, older adults may view their experiences as failures, and feel a sense of despair. They may fear death and struggle to find their purpose. However, older adults who successfully pass through this stage will look back on life with contentment and fulfillment.

What Is Behavior?

When people talk about **behavior**, they are referring to actions that are responses to a stimulus (something that causes the action). Behavior differs from attitude. In Chapter 1, you learned that an *attitude* is a way of feeling or thinking about a person, object, or situation. When these feelings and thoughts are acted on, they become behaviors.

Most behaviors are **overt**, or open to view. Examples of overt behaviors are smiling or opening a door. Behaviors can also be **covert**, or internal and not shown openly. An example is a resident saying he is afraid of a procedure but there are no observable physical signs of fear. The fear is real for the resident, however.

Behaviors change throughout a person's life. Some behaviors are a result of a person's developmental stage. Behavioral differences can also occur as people learn or their goals change, or as a result of generational differences. Research shows that each *generation*, or group of people who are born during the same time, has its own special attitudes, behaviors, expectations, and habits. Each member of a generation experiences similar important events within his or her lifetime. Specific ideas and experiences motivate the members of a generation. Because members of a generation are around the same age, each generation's members seem to have similar ideas, problems, and attitudes.

Culture may also affect behavior. As you learned in Chapter 1, *culture* is the traditions, beliefs, rituals, customs, and values that are specific to a group of people. Cultural differences that impact behavior affect how people communicate, eat, dress, and carry out their traditions.

How Do Generational Differences Affect Behavior and Attitudes?

A *generation gap* occurs when people from different generations have trouble communicating because of differences in traditions, attitudes, or beliefs. For example, older generations may talk more formally than your generation does.

Understanding the behaviors of other generations is helpful, but do not focus too much attention on differences. Doing so might cause you to believe *stereotypes* (simplifications or biases) about a particular generation. Believing stereotypes can prevent you from getting to know a resident. Rather, talk openly with people to learn about generational differences and value the qualities of each generation.

Understanding residents' generations will help you build *rapport* (mutual understanding in relationships) and communicate more effectively (**Figure 7.3**):

- **The silent generation (1928–1945):** having lived through World War II and the Great Depression, this generation tends to have strong feelings of patriotism (love for their country), are often hard workers, prefer to save their money, and value security and comfort.
- **The baby boomers (1946–1964):** this generation enjoyed a strong economy when they first entered the workforce (began working as adults). They tend to value hard work; are motivated to achieve professional goals; and are often independent, optimistic (having a positive attitude), confident, and patriotic.
- **Generation X (1965–1976):** as children of working parents, this generation is often defined by its independence. People of this generation tend to be well educated and feel comfortable starting their own businesses.

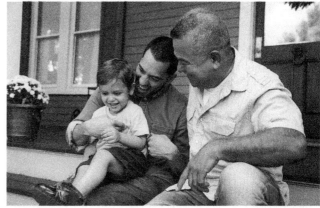
MBI/Shutterstock.com

Figure 7.3 Positive intergenerational relationships are built on understanding and good communication.

- **Millennials (1977–1995):** this generation is very comfortable using technology, having experienced its rapid growth during their youth. They are often comfortable with changing fashion, are flexible, and value exercise and travel. Many also volunteer or give to causes (charities) in which they believe.

- **Generation Z (1996–2004):** advancements in technology have greatly impacted this generation, causing them to have high expectations of technology and strong multitasking abilities (can perform more than one task at a time). This generation may be independent, less focused, and will take more risks than others.

SECTION 7.1 Review and Assessment

Key Terms Mini Glossary

behavior a manner of acting; the way a person responds to stimulation.

covert not shown openly; hidden.

empathy understanding for another person's feelings and emotions.

generation a group of people who are born and who live during the same time.

generation gap a lack of communication between one generation and another; often due to differences in customs, attitudes, and beliefs.

genuine honest, open, and sincere in communication and relationships.

homeostasis an internal balance in the human body.

motivation choosing to act on something a person wants.

overt open to view; observable.

rapport mutual understanding in a relationship.

respect a feeling of appreciation and admiration for another person.

self-actualization a person's belief that he or she has developed to full potential.

self-esteem a person's confidence and regard for himself or herself.

self-respect a person's appreciation and acceptance of himself or herself.

stereotypes simplifications or biases about a group that shape the treatment of all group members.

Apply the Key Terms

Write a sentence using each key term properly.

1. behavior
2. empathy
3. generation gap
4. motivation
5. stereotype

Know and Understand the Facts

1. Explain the differences between extrinsic and intrinsic motivation.
2. Describe the five levels in Maslow's hierarchy of needs.
3. What is the difference between an attitude and a behavior?
4. Describe three similarities and three differences between two of the generations discussed in this section.

Analyze and Apply Concepts

1. Why is it helpful for holistic nursing assistants to understand Maslow's hierarchy of needs?
2. Explain how you can assist residents in meeting a particular need, such as safety and security.
3. Name two reasons why there are differences in people's behavior.

4. Give one example of a situation in which you could communicate more effectively with residents of a different generation.

Think Critically

Read the following care situation. Then answer the questions that follow.

When you enter Mrs. D's room in your community's assisted living facility, you find Mrs. D sitting in a chair. Mrs. D is still in her pajamas and is looking out the window. You ask if Mrs. D would like to go to breakfast and you offer to assist her to the dining room. Mrs. D doesn't smile and shakes her head saying "no." This is not her usual behavior—Mrs. D is always ready to go for meals and seems to enjoy eating with her friends. You know that yesterday Mrs. D's daughter visited and was crying. After the visit, Mrs. D also cried and did not sleep well.

1. What do you think might have caused the change in Mrs. D's behavior?
2. In your opinion, what level of Maslow's hierarchy of needs has Mrs. D achieved?
3. What can you do to respect Mrs. D's not wanting to go to the dining room while still being sure her needs are met?

Body, Mind, and Spirit

Objectives

To achieve the objectives for this section, you must successfully:

- **explain** the body, mind, and spirit and how they relate to holistic relationships and care.
- **examine** the impact the body, mind, and spirit have on your self-image, health, and wellness.
- **describe** how recognizing and being aware of the connection between body, mind, and spirit can influence caregiving.

Key Terms

Learn these key terms to better understand the information presented in the section.

autonomy

conscious

parasympathetic nervous
   system (PNS)

self-image

subconscious

sympathetic nervous
   system (SNS)

Questions to Consider

- Were you aware that the body, mind, and spirit are all connected?
- Have you noticed this connection in your own life? For example, when you feel stressed (this comes from the mind), do you also get a headache (the body's reaction)? When you no longer want to do something (influenced by the spirit), do you find reasons not to (this comes from the mind)?

What Is the Relationship among Body, Mind, and Spirit?

A person's body, mind, and spirit are constantly interacting with each other. These three elements are connected. This means that people live their lives with all three influencing what they do (**Figure 7.4**).

Body

You already know that the body requires food and water, which are basic needs. The human body is a highly complex system. Each person's body performs the same functions, but each body is also unique. How the body responds to its basic needs and how the body's needs affect a person's mind can be different. These interactions are what make each of us a special, interconnected system.

Mind

Your *mind* is constantly thinking, questioning, and directing your behavior based on your perception of the world. Your mind becomes aware of situations through your senses of hearing, sight, taste, smell, and touch. Your thoughts can be either **conscious** (aware) or **subconscious** (unaware).

The connection between the mind and body is demonstrated when a thought prompts a physical reaction in the body. For example, it is possible to lessen feelings of anxiety by using deep breathing to calm yourself. When you stop thinking about your anxiety and focus instead on your breathing, your body begins to relax. This relaxation is felt especially in the abdominal region where tension and anxiety are held. Breathing also has the ability to relax the nervous system. Once you begin deep-breathing exercises, the ***parasympathetic nervous system (PNS)*** (a part of the body's nervous system that controls the automatic daily functions of the cardiovascular, respiratory, and gastrointestinal systems) takes over and returns your body to a homeostatic (balanced) state. You begin to feel calm and more open to problem solving and decision-making.

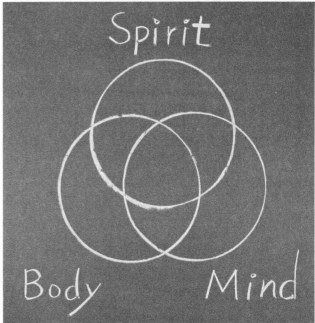

Anson0618/Shutterstock.com

Figure 7.4 The body, mind, and spirit interact, creating a connection so that people can live their lives with all three influencing what they do.

The opposite happens when the **sympathetic nervous system (SNS)**, (another part of the body's nervous system) sets off the fight-or-flight response. In the *fight-or-flight response*, increased blood flow to the lungs and heart prepare a person to react to the situation by either running or fighting. At this time, the brain is not functioning at its best. It is hard for the mind to be optimistic and see possibilities, and it is difficult to make decisions (**Figure 7.5**).

Spirit

The spirit is also connected to the body and mind. Your *spirit* consists of your inner qualities. When a person is said to have *spirituality*, he or she is typically seen as honest, loving, caring, wise, imaginative, and compassionate (kind).

Sometimes, when spirit is discussed, only a person's religion is considered, but the spirit is more than this. The spirit is a person's *higher self*, or the inner qualities that help a person feel whole and achieve inner peace and harmony (balance). Some ways to get to know your spirit are through meditation, prayer, poetry, music, and talks with friends. These activities are proven to calm the body and mind. This feeling of calm can create a connection between the body and mind. As the body and mind influence each other, many have a better sense of well-being and peace.

Positive connections between the body, mind, and spirit help create a healthy lifestyle. Some exercises and activities you can do to strengthen these connections include walking, participating in yoga or tai chi, weight lifting, and hiking (**Figure 7.6**). Eating a nutritious diet (including four or five cups of fruits and vegetables a day), spending time with friends and family, writing in a journal, or doing some creative activity will also help promote positive connections between your body, mind, and spirit.

How Does the Body-Mind-Spirit Connection Influence Caregiving?

Connections between the body, mind, and spirit greatly influence the quality of care you give to others. Not only is it important to understand your own body-mind-spirit connection, but it is also important that you are aware of how these connections affect others.

Your Body-Mind-Spirit Connection

When your body, mind, and spirit are connected, your body is as healthy as it can be, your mind is clear, and your spirit is in harmony with your body and mind. This connection will help you feel strong and confident. It will also help you develop a positive **self-image** (view of yourself).

When you have a strong body-mind-spirit connection, you will have a positive presence and will have the ability to be gentle and caring. You will be able to sense when others are stressed and help them use calming breaths. You will understand the importance of a healthy lifestyle.

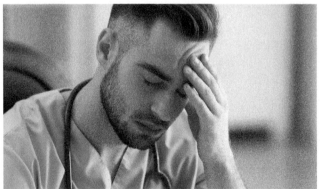

Africa Studio/Shutterstock.com

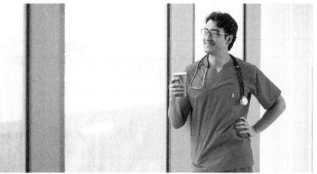

Elnur/Shutterstock.com

Figure 7.5 Look at the two images in this figure. Which part of the nervous system (sympathetic or parasympathetic) is set off in each image?

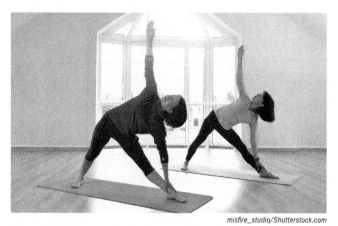

misfire_studio/Shutterstock.com

Figure 7.6 Many people find yoga to have both mental and physical health benefits.

The Body-Mind-Spirit Connection and Caregiving

The body-mind-spirit connection not only affects you personally, but also impacts your caregiving. When you understand your own body-mind-spirit connection, your approach to residents will be helpful, you will use supportive communication, and you will be better able to build mutual respect. You will also be able to focus on the unique needs and desires of those in your care and promote resident *autonomy* (personal independence). Encouraging residents to be as independent as possible will help them maintain strong body-mind-spirit connections.

Remember that the way you deliver holistic care is an extension of who you are as an individual. Only you can build a strong connection between yourself and those in your care.

Holistic care begins when you first meet a resident. This is the resident's first impression of you, and you only get one first impression. Pay close attention to the way you walk into the room, the tone of your voice, and the way you make contact. Remember that the resident's room is his or her personal space. Create trust by looking directly at the resident, being attentive (interested), and showing appropriate concern. Be respectful and use the resident's title and last name, such as *Mr. Antar*.

It is important to always explain what care you will provide. Create rapport with residents by taking time to listen to them (**Figure 7.7**). Avoid interrupting or making judgmental statements, such as "You don't look well today." Listening helps develop positive regard, trust, and mutual respect between the nursing assistant and resident. When you listen well, your communication will be caring and sincere. In addition to listening, always try to answer any

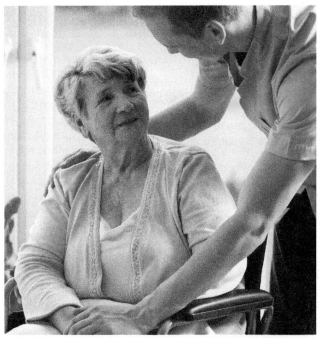

Phtographee.eu/Shutterstock.com

Figure 7.7 With the resident's permission, you can use touch to communicate that you are listening.

BECOMING A HOLISTIC NURSING ASSISTANT

Assessing Your Own Body, Mind, and Spirit

How does a person learn more about connections between the body, mind, and spirit? One important way to learn more about this is to become aware of your own body, mind, and spirit. Gaining this awareness can strengthen your body-mind-spirit connection.

The following statements represent qualities of strong connections between the body, mind, and spirit. Consider which statements are true for you. The more statements that are true for you, the stronger your connections are in that area.

Are you aware of your body? Which statements are true for you?

- I eat between four and five cups of fruits and vegetables daily.
- I exercise regularly.
- I sleep between seven and nine hours every night.

Are you aware of your mind? Which statements are true for you?

- I find time during the day to relax, even if only for a few minutes at a time.

- I communicate well with all types of people and am a good listener.
- I have written goals that will help me achieve my life and career goals.

Are you aware of your spirit? Which statements are true for you?

- I enjoy the environment and regularly walk or play outside.
- I would describe myself as a happy person.
- I have positive relationships with my family and friends.
- I like what I am currently doing—for example, going to school or a job.

Apply It

1. How many statements were true for you in each category?

2. If there were some statements that were not true for you, what can you do to change this?

questions residents have. You may also want to use touch, if appropriate, such as a handshake or pat on the arm, when communicating.

The holistic nursing assistant's role in giving care is always to build rapport, positive regard, and trust through the use of empathy, respect, being genuine (real), and effective communication. Relationships are built on respect and trust. Respect and trust are choices people make. When you give respect and build trust, you will get them in return. The saying "Treat others how you want to be treated" applies to holistic nursing care.

SECTION 7.2 Review and Assessment

Key Terms Mini Glossary

autonomy the personal independence and freedom to determine one's own actions and behavior.

conscious aware of feelings, actions, and outside surroundings.

parasympathetic nervous system (PNS) a part of the body's nervous system that controls the automatic daily functions of the cardiovascular, respiratory, and gastrointestinal systems; helps the body return to a homeostatic state after experiencing pain or stress.

self-image the way a person thinks about himself or herself, abilities, and appearance.

subconscious not fully aware of feelings, actions, and outside surroundings.

sympathetic nervous system (SNS) a part of the body's nervous system; sets off the fight-or-flight response.

Apply the Key Terms

An incorrect key term is used in each of the following statements. Identify the incorrect key term and then replace it with the correct term.

1. Self-image is personal independence and freedom to determine one's own actions and behavior.
2. The subconscious is awareness of feelings, actions, and outside surroundings.
3. The sympathetic nervous system (SNS) is a part of the body's nervous system that controls the automatic daily functions of the cardiovascular, respiratory, and gastrointestinal systems. It also helps the body return to a homeostatic state after experiencing pain or stress.
4. Autonomy is the way a person thinks about his or her self, abilities, and appearance.
5. The subconscious sets off the fight-or-flight response.

Know and Understand the Facts

1. In your own words, explain the connection between the body, mind, and spirit.
2. What is the difference between conscious and subconscious thoughts?
3. Describe two ways you can develop holistic relationships that connect the body, mind, and spirit.

Analyze and Apply Concepts

1. Describe three ways you can strengthen your spirit.
2. How can understanding the body, mind, and spirit help you deliver resident-centered care?

Think Critically

Read the following care situation. Then answer the questions that follow.

Mr. B is a retired army officer. He has been in a nursing home for the past month due to complications (problems) from an ulcer. Although Mr. B is in a lot of pain, he is very outspoken about wanting to go home. When Mr. B communicates with staff, his responses are very short and sometimes rude. This morning, Sarah, a nursing assistant, is assigned to help him wash, clean his dentures (artificial teeth), and get dressed.

1. What can Sarah do to help make the connection between her body, mind, and spirit strong so she can best care for Mr. B?
2. What can Sarah do to build a strong holistic relationship with Mr. B?

Work-Life Balance

Objectives

To achieve the objectives for this section, you must successfully:

- **identify** stressors.
- **describe** ways to manage stress.
- **discuss** ways to improve your work-life balance.

Key Terms

Learn these key terms to better understand the information presented in the section.

distress
energy
eustress
hormones

prioritizing
stress management
work-life balance

Questions to Consider

- Have you ever felt stressed because of a situation or person? What do you think caused the stress?
- How do you experience stress? Do you get a headache or stomachache? Does your heart beat faster or do you feel short of breath? Do you feel that you are running out of time and can't get anything done? What effect does your stress have on others in your life?
- How do you manage the stress in your life? Does the way you manage stress help you balance school, work, and other parts of your life?

What Is Stress?

Stress is a physical or mental response to a situation that causes worry or tension. Everyone experiences stress. It is considered normal and it affects each person differently. Some people get headaches, have trouble sleeping, experience sore muscles, or may even become depressed.

There are many possible sources of stress. Stress can come from external (outside) factors, such as the environment or social situations. Stress can also be the result of an illness or medical procedure.

Eustress vs. Distress

Some stress can be good. *Eustress*, or good stress, can motivate you to do new or challenging tasks such as studying hard to do well on an upcoming test or to apply for a job you have been wanting. Stress that remains at a high level, lasts for a long time, or gets out of control can turn into bad stress, or *distress*.

When someone is in distress, his or her body may not function properly, and he or she may have unhealthy feelings and emotions. When people are stressed, they release *hormones*, which are chemical substances that regulate (control) body processes. Hormones help protect the body and prepare the body for the challenges of stress. At this time, the sympathetic nervous system (SNS) also sets off the fight-or-flight response. During the fight-or-flight response, the heart may beat faster, the person may start to sweat, the stomach may stop digesting food, and sometimes the immune system fails. This response helps people focus and be alert in case they need to defend themselves. If this response continues over time, it can harm physical and emotional health.

Signs and Symptoms of Stress

There are several signs and symptoms of stress. These signs and symptoms can affect mental, emotional, physical, and behavioral health:

- **Mental symptoms:** inability to concentrate, constant worry, or seeing only the negative
- **Emotional symptoms:** moodiness, short temper, agitation, loneliness, or depression
- **Physical symptoms:** aches and pains, dizziness, nausea, rapid heartbeat, or frequent colds
- **Behavioral symptoms:** procrastination (putting things off), isolation, nervous habits, or the use of alcohol or drugs to relax

It is not possible to completely eliminate all stress from your life. Typically, people have their own unique reactions to stressors. For example, some people may get headaches, others may need more sleep, and some may become tense and angry. Recognizing stressors is the first step to getting them under control and being able to recognize them in others. Stress can also interfere with residents' abilities to achieve wellness. Be sure to report any signs or symptoms of stress in residents to the licensed nursing staff. This is very important information.

How Can Stress Be Managed?

Stress management includes strategies to handle and control stress. These strategies are important not only for yourself, but also for your work as a holistic nursing assistant. Understanding how to manage stress will improve how you work with others and care for residents. When you manage stress, you will also find your work environment more enjoyable and productive.

Identifying Stressors

The first way to manage stress is to identify stressors before they cause strong reactions. To do this, take a breath to relax your body and begin to identify any sources of stress. Focus on relaxing so you can identify any stressors that are making you feel tight or tense.

Identifying each stressor will help you decide if your stressors are important. You may feel stressed about something that has not happened yet, or you may feel stress from external pressures. If you practice identifying your important stressors, you may be able to stop strong stress responses before you and your body react to them.

As a holistic nursing assistant, you should also try to identify stressors that affect residents in your care. Residents may feel worried and stressed about not having any visitors, becoming forgetful, or losing people they love. You can help residents identify these stressors and determine if stressors are important to them. For example, you may care for a resident who is worried that he will not have visitors. Explore the reality of this situation with the resident by asking when he last had visitors and who those visitors were. Ask when these visitors said they would return. You may find that the resident is concerned only about who is visiting today, not about never having visitors.

Changing Focus

Another stress-management strategy is to shift focus away from a stressor and onto something that is not stressful—for example, a sport, book, candle, deep breathing, a saying, or a game. Focusing on something that is not stressful will give you and your body a break. For example, if you are feeling stressed, you may want to take a walk to release tension. As you walk, focus on your surroundings

---

THINK ABOUT THIS

In a recent survey, 89 percent of people interviewed said they had experienced serious stress in their lives. According to the American Academy of Family Physicians, two-thirds of office visits to family doctors are for stress-related symptoms.

---

or your breathing. Humor is another way to relieve stress. Even just smiling creates a relaxation response in the body. Laughing is very good for the body and spirit as well. By doing this, you and your body will learn how it feels to be relaxed and not stressed. Once you experience not being stressed, you will want more of this feeling, and so will those in your care (**Figure 7.8**).

Using Support from Others

Relying on strong support from family and friends is another stress-management strategy. Often, family and friends can provide the assistance needed during difficult times and can help you feel more positive and optimistic (hopeful). Studies have shown that when people are supported by caring family and friends, recovery time is reduced.

Managing Time and Energy

Using your time and *energy* (power and drive) wisely is another important strategy for managing stress. Being aware of time and planning your day will allow you to get your work done more easily. The same is true for energy. If you are aware of your energy levels and understand how you can increase them, you will not only get your work done, but you will also feel good about what you are doing. One of the first steps in properly managing your time is analyzing how you spend it. One way to do this is to write down what you did last week, including specific details about how each day was spent. Make sure the week you analyze is representative of a typical week in your routine schedule.

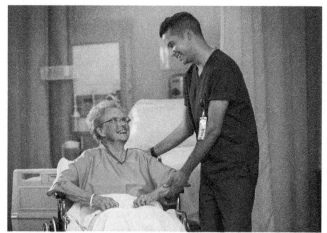
© Tori Soper Photography

Figure 7.8 Laughter and humor can help you reduce and manage stress.

Once you have written down exactly how you spend your time, you can decide what changes, if any, you would like to make. Maybe you would like to spend less time watching television or playing on your phone, and more time reading. Once you decide what changes you want to make, you can list them from most to least important. Then make the changes by taking action. Other time-management strategies you can use include:

- Use your time effectively. Be aware of whether you are wasting time or checking your phone too often (**Figure 7.9**).
- Break large projects up into small tasks. For example, when you work on a paper, first create an outline of the paper's topics. Then use the outline to begin your draft.
- Say *no* or ask for more time when you do not have the necessary time to complete a task properly. This is a way to respect yourself and others.

Be aware of how you use your personal energy during the day. If you are a morning person and have more energy in the morning, complete difficult or time-consuming work during the morning hours. If you have more energy during the evening hours, use that time to complete more challenging tasks. Also, pay attention to other people's energy levels and the effect they have on you. If another person's energy is low, this may lower your energy level. Understand that those in your care may have low energy levels due to illness. You may have to lessen your energy level to match that of others. Protect yourself against distracting or negative energy, such as another person's negative attitude. Try not to let this attitude affect you. Stressful or difficult events may leave you feeling tired. When this happens, you can restore your energy by relaxing or by refocusing on your responsibilities and the tasks required of you.

The key to effective time and energy management is to be mindful of what needs to be done and how it can be done. This can make your day and what you do satisfying and nurturing for yourself and, if possible, for others.

Establishing Priorities

One stress management strategy that is especially helpful to keep work challenges under control is **prioritizing**, or organizing responsibilities or tasks so that the most important tasks are completed first. Prioritizing is also an important time-management strategy, especially when you need to complete many routine tasks for residents.

When you set priorities, you determine which tasks are most important and should come before others. Some people are comfortable using *to-do lists* to prioritize. You can even create a quick written to-do list at work once you are given an assignment. The best way to set priorities is to use either your personal to-do list or an assignment sheet. On the list or sheet, write an *A* next to tasks that are high-priority and that need to be done that day. Write a *B* next to items that can wait until after A-level tasks are completed. Write a *C* next to tasks that you would like to get done, but can complete after A and B tasks are completed (**Figure 7.10**).

As you prioritize, think about how much time each task might take. Always allow extra time to solve any problems that may occur. Be flexible, when possible.

You may finish a task early. If you do, then just move on to the next item on your list. Be sure to leave time for routine breaks where you can relax and take time for yourself. Also figure in time-outs if you are at a computer or are sitting for long periods of time. When using a to-do list at work, be sure to review your priorities with the licensed nursing staff. You will need to complete all of the A-level tasks on your list. Check the list often to make sure you are on track. Feel free to reprioritize tasks if there is a change in a resident's condition or in your assignments. Remember to mark any tasks completed. This will give you a sense of accomplishment.

Prioritizing is meant to decrease stress, not to cause it. Therefore, be sure your priorities are organized and realistic. Understanding how to set priorities can be a very valuable skill for holistic nursing assistants. Prioritizing will help you get more done than you usually would in the same time period.

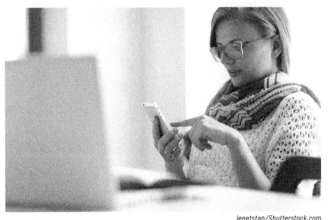

lenetstan/Shutterstock.com

Figure 7.9 In today's world, your smartphone can be a distraction, preventing you from effectively managing your time.

Priority	Mr. D	Mrs. S	Ms. D	Mr. F	Mrs. G
A	Assist with ambulation with new cane two times for 20 minutes	Measure intake and output	Apply warm compress to right foot for 20 minutes	Fall risk; remind him to ask for help to the bathroom	Turn and position every two hours
B	Assist with dressing change	Assist with shower	Frequently check pain levels during shift	Assist with eating breakfast and lunch	Give a partial bed bath and pay special attention to perineal care
C	Assist with shaving	Urinary leg bag change	Keep fresh water available to encourage fluids	Take him to afternoon facility activities	Provide snacks two times during shift

Goodheart-Willcox Publisher

Figure 7.10 This is an example of a priority list for a nursing assistant for one shift.

What Is the Best Way to Create a Work-Life Balance?

When you begin working as a holistic nursing assistant, you will find that achieving a positive *work-life balance* is another way to manage stress. Work-life balance describes the state of a person's time and energy contributions to career, work, and family commitments (**Figure 7.11**). When you are stressed at work, that stress may interfere with your ability to provide quality care to residents. Work-related stress can also affect your home life. A positive work-life balance allows you to be mentally present at home when you are home and to focus on your work responsibilities when you are at work. Doing this can help you feel more in control, which can reduce stress levels.

The best way to determine whether you have a positive work-life balance is to think about how you would answer the following questions:

- Do you think of yourself as healthy?
- Are your relationships strong, supportive, and caring?
- Are you aware and respectful of your environment?
- Are you able to rest and relax?
- Do you spend time on your own personal development?

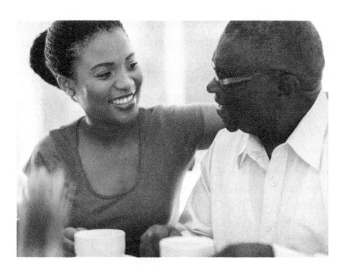
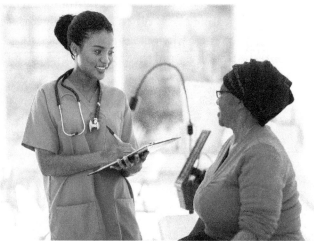

michaeljung/Shutterstock.com

Figure 7.11 Spending time with family can be a positive way to relieve stress, improving your ability to provide quality care while at work.

- Do you have enough money for your current and future needs?
- Are you happy with your career? If you are not, do you have a plan to get more education and training?
- Do you have passion or enthusiasm for what you are currently doing?

If your answer to each of these questions is *yes,* this shows that you have the potential for an outstanding work-life balance. This is not realistic, however. Everyone has one or more areas that need work. Identify those areas and determine how you will strengthen them. In each area that is strengthened, your work and life will become more balanced. This will make each day less stressful as you work.

SECTION 7.3 **Review and Assessment**

Key Terms Mini Glossary

distress bad stress; causes bodily symptoms that can lead to disease and poor coping and decision making.

energy the power and drive to make decisions and complete tasks.

eustress good stress; helps people become motivated and productive.

hormones chemical substances that are produced in the body and that control and regulate specific body processes.

prioritizing organizing responsibilities or tasks so that the most important tasks are completed first.

stress management the process of taking actions to lessen or remove reactions to stress and stressful events.

work-life balance the state of a person's time and energy contributions to career, work, and family commitments.

Apply the Key Terms

Use the appropriate key term to complete each sentence.

1. A holistic nursing assistant was able to use _____ to lessen or remove reactions to stress and stressful events she experienced at work.
2. There are two types of stress. One type is _____, or good stress, which helps people become motivated and productive.
3. Another type of stress is _____, or bad stress, which causes physical symptoms that can lead to disease and poor coping and decision making.
4. One way to manage time is _____, in which responsibilities or tasks are organized so that the most important tasks are completed first.
5. _____ is the state of a person's time and energy contributions to career, work, and family commitments.

Know and Understand the Facts

1. Name one physical and one mental effect of stress.
2. Identify two sources of stress.
3. What are three possible symptoms of stress in residents?

Analyze and Apply Concepts

1. What are two ways holistic nursing assistants can manage their stress?
2. What can holistic nursing assistants do to help reduce the stress of residents in their care?
3. Describe how to prioritize work tasks and responsibilities.
4. What might cause a negative work-life balance, and what can you do to fix this balance?

Think Critically

Read the following care situation. Then answer the questions that follow.

Mrs. P, one of the residents on your unit, is sweating and appears anxious. She is trying to find her glasses but cannot. Mrs. P seems to be upset with herself for losing her glasses. She wants to be independent, so she doesn't feel she should ask for help. When you come into Mrs. P's room to help her with morning care, you hear her quietly repeating that she cannot find her glasses.

1. What signs do you observe that might show that Mrs. P is stressed?
2. What can you do to help Mrs. P manage her stress?

Key Points

Reviewing the key points for this chapter will help you practice more safely and competently as a holistic nursing assistant and will help you prepare for the certification competency examination.

- When people are motivated, they are more likely to choose to act on something they want.
- When delivering care, you must understand the basic human needs all people have. According to Maslow's hierarchy of needs, needs go from low-level needs (basic needs such as food, water, sleep, and elimination) to the highest-level needs (self-actualization).
- People develop physically, mentally, emotionally, and socially based on their unique characteristics (traits).
- Caring for different generations is an opportunity to learn and grow. Understanding generational differences can help you better communicate with residents and provide quality holistic care.
- A strong body-mind-spirit connection will help you see yourself more effectively and build a strong connection between yourself and those in your care.
- Stress is something we all experience. We sometimes have bad stress (distress) and good stress (eustress). Stress can often be lessened by identifying stressors, changing focus, relying on a support system, managing time and energy, and establishing priorities.

Action Steps to Holistic Care

Review the information in this chapter. Complete the following activities.

1. With a partner, prepare a poster that shows two challenges people of different generations face.
2. Find pictures in a magazine, in a newspaper, or online that best demonstrate providing holistic care to a resident. Describe each image and explain why it was selected.
3. Research one growth and development model not discussed in this chapter. Write a brief report that summarizes the theory or model.
4. With a partner, prepare a poster or digital presentation that shows how the body, mind, and spirit interact with each other when a person is happy, sad, stressed, fearful, and tired.

Building Math Skill

Kate planned her tasks and meals for her 7 a.m. to 3 p.m. shift at the long-term care center so she would not feel stressed. She planned 3 hours for hygiene care, 50 minutes for lunch, and 10 minutes for one break. She also knew she would need 1 hour to assist in feeding two residents, 2 hours for special procedures, and 1 hour for shift report and charting. What percent of the shift did she assign to each task and meals?

Preparing for the Certification Competency Examination

To prepare for the nursing assistant certification competency examination, you will need to know content found in this chapter. This content may be tested in the knowledge (written or oral) and skills (hands-on demonstration) portions of the exam. The following areas will be emphasized:

- basic human needs across the life span
- human growth and development
- supportive communication
- behavior that is positive and nonthreatening
- the nursing assistant's role in accommodating spiritual differences
- sources of stress
- appropriate stress-relieving techniques
- signs and symptoms of stress
- time-management skills

These sample test questions are similar to ones you will find on the certification competency exam. See how well you can answer them. Be sure to select the *best* answer.

1. Which of the following is *not* an intrinsic motivational factor?
   A. a desire to help others
   B. a desire for recognition
   C. an award
   D. a challenge
2. What qualities are needed to develop a positive relationship?
   A. being in control
   B. knowing all the answers
   C. being caring and professional
   D. showing sympathy

3. A resident sometimes gets mad and yells at the nursing staff. He is very proud and does not want to be in the facility. What would be the best approach to use when you first meet him?
   A. go inside and introduce yourself, and then sit down for a moment and listen to him
   B. tell the resident that no one wants to take care of him
   C. observe the resident in a nonjudgmental way and slowly start taking care of him
   D. go into the room smiling and begin to prepare him for his morning meal

4. As you approach Mrs. S's room, you hear her crying. What should you do?
   A. don't go in; ask someone else to go in and check on her
   B. take a breath, knock, go in, approach Mrs. S, gently touch her shoulder, and ask if you can help
   C. go away, wait for an hour, and then come back to see Mrs. S
   D. go in and tell Mrs. S to stop crying, reminding her that things could be worse

5. Mr. C shares with you that no one cares about him anymore. You've noticed that he has not had visitors this past month. What need is Mr. C expressing?
   A. self-esteem
   B. self-actualization
   C. basic and physiological
   D. love and belonging

6. Mrs. M recently had a hip fracture (break) that required surgery. When you encourage Mrs. M to get up and use her walker to go to the restroom, she refuses. What question should you be asking yourself?
   A. Is Mrs. M having pain or discomfort?
   B. Is Mrs. M angry about her hip surgery?
   C. Is Mrs. M giving you trouble because she doesn't like you?
   D. Is Mrs. M just being difficult because she wants sympathy?

7. Which of the following is one way to create a healing environment that is aware of the body, mind, and spirit?
   A. use behaviors that communicate that residents will get better soon
   B. be present and listen to residents whenever it is appropriate and helpful
   C. talk about ways residents will be able to take care of themselves when they get home
   D. keep busy in residents' rooms and get as much done as you possibly can

8. Which of the following generations is most likely to work very hard?
   A. the baby boomers
   B. millennials
   C. the silent generation
   D. generation Z

9. Mr. E is a 73-year-old man who recently had one leg amputated (surgically removed). He appears very nervous. Which of the following would be the best way to approach him?
   A. feel sorry for Mr. E
   B. encourage Mr. E to try taking deep calming breaths, if he agrees
   C. tell Mr. E to try to think about happy things in his life
   D. reassure Mr. E that there are people who have it worse

10. A nursing assistant wants to help a resident having difficulty with his physical therapy. Which of the following should she do?
    A. observe the resident and talk about what his job was in the service
    B. tell the resident he does not have a good self-image and needs to focus
    C. ask the resident if there is an exercise he used to do that could be changed
    D. get upset and tell the resident he needs to exercise to feel better

11. Which need is fulfilled when a person feels satisfied with his or her state of health, property, and home?
    A. basic needs
    B. love and belonging
    C. self-esteem
    D. safety and security

12. Which part of the nervous system sets off the fight-or-flight response?
    A. central
    B. sympathetic
    C. parasympathetic
    D. subconscious

13. Which of the following would help you achieve a positive work-life balance?
    A. achieving harmony in your life by using stress-management tools
    B. letting your work affect your emotions and home life
    C. ignoring your emotions because they won't affect your work
    D. identifying that work is stressful and realizing that is just the way it is

14. Which of the following statements about stress is *true*?
    A. Everyone reacts to stress in the same way.
    B. Stress management is easy to include in your life.
    C. Stress cannot be managed; instead, it manages you.
    D. Stress is different for everyone.

15. A nursing assistant in an assisted living facility is responsible for 20 residents. He cannot find enough time to care for all of the residents. He is feeling frustrated and doesn't know what to do. Which of the following should you do to help him?
    A. tell him to complain that he has too much work
    B. agree that it is just too much work for the time he has left on the shift
    C. tell him to quit his job since this is just unfair and it is not the right job for him
    D. ask him if he has set the right priorities for his work

Did you have difficulty with any of the questions? If you did, review the chapter to find the correct answer(s).

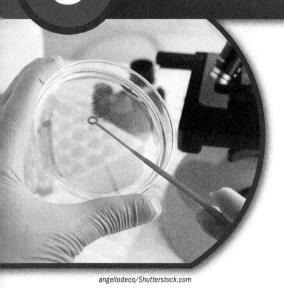

angellodeco/Shutterstock.com

Chapter Outline

Section 8.1
Body Defenses
and Infection

Section 8.2
Standard and
Transmission-Based
Precautions

Section 8.3
Wound Care

Welcome to the Chapter

One of your most important responsibilities as a nursing assistant is to help prevent and control infection. To do so, you must understand how the body protects itself from infection, how infection spreads, and what you can do to prevent it from spreading. In this chapter you will learn about the body's defenses, including immunity, or resistance to disease. You will also learn about the chain of infection and how breaking this chain can help prevent and control infections in healthcare facilities. Important skills related to infection prevention and control are also discussed. These skills include following proper hand hygiene practices, using personal protective equipment (PPE), double-bagging biohazardous waste, transporting residents to and from isolation, and following exposure control plans. You will also learn about types of wounds and wound care, ways to maintain a sterile field, and the nursing assistant's responsibilities during dressing changes.

The information and procedures presented in this chapter will help you build the knowledge and skills needed to become a holistic nursing assistant. Check with your instructor to ensure that these procedures are within your state's regulations for nursing assistant practice. The topics discussed in the chapter are highlighted on the Providing Holistic Care Framework.

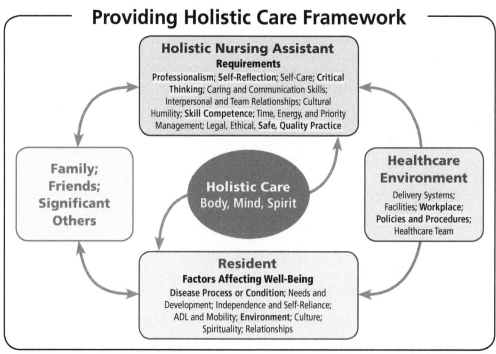

Providing Holistic Care Framework

Holistic Nursing Assistant
Requirements
Professionalism; **Self-Reflection; Self-Care; Critical Thinking;** Caring and Communication Skills; Interpersonal and Team Relationships; Cultural Humility; **Skill Competence;** Time, Energy, and Priority Management; Legal, Ethical, **Safe, Quality Practice**

Family; Friends; Significant Others

Holistic Care
Body, Mind, Spirit

Healthcare Environment
Delivery Systems; Facilities; **Workplace; Policies and Procedures;** Healthcare Team

Resident
Factors Affecting Well-Being
Disease Process or Condition; Needs and Development; Independence and Self-Reliance; ADL and Mobility; **Environment;** Culture; Spirituality; Relationships

Goodheart-Willcox Publisher

Body Defenses and Infection

Objectives

To achieve the objectives for this section, you must successfully:

- **describe** the natural lines of defense against disease in the human body.
- **explain** the immune response, immunity, and risk for infection and disease.
- **identify** the four types of microorganisms.
- **describe** the six links of the chain of infection.
- **explain** modes and methods of transmission, signs and symptoms of infection, and general treatment.
- **identify** the reasons healthcare-associated infections (HAIs) occur.

Key Terms

Learn these key terms to better understand the information presented in the section.

antibodies	inflammation
antigens	microorganisms
bacteria	mucus
catheter	noncommunicable
cell	diseases
chlorophyll	pathogens
communicable diseases	phagocytosis
culture	photosynthesis
dormant	tissue
dressing	toxins
enzymes	viruses
infection	

Questions to Consider

- Do you remember receiving vaccinations when you were a child? Did anyone object to the vaccinations you received?
- Have you ever had a childhood disease, such as the measles or chickenpox? What was this experience like?
- Have you recently received any adult vaccinations? Did you have any side effects from a vaccination?

What Are Microorganisms and Pathogens?

No matter where you are, very small organisms live around and with you. These organisms are so small that they are only visible through a microscope. As a result, they are called *microorganisms*, or *microbes*.

Microorganisms can be found in many places—in the air, water, and soil and on plants, animals, and people. Some microorganisms are useful and do not cause disease. These are called *normal flora*. Normal flora do not cause problems if they do not travel to new locations. Normal flora can cause disease if they move away from the place where they live. When this occurs, normal flora become **pathogens** and are sometimes called *germs*.

What Are the Types of Microorganisms?

Several types of microorganisms can cause infections in humans. The four basic types of microorganisms are bacteria, viruses, fungi, and parasites.

Bacteria

Bacteria are single-celled microorganisms that are often harmless, but can also cause **infections** (the invasion and growth of harmful pathogens in the body). The human body must constantly protect itself from infection and disease in any part of the body. If bacterial infections are not treated, they may spread.

Bacteria can enter the body through the skin, nose, mouth, eyes, ears, lungs, urethra, and vagina, among other places. Once bacteria get in, they multiply (reproduce) quickly, causing infection. Bacterial infection can destroy tissues and cells; bacteria may also overpower the body and prevent it from functioning properly. An example of a bacterial infection is strep throat.

Bacterial infections are most commonly treated with antibiotics. Antibiotics may be taken by mouth, applied to the skin, or injected intramuscularly (into a muscle) or intravenously (into a vein). One challenge of the widespread use of antibiotics is the development of antibiotic resistance.

Antibiotic resistance develops when bacteria change to resist the effects of an antibiotic. Bacteria that survive an antibiotic treatment multiply into bacteria that are resistant to (or unaffected by) that antibiotic. Bacteria that are resistant to more than one antibiotic are called *multidrug-resistant organisms (MDROs)*. Examples of MDROs are methicillin-resistant *Staphylococcus aureus* (MRSA) and vancomycin-intermediate or vancomycin-resistant *Enterococcus* (VRE). Antibiotic resistance has negative consequences (outcomes) for those who have infections. For example, when a person has an infection that is antibiotic resistant, recovery time can be very slow. In some cases, death can occur if the infection cannot be treated. Good hygiene, cleanliness, and the careful use of antibiotics can help prevent antibiotic resistance. Some facilities have antibiotic policies and guidelines about the use of antibiotics and ways to manage antibiotic resistance.

Viruses

Viruses are the smallest microorganisms. They are 100 times smaller than bacteria and cannot grow or multiply by themselves. Instead, viruses take over another living cell called a *host cell* (usually plant or animal cells). The virus takes over the host cell, including all of its functions. The host cell, now infected with the virus, reproduces the virus, causing it to spread. Some viruses spread through saliva, coughing, sneezing, sexual contact, or through the *fecal-oral route* (through water or food contaminated with feces). The common cold and influenza (commonly called the *flu*) are both viral infections.

Another example is SARS-COV-2, which is the virus that causes COVID-19 (CO = corona, VI = virus, and D = disease). This is a novel virus that has not been seen before in humans.

According to the CDC and the World Health Organization (WHO), COVID-19 spreads when an infected person coughs, sneezes, sings, talks, or breathes. Particles are inhaled into the nose, mouth, airways, and lungs of other people, causing the infection. These particles can travel distances of 6 feet (2 arm lengths) and beyond and can remain in the air for a long time. They can also land on surfaces or objects and stay there for hours, causing possible transfer when other people touch those surfaces or objects and then touch their mouth, nose, or eyes. COVID-19 seems to spread easily in communities; people who live in the same area become infected with the virus through a process called community spread. This is one of the reasons why *contact tracing* occurs. Contract tracing is the identification and follow-up of people who may have come into contact with a communicable disease.

Viral infections cannot be treated with antibiotics. They are treated with antiviral prescription medications. Like antibiotics, antiviral medications are specific to particular viruses, but rather than destroying a virus, they slow virus development even if the virus has been recently contracted (caught). Vaccinations exist for viral pneumonia, the flu, COVID-19, polio, measles, mumps, rubella, and smallpox.

Fungi

A fungus is an organism that lacks **chlorophyll** (a substance found in plants that absorbs and transfers light). Fungi reproduce through *spores*, which are single-celled and capable of reproducing on their own. Fungi must digest food to live, since they are incapable of **photosynthesis** (the process of converting energy from the sun into chemical energy). Types of fungi include mushrooms, molds, yeasts, and parasitic fungi.

Fungi are common. In fact, people breathe in or come into contact with fungal spores daily without getting sick. The human body naturally contains some fungi, including yeasts and parasitic fungi. Yeast infection can occur when the amount of yeast in the body becomes imbalanced. Opportunistic (develops only under certain circumstances) fungi can also cause infection by attacking a weak immune system. Examples of fungal infections include athlete's foot, vaginal yeast infections, and ringworm. Fungal infections are typically treated using over-the-counter or prescription antifungal creams, ointments, or medications.

Parasites

Parasites are organisms that live on or in other organisms, or *hosts*. Parasites feed on the host. Some parasites do not affect the host, while other parasites make the host sick.

Parasites can be spread through contaminated water, waste, fecal matter, blood, sexual contact, and mishandled or undercooked food. Some parasitic infections are spread by insects, which carry the disease and transmit it while feeding on the host. One example is malaria, which is spread by mosquitos.

Not all parasitic infections can be treated, although antibiotics and other medications (such as lotions or creams) can be helpful for treating particular infections. Treatment should also include removal of the infestation (for example, bedbugs or lice).

What Are the Barriers to Infection?

The body's first line of defense against infection includes physical and chemical barriers in different parts of the human body. Structures and substances of the human body protect it and prevent pathogens from getting inside. The skin, for example, is one of the body's best defenses because it creates a physical barrier between the inner structures of the body and the outside environment. The skin also releases *enzymes* (chemical substances that cause specific reactions) when it is cut or torn. These enzymes are chemical barriers that kill bacteria that may try to enter the body. Another example of a barrier is the nasal passages of the respiratory system. These are lined with membranes that contain *mucus* (a thick, slippery fluid that moistens and protects parts of the body), and tiny hairs that trap microorganisms that may cause infection or disease.

What Is the Immune Response?

The body's second line of defense, the immune response, is a cellular and chemical response that helps fight against infection. In the immune response, the body looks for differences between its own *cells* (the smallest structural unit of the body) and *tissues* (specialized cells that act together to perform specific functions) and foreign (outside) substances. Foreign substances are known as *antigens* and may include *toxins* (poisons).

As part of the immune response, cells with foreign antigens and toxins are identified by *antibodies*. Antibodies are proteins in the blood that attach themselves to antigens and mark them for destruction by the immune system. These antigens are then destroyed through a process called *phagocytosis* (**Figure 8.1**). The immune system remembers each antigen it meets, and if an antigen appears again, the body is prepared to respond. Each time a new antigen enters the body, the body must develop a new set of antibodies for that specific

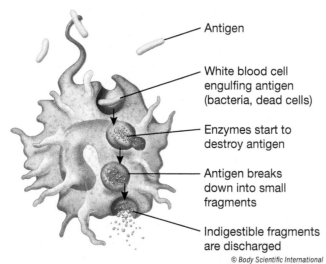

- Antigen
- White blood cell engulfing antigen (bacteria, dead cells)
- Enzymes start to destroy antigen
- Antigen breaks down into small fragments
- Indigestible fragments are discharged

© Body Scientific International

Figure 8.1 During phagocytosis, white blood cells engulf antigens and destroy them. Antibodies mark antigens for destruction.

antigen. The human body can develop around 100 million types of antibodies.

For example, people who get mumps can build enough antibodies that they are unlikely to get the disease again. If these people do get mumps again, they will usually have a milder case.

How Does Vaccination Create Immunity?

Vaccines can also build immunity. As you learned in Chapter 2, a *vaccine* is a mixture that usually contains a very mild form of a disease so the body builds antibodies against that disease. Vaccines are created to prevent or reduce the severity of diseases. An example of a common vaccine is the annual flu shot. People who receive a flu vaccine are injected with a mixture that contains a flu antigen that has been weakened or killed. Introducing this weakened or killed antigen tells the body to develop antibodies specific to that antigen. As a result, the body will attack and destroy that antigen if exposed to it again. If exposed to that flu antigen, the vaccinated person will usually not get sick or will have a milder case if he or she does get sick. Vaccinating a large number of people against a disease helps control the spread of that disease. When the majority of a population is immune, this is called *community immunity* or *herd immunity*.

Sometimes vaccinations are given once. Other vaccines require more doses, called *boosters*, after the initial vaccine. Specific vaccinations are often recommended or even required when a person is traveling to another country. Vaccinations are also required for people who work in certain professions, such as healthcare. The goal of vaccination is protection for yourself and others.

What Is the Inflammatory Response?

Other body responses also defend against infection. The *inflammatory response* causes *inflammation* (swelling and redness that occurs as the body's response to an infection). Inflammation occurs when body tissues secrete chemicals that cause swelling (puffiness) around the damaged area. Inflammation can also make the affected area warm to the touch and red. It may also cause a fever (increased body heat), which destroys antigens or toxins. The inflammatory response lets white blood cells (which fight infection) and other cells know to travel to the injured area of the body and attack toxins. Sometimes *pus*, a product of the immune response, can be found at the site of injury. Pus contains tissue, dead antigens, and white blood cells (**Figure 8.2**).

As a holistic nursing assistant, you will observe and report inflammation. If you observe inflammation, you might document that "the area around the wound on the upper arm was red, swollen, and warm to the touch." Often, pressure from swelling and the increased body heat resulting from the inflammation causes pain.

What Increases the Risk for Infection?

Risks for infection and disease are everywhere, but some people are more vulnerable to these risks than others. People who are older have more difficulty avoiding infection, particularly during flu season or during extremely hot or cold weather. Older adults often have less resistance to infection because acute or chronic illness can slow the metabolism.

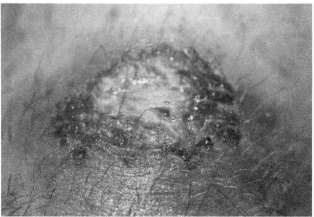

Kondor83/iStock/Getty Images Plus via Getty Images

Figure 8.2 Inflammation and pus indicate the presence of an infection.

People in poor health (for example, people with respiratory or cardiovascular conditions) have limited resistance to colds and flu. These people often experience more severe symptoms. People with autoimmune disorders or human immunodeficiency virus (HIV) may have chronic conditions that lower immunity. Also at increased risk are residents who have been in a healthcare facility for a long time.

Residents in long-term care facilities are susceptible to infection, particularly if they have a *catheter* (a flexible tube that is inserted through a narrow opening into the body). Urinary catheters and IVs increase risk for infection because they are foreign objects placed inside the body. Increased risk for infection has become a major problem in healthcare facilities. Infections acquired within healthcare facilities are called *healthcare-associated infections (HAIs)*. You will learn more about HAIs later in this chapter.

What Are Different Types of Infections?

Infections can be local, systemic, or opportunistic:

- **Local infections:** confined, or limited, to one area of the body. Signs and symptoms of a local infection include fever; redness, heat, pain, and swelling at the site; and pus or discharge that may be foul smelling.
- **Systemic infection:** widespread and travels throughout the body in the bloodstream. The signs and symptoms of a systemic infection include aches, sometimes chills and fever, nausea and vomiting, and general overall weakness. A viral flu is an example of a systemic infection.

- **Opportunistic infections (OIs):** develop only under certain circumstances, as a result of a weakened immune system. The opportunistic infection takes advantage of the weakened immune system and creates a second infection. For example, pneumocystis pneumonia is a common opportunistic infection in people who have HIV/AIDS.

- **Healthcare-associated infections (HAIs):** an infection that occurs in a healthcare facility (also called a *nosocomial infection*). *Clostridium difficile* (*C. difficile*) is an example of an HAI. Catheter-associated urinary tract infections (CAUTIs) are also examples of HAIs. Older adults and people with diseases or conditions that require the long-term use of antibiotics are at greater risk of getting this infection. *C. difficile* bacteria are spread by surfaces or instruments contaminated with infected feces (for example, commodes, bathtubs, and rectal thermometers).

What Is the Chain of Infection?

For an infection to develop, a certain order of events must occur that leads to infection. This is called the

chain of infection. There are six links in the chain of infection (**Figure 8.3**):

1. **Infectious agent:** An infectious agent, or *pathogen*, must be present to cause infection. The pathogen might be a bacterium, virus, fungus, or parasite. It must have the ability to cause disease, multiply and grow, and enter the body.

2. **Reservoirs:** The pathogen needs a *reservoir*, or a place, where it can live and reproduce. Reservoirs can be environmental or human. A potential reservoir for infection might be a toilet seat or feces.

3. **Portal of exit:** Pathogens need a *portal of exit*, or a way to leave the reservoir. A portal of exit can be through a sneeze, a cough, blood, or feces.

Chain of Infection

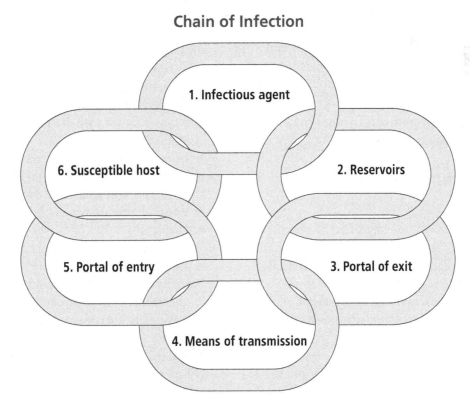

Goodheart-Willcox Publisher

Figure 8.3 The chain of infection consists of six links: the infectious agent, reservoirs, portal of exit, means of transmission, portal of entry, and susceptible host.

4. **Means of transmission**: There must be a means of transmission, or a *carrier*, for the pathogen to move from one place to another. Pathogens can be transmitted directly (between two people, such as through a sneeze or cough) or indirectly (from a contaminated piece of equipment). Sometimes human carriers can incubate, or hold and allow a disease to grow and be harmful to others, even if they are not sick themselves.
5. **Portal of entry**: A *portal of entry* must exist for the pathogen to enter a person. The portal of entry could be the nose (pathogens can be breathed in), the mouth (through eating contaminated food), or an open wound.
6. **Susceptible host**: A susceptible host that cannot resist the pathogen will become ill. Whether an infection forms depends on several risk factors, including the host's age, existing diseases and conditions, and the amount of infectious agent.

The purpose of infection control is to break the links in the chain of infection.

How Do Communicable Diseases Spread?

Diseases and infections can be identified by how they are transmitted, or spread. Diseases that cannot be transmitted between people, objects, and animals are *noncommunicable*, or not contagious. Examples of **noncommunicable diseases** include genetic (inherited) diseases, cancers, mental disorders, and heart disease.

Communicable diseases are contagious and can be transmitted between people and animals, and to objects. Communicable diseases can spread through the air, through contact, by swallowing contaminated food or water, from an insect bite, and through bloodborne pathogens. These diseases can also develop opportunistically or due to the reactivation (awakening) of a **dormant** organism (an organism whose functions have slowed or stopped). Methods of transmission include:

- **Airborne transmission:** occurs when microscopic pathogens move in the air or become trapped in dust; also called *droplet transmission*. If these pathogens are inhaled (breathed in) by a susceptible host, they can cause illness. Airborne transmission can occur when someone who is ill coughs, sneezes, talks, laughs, sings, or spits.
- **Contact transmission:** occurs when an infectious agent or reservoir containing a pathogen comes into contact with a host. Contact can be direct—through touch, sexual contact, blood, or body fluids (such as urine, feces, or vomit). Contact can also be indirect—through contaminated items such as soiled (dirty) linen, clothing, a **dressing** (bandage) soaked with drainage, or used specimen containers.
- **Vehicle transmission:** occurs when an infectious agent is ingested (taken into the body) through contaminated food or water. An example of a disease spread by vehicle transmission is *dysentery*.
- **Vector transmission:** occurs when an infection is the result of an animal or insect bite. This can be caused by a break in the skin or transmitted by the vector's mucous membrane (the lining of a body cavity or passageway). The mosquito is a common vector and can carry diseases such as malaria, Zika virus, and West Nile virus (**Figure 8.4**). Ticks, fleas, and other insects are also vectors for disease.

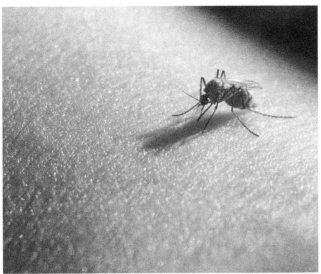

Alexander Penyushkin/Shutterstock.com

Figure 8.4 Mosquitoes are common vectors of many diseases.

- **Bloodborne pathogens:** as you learned in Chapter 4, bloodborne pathogens are disease-causing microorganisms found in an infected person's blood. Bloodborne pathogens can be transmitted through exposure to human blood and other potentially infectious body fluids, sharps-related injuries and needlesticks, and other injuries that break the skin. Bloodborne pathogens are very dangerous in healthcare settings, where healthcare staff members may be exposed to blood.

How Do You Know When Someone Has an Infection?

A person who thinks he or she has an infection should get medical attention from a doctor. Observing signs and symptoms of an infection can lead to its identification. An infection can also be detected using laboratory tests and X-rays.

Typically, the first tests done are blood tests. A common blood test to identify infection is a white blood cell count. The body releases more white blood cells into the bloodstream when an infection is present. As a result, an elevated (raised) white blood cell count may be a sign of an infection.

Blood or fungi *cultures* (the process of growing cells in a favorable environment) may be used to determine the type of microorganism causing the infection. These cultures also help determine what type of treatment is needed.

Specific infections may require additional tests. A urinary tract infection (UTI), for example, is tested using urine samples and a urine culture. To diagnose pneumonia, a doctor may order an X-ray of the lungs and a sputum test. Skin tests can also be used to identify specific infections. Some of these tests will be discussed in Chapter 16.

BECOMING A HOLISTIC NURSING ASSISTANT
Caring for Residents with Infections

When caring for residents with infections, holistic nursing assistants must remember several important things. Often, the focus of care is stopping the infection as quickly as possible. It is also important, however, to consider the psychosocial aspects of care.

When providing holistic care, be aware of and sensitive to the resident's fear or guilt surrounding an infection. Perhaps the resident knew someone who died from an infection; perhaps the resident did not keep a wound clean enough. It is important to recognize pain that can occur with an infection. Being sensitive to, observing, and reporting levels of pain will help relieve pain and promote healing.

Some people may be embarrassed by the odor associated from wound seepage (discharge) or rashes. As a holistic nursing assistant, help maintain good

hygiene and keep any dressings clean and fresh. This will help eliminate the smell and any embarrassment.

Finally, realize that personal protective equipment (PPE) and the processes used in infection control may be frightening to residents. The sight of a mask and gown can be upsetting for older adults. Provide advance notice about the use of PPE and explain why PPE is necessary. You will learn more about PPE in the next section.

Apply It

1. Think back to a time when you were sick with an infection. Did you find your symptoms embarrassing or painful? What made you feel more at ease?
2. Some people find caring for a resident with an infection difficult, fearful, or unpleasant. What actions might a holistic nursing assistant take to be sure he or she feels able to provide this care?

SECTION 8.1 **Review and Assessment**

Key Terms Mini Glossary

antibodies proteins in the blood that attach themselves to antigens and mark them for destruction by the immune system.

antigens substances foreign to the body that trigger the production of antibodies.

bacteria single-celled, microscopic pathogens that can cause infection.

catheter a flexible tube that is inserted through a narrow opening into the body.

cell the smallest and most basic structural and functional unit of the human body.

chlorophyll a green substance found in plants; absorbs light and transfers it through the plant during photosynthesis.

communicable diseases diseases that can be transmitted between people and animals, and to objects; also called *contagious diseases* or *infectious diseases*.

culture the process of cultivating (growing) living cells in a substance favorable to their growth.

dormant having slowed or stopped functions.

dressing a protective material placed on a wound; also called a *bandage*.

enzymes chemical agents that can cause specific biochemical reactions.

infection the invasion and growth of harmful pathogens in the body; leads to disease.

inflammation the protective response of body tissue to irritation, injury, or infection; causes swelling and redness.

microorganisms living things, or *organisms*, that are so small they can only be seen through a microscope.

mucus a thick, slippery fluid that moistens and protects parts of the body.

noncommunicable diseases diseases that are not contagious and cannot be transmitted between people and animals or to objects.

pathogens disease-causing microorganisms.

phagocytosis the process by which a white blood cell engulfs (surrounds) and destroys foreign antigens.

photosynthesis the process by which plants and other organisms convert light energy from the sun into chemical energy; allows plants and other organisms to function.

tissue a collection of specialized cells that act together to perform specific functions.

toxins poisons.

viruses the smallest microorganisms; viruses cannot grow or multiply by themselves; instead, they take over another living or host cell.

Apply the Key Terms

Write a sentence using each key term properly.

1. antibody
2. bacteria
3. infection
4. antigen
5. toxin

Know and Understand the Facts

1. Describe the immune response.
2. What is a vaccine?
3. What does community or herd immunity accomplish?
4. List the six links in the chain of infection.
5. Identify and describe one method of infection transmission.
6. What does *HAI* mean?

Analyze and Apply Concepts

1. What happens when inflammation occurs?
2. Explain why age might increase an older person's risk for infection.
3. Describe the sequence of events that must occur to create a chain of infection.

4. Explain the difference between communicable and noncommunicable diseases. Give one example of each.

Think Critically

Read the following care situation. Then answer the questions that follow.

Mr. S, who is 80 years old, fell last week at home and now has a bacterial infection in his lower leg. He fell during the evening while going to the bathroom and suffered a deep cut. His daughter, who lives with him, stopped the bleeding and cleaned the wound. She put a bandage on it. Two days later, Mr. S complained that his leg really hurt, that stuff was coming out of the wound, and that he felt hot. His daughter took his temperature and found he had a high fever and the wound was very swollen with pus coming out of it.

1. What signs and symptoms show the presence of an infection?
2. What might be the reason Mr. S was at risk for an infection?
3. If you were caring for Mr. S, what holistic care considerations should you be aware of?

Standard and Transmission-Based Precautions

Objectives

To achieve the objectives for this section, you must successfully:

- **explain** the principles and procedures required in standard and transmission-based precautions.
- **describe** the parts of an exposure control plan.
- **explain** how to perform proper hand hygiene.
- **identify** the steps needed to correctly put on and remove personal protective equipment (PPE).
- **describe** double-bagging and proper transport to and from isolation.

Key Terms

Learn these key terms to better understand the information presented in the section.

alcohol-based
  hand sanitizer
asepsis
epidermis
excretions
friction

isolation
quarantine
secretions
sterile
World Health
  Organization (WHO)

Questions to Consider

- How many times do you wash your hands each day? Do you wash your hands only in certain situations, such as before eating, after you have coughed or sneezed, or after going to the bathroom?
- Think about why you wash your hands. Do you wash your hands to be clean, out of habit, or because someone said you should? When you wash your hands, do you think about your own cleanliness or the health of others?

What Is Asepsis?

As a nursing assistant, you will be responsible for helping prevent the spread of infection in a healthcare facility. One way nursing assistants prevent infection is by helping maintain *asepsis* (the absence of infections or infectious material). In healthcare, the terms *clean* and *dirty* are used when talking about asepsis. Items such as equipment that have come in contact with potential pathogens are considered *dirty*. Items that have *not* come in contact with potential pathogens are considered *clean*.

When giving care, work with clean surfaces and then move to dirty surfaces. Following these guidelines will help prevent *touch contamination* (the transfer of

potential pathogens from a dirty to a clean surface or object). Always touch clean body parts or surfaces before touching those that are dirty or contaminated. Never touch your own face, nose, or eyeglasses before touching a resident.

There are two types of asepsis. *Medical asepsis* is a clean technique used to reduce the number and spread of microorganisms. This, in turn, prevents and controls infection. Medical asepsis procedures include hand hygiene, the use of personal protective equipment (PPE), and isolation. PPE includes specialized clothing and accessories (such as gloves, gowns, masks, and goggles) that protect against infection or injury. *Surgical asepsis* is a sterile process that completely eliminates microorganisms from the surface of an object. This is always used to maintain a sterile field (area) during surgery. It may also be used for certain wounds or procedures.

What Are Standard Precautions?

To achieve medical asepsis, healthcare staff members follow standard and transmission-based precautions (actions taken to prevent harm). *Standard precautions* are basic infection prevention and control practices used to prevent the spread of disease. *Transmission-based precautions* are done in addition to standard precautions to prevent the spread of disease from direct contact with pathogens, droplets of infectious microorganisms, and airborne pathogens. In the United States, these measures are guided by the Centers for Disease Control and Prevention (CDC) and are supported by evidence-based research. You will learn more about transmission-based precautions later in this section.

Standard precautions protect staff, residents, family members, and visitors from diseases that can be spread through contact with blood, body fluids, breaks in the skin (including rashes), and mucous membranes. Standard precautions include hand hygiene, the use of PPE, respiratory hygiene, cough etiquette, safe injection practices, safe handling of sharps to prevent injuries, and careful management of potentially contaminated equipment and surfaces. Standard precautions should be used appropriately and consistently with every resident.

Hand Hygiene

The role of hand washing in preventing the spread of infection was discovered in the nineteenth century and is a very important infection control practice today. *Hand hygiene* includes hand washing with soap (sometimes antimicrobial, which kills microorganisms or stops their growth) and water or the use of an **alcohol-based hand sanitizer**. An alcohol-based hand sanitizer is a liquid, gel, or foam preparation that kills most bacteria and fungi and stops some viruses found on the skin (**Figure 8.5**). The CDC and the **World Health Organization (WHO)** are leaders in setting hand hygiene guidelines. The WHO is an agency of the United Nations that focuses on international public health.

The **epidermis** (the outer surface of the skin) on the hands is tough and is composed of 10–20 layers of cells. These cells are constantly being replaced by new cells. The old cells and many microorganisms picked up during routine daily activities can remain on the hands (**Figure 8.6**). Unless microorganisms are removed, they can survive 30–180 minutes on the hands. Therefore, hand hygiene is critical. When

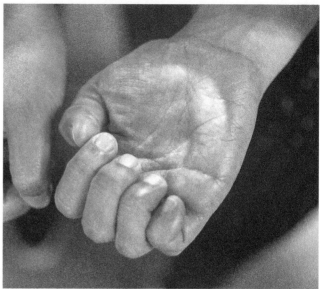

Pompak Khunatorn/iStock/Getty Images Plus via Getty Images

Figure 8.6 The hands in this image have been lit with a UV light to show the areas (in light blue) that have not been adequately washed and that still contain microorganisms.

working in a healthcare facility, nursing assistants should follow facility policy on how to perform hand hygiene. Hand hygiene must occur often and whenever hands are visibly soiled. In addition, hand hygiene should be performed before and after certain events and activities (**Figure 8.7**).

When to Perform Hand Hygiene

Before...
• going on break or eating a meal
• leaving a shift
• entering a resident's room
• putting on gloves
• handling a meal tray
• getting clean linens
• procedures
After...
• first entering a healthcare facility
• using the restroom
• leaving a resident's room
• touching a resident
• taking off gloves
• exposure to bodily fluids
• picking up an object from the floor or a dirty surface

Goodheart-Willcox Publisher

Figure 8.7 Nursing assistants must always perform hand hygiene before and after these activities.

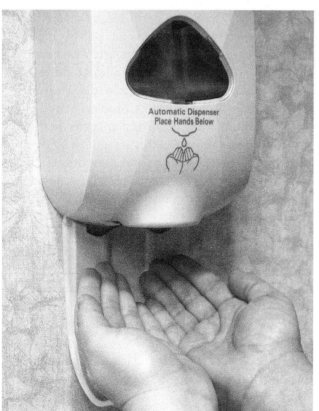

Paul Velgos/Shutterstock.com

Figure 8.5 In a healthcare facility, alcohol-based hand sanitizer can be found in hand sanitizer dispensers.

Alcohol-based hand sanitizers can be purchased easily and are often found in dispensers in healthcare facilities, grocery stores, and other public places. Effective hand sanitizers usually contain at least 60–95 percent alcohol.

While hand washing or using hand sanitizer, *friction* (resistance produced by rubbing two surfaces) helps remove microorganisms. Remember that wearing gloves is not a substitute for proper hand hygiene. Knowing how to effectively perform hand hygiene procedures is important for infection prevention and control.

Procedure

Hand Washing

Rationale

Standard precautions require routine and proper hand washing to remove and prevent the spread of microorganisms.

Preparation

1. Locate a sink near the place you will give care. There must be:
   - a sufficient supply of antimicrobial soap
   - a sink with warm, running water
   - clean paper towels in a dispenser
   - an appropriate waste container nearby
2. If your sleeves are long, use a clean, dry paper towel to push them up your arms until they are close to your elbows.
3. Remove any watches or rings. If you cannot remove a watch, use a clean, dry paper towel to push it up your arm away from your hand. If you cannot remove your rings, you will have to lather (spread) soap underneath them.

   Best Practice: The sink is always contaminated. Stand far enough away from the sink that your clothing does not touch it (**Figure 8.8**). Do not touch the inside of the sink at any time. Always rewash your hands if they touch the sink at any time.

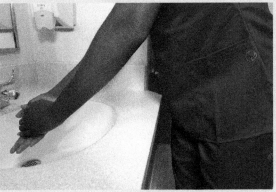

Figure 8.8   *Wards Forest Media, LLC*

The Procedure

4. Using a clean, dry paper towel, turn on the faucet. Do not turn on the faucet with your bare hands. Adjust the water temperature until the water is warm. Be sure the water does not splash on your scrubs.
5. Thoroughly wet your hands, wrists, and the skin 1–2 inches above your wrists.
6. Remove your hands from the water. Apply enough soap and work it into a thick lather over your hands, wrists, and the skin at least 1–2 inches above your wrists (**Figure 8.9**). If you have not removed your rings, lather soap underneath them.

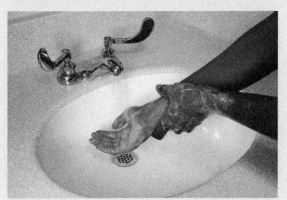

Figure 8.9   *Wards Forest Media, LLC*

   Best Practice: When washing your hands, keep your hands and forearms below your elbows. Water should flow down off your fingertips, never up your arms.

7. Rub your palms together in a circular, counterclockwise motion.
8. Push the fingers of the right hand between the fingers of the left hand and rub up and down.
9. Push the fingers of the left hand between the fingers of the right hand and rub up and down.
10. With fingers interlaced, rub the palms together from side to side.

(continued)

Hand Washing *(continued)*

11. Bend your fingers and interlock them. The backs of your fingers should touch the opposite palm. Rub from side to side (**Figure 8.10**). Clean under your fingernails by rubbing them against the other palm and forcing soap underneath them. Continue rubbing to clean around the tops of your nails. Reverse hands and repeat this step.

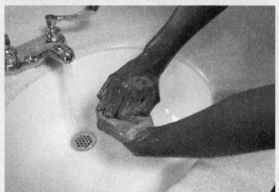

Figure 8.10   *Wards Forest Media, LLC*

12. Hold the left thumb in the palm of the right hand. Rub in a circular, counterclockwise motion.
13. Hold the right thumb in the palm of the left hand. Rub in a circular, counterclockwise motion.
14. Hold the fingers of the right hand together and place them in the middle of the left palm. Rub in a circular, counterclockwise motion.
15. Hold the fingers of the left hand together and place them in the middle of the right palm. Rub in a circular, counterclockwise motion.

> **Best Practice:** Work up a good foam as you wash over every part of your hands and wrists.

16. Wash your hands for a minimum of 20 seconds. You can use different methods to be sure you reach the 20-second minimum. For example, you could sing the "Happy Birthday" song twice from beginning to end.
17. Hold your hands under the running water with your fingers pointing downward (**Figure 8.11**). Rinse your wrists and hands thoroughly.

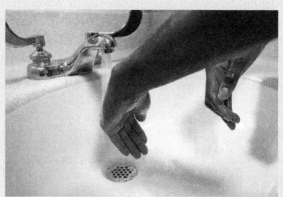

Figure 8.11   *Wards Forest Media, LLC*

18. Using a clean, dry paper towel, dry your hands and then your wrists, moving from your clean hand up toward the dirty forearm. Grab only one paper towel from the dispenser. Do not touch the dispenser and do not shake water from your hands.
19. Drop the used paper towel into the waste container. If another paper towel is needed, use the same procedure. Never touch the waste container.

Follow-Up

20. Use a clean, dry paper towel to turn off the sink faucet (**Figure 8.12**). Your bare hand should not touch the sink faucet. The faucet is always considered contaminated.

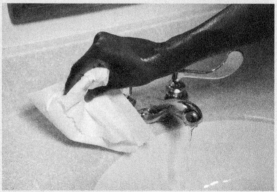

Figure 8.12   *Wards Forest Media, LLC*

21. Discard the paper towel into the waste container. Never touch the waste container.

Reporting and Documentation

This is an accepted, standard procedure. It does not need to be reported or documented.

Procedure

Using Hand Sanitizer

Rationale

Standard precautions require routine and proper hand hygiene. Using an alcohol-based hand sanitizer can help remove and prevent the spread of microorganisms.

Preparation

1. Locate the nearest hand sanitizer dispenser.
2. If your sleeves are long, use a clean, dry paper towel to push them up your arms until they are close to your elbows.
3. Remove any watches or rings. If you cannot remove a watch, use a clean, dry paper towel to push it up your arm away from your hand. If you cannot remove your rings, you will have to cover the rings with hand sanitizer.

The Procedure

4. Squeeze hand sanitizer from the dispenser into the cupped palm of one hand. Use enough hand sanitizer, usually one full pump, to cover the surfaces of the palms and fingers and perform the entire procedure.

   Best Practice: This procedure should take at least 20 seconds. Add more hand sanitizer to your hands, if needed.

5. Rub your palms together in a circular, counter-clockwise motion (**Figure 8.13**).

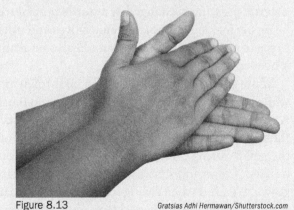

Figure 8.13   *Gratsias Adhi Hermawan/Shutterstock.com*

6. Push the fingers of the right hand between the fingers of the left hand and rub up and down (**Figure 8.14**).

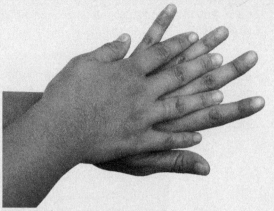

Figure 8.14   *Gratsias Adhi Hermawan/Shutterstock.com*

7. Push the fingers of the left hand between the fingers of the right hand and rub up and down.
8. With fingers interlaced, rub the palms together from side to side (**Figure 8.15**).

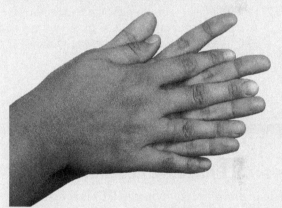

Figure 8.15   *Gratsias Adhi Hermawan/Shutterstock.com*

9. Bend your fingers and interlock them. The backs of your fingers should touch the opposite palm (**Figure 8.16**). Rub from side to side. Reverse hands and repeat this step.

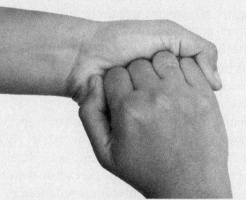

Figure 8.16   *Gratsias Adhi Hermawan/Shutterstock.com*

(continued)

Using Hand Sanitizer *(continued)*

10. Hold the left thumb in the palm of the right hand. Rub in a circular, counterclockwise motion (**Figure 8.17**).

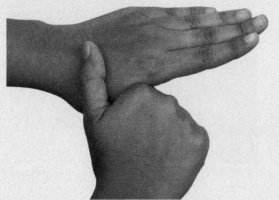

Figure 8.17 — *Gratsias Adhi Hermawan/Shutterstock.com*

11. Hold the right thumb in the palm of the left hand. Rub in a circular, counterclockwise motion.
12. Hold the fingers of the right hand together and place them in the middle of the left palm. Rub in a circular, counterclockwise motion (**Figure 8.18**).

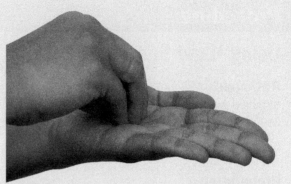

Figure 8.18 — *Gratsias Adhi Hermawan/Shutterstock.com*

13. Hold the fingers of the left hand together and place them in the middle of the right palm. Rub in a circular, counterclockwise motion.
14. Continue to rub your hands for the full 20 seconds.

> **Best Practice:** Creating friction is just as important when using hand sanitizer as it is when washing the hands.

Follow-Up

15. When the hands feel dry, the procedure is complete.

Reporting and Documentation

This is an accepted, standard procedure. It does not need to be reported or documented.

Personal Protective Equipment (PPE)

Personal protective equipment (PPE) is specialized clothing and accessories that protect the wearer from exposure to infectious materials. PPE creates barriers that prevent microorganisms from making contact with the wearer's skin or mucous membranes. PPE also protects residents with compromised (weakened) immune systems from caregivers. PPE includes gloves, gowns, face protection (masks, respirators, goggles, face shields), and in some cases, head covers and protective gear for the feet (such as booties). To be effective, PPE must be put on (*donned*) and taken off (*doffed*) according to procedure.

Depending on the circumstances, you may sometimes need to wear one, two, or all types of PPE when giving care (**Figure 8.19**). For example, all types of PPE are required if the procedure requires contact with *secretions* (substances produced by cells or organs) or *excretions* (waste products expelled from the body). You will need to use *sterile* gloves that are completely free of living microorganisms if a sterile dressing is changed or a sterile procedure is being performed. Hypoallergenic gloves and other types of nonallergenic gloves should also be available, if needed.

Some gowns are disposable (can be thrown away), while others can be laundered (washed) and reused. A gown should be selected based on its resistance to fluids. For example, if fluid is likely to leak through the gown during care, a fluid-resistant gown should be used. Clean and sterile gowns also exist. Clean gowns are used when caring for residents in isolation. A sterile gown is usually necessary during an invasive procedure (a procedure that enters the body) such as surgery.

Face protection is necessary for certain procedures, conditions, and types of care. For example, face protection is required if splashes or sprays of blood, body fluids, or secretions are expected, if the resident is in an isolation room or if there is a potential for the

When to Wear PPE

Disposable, Nonsterile Gloves
• when touching blood, body fluids, mucous membranes, secretions, excretions, breaks in the skin, or contaminated items • if the resident has open or seeping sores or rashes • if the resident's disease or condition requires them • when changing a nonsterile dressing • if handling soiled linens • if the caregiver has scrapes, scratches, or chapped skin
Gowns
• if in contact with blood, body fluids, secretions, or excretions • when giving care in an isolation room • during an invasive procedure
Face Protection
• during procedures when splashes or sprays of blood, body fluids, or secretions are possible

Goodheart-Willcox Publisher

Figure 8.19 Nursing assistants must always wear PPE such as gloves, gowns, and face protection when performing certain activities.

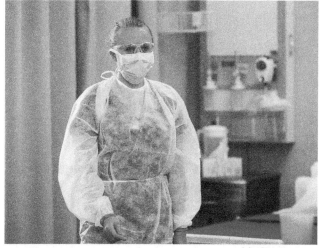

© Tori Soper Photography

Figure 8.20 This nursing assistant is wearing goggles and a mask for face protection.

transmission of microorganisms. There are different types of face protection (**Figure 8.20**):

- **Goggles**: the most reliable and practical eye protection against splashes, sprays, and respiratory droplets but does not protect other parts of the face. Personal or safety eyeglasses are not substitutes for goggles.
- **Face shield**: protects the face from the chin to the forehead and sometimes over the top of the head. It should wrap around the face to the ear to reduce any splashes going around the edge of the shield and reaching the eyes.

- **Mask**: protects the nose and mouth from splashes or sprays of blood or body fluids, prevents droplets from being transmitted by close contact, and prevents the contamination of a resident's wounds by mucus and saliva (spit). Masks do not fit snugly (securely) on the face or provide a tight seal, so they are not a totally reliable protection against airborne transmission. Masks may also be given to residents to limit the spread of their infectious respiratory secretions.
- **Respirator**: protects the nose and mouth and filters the air to prevent breathing in micro-organisms. A respirator must fit the wearer's face and provide a tight seal to be effective. Types of respirators include disposable respirators; surgical N95 (medical) respirators; powered, air-purifying respirators (PAPRs); and self-contained breathing apparatus (SCBA) respirators.

Procedure

Putting On and Removing Disposable Gloves

Rationale
Standard and transmission-based precautions require the use of disposable, nonsterile gloves for a variety of procedures. Putting on and removing gloves properly helps ensure infection prevention and control.

Preparation

Best Practice: Perform the following procedure only when putting on or removing disposable gloves in a resident's room.

1. Bring two pairs of disposable gloves in the correct size into the resident's room and place them on a clean surface. A box of disposable gloves may already be in the room. If a box is available, be sure the gloves are the correct size.

(continued)

Putting On and Removing Disposable Gloves *(continued)*

2. Before putting on the gloves, inspect (check) them for cracks, holes, tears, or any discoloration. Rings and fingernails may puncture (poke a hole in) gloves; avoid these to protect yourself and the resident. Discard damaged gloves.

3. If a gown is required, put on the gown before putting on the gloves.

The Procedure: Putting On Disposable Gloves

4. Wash your hands or use hand sanitizer to ensure infection control.

5. Your hands should be dry. Gloves are easier to put on dry hands.

6. Pick up one glove by its cuff (**Figure 8.21**).

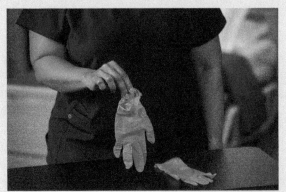

Figure 8.21   © Tori Soper Photography

7. Pull the glove onto your hand (**Figure 8.22**). The outside of a nonsterile glove is always considered contaminated, so keep your gloved hands away from your clothing and other areas.

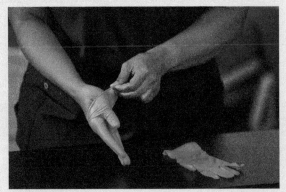

Figure 8.22   © Tori Soper Photography

8. Repeat steps 6 and 7 with the glove for your other hand.

9. Interlace your fingers to adjust the gloves on your hands.

10. If you are wearing a gown, pull the cuffs of the gloves up over the sleeves of the gown (**Figure 8.23**).

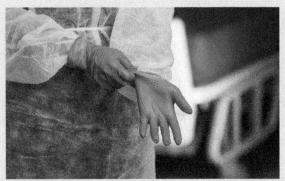

Figure 8.23   © Tori Soper Photography

Best Practice: Always remove gloves if they become torn or soiled during a procedure. Then wash your hands or use hand sanitizer to ensure infection control and put on another pair of gloves using the same procedure.

The Procedure: Removing Disposable Gloves

11. To remove your gloves, use the gloved fingers of one hand to grasp the glove on the other gloved hand just below the cuff.

12. Pull the cuff of the glove down, drawing it over your hand and turning it inside out (**Figure 8.24**).

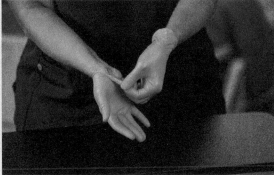

Figure 8.24   © Tori Soper Photography

13. Pull the glove off your hand and hold it in the palm of the other gloved hand (**Figure 8.25**).

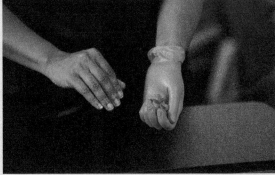

Figure 8.25   © Tori Soper Photography

14. Insert the fingers of the ungloved hand under the cuff of the remaining glove on the other hand.
15. Slowly pull the glove off, turning it inside out and drawing it over the first glove.
16. Drop both gloves into the appropriate waste container.

> **Best Practice:** Never wash or reuse disposable gloves.

Follow-Up
17. Wash your hands to ensure infection control.

Reporting and Documentation
This is an accepted, standard procedure. It does not need to be reported or documented.

Procedure

Putting On and Removing Gowns

Rationale
Standard and transmission-based precautions require that healthcare staff members wear gowns during procedures in which they might be exposed to or transmit microorganisms. Gowns create barriers that protect healthcare staff and residents. In some situations, such as caring for residents in isolation, gowning must occur before entering the room.

Preparation
1. Select the appropriate gown.
2. Remove any watches or jewelry.
3. If wearing long sleeves, roll them up above your elbows.

> **Best Practice:** As often as possible, carry out all procedures that require a gown at one time. This avoids regowning for multiple entries into and exits from the same room.

The Procedure: Putting On a Gown
4. Wash your hands or use hand sanitizer to ensure infection control.
5. Hold the gown by the shoulders out in front of you. The back of the gown should face you.
6. Unfold the gown carefully. Do not shake it open.
7. Slide your hands and arms into each of the sleeves of the gown (**Figure 8.26**).

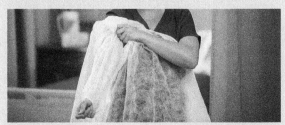

Figure 8.26   © Tori Soper Photography

8. Pull the top of the gown around your neck to cover your scrubs.
9. Reach behind the gown and tie the neck ties using a simple shoelace bow.
10. Reach behind the gown again. Grab the open edges of the gown and pull them together so they overlap. Your clothing should be covered completely.
11. Tie the waist ties in the back using a simple shoelace bow (**Figure 8.27**).

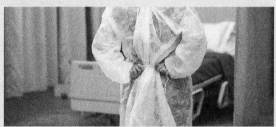

Figure 8.27   © Tori Soper Photography

12. Put on disposable gloves. Always put on gloves after putting on a gown. Pull the gloves up over the cuffs of the gown sleeves.

The Procedure: Removing a Gown
13. Before removing your gown, first remove and discard your gloves. Be careful not to contaminate yourself.

> **Best Practice:** Do not touch the outside of the gown as you remove it.

14. Reach behind the gown and untie both the neck and waist ties.
15. Slide your hands back into the sleeves of the gown. Using one hand (still inside the sleeve), hold the cuff of the opposite sleeve and begin pulling your arm out of that sleeve (**Figure 8.28**). Be careful not to touch the outside of the gown.

(continued)

Putting On and Removing Gowns *(continued)*

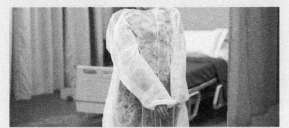

Figure 8.28 © Tori Soper Photography

16. Repeat step 15 to begin pulling the other arm out of its sleeve. Do not touch the outside of the gown with your hands as you pull the gown down off your shoulders and arms.

17. Turn the gown inside out as you remove it (**Figure 8.29**).

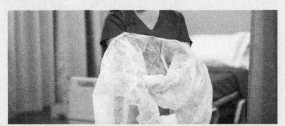

Figure 8.29 © Tori Soper Photography

18. Hold the gown, turned inside out, away from your clothing.

19. Roll the gown so the contaminated outside faces inward toward the gown (**Figure 8.30**).

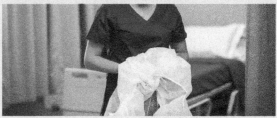

Figure 8.30 © Tori Soper Photography

20. The gown is now considered infectious waste. Dispose of the gown in the appropriate waste container before leaving the room. Do not wear the gown again. If the gown is a reusable cloth gown, it should be worn only once and should be handled as contaminated linen according to facility policy.

Follow-Up

21. Wash your hands to ensure infection control.

Reporting and Documentation

This is an accepted, standard procedure. It does not need to be reported or documented.

Procedure

Wearing Face Protection

Rationale

Properly applying a mask, respirator, goggles, or face shield provides a barrier that protects those who are giving and receiving care. In some situations, such as working with residents in isolation, this PPE must be put on outside the room.

Preparation

1. Assemble the needed equipment (the mask, respirator, goggles, or face shield).
2. Wash your hands or use hand sanitizer to ensure infection control.

The Procedure: Putting On a Mask or Respirator

3. Pick up the mask or respirator by its ties or elastic band. Place the mask or respirator over your nose, face, and chin. Secure the ties or elastic band of the mask or respirator behind your head and neck or behind your ears (**Figure 8.31**).

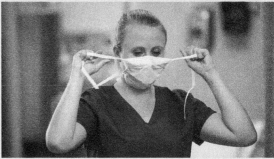

Figure 8.31 © Tori Soper Photography

4. Do not touch the portion of the mask or respirator that will cover your face. Only handle the ties or elastic band.
5. Adjust the mask or respirator over your nose, mouth, and chin by pinching the flexible portion over the bridge of the nose. The mask or respirator should fit snugly over the nose and under the chin. If you wear eyeglasses, the mask must also fit snugly under the bottom of your eyeglasses.

6. Check that the mask or respirator fits properly and seals tightly on your face.
7. Try to avoid coughing, sneezing, and unnecessary talking while wearing the mask or respirator to prevent contamination. If the mask or respirator becomes moist (wet), contaminated, or damaged, replace it.

> **Best Practice:** When talking with the resident, smile behind your mask and continue to smile whenever you can. Even if your mask covers your mouth, your smile will be seen in your eyes. It will go a long way to help the resident feel comfortable and accepted.

8. Do not let the mask or respirator hang around your neck when not in use.

The Procedure: Removing a Mask or Respirator

9. If you are wearing gloves, remove and discard them. Be careful not to contaminate yourself.
10. Before removing the mask or respirator, wash your hands or use hand sanitizer to ensure infection control.
11. Untie the ties or remove the elastic band of the mask or respirator. Start with the ties or elastic band at the bottom of the mask or respirator and then untie or remove the ties or elastic band at the top.
12. Grasp the mask or respirator by its ties or elastic band. Use both hands to pull the mask or respirator away from the face. Dispose of the contaminated mask or respirator according to facility policy.

The Procedure: Putting On Goggles or a Face Shield

13. Place the goggles or face shield on your face and eyes and adjust them so they protect the face and eyes.

> **Best Practice:** Personal eyeglasses or contact lenses are not adequate eye protection.

14. Try to avoid coughing, sneezing, and unnecessary talking while wearing a face shield to prevent contamination. If the goggles or face shield become moist, contaminated, or damaged, replace them.
15. Do not let the goggles or face shield hang around your neck when not in use.

The Procedure: Removing Goggles or a Face Shield

16. If you are wearing gloves, remove and discard them. The outside of the goggles or face shield is contaminated, so do not touch it with your bare hands.
17. Wash your hands or use hand sanitizer to ensure infection control.
18. With ungloved, clean hands, remove your goggles or face shield by grasping the clean earpiece with both hands and lifting the goggles or face shield away from your face.
19. Discard the goggles or face shield in the appropriate waste container, according to facility policy.

Follow-Up

20. Do not reuse any disposable face protection.
21. Wash your hands to ensure infection control.

Reporting and Documentation

This is an accepted, standard procedure. It does not need to be reported or documented.

Respiratory Hygiene and Cough Etiquette

In addition to hand hygiene and the use of PPE, respiratory hygiene and cough etiquette are also standard precautions that protect others from the spread of infection from respiratory secretions (such as saliva or nasal mucus) of residents who show signs and symptoms of a respiratory infection. The facility may require additional procedures. These actions include:

- covering your mouth and nose with a tissue when coughing or sneezing
- coughing or sneezing into your upper sleeve or elbow (not into your hands) if a tissue is not available (**Figure 8.32**)
- using the nearest waste container to dispose of a tissue after its use
- washing your hands or using hand sanitizer after contact with respiratory secretions and contaminated objects or materials
- placing a napkin over a resident's mouth if he or she coughs during mealtime to prevent droplet contamination of other residents' food
- providing tissues and no-touch waste containers for tissue disposal
- placing hand sanitizer dispensers, tissues, and waste containers in convenient, public areas
- providing soap dispensers and clean paper towels next to sinks
- Wearing a mask and offering a mask to people with respiratory symptoms, depending on conditions.
- Keeping at least six feet between you and others and not gathering in small, crowded areas, depending on conditions or local ordinances.

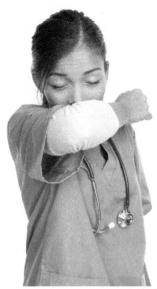

Figure 8.32 If you do not have a tissue, cough or sneeze into your elbow, not your hands.

Maridav/Shutterstock.com

One way to encourage respiratory hygiene and cough etiquette is to hang informational posters where they can be seen by visitors, family members, and residents. Posters should be written in languages appropriate to the geographic area.

Potentially Contaminated Equipment or Surfaces

All equipment and surfaces have the potential to become contaminated. For example, hands and gloves can easily pick up microorganisms after contact with contaminated surfaces and equipment and can transfer microorganisms to residents and to other surfaces. As a result, all equipment and working surfaces must be cleaned and decontaminated (to reduce the number of pathogens and prevent transmission) after contact with blood or other potentially infectious materials.

The first step in eliminating microorganisms from contaminated surfaces and equipment is cleaning. During *cleaning*, foreign materials are removed from surfaces and equipment. Cleaning must always come before disinfection and sterilization procedures. Healthcare facilities usually have schedules and procedures for cleaning and specific methods for decontamination. Cleaning is usually done with water, scrubbing, and detergents. Sometimes products containing natural enzymes are more effective than detergents on stubborn stains or waste.

During *disinfection*, germicides known as *disinfectants* prevent microorganisms from spreading and destroy many microorganisms, depending on their strength. Disinfectants are available in wipes or sprays. *Sterilization* completely eliminates all forms of microorganisms using extreme physical or chemical processes, such as steam under pressure or liquid chemicals. Gloves must always be worn during cleaning, disinfection, and sterilization procedures.

All disposable equipment can be used only once and then must be thrown away. Contaminated equipment, nondisposable clothing, and supplies are double-bagged in biohazard waste bags for proper handling and disposal.

Procedure

Double-Bagging

Rationale
The proper removal and disposal of infectious waste from an isolation room protects healthcare staff and prevents contamination of the environment.

Preparation
1. This procedure requires two healthcare staff members. One staff member should stand inside the isolation room, and the other should stand outside the room. The procedure requires:
   - disposable gloves for staff outside the isolation room
   - appropriate PPE for staff inside the isolation room
   - 2 leakproof, plastic biohazard waste bags (**Figure 8.33**)

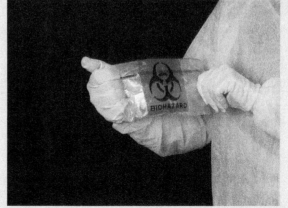

Figure 8.33

Timothy OLeary/Shutterstock.com

The Procedure: Inside the Isolation Room

2. Wearing disposable gloves and other appropriate PPE, stand in the room by the doorway with the full bag of waste. Be sure the contaminated biohazard waste bag is closed tightly.
3. Wait until the staff member outside the room folds the top of a clean biohazard waste bag into a cuff.
4. Place the contaminated biohazard waste bag inside the clean biohazard waste bag (**Figure 8.34**).

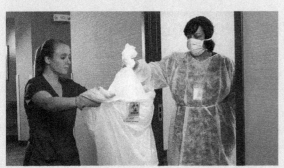

Figure 8.34 © Tori Soper Photography

Best Practice: Do not touch the outside of the clean biohazard waste bag when placing the contaminated biohazard waste bag inside.

The Procedure: Outside the Isolation Room

5. Wearing disposable gloves, stand outside the doorway with a clean biohazard waste bag.
6. Fold the top of the clean biohazard waste bag into a cuff. The cuff protects your hands from contamination.
7. Hold the clean biohazard waste bag wide open.
8. Remain standing outside the doorway while the staff member inside the room places the contaminated biohazard waste bag inside the clean biohazard waste bag.
9. Tie the clean biohazard waste bag with the biohazard waste and take it to the appropriate department for disposal, disinfection, or sterilization.

Follow-Up: Inside the Isolation Room

10. Remove your PPE before leaving the room.
11. Wash your hands to ensure infection control.

Follow-Up: Outside the Isolation Room

12. Remove and discard your gloves.
13. Wash your hands to ensure infection control.

Reporting and Documentation

This is an accepted, standard procedure. It does not need to be reported or documented.

In addition to handling potentially contaminated equipment or surfaces, holistic nursing assistants also make sure that rooms are cleaned after discharge (sometimes called *terminal cleaning*). This type of cleaning prepares rooms that are free from soil and microorganisms for the next resident. Depending on facility policy, this procedure may be carried out by a nursing assistant, shared with the housekeeping department, or completed only by housekeeping staff. If asked to clean a room after discharge, be sure to follow the facility procedure.

What Are Transmission-Based Precautions?

Transmission-based precautions are performed in addition to standard precautions. They are used for residents who are known or suspected to be infected with specific pathogens. Transmission-based precautions include contact precautions, droplet precautions, and airborne precautions. One example of a transmission-based precaution is wearing goggles or face shields during contact, not just when splashes or sprays are expected.

Contact Precautions

Contact precautions are used when microorganisms may be spread by direct or indirect contact (for example, contact with draining wounds, feces, vomit, head lice, or body fluids). Contact precautions require that gloves and a gown be worn upon entering a room and when coming into contact with residents, surfaces, or objects in the room (**Figure 8.35**). Contact precautions also require that reusable items be cleaned or disinfected and that nonreusable items be discarded immediately after use.

Droplet Precautions

Droplet precautions are used when an infection can be spread by respiratory droplets or by contact with mucous membranes. Examples of these infections include influenza, COVID-19, and pertussis (whooping cough). Respiratory droplets can travel six feet or more. When following droplet precautions, put on a face mask or respirator before entering the room. Your facility may also require you to wear a face shield and goggles. These precautions are very important if the resident has a fever.

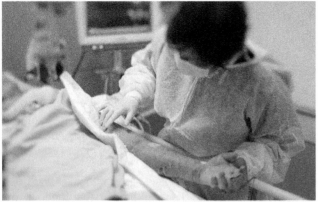

PongMoji/iStock/Getty Images Plus via Getty Images

Figure 8.35 Contact precautions prevent direct contact with contaminated objects. These precautions include wearing a gown and gloves. This nursing assistant is also wearing a mask to prevent the spread of infection via respiratory droplets.

Airborne Precautions

Airborne precautions are required when a disease can be spread by microorganisms in the air. An example of such a disease is tuberculosis. You should follow airborne precautions when entering the room of a resident suspected or known to have such a disease.

Airborne precautions typically require the use of a respirator, often one certified by the National Institute of Occupational Safety and Health (NIOSH). In some cases, a high-efficiency particulate air (HEPA) filtration unit may also be used to filter out airborne pathogens in the room.

Enteric, Wound, and Skin Precautions

In healthcare, you may also have to use other specific precautions. *Enteric precautions* help control diseases that can spread through direct or indirect oral contact with infected feces or contaminated articles. *Wound* and *skin precautions* help prevent the spread of microorganisms found in infected wounds and heavy secretions.

Bloodborne Pathogen Precautions

Special Occupational Safety and Health Administration (OSHA) safety standards apply to bloodborne pathogens such as HIV, hepatitis B and C, the *Plasmodium* parasite (which causes malaria), *Treponema pallidum* bacteria (which cause syphilis), and the Ebola virus. Bloodborne pathogen precautions protect healthcare staff and others who come into contact with blood and other potentially infectious materials (OPIM), such as semen and vaginal secretions. Contact may occur through needlesticks; cuts from

procedures; or direct contact between infected blood or secretions and broken skin, mucous membranes, or the eyes. The use of OSHA safety standards prevents exposure to bloodborne pathogens and reduces the chance of infection if contact accidentally occurs. These standards also require that facilities develop and use an *exposure control plan*, which includes specialized requirements, procedures, and training for staff members who are exposed to blood and OPIM.

Isolation and Quarantine

When transmission-based precautions are in place, a resident may be placed in **isolation**, which uses specific preventive measures to limit or eliminate the spread of microorganisms from an infected person to others. Isolation is different than quarantine. **Quarantine** is an action taken to separate and restrict the movement of people believed to be exposed to a communicable disease from others who have not been exposed. This is done to prevent spread.

Isolation protects both residents and healthcare staff, and isolation rooms are labeled with a sign on the door (**Figure 8.36**). Be sure the resident and the resident's family members understand why isolation and precautions are necessary and that the resident's rights are maintained, even during isolation.

Staff members entering an isolation room must wear masks, gowns, gloves, and any other required PPE. Because isolation requires the use of a mask, gown, and gloves, always check with the resident before leaving the room to determine if there is more you can do for him or her. This reduces the number of

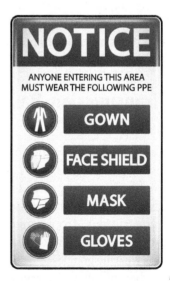

Idea.s/Shutterstock.com

Figure 8.36 Signs should mark isolation rooms and the type of isolation.

times you will have to reenter the room. Reentering the room requires masking, gowning, and gloving and increases the risk for cross-contamination.

Isolation includes additional guidelines for cleaning and disinfecting equipment and disposing of trash in proper waste containers. There are several categories of isolation, which depend on the disease's mode of transmission and isolation requirements:

1. **Strict isolation**: used to prevent the transmission of all highly communicable diseases spread by contact or through the air.

2. **Respiratory isolation**: used to prevent the transmission of microorganisms spread by droplets that may be sneezed out or breathed in; may use special ventilation (air flow) and filtration systems.

3. **Protective isolation**: used to protect people who are vulnerable to pathogenic microorganisms due to lowered immunity (for example, residents with leukemia and those receiving treatments that decrease resistance to disease).

Procedure

Transporting to and from Isolation

Rationale

There are times when transport is needed to or from an isolation room for diagnostic tests or procedures. Contact precautions should be followed during transport. Use of PPE is determined by facility policy, the type of isolation, and precautions.

Preparation

1. Ask the licensed nursing staff if there are doctor's orders for the procedure, if there are any specific instructions listed in the plan of care, and if the resident can be moved into the positions required for this procedure.
2. Notify the department that will receive the resident from isolation.
3. Wash your hands or use hand sanitizer to ensure infection control.
4. Put on PPE as required by the type of precautions in place.
5. The door will be closed, so knock before entering the room, letting the resident know you are entering.
6. Introduce yourself using your first or preferred name and title. Explain that you work with the licensed nursing staff and will be providing care.
7. Greet the resident and ask the resident to state his or her full name, if able. Then check the resident's identification bracelet.
8. Use Mr., Mrs., or Ms. and the resident's last name when conversing.
9. Explain the procedure in simple terms, even if the resident is not able to communicate or is disoriented. Ask permission to perform the procedure.

10. Bring the necessary equipment into the room. Place the following items in an easy-to-reach place:
    - transport vehicle, such as a wheelchair or stretcher
    - clean sheet(s)
    - bath blanket(s)
    - mask for the resident, if needed
11. Maintain safety by asking for assistance. If using a stretcher, ask another staff member to assist you.
12. Cover the stretcher or wheelchair with a clean sheet. Do not let the sheet touch the floor.

The Procedure

13. Provide privacy by closing the curtains, using a screen, or closing the door to the room.
14. Raise or lower the bed to the appropriate position for the transport vehicle. The bed should be in the low position for the wheelchair or should be raised to the height needed for a stretcher.
15. Lock the wheels on both the bed and the transport vehicle.
16. Maintain safety during the procedure. If there are side rails, raise and lock the rails on the opposite side of the bed from where you will be working. Lower the rail on the side where you are working.
17. Put a mask on the resident, if instructed and according to facility policy.
18. Help the resident into the wheelchair or onto the stretcher. Allow him or her to do as much as possible.
19. If using a wheelchair, wrap a sheet or bath blanket around the resident and then cover the resident with another sheet or bath blanket. Make sure the sheet or bath blanket does not touch the floor. If using a stretcher, cover the resident with a sheet or bath blanket.

(continued)

Transporting to and from Isolation *(continued)*

20. If appropriate to facility policy, the type of isolation, and precautions, remove your PPE and wash your hands or use hand sanitizer to ensure infection control.
21. Open the door, unlock the wheels of the transport vehicle, and move the resident out of the isolation unit.
22. To return the resident to isolation, place the wheelchair or stretcher near the door of the room. Put on PPE before entering the isolation room.
23. Enter the isolation room, lock the wheels, and unwrap the resident. Remove the resident's mask, if used.
24. Discard the mask in the biohazard waste container located in the room.
25. Check to be sure the bed wheels are locked, then assist the resident from the wheelchair or stretcher back to bed.
26. Reposition the resident and lower the bed.
27. Follow the plan of care to determine if the side rails should be raised or lowered.
28. Remove, clean, and store equipment in the proper location. Remove soiled linens and discard disposable equipment.

Follow-Up

29. Make sure the resident is comfortable and place the call light and personal items within reach.
30. Conduct a safety check before leaving the room. The room should be clean and free from clutter or spills.
31. Remove your PPE before leaving the room.
32. Wash your hands or use hand sanitizer before leaving the room.
33. Remove the transport vehicle from the isolation room. Clean and store the transport vehicle according to facility policy.

Reporting and Documentation

34. Report any specific observations, complications, or unusual responses to the licensed nursing staff. Document this information, along with the care provided, in the chart or EMR.

What Is an Exposure Control Plan?

OSHA guarantees the right to a safe workplace to all staff, and particularly to staff who may be exposed to contaminated blood or body fluids. Healthcare facilities must provide annual, cost-free training during work hours about the hazards, risks, and measures of protection related to exposure. Healthcare facilities must also provide all necessary equipment and a system for reporting exposure. If a healthcare staff member is exposed to blood or body fluids, he or she should follow the facility's *exposure control plan*. In addition, healthcare facilities must provide free hepatitis B vaccines and immediate, confidential medical evaluation and follow-up for anyone exposed to blood or body fluids.

Healthcare staff members also have responsibilities in preventing exposure. They must always follow standard precautions, be immunized against hepatitis B, report all exposures immediately, and follow recommended post-exposure treatment. Healthcare staff members should also support others who have been exposed and maintain their confidentiality.

A written exposure control plan should include:
- a list of all job positions at risk for exposure
- requirements for hepatitis B vaccination
- policies related to standard precautions, including hand hygiene practices and the use of PPE
- the number of people allowed in a resident's room
- safe management and disposal of sharps
- procedures for isolation and the management of isolation care
- hazard communication, including common and clear classifications of any chemicals used, hazard information on labels, and training
- procedures for transferring residents with suspected or confirmed infections to isolation rooms
- specific precautions to be taken before and during transfer to and from isolation
- procedures for cleaning and disinfecting contaminated equipment and surfaces
- waste-management procedures
- postexposure follow-up
- work practices that reduce or eliminate exposure to blood and OPIM (for example, not eating or drinking in potentially contaminated areas)

If exposure does occur, healthcare facility procedures must be followed. These procedures may include washing needlesticks or cuts with soap and water; flushing any splashes to the nose, mouth, or skin with water; washing the eyes with clean water, saline, or sterile solutions (**Figure 8.37**). You should also report the exposure incident immediately so that instructions for treatment (along with any possible risks) can be provided and started as soon as possible.

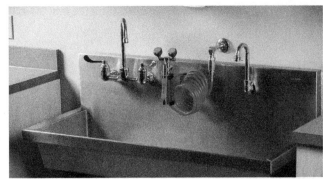

© Tori Soper Photography

Figure 8.37 An exposure control plan must include procedures for using emergency eye-wash equipment.

SECTION 8.2 **Review and Assessment**

Key Terms Mini Glossary

alcohol-based hand sanitizer a liquid, gel, or foam preparation containing alcohol; kills most bacteria and fungi and destroys some viruses found on the skin.

asepsis the absence of infection or infectious material; also called sterile.

epidermis the outermost layer of the skin; contains keratin and melanin.

excretions waste products expelled from the body.

friction the resistance between two objects or surfaces rubbing against each other.

isolation specific preventive measures that limit or eliminate the spread of pathogens from an infected person to others.

quarantine an action taken to separate and restrict exposed people from those who have not been exposed to prevent the spread of a communicable disease.

secretions substances produced and released by cells or organs.

sterile free of living microorganisms.

World Health Organization (WHO) an agency of the United Nations that focuses on international public health.

Apply the Key Terms

Identify the key term used in each sentence.

1. Mr. B was put in an isolation room to limit or eliminate the spread of pathogens from him to others.
2. A nursing assistant noticed that increased oral secretions were produced when she was feeding the resident she was caring for.
3. One way to carry out hand hygiene is to use alcohol-based hand sanitizer, which is a liquid, gel, or foam preparation containing alcohol that kills most bacteria and fungi and destroys some viruses found on the skin.
4. Feces are a waste product expelled from the body; also called excretion.
5. An important part of the procedure for hand hygiene is using friction to create resistance between the hands by rubbing them against each other.

Know and Understand the Facts

1. List three standard precautions.
2. Identify three transmission-based precautions.
3. Identify three actions that show proper respiratory hygiene and cough etiquette.
4. List four parts of an exposure control plan.

Analyze and Apply Concepts

1. List three situations when disposable, nonsterile gloves should be worn.
2. Explain the procedure for hand washing.
3. Describe the proper procedure for putting on and taking off a gown.

Think Critically

Read the following care situation. Then answer the questions that follow.

Keiko, a new nursing assistant, was asked to take care of Mr. D, a resident who is in isolation with hepatitis B. Mr. D has several decubitus ulcers (bedsores) that are draining. This is the first time Keiko is taking care of Mr. D.

1. What specific precautions are necessary when caring for Mr. D?
2. What PPE should Keiko wear?
3. To provide holistic care, what approach should Keiko take when she enters Mr. D's room?

Wound Care

Objectives

To achieve the objectives for this section, you must successfully:

- **describe** the characteristics of penetrating and nonpenetrating wounds.
- **explain** the steps in assisting with the changing of a nonsterile dressing.
- **identify** the requirements to maintain a sterile field.
- **list** the steps for putting on and removing sterile gloves.

Key Terms

Learn these key terms to better understand the information presented in the section.

abrasions
contusions
exudate
frostbite
lacerations

nonpenetrating wounds
penetrating wounds
sterile field
wound

Questions to Consider

- What types of wounds have you, a friend, or a family member had? Was the wound a result of an accident at home, in a car, or because of surgery?
- Did the wound bleed a lot or require stitches? How quickly did it heal?
- Did you get an infection with the wound? If so, how was the infection treated?

How Are Wounds Categorized?

A *wound* is an injury to body tissue that is caused by a cut, blow, or other force. There are two major categories of wounds: penetrating wounds and nonpenetrating wounds. *Penetrating wounds* are characterized by a break in the skin. *Nonpenetrating wounds* do not break through the skin.

Penetrating Wounds

Penetrating wounds break through the skin and are sometimes deep enough to cut through body tissues and organs. Some examples of penetrating wounds include:

- simple cuts that cause an opening in the skin and bleeding
- decubitus ulcers that wear through the skin's surface
- stab wounds from a sharp object, such as a knife or a needle
- gunshot wounds
- wounds from a surgical procedure

Nonpenetrating Wounds

Nonpenetrating wounds are caused by rubbing or friction on the surface of the skin. They do not break through the skin. These wounds include:

- *abrasions* that result from being hit by or falling against a blunt (unsharpened) object
- decubitus ulcers that do not penetrate the skin
- *lacerations*, or tear-like wounds that have ragged edges and may be caused by being cut with a sharp object
- *contusions*, or swollen bruises that are caused by broken blood vessels and may result from falling or being hit by a blunt object (**Figure 8.38**)
- concussions, which cause no visible external wounds to the skin, but cause internal damage to the brain and brain tissue

Other Types of Wounds

Other types of wounds include a bite or a sting from an insect or animal or *thermal wounds* from exposure to extreme temperatures. Examples of thermal wounds

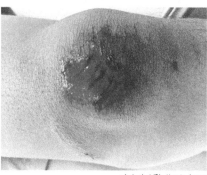
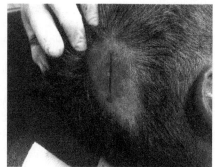
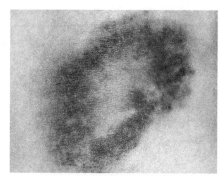

chatuphot/Shutterstock.com

Zetar Infinity/Shutterstock.com

Lukiyanova Natalia frenta/Shutterstock.com

A   **B**   **C**

Figure 8.38 Illustrated here are an abrasion (A), laceration (B), and contusion (C).

include sunburn, burns from a fire, and *frostbite* (a condition in which extreme cold temperatures cause freezing and damage to body tissues). *Chemical wounds* can result from breathing in or touching chemical substances, and can cause skin or lung damage (**Figure 8.39**). In *electrical wounds*, high-voltage electrical currents enter the body and cause serious internal damage, even if the skin only has a minor burn.

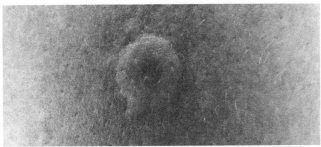

Linda Bestwick/Shutterstock.com

A

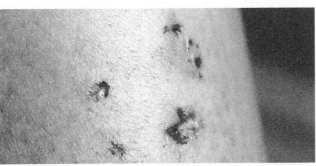

RapidEye/iStock/Getty Images Plus via Getty Images

B

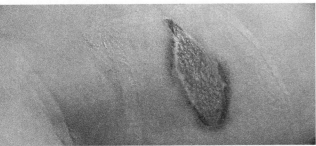

Anukool Manoton/Shutterstock.com

C

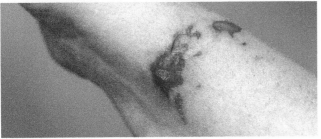

Rashid Valitov/Shutterstock.com

D

Figure 8.39 Illustrated here are a wasp sting (A), dog bite (B), thermal burn (C), and chemical burn (D).

What Should Be Observed and Reported about Wounds?

As a nursing assistant, you should be able to observe, report, and document the condition of a wound. For example, if the edges of the wound are red and swollen, this may be a sign of a possible infection. Also report and document the color, amount, and smell of drainage from a wound. Drainage that is thin, watery, and slightly yellow or colorless is called *clear* or *serous drainage*. Other types of drainage may be thin, watery, and slightly pink from blood. These types of drainage are usually considered normal early in the healing process.

Drainage of an abnormal color might be tinged (colored) with large amounts of blood (sanguinous) or be mostly blood. Another abnormal type of drainage is *purulent drainage*, which is filled with pus. Purulent drainage is typically gray, green, or yellow and is often thick in consistency. This type of drainage is usually a sign of an infection.

Some drainage is always expected during wound healing, and a small to moderate amount of drainage is usually normal. If drainage soaks a dressing, however, this needs to be reported immediately. The odor of a wound is usually not as important as the color and amount of drainage, though a very strong or foul (bad) odor might be an infection. Some wounds, particularly wounds from a surgery, will have a drain, or small tube, surgically inserted within or underneath the wound (**Figure 8.40**). The drain makes sure fluid can empty easily from the wound. You will learn more about how to report and document care in Chapter 13.

What Types of Dressings Are Commonly Used?

Many residents have wounds that are covered with dressings. Dressings are used to protect wounds, absorb drainage, and promote comfort and healing. Several factors help or hinder (prevent or slow) the wound healing process. These include the health and age of the resident, nutritional and respiratory status, medications, cultural and socioeconomic factors, and diseases. For example, residents with diabetes often have slower healing due to poor blood circulation.

The dressing material is selected based on what is needed for the wound to heal effectively. There are many kinds of dressing materials. Gauze dressings which come in different sizes (for example 2 inches by 2 inches; called *2×2s*) are used most often. Dressings

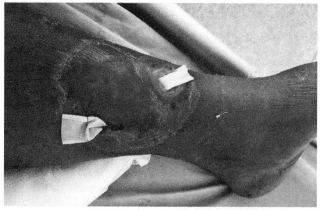

Tewan Banditrukkanka/Shutterstock.com

Figure 8.40 Drainage tubes help wounds drain and heal.

may also be made of other materials such as transparent adhesive film. Some dressings are held in place by bandages. For example, Montgomery ties or straps are often paired with adhesive tapes applied to either side of a wound (usually an abdominal wound). Montgomery ties or straps have perforated edges that do not require removal and reapplication of tape during every dressing change.

Dry dressings are applied in several layers to absorb drainage. Wet dressings are saturated with a prescribed solution to promote healing. They are usually covered with dry dressings. Dressings may be nonsterile or sterile.

Nonsterile Dressings

Nonsterile dressings protect open wounds from contamination and absorb *exudate,* or drainage. Nonsterile dressings are routinely changed and are changed more often if there are large amounts of drainage. Licensed nursing staff members may ask nursing assistants to assist with these dressing changes. This is an important responsibility. During dressing changes, hand hygiene and careful observation of the wound and drainage are very important.

Procedure

Assisting with Nonsterile Dressing Changes

Rationale

Using the correct procedure to assist with changing a nonsterile dressing will help prevent infection and promote healing.

Preparation

1. Ask the licensed nursing staff if there are doctor's orders for the procedure, if there are any specific instructions listed in the plan of care, and if the resident can be moved into the positions required for this procedure.
2. Wash your hands or use hand sanitizer before entering the room.
3. Knock before entering the room.
4. Introduce yourself using your first or preferred name and title. Explain that you work with the licensed nursing staff and will be providing care.
5. Greet the resident and ask the resident to state his or her full name, if able. Then check the resident's identification bracelet.
6. Use Mr., Mrs., or Ms. and the resident's last name when conversing.
7. Explain the procedure in simple terms, even if the resident is not able to communicate or is disoriented. Ask permission to perform the procedure.

8. Bring the necessary equipment into the room. Place the following items in an easy-to-reach place:
   - at least four pairs of disposable gloves
   - PPE, as needed
   - tape or Montgomery straps
   - dressing supplies or a dressing changing kit used in the facility, as directed by the licensed nursing staff (**Figure 8.41**)

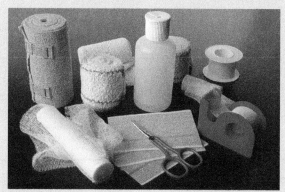

Figure 8.41   *thodonal88/Shutterstock.com*

   - saline solution or cleaning solution, as directed by the licensed nursing staff
   - tape-adhesive remover
   - plastic bag or a biohazard waste bag, if needed
   - bath blanket
   - disposable protective pad
   - waterproof drape

> **Best Practice:** Arrange your equipment on the overbed table so you do not have to reach over or turn your back on your work area.

The Procedure

9. Provide privacy by closing the curtains, using a screen, or closing the door to the room.
10. Lock the bed wheels and then raise the bed to hip level.
11. Maintain safety during the procedure. If there are side rails, raise and lock the rails on the opposite side of the bed from where you will be working. Lower the rail on the side where you are working.
12. Assist the resident into a comfortable position.
13. Place a bath blanket over the top linens. Then fanfold the linens (fold them back on themselves) underneath to prevent exposing the resident.
14. Expose only the affected body part and place the waterproof drape (if available) around it. If a waterproof drape is not available, use a disposable protective pad.
15. Make a cuff at the top of the plastic bag and place it within reach.
16. Wash your hands or use hand sanitizer to ensure infection control.
17. Put on disposable gloves and PPE, as required.
18. Remove tape or Montgomery straps to expose the existing dressing.
19. If needed, wet a 4×4 dressing with tape-adhesive remover and clean around the tape for easier removal. Always wipe away from the dressing.
20. Remove each layer of the existing dressing, starting with the top dressing. A licensed nursing staff member may also perform this task. Place the used dressings in the plastic bag.

> **Best Practice:** Avoid allowing the resident to see the soiled side of the dressing, as this may make him or her feel uncomfortable.

21. Very gently remove the dressing that covers the wound. A licensed nursing staff member may also perform this task. If the dressing sticks to the wound or to the drain site, moisten the dressing with saline before removing it. Place the used dressing in the plastic bag.
22. Observe the wound, wound drainage, and the drain site. A licensed nursing staff member will likely inspect the wound.
23. Remove your gloves and place them in the plastic bag.
24. Wash your hands or use hand sanitizer to ensure infection control.
25. Put on a new pair of disposable gloves.

26. Open new dressings and cut the length of tape needed.
27. Clean the wound with saline or another solution, as directed by the licensed nursing staff. Start cleaning at the top of the wound and work your way down to the bottom. Clean by stroking out and away from the wound toward the surrounding skin. Use a new piece of gauze for each stroke. Place soiled gauze in the plastic bag.
28. Apply clean dressings as directed by the licensed nursing staff. Do not touch the side of the dressing that will cover the wound.
29. Secure the dressings in place using tape or Montgomery straps. Nonallergenic tape is available if the resident has an allergy.
30. Remove your gloves and place them in the plastic bag.
31. Wash your hands or use hand sanitizer to ensure infection control.
32. Put on a new pair of disposable gloves.
33. Cover the resident with the top linens and remove the bath blanket by rolling it up, with the resident side facing inward, underneath the top linens.
34. Discard used supplies in the plastic bag. Ask the licensed nursing staff member if he or she would like to see the soiled dressing. Tie the plastic bag and discard it according to facility policy.
35. Remove and discard your gloves.
36. Wash your hands or use hand sanitizer to ensure infection control.
37. Put on a new pair of disposable gloves.
38. Check to be sure the bed wheels are locked, then reposition the resident and lower the bed.
39. Follow the plan of care to determine if the side rails should be raised or lowered.
40. Remove, clean, and store equipment in the proper location. Remove soiled linens and discard disposable equipment.

Follow-Up

41. Remove and discard your gloves.
42. Wash your hands to ensure infection control.
43. Make sure the resident is comfortable and place the call light and personal items within reach.
44. Conduct a safety check before leaving the room. The room should be clean and free from clutter or spills.
45. Wash your hands or use hand sanitizer before leaving the room.

Reporting and Documentation

46. Report any specific observations, complications, or unusual responses to the licensed nursing staff. Document this information, along with the care provided, in the chart or EMR.

Sterile Dressings

Sterile dressings are applied in a sterile field. A *sterile field* is an area that is free from living microorganisms. A sterile field may also be required for changing the dressing of a wound with microorganisms or for performing specific procedures. Only equipment and supplies that have been sterilized can be placed or used in a sterile field, such as sterile gloves and drapes for an examination.

As a nursing assistant, you may be asked to wear sterile gloves to help maintain a sterile field or assist with sterile procedures or dressing changes.

Procedure

Putting On and Removing Sterile Gloves

Rationale

Only sterile items can touch other sterile items. Therefore, sterile gloves must be worn when performing any sterile procedure. Any time a sterile item or the sterile field has been contaminated, the contaminated item must be removed and the procedure started over with sterile supplies.

Preparation

1. Locate a package of sterile gloves in the correct size. Sterile gloves should have both an outer and inner package. Check that the gloves have not expired. Inspect the package to be sure it is dry and free from tears, holes, punctures, or water stains.
2. Arrange the area in which you will be putting on the sterile gloves. Be sure you have enough room to maintain a sterile field.
3. Prepare the work surface so it is at waist level and within your sight.
4. Clean and dry the work surface.

   > **Best Practice:** Do not turn your back on the sterile field or leave the sterile field unattended. Do not cough, sneeze, talk, or laugh during this procedure. Airborne microorganisms can contaminate sterile items or the sterile field.

5. Wash your hands or use hand sanitizer to ensure infection control.
6. If a gown is required, put the gown on before putting on the gloves.

The Procedure: Putting On Sterile Gloves

7. Open the outer package of the gloves by grasping and gently peeling back the flaps.
8. Remove the inner package. Place it on the work surface.

9. Read the manufacturer's instructions on the inner package. The package should be labeled with directional terms such as *right*, *left*, *up*, and *down*.
10. Arrange the inner package on the work surface so that the right glove lies near your right hand and the left glove lies near your left hand. The cuffs of the gloves should lie near you, and the fingers of the gloves should point away from you.
11. Using the thumb and index finger of each hand, grasp the folded edges of the inner package.
12. Fold back the inner package to expose the gloves (**Figure 8.42**).

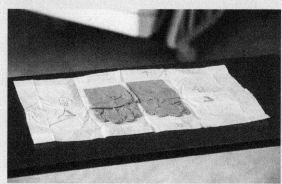

Figure 8.42   © Tori Soper Photography

> **Best Practice:** The inside of the sterile package is a sterile field. Do not touch or otherwise contaminate the inside of the package or the gloves.

13. Each glove has a cuff about 2–3 inches wide. The cuffs and insides of the gloves are *not* considered sterile.
14. Pick up one glove at the cuff with your thumb, index finger, and middle finger. If you are right-handed, put on the right glove first. If you are left-handed, put on the left glove first. Always pick up a glove with the opposite hand.
15. Turn your hand so that the palm side of the glove faces up. Lift the cuff up and slide your fingers and hand into the glove (**Figure 8.43**).

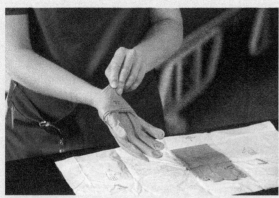

Figure 8.43   © Tori Soper Photography

16. Pull the glove up over your hand. If some of your fingers get stuck, leave them that way until you put on the other glove. Do not use your ungloved hand to straighten the glove.

   Best Practice: Do not let the outside of the glove touch any nonsterile surface.

17. Leave the cuff turned down on the second glove.

18. Reach under the cuff of the second glove using the four fingers of your gloved hand (**Figure 8.44**). Be careful not to contaminate your thumb.

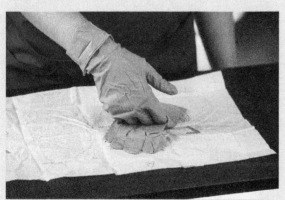

Figure 8.44   © Tori Soper Photography

19. With your fingers under the cuff, put on the second glove. Your gloved hand should not touch the cuff itself or any surface.

20. Adjust each glove for comfort with the opposite hand.

21. Slide your fingers under the cuffs to pull them up.

22. Touch only sterile items while wearing sterile gloves.

   Best Practice: Keep your gloved hands and the sterile field above your waist. To avoid possible contamination, interlace your fingers away from your scrubs while waiting for the procedure.

The Procedure: Removing Sterile Gloves

23. Grasp one gloved hand just below the cuff with the gloved fingers of your other hand.

24. Pull the cuff of the glove down, drawing it over your hand and turning it inside out.

25. Pull the glove off your hand and hold it in the palm of your other, gloved hand.

26. Insert your ungloved fingers under the cuff of the remaining glove.

27. Slowly pull the glove off, turning it inside out and drawing it over the first glove.

28. Drop both gloves into the appropriate waste container.

   Best Practice: Never reuse sterile gloves.

Follow-Up

29. Wash your hands to ensure infection control.

Reporting and Documentation

This is an accepted, standard procedure. It does not need to be reported or documented.

SECTION 8.3 **Review and Assessment**

Key Terms Mini Glossary

abrasions scraping of the outer layer of skin.

contusions bruises caused by damaged or broken blood vessels; may cause swelling.

exudate a liquid or semisolid discharge from body tissues or a blood vessel; drains from a wound and is caused by tissue damage.

frostbite a condition in which extremely cold temperatures cause freezing and damage to body tissues, such as the skin on the fingers, toes, nose, ears, cheeks, and chin.

lacerations wounds that tear body tissue and result in ragged edges.

nonpenetrating wounds wounds that do not enter into or through the skin; are caused by rubbing or friction on the surface of the skin.

penetrating wounds wounds that enter into or through the skin.

sterile field an area that is free from living pathogenic microorganisms.

wound an injury to body tissue; can be caused by a cut, blow, or other force.

Apply the Key Terms

Think about the definitions of the following key terms. Describe one difference between each pair of key terms.

1. contusions and lacerations
2. wound and exudate
3. nonpenetrating wounds and lacerations
4. frostbite and contusion
5. penetrating wound and sterile field

Know and Understand the Facts

1. What is the difference between a penetrating and nonpenetrating wound? Give two examples of each.
2. Name two types of wounds that are not penetrating, or nonpentrating.
3. What are three things that should be observed, reported, and documented about wound drainage?
4. List three ways a sterile field can be maintained when putting on sterile gloves.

Analyze and Apply Concepts

1. List the steps for changing a nonsterile dressing.
2. Describe the type of wound drainage that may be a sign of the presence of an infection.
3. What should be done if a sterile field becomes contaminated?
4. Explain the correct procedure for putting on and removing sterile gloves.

Think Critically

Read the following care situation. Then answer the questions that follow.

Mr. Y was admitted to a skilled care facility with a large wound on his left arm. He is Asian-American, 78 years old, and frail. He has had this wound on and off for the past year, and his doctor feels that regular, supervised dressing changes will improve healing. Amelia, a nursing assistant, is assigned to Mr. Y's care. When Amelia enters Mr. Y's room, she observes that Mr. Y is holding his arm close and breathing quickly. When Amelia asks if Mr. Y is in pain, he smiles and says, "No." Amelia is assigned to change Mr. Y's first nonsterile dressing.

1. What should Amelia do to follow up on her observations about Mr. Y's pain prior to the dressing change?
2. Should Amelia change the dressing even if she believes Mr. Y is in pain? Explain your answer.
3. What questions should Amelia ask the licensed nursing staff about Mr. Y's wound before changing the dressing?
4. Describe how Amelia should clean the wound during the dressing change.

Key Points

Reviewing the key points for this chapter will help you practice more safely and competently as a holistic nursing assistant and will help you prepare for the certification competency examination.

- Antibodies fight infection by identifying and destroying foreign substances (antigens and toxins) through a process called *phagocytosis*.
- Microorganisms that can cause disease are called *pathogens*. There are four types of pathogens: bacteria, viruses, fungi, and parasites.
- Infections can be local, systemic, or opportunistic. Healthcare-associated infections (HAIs) may happen as result of a person's stay in a healthcare facility.
- The chain of infection includes six links: an infectious agent, reservoir, portal of exit, means of transmission, portal of entry, and susceptible host.
- Asepsis, or the absence of microorganisms, is important for preventing the spread of infection.
- Standard precautions and transmission-based precautions prevent and control infection.
- Dressings may be wet or dry, sterile or nonsterile.

Action Steps to Holistic Care

Review the information in this chapter. Complete the following activities.

1. With a partner, practice the procedures for donning and doffing personal protective equipment (PPE). Use disposable gloves, a gown, face mask and goggles. Take turns practicing the procedures and evaluating each other's performance. Observe for any steps in the procedures that your partner performed incorrectly or forgot. Afterwards, review the procedures to identify any steps you may have performed inaccurately or forgotten.
2. With a partner, prepare a poster about taking care of a resident in isolation. Include infection control, transmission-based precautions, and supportive approaches and actions.
3. With a partner, prepare a poster discussing one category of infection, including a specific example and its location. Also include the signs and symptoms and possible treatment.
4. Research current scientific information about vaccinations. Write a brief report describing three current facts about vaccinations not covered in this chapter.

Building Math Skill

Jamie, a new nursing assistant, is asked to change Mrs. S's dressing. This is his second time doing a dressing change. You remind him that he will need to use appropriate hand hygiene throughout the procedure, and that he will be putting on new and taking off used pairs of disposable gloves multiple times during the dressing change: putting on a pair of new gloves when starting the procedure, taking off the pair of soiled gloves after removing the current dressing, putting on a new pair of gloves to put on the new dressing, taking off the pair of gloves after completing the new dressing change, and putting on a new pair of gloves to clean up after the dressing change. How many pairs of new disposable gloves should he have in Mrs. S's room for his use during the procedure?

Preparing for the Certification Competency Examination

To prepare for the nursing assistant certification competency examination, you will need to know content found in this chapter. This content may be tested in the knowledge (written or oral) and skills (hands-on demonstration) portions of the exam. The following areas will be emphasized:

- types of microorganisms
- the immune response, immunity, and vaccination
- people at risk for infection and the infectious process
- chain of infection and modes and methods of transmission
- signs and symptoms of infection
- bloodborne pathogens and healthcare-associated and nosocomial infections
- standard precautions, including hand hygiene and PPE
- transmission-based precautions and bloodborne pathogen standards
- respiratory hygiene and cough etiquette
- sterile dressings and maintenance of sterile fields
- procedure for putting on and removing sterile gloves
- exposure control plan and reporting

These sample test questions are similar to ones you will find on the certification competency exam. See how well you can answer them. Be sure to select the *best* answer.

(Continued)

1. Which of the following is a microorganism that causes infection?
   A. culture
   B. chlorophyll
   C. pus
   D. pathogen

2. Which of the following are links in the chain of infection?
   A. host and parasite
   B. reservoir and source
   C. portal of exit and portal of entry
   D. transmission and virus

3. Standard precautions include which of the following?
   A. isolation techniques
   B. the use of sterile gloves
   C. cleansing draining wounds
   D. proper hand washing

4. Which of the following people are most at risk for getting an infection?
   A. Janie, 16 years old
   B. Mrs. F, 85 years old
   C. Lester, 8 years old
   D. Ms. W, 45 years old

5. When nursing assistants are exposed to a blood spill or splash, what is the first thing they should do?
   A. put on a pair of new gloves and a mask
   B. follow the healthcare facility's exposure control plan
   C. keep working until finished and then tell a member of the licensed nursing staff
   D. wipe off the blood with a sterile dressing

6. Transmission-based precautions include
   A. infection precautions
   B. pathogen precautions
   C. contact precautions
   D. respiratory precautions

7. When a body part is warm to the touch, red, swollen, and has pus, these are signs of a(n)
   A. systemic infection
   B. regional infection
   C. local infection
   D. area infection

8. Which type of microorganism most commonly causes infection?
   A. fungus
   B. microbe
   C. virus
   D. bacterium

9. A nursing assistant is helping care for a resident when she observes that a blood-soaked dressing has fallen onto the bed linens. This resident has hepatitis. The nursing assistant tells the licensed nursing staff member about the fallen item. She has just prevented a possible infection from
   A. fungal pathogens
   B. bloodborne pathogens
   C. normal flora
   D. protozoan pathogens

10. During vaccination, people are injected with a(n)
    A. biological preparation of an antigen that has been weakened or killed
    B. antibiotic that will kill antigens in the body
    C. antiviral medication that will decrease the toxicity of the host
    D. microscopic preparation of an antibody that is ready to kill an antigen

11. Which of the following *best* shows the presence of inflammation?
    A. There are visible sores and swelling.
    B. There is pus, the area is cool to the touch, and the patient is feverish.
    C. The area is swollen, cool to the touch, and red.
    D. The area is swollen, warm to the touch, and red.

12. Hand hygiene must be used
    A. before handling a meal tray
    B. after charting
    C. before going to a meeting
    D. after eating a meal

13. Ms. N has an infection. In the chain of infection, she is which link?
    A. reservoir
    B. susceptible host
    C. portal of exit
    D. portal of entry

14. A resident has a wound that is swollen and bruised. What is this called?
    A. laceration
    B. contusion
    C. concussion
    D. abrasion

15. Which of the following is a guideline for proper hand hygiene?
    A. use a hand sanitizer for at least 20 seconds
    B. dry your hands thoroughly after turning off the faucet
    C. wash your hands for at least 10 seconds
    D. use only very hot water and alcohol-based soap

Did you have difficulty with any of the questions? If you did, review the chapter to find the correct answer(s).

9 The Body's Anatomy and Physiology

Welcome to the Chapter

When providing care as a holistic nursing assistant, you will need to understand the structure of the healthy human body and the way the human body functions at its highest level. This knowledge is important because many of the procedures you will perform affect the body in different ways. This chapter covers the structure of the body, from microscopic cells to the structure and function of the 12 body systems. You will learn not only how the body systems work, but also how they are affected by lifestyle choices and aging. You will also learn the importance of medical terminology, the structure of medical terms, and medical terms related to specific body structures and functions.

What you learn in this chapter will help you develop your knowledge and skills to become a holistic nursing assistant. The topics discussed in the chapter are highlighted on the Providing Holistic Care Framework.

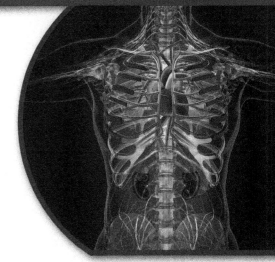
Yevhen Vitte/Shutterstock.com

Chapter Outline

Section 9.1
Medical Terminology and Body Structures

Section 9.2
Body Systems

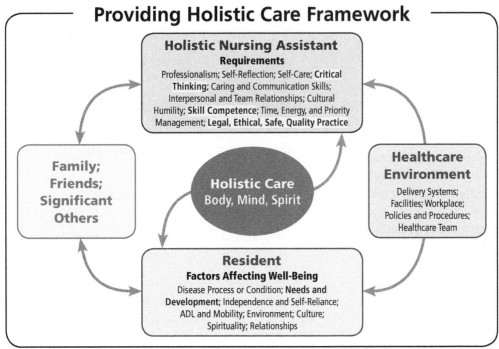

Providing Holistic Care Framework

Holistic Nursing Assistant
Requirements
Professionalism; Self-Reflection; Self-Care; **Critical Thinking;** Caring and Communication Skills; Interpersonal and Team Relationships; Cultural Humility; **Skill Competence;** Time, Energy, and Priority Management; **Legal, Ethical, Safe, Quality Practice**

Family; Friends; Significant Others

Holistic Care
Body, Mind, Spirit

Healthcare Environment
Delivery Systems; Facilities; Workplace; Policies and Procedures; Healthcare Team

Resident
Factors Affecting Well-Being
Disease Process or Condition; **Needs and Development;** Independence and Self-Reliance; ADL and Mobility; Environment; Culture; Spirituality; Relationships

Goodheart-Willcox Publisher

Medical Terminology and Body Structures

Objectives

To achieve the objectives for this section, you must successfully:

- **form** medical terms using root words, combining vowels, combining forms, prefixes, and suffixes.
- **recognize** medical abbreviations.
- **identify** the medical terminology used to describe body positions, directions, cavities, and movements.
- **explain** cell structure and function.
- **describe** the four types of body tissues, the body membranes, and the actions of these structures.

Key Terms

Learn these key terms to better understand the information presented in the section.

acronyms	neurons
atrophy	nutrients
body cavities	organs
Fowler's position	prone position
lateral position	supine position
medical terminology	tumors
membranes	

Questions to Consider

- Think about your body and about how it looks and functions. You might want to view yourself in a mirror as you are doing this. In what ways is your body similar to the bodies of others?
- What about your body is different from others' bodies? Why do you think these similarities and differences exist?

What Is Medical Terminology?

Medical terminology is the language of medicine. It is a standard way to communicate the structure, processes, functions, diseases, and conditions of the human body. You will use medical terminology every day as a holistic nursing assistant. Correct pronunciation and spelling are very important when providing and documenting care and when communicating with others in the healthcare facility.

Learning medical terminology requires more than recognizing medical terms. You must also learn to use medical word parts to build new terms. A strong understanding of medical word parts will let you to break down unfamiliar terms and learn their meanings.

Medical Word Parts

Five word parts can be used to form a medical term:

- **Root word:** usually derived from Greek or Latin, it is always part of a medical term. The root word never stands on its own.
- **Combining vowel:** a vowel (*a, e, i, o,* or *u*) attached to the end of the root word that links word parts for easier pronunciation. A combining vowel is *not* used between a root word and a suffix when the suffix begins with a vowel.
- **Combining form:** the root word plus its combining vowel. For example, the root word *cardi* and the combining vowel *o* make the combining form *cardi/o.*
- **Prefix:** attached to the beginning of a root word, prefixes usually identify a location, time, or number.
- **Suffix:** attached to the end of a root word, suffixes usually identify a condition, disease, diagnosis, surgical procedure, or therapy.

The Structure of Medical Terms

You can form many different medical terms using just one root word and various combining forms, prefixes, and suffixes. For example, the following medical terms use the root words *cardi* and *card*:

P = Prefix
RW = Root Word
S = Suffix
CV = Combining Vowel

tachy- / card / -ia = fast heart rate
P + RW + S

cardi / o / -pathy = heart disease
RW + CV + S

cardi / -ac = pertaining to the heart
RW + S

cardi / o / -logy = study of the heart
RW + CV + S

peri- / card / -itis = inflammation of the lining
P + RW + S   around the heart

As with most English words, many medical terms can be made plural by adding an *-s* or *-es*. There are different rules for creating plural forms for terms that come from Greek or Latin. For example, the singular term *bronchus* becomes *bronchi* when plural. In the same way, the term *diagnosis* becomes *diagnoses* when plural.

In Appendix A, you will find a glossary of common combining forms, prefixes, and suffixes. Studying these word parts will help you begin to form medical terms and start using medical terminology. This resource will also help you prepare for the certification competency exam and begin working as a holistic nursing assistant.

Medical Abbreviations

Medical terminology includes *abbreviations*, which are used to speed up communication in healthcare facilities. Abbreviations are usually short combinations of letters used to represent longer words. For example, the abbreviation *AM* stands for "morning," and the single letter *q* represents the word *every*. Medical terminology also uses ***acronyms***, which are formed from the first letters or groups of letters in a phrase. An example of an acronym is *BP* for "blood pressure."

Figure 9.1 lists many of the common abbreviations and acronyms you will hear, read, and use when working as a nursing assistant. Other abbreviations and acronyms are also included throughout this textbook. Abbreviations for common diseases and conditions are discussed in Chapter 10.

How Is the Human Body Described?

Many terms are used to describe the body positions, directions, and movements. You will not be able to provide safe, quality care if you do not understand these terms.

Medical Abbreviations and Acronyms

Abbreviation or Acronym	Meaning	Abbreviation or Acronym	Meaning	Abbreviation or Acronym	Meaning
ABC	airway, breathing, circulation	BLS	basic life support	COPD	chronic obstructive pulmonary disease
abd	abdomen	BM	bowel movement	CPR	cardiopulmonary resuscitation
ac; a.c.	before meals	BMR	basic metabolic rate	CSF	cerebrospinal fluid
ACLS	advanced cardiac life support	BP; B/P	blood pressure	CT Scan	computerized axial tomography scan
Ad Lib	as desired	bpm	beats per minute	CVA	cerebrovascular accident (stroke)
ADLs	activities of daily living	BRP	bathroom privileges	D/C	discontinue
ADM	admission	BS	breath sounds	DNR	do not resuscitate
AM	in the morning	c̄	with	DOA	dead on arrival
AMA; a.m.a.	against medical advice	cap	capsule	DOB	date of birth
Amb	ambulatory	CATH	catheter	Dx	diagnosis
AMT	amount	CBC	complete blood count	ED	emergency department
AS	left ear	CHF	congestive heart failure	EKG; ECG	electrocardiogram
AU	each ear	CNS	central nervous system	ENT	ear, nose, throat
BID; b.i.d.	twice a day	c/o	complains of	ER	emergency room

(continued)

Goodheart-Willcox Publisher

Figure 9.1 Different healthcare facilities use different abbreviations. Always check a healthcare facility's policies and procedures to learn about which abbreviations are used.

Abbreviation or Acronym	Meaning	Abbreviation or Acronym	Meaning	Abbreviation or Acronym	Meaning
FB	foreign body	NG; ng	nasogastric	R	respiration
FH	family history	NKA	no known allergies	R/O	rule out
Fx	fracture	NPO; n.p.o.	nothing by mouth	ROM	range of motion
GB	gallbladder	N/V	nausea, vomiting	Rx	prescribed medication; treatment
GI	gastrointestinal	OD	right eye; overdose	s̄	without
GTT; gtt	drops	OP	outpatient	SOB	shortness of breath
Hgb; hgb	hemoglobin	OR	operating room	S/S	signs and symptoms
H&P	history and physical	OS	left eye	STAT	immediately
hs	hour of sleep; bedtime	OTC	over the counter	Sx	symptom
Hx; hx	history	OU	both eyes	T	temperature
IM	intramuscular	P	pulse	Tab	tablet
I&O	intake and output	p.c.; pc	after meals	TID; t.i.d.	three times a day
IV	intravenous	PO; po; p.o.	by mouth	TPR	temperature, pulse, respiration
LOC	level of consciousness	P/O; postop	postoperative	Tx	treatment
mg	milligrams	preop	before surgery	UA	urinalysis
MRI	magnetic resonance imaging	PRN; p.r.n.	as needed	VS	vital signs
MRSA	methicillin-resistant *Staphylococcus aureus*	q	every	wt	weight
NEG	negative	QID; q.i.d.	four times a day		

Goodheart-Willcox Publisher

Figure 9.1 *(Continued)*

Body Positions

As a nursing assistant, you will be asked to place residents into different body positions for a variety of reasons, including examinations, treatments, and assistance with ADLs. For example, you might place a resident into Fowler's position if the resident is eating a meal in bed or if you are performing oral care.

The most common body positions you will be asked to do as a nursing assistant are Fowler's position, lateral position, prone position, and supine position (**Figure 9.2**):

- *Fowler's position*: the person is seated in bed, and the backrest of the bed is at a 45° angle; the legs are extended flat.
- *Lateral position*: the person lies on his or her side with arms free and knees slightly bent.
- *Prone position*: the person lies on his or her abdomen with arms and hands at each side, feet comfortably positioned, and head turned to the side.
- *Supine position*: the person lies flat on his or her back with the arms at each side.

Other positions will be discussed in later chapters of this textbook.

Directional Terms

Specific anatomic directional terms describe different body and body part positions and their locations

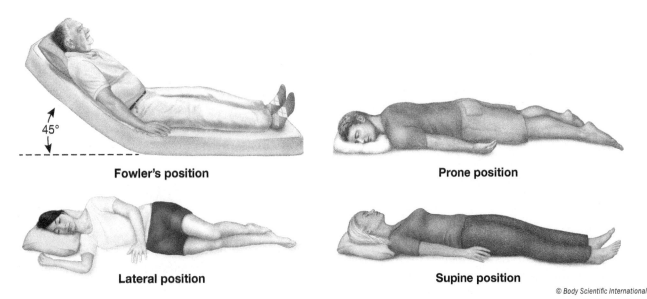

Fowler's position

Prone position

Lateral position

Supine position

© Body Scientific International

Figure 9.2 These are the four most common body positions used. Pillows provide comfort and support.

(**Figure 9.3**). Healthcare providers, such as doctors, often write orders or give instructions using these terms. Holistic nursing assistants must also perform procedures following directions that use these terms. For example, a doctor's order might ask that you place a warm compress on a resident's knee, which is on the *anterior* or ventral side of the body. A licensed nursing staff member might also direct you to look at a dressing located on a resident's back, which is on the *posterior* or dorsal side of the body.

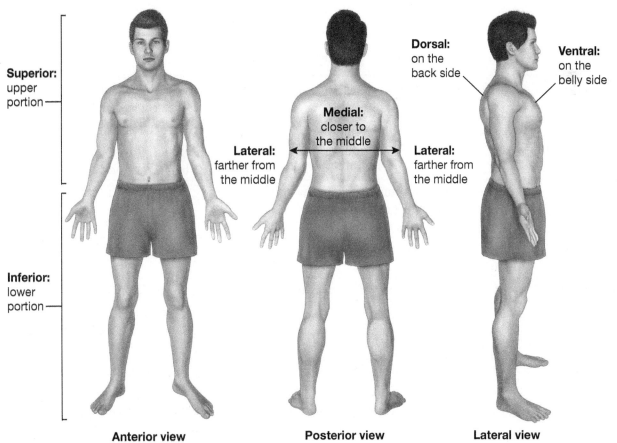

Superior: upper portion

Inferior: lower portion

Lateral: farther from the middle

Medial: closer to the middle

Lateral: farther from the middle

Dorsal: on the back side

Ventral: on the belly side

Anterior view

Posterior view

Lateral view

© Body Scientific International

Figure 9.3 These directional terms help describe locations on the body.

CULTURE CUES

Perceptions of the Body

People have a variety of their own perceptions about their body and its functions. These perceptions are influenced by culture, family values about health and wellness, and experiences with health and body functions. For instance, if someone comes from a culture in which talking about a particular body function is not acceptable, that person may not communicate the necessary information to healthcare providers.

Apply It

1. What two perceptions do you have about your health and body functions? How have these perceptions affected your health and wellness?
2. How could you, as a holistic nursing assistant, learn about residents' perceptions about their body functions?

Body Cavities

The human body is divided into *body cavities*, which are spaces in the body that contain organs. *Organs* are made up of groups of tissues that have specific structures and functions, which you will learn more about later in this chapter.

- **Cranial cavity**: contains the brain (cerebrum), and its blood vessels and nerves
- **Spinal cavity**: contains the spinal cord, spinal column, and vertebrae
- **Thoracic cavity**: contains the lungs, heart, trachea, pharynx, larynx, and bronchial tubes

- **Abdominal cavity**: contains the liver, gallbladder, stomach, pancreas, intestines, spleen, and kidneys
- **Pelvic cavity**: contains the sigmoid colon, rectum, anus, urinary bladder, urethra, ureters, and male and female reproductive organs

Body Movements

Medical terms are also used to describe body movements (**Figure 9.4**). You will see terms related to movement when you provide active and passive range-of-motion (ROM) exercises for residents' joints and limbs.

Body Movements

Movement	Description	Example
flexion	the act of bending a joint	bending the arm at the elbow
extension	the act of straightening a joint	straightening the arm at the elbow
hyperextension	an exaggerated, or extreme, extension	moving the arm from the side so that it extends behind the body
abduction	lateral (sideways) movement away from the midline (an invisible line running vertically through the body)	moving the leg away from the body
adduction	lateral movement toward the midline of the body	moving the leg toward the body
rotation	turning of a body part around an axis, or fixed point	rotating the ankle outward so that the foot moves away from the body
circumduction	rotating a body part in a complete circle	moving the pointer finger in a circular motion
supination	rotating a body part away from the body	rotating the forearm so that the palm faces upward
pronation	rotating a body part toward the body	rotating the forearm so that the palm faces downward

Goodheart-Willcox Publisher

Figure 9.4 Review the terms used, descriptions, and examples for body movement.

What Roles Do Cells, Tissues, and Membranes Play in Body Structure?

Three important internal structures are the basis of life in the human body: cells, tissues, and membranes. Tissues and membranes are made up of groups of cells with similar structures and functions.

Cells

The cell is the structural and functional unit of the human body. There are about 37 trillion cells in the human body and between 200 and 300 different types of cells.

Even though cells have different functions, most cells contain the same basic structures, which are called *organelles* (**Figure 9.5**). The *nucleus* directs all cell activities and is found in every type of cell except mature red blood cells. The outer layer of the cell, called the *cell membrane*, decides what can and cannot enter and exit the cell. Inside the cell, the *cytoplasm* is a jelly-like substance that includes all of the organelles. *Ribosomes* build the proteins the cell needs, while *mitochondria* create the energy the cell needs.

Mature cells exist in bone, muscle, and blood. Mature cells come in a variety of different shapes—from long, thin cells to cells shaped like round discs. All cells can maintain their shape, reproduce by dividing and multiplying, use oxygen and **nutrients** (substances needed for normal body function), produce energy, and eliminate waste. Cells can also:

- *atrophy*, or shrink or decrease in size
- enlarge due to an increase in proteins in the cell membrane (called *hypertrophy*)

- increase rates of cell division, causing more cells to reproduce often to make up for loss of cells (called *hyperplasia*)
- become abnormal in their sizes, shapes, or organization (called *dysplasia*)
- grow into unusual shapes, called **tumors** or neoplasms

When examined, the cells in a tumor may be *benign*, or normal. The cells in a tumor may also be *malignant*, or abnormal with growth that is out of control

Tissues

As you learned in Chapter 8, tissues are groups of similar cells that perform a common function. There are four types of tissue, and each performs unique functions:

- **Connective tissue:** connects or supports body tissues, structures, and organs, providing strength and flexibility. Cartilage, bone, and blood are all types of connective tissue.
- **Epithelial tissue:** provides a covering for external body parts and lines internal organs. Epithelial tissue can be found in the skin and also in the intestines.
- **Muscle tissue:** contracts, or shortens, to produce movement. There are three types of muscle tissue: *skeletal*, *smooth*, and *cardiac*.
- **Nerve tissue:** composed of nerve cells, called **neurons**. Neurons carry electrochemical messages to and from various parts of the body to produce sensation (feeling), movement, and mental activity.

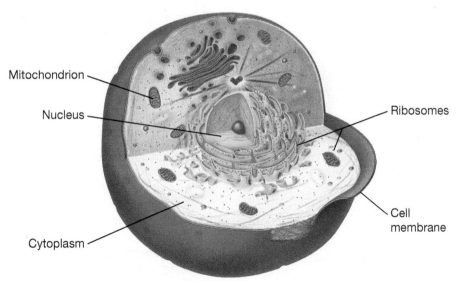

Mitochondrion

Nucleus

Ribosomes

Cell membrane

Cytoplasm

© Body Scientific International

Figure 9.5 These are the basic structures of a human cell.

Membranes

Body *membranes* are thin, soft, and flexible structures that support and protect body surfaces, organs, and joints. The major categories of body membranes are epithelial and connective. *Epithelial membranes* coat and protect the surfaces of the body and internal organs. There are three types of epithelial membranes: cutaneous membranes (skin), mucous membranes (can be found in the nose), and serous membranes (cover the heart and lung muscles). Connective tissue membranes prevent friction and help joints move, and cover and protect the brain and spinal cord.

SECTION 9.1 Review and Assessment

Key Terms Mini Glossary

acronyms words formed from the first letters or groups of letters in a phrase.

atrophy to shrink or decrease in size.

body cavities spaces in the human body that contain organs.

Fowler's position a body position in which a resident lies with legs extended on an examining table or bed; the head of the bed is raised to a 45° angle.

lateral position a body position in which a resident lies on his or her side with arms free and knees slightly bent.

medical terminology the standard way to communicate structure, processes, functions, diseases, and conditions of the human body; the language used in healthcare.

membranes thin, soft, flexible structures that cover, line, or act as boundaries for cells or organs.

neurons cells of the nervous system that transmit information throughout the body in the form of electrochemical messages (neural impulses); each neuron is composed of a cell body, dendrites, and axons.

nutrients substances the body needs to function normally; include water, protein, carbohydrates, fats, minerals, and vitamins.

organs collections of tissues that have specific structures and functions.

prone position a body position in which a resident lies on his or her abdomen with arms and hands at each side, feet comfortably positioned, and head turned to the side.

supine position a body position in which a resident lies flat on his or her back with the arms at each side.

tumor an abnormal growth of tissue that has no function in the body; can be benign (noncancerous) or malignant (cancerous).

Apply the Key Terms

Think about the definitions of the following key terms. Describe one difference between each pair of key terms.

1. prone position and supine position
2. Fowler's position and lateral position
3. acronyms and medical terminology
4. neurons and membranes
5. atrophy and tumor

Know and Understand the Facts

1. Identify the five word parts that can be used to form a medical term.
2. Describe two body positions and one body direction.
3. List two types of body movement.
4. Describe one structure and its function in a human cell.
5. What are the four types of body tissue?

Analyze and Apply Concepts

1. Form and define five medical terms that use a root word, combining vowel, and suffix.
2. Form and define five medical terms that use a prefix, root word, and suffix.

3. Working with a partner, demonstrate adduction and abduction of the leg. Evaluate your partner's performance.
4. Working with a partner, demonstrate the supine and prone positions. Evaluate your partner's performance.

Think Critically

Read the following care situation. Then answer the questions that follow.

Josie, a nursing assistant, has been asked to put Mr. T in Fowler's position because he has pneumonitis. Josie has also been asked to take Mr. T's B/P, P, and R. Josie finds that Mr. T has a very fast heart rate and is having trouble breathing.

1. Explain how Josie should place Mr. T in a Fowler's position.
2. Identify the word elements for *pneumonitis*. What does the term *pneumonitis* mean?
3. What do the medical abbreviations *B/P, P,* and *R* mean?
4. What are the medical terms used for a fast heart rate and difficulty breathing? Use the table of medical word parts in Appendix A to assemble the words.

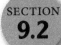
Body Systems

Objectives

To achieve the objectives for this section, you must successfully:
- **describe** the structure of each body system.
- **explain** the primary functions of each body system.
- **discuss** the impact lifestyle choices and the aging process have on body systems.

Key Terms

Learn these key terms to better understand the information presented in the section.

alimentary canal
anatomy
appendicular skeleton
autonomic nervous
  system (ANS)
axial skeleton
central nervous
  system (CNS)
deoxyribonucleic
  acid (DNA)
ducts
endocrine glands
exocrine glands
gland

ligaments
peripheral nervous
  system (PNS)
physiology
plasma
platelets
receptors
red blood cells
somatic nervous system
sperm
sphincter
tendons
white blood cells

Question to Consider

- Think about situations in which your body systems worked together. In these situations, which body systems were working together?

What Are Anatomy and Physiology?

Human bodies are made up of systems that have particular organs, structures, and functions. These *body systems* work both independently and together to make sure the body operates effectively. In this section, you will learn about *anatomy*, or the structure of the human body, and about *physiology*, the function of the human body. You will learn about the anatomy and physiology of the following body systems:

- integumentary system
- skeletal system
- muscular system
- nervous system

- sensory system
- endocrine system
- cardiovascular system
- respiratory system
- immune and lymphatic systems
- gastrointestinal system
- urinary system
- reproductive systems

There is an important relationship between human anatomy and physiology. The structure (anatomy) of the body is designed to accomplish specific functions (physiology) within each body system. As you learned in Chapter 7, maintaining homeostasis requires a balance of functions. This balance is achieved using the relationship between the body's anatomy and physiology. When body systems are structured properly and function effectively, the outcome is a healthy body. Disease occurs when a structure or system in the body is injured, altered, or is badly formed, impacting its function.

How Does the Integumentary System Protect the Body?

The *integumentary system* is composed of the skin; subcutaneous lipocytes (fat cells); nerves; blood vessels; and accessory (additional) organs, including sweat and sebaceous glands, hair, hair follicles (small sacs or cavities), nails, and nail follicles. The skin is the largest organ in the human body.

The Skin

The skin is considered the body's greatest line of defense because it prevents disease-causing microorganisms from entering the body. The skin also protects the body from exposure to ultraviolet (UV) rays from the sun and produces vitamin D in response to sunlight. Vitamin D makes it possible for the body to develop and maintain strong bones and a healthy immune system. The elasticity (flexibility) of skin permits growth and movement, as well as self-repair.

The skin contains the majority of the body's *receptors*, or sensory nerve endings, for touch, pressure, temperature, pain, and itch. The skin also regulates or controls body temperature. When the body is too hot, glands in the skin produce sweat, which cools the body as it evaporates off the skin. *Capillaries* (small blood vessels) in the skin also expand to release body heat and contract to trap heat within the body. Hair follicles attached to tiny muscles cause hair on the skin to stand up and trap heat when the body is cold. Blood vessels remove waste and pass nutrients through the layers of the skin, and nerves send signals to the brain so you know how something feels.

Layers of the Skin

The skin is a *cutaneous membrane* and consists of two major layers (**Figure 9.6**). The outer layer is called the epidermis. The inner, thicker layer is called the dermis.

The epidermis is made up of cells containing *keratin*, a protein that makes the skin durable and waterproof. New cells are produced in the deepest layer of the epidermis, and as cells age, they move toward the surface of the skin and then shed (fall off). This process takes about four weeks. The epidermis also contains *melanin*, which determines skin's color and protects the body from the sun's UV rays.

The dermis is a fibrous connective tissue made up of tough, thin threads. The dermis contains the proteins *collagen* and *elastin*, which keep skin in place and allow flexibility. Sensory nerve receptors that cause us to feel pressure, pain, and temperature are located in the dermis. Hair and nail follicles are found in the dermis, as are sweat and sebaceous glands.

Below the dermis is the *hypodermis*, which is not technically part of the integumentary system. This subcutaneous layer is made up of loose connective tissue, or *adipose tissue*, that consists mainly of fat cells. This layer provides padding and insulation, keeps the body warm, and connects the skin to the muscles beneath.

Sweat Glands and Sebaceous Glands

A **gland** is a group of specialized cells that secrete substances. *Sweat glands* are tiny, coiled glands that appear as pores (small holes) on the surface of the skin. The palms of the hands and soles of the feet contain the most sweat glands. Sweat glands secrete *perspiration*, or sweat. Perspiration is mostly made of water and moistens the surface of the skin to cool down the body.

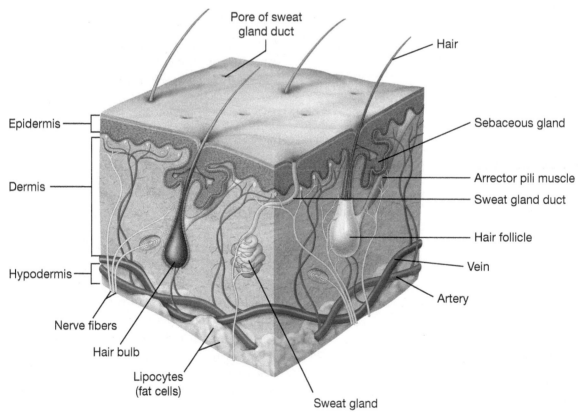

© *Body Scientific International*

Figure 9.6 The skin, a cutaneous membrane, has an outer layer called the *epidermis* and a thicker inner layer, called the *dermis*.

Sebaceous glands produce an oily substance called *sebum*. Sebum keeps the skin lubricated, which prevents infectious organisms from entering the body. It also keeps the skin smooth and soft. Sebum is released through **ducts** (tubes for conveying substances) located in hair follicles.

Hair and Fingernails

The hair and fingernails are made of the protein keratin and epithelial cells. Hair is mostly dead cells that fuse together and grow in strands from a root in the hair follicle. Hair keeps the body warm and covers the entire body, with the exceptions of the palms of the hands, soles of the feet, lips, eyelids, and scar tissue.

Each fingernail has a *nail plate*, a hard surface due to the presence of keratin. The *cuticle* of a nail is a band of tissue at the sides and base of the nail plate. The *nail root* anchors the nail plate. The pink color of the nail comes from blood vessels directly underneath the nail plate. The moon-shaped area on the nail is a thicker layer of cells that grow at the nail base. Nails help protect the ends of fingers and toes.

How Does the Skeletal System Support the Body?

At birth, the human body has 270 bones. As an infant grows, some bones fuse together; the adult skeleton has 206 bones.

The *skeletal system*:
- provides structure and shape for the body
- acts as levers for muscular action
- protects internal organs by shielding them with bony structure
- stores calcium and phosphorus needed for regulatory functions
- forms red and white blood cells and platelets in the bone marrow through *hematopoiesis*

Types of Bones

Bones make up the majority of the skeletal system. They come in a variety of sizes and shapes:
- **Long bones**: found in the legs or arms (extremities)
- **Flat bones**: found in the skull and breastbone
- **Short bones**: found in the hands and feet
- **Irregular bones**: found in the jaw and spinal column

- **Sesamoid bones**: found in the kneecap, wrist, and feet

Bone Composition

Bones are made up of two types of bone tissue: compact bone and spongy bone. Compact bone tissue is dense, hard, and strong. It is located in the outer layer of the bone and is mainly found in the shaft of long bones. Spongy bone tissue is less dense and is usually found at the ends of long bones. Spaces inside spongy bone tissue contain red bone marrow. **Red blood cells**, **white blood cells**, and **platelets** are formed in red bone marrow. Red blood cells help with oxygen and carbon dioxide exchange throughout the body, white blood cells fight infection, and platelets aid in clotting.

Bones have rough, exterior openings, grooves, and depressions that provide structure for the attachment of muscles and tendons, for the passage of blood vessels and nerves, and for joints.

Tendons, Ligaments, and Joints

Tendons are tough, flexible bands of fibrous connective tissue that connect muscles to bones. Joints are locations where two or more bones connect. Bones are linked together by **ligaments**, which are also bands of connective tissue. Ligaments have a membrane that produces synovial fluid to lubricate joints. Tendons and ligaments help stabilize joints and allow movement.

The type of joint determines the extent and direction of movement. Some joints do not allow any movement, while others let a limb move freely. There are three types of joints:
- unmovable joints, such as the sutures (immovable joints) in the cranium
- slightly movable joints, such as the ribs
- freely movable joints, including gliding, hinge, pivot, condylar, saddle, and ball-and-socket joints (**Figure 9.7**)

The Axial and Appendicular Skeletons

The skeletal system has two major divisions—the **axial skeleton** and the **appendicular skeleton**. The axial skeleton provides stability, while the appendicular skeleton allows the body to move (**Figure 9.8**).

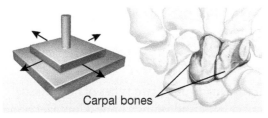

Gliding joint (intercarpal)

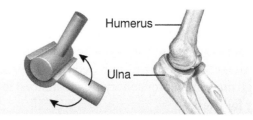

Hinge joint (humeroulnar)

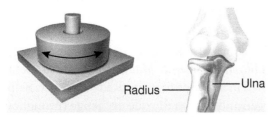

Pivot joint (radioulnar)

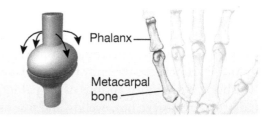

Condylar joint (metacarpophalangeal)

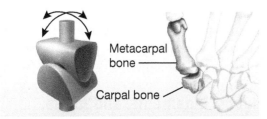

Saddle joint (trapeziometacarpal)

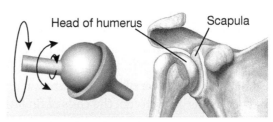

Ball-and-socket joint (humeroscapular)

© Body Scientific International

Figure 9.7 There are six types of freely movable joints.

How Does the Muscular System Enable Movement?

The *muscular system* is made up of more than 600 muscles and accounts for 40–50 percent of the body's weight (**Figure 9.9**). The muscular system works with many other body systems to help the body move, respond to external stimuli (something that causes a response), and produce heat. Specific functions of the muscular system include:

- contracting and relaxing of the muscles to move the body's skeleton
- using the muscles and muscle tone to hold body parts in proper position
- providing a protective covering for internal organs
- producing the majority of heat, through movement, needed to keep the body warm
- moving food through the gastrointestinal system and transporting blood and fluids through the body's vessels

Muscle tissue must be able to contract, be elastic and stretchable, and have the ability to receive and respond to neural messages.

Muscles are covered by fascia, a fibrous connective tissue that attaches muscles to tendons. As you have learned, tendons connect muscle to bone. Both ends of a muscle are connected to bone. Within each muscle are thousands of *muscle fibers*, each with its own motor nerve ending that sends and receives signals through the nervous system. There are three types of muscle:

- **Skeletal muscles:** (also called *striated muscles*) connect to bones and move the skeleton by contracting and relaxing. Because skeletal muscles are consciously controlled, they are considered *voluntary muscles*. These muscles are found in the scalp, face, mouth, arms, hands, abdomen, legs, and feet.
- **Smooth muscles:** (also called *visceral muscles*) contract and relax without a person's awareness. Smooth muscles are found in the walls of organs. As they contract and relax, these muscles move the contents inside an organ. An example of smooth muscles at work is the involuntary process of peristalsis, in which muscle contractions move food through the gastrointestinal tract.

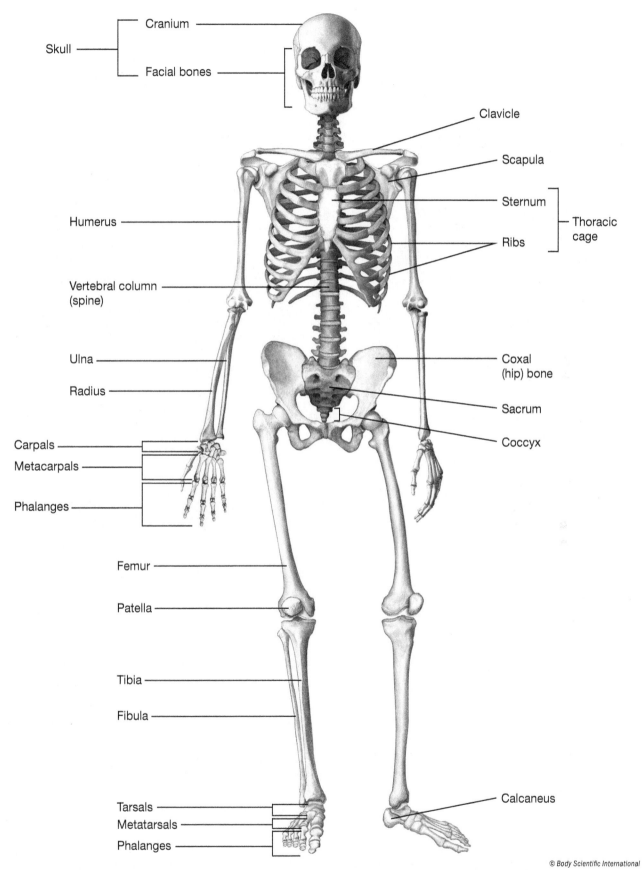

Skull
- Cranium
- Facial bones

Clavicle

Scapula

Sternum

Thoracic cage

Humerus

Ribs

Vertebral column (spine)

Ulna

Radius

Coxal (hip) bone

Sacrum

Coccyx

Carpals

Metacarpals

Phalanges

Femur

Patella

Tibia

Fibula

Tarsals

Metatarsals

Phalanges

Calcaneus

© Body Scientific International

Figure 9.8 The axial skeleton (shown here in magenta) is made up of the head and trunk, which provide stability for the body. The appendicular skeleton is made up of the appendages (arms, shoulders, and legs), which allow the body to move.

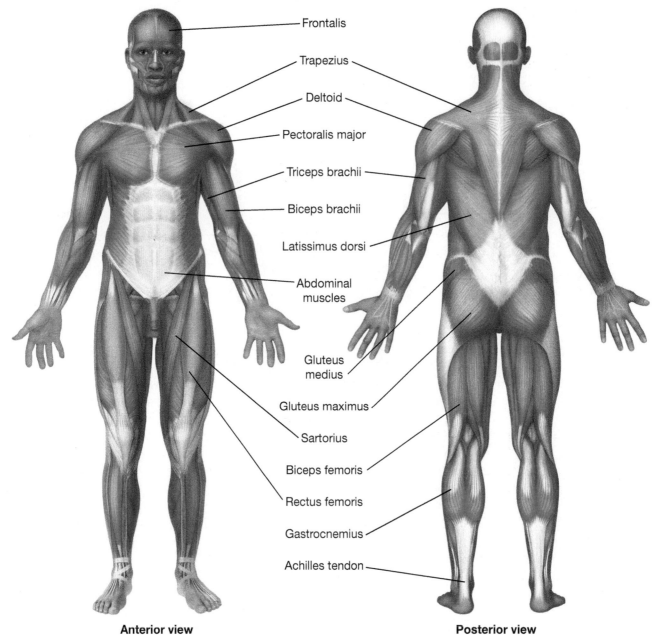

Figure 9.9 There are more than 600 muscles to help the body move, hold body parts in place, provide protection for organs, and produce heat.

© Body Scientific International

- **Cardiac muscle:** found only in the heart and makes up most of the heart wall. It is a striated muscle and causes the heart to contract, or *beat*. These smooth muscle contractions occur involuntarily.

THINK ABOUT THIS

The muscle that lets your eye blink is the fastest muscle in your body. It allows you to blink five times per second. On average, you blink 15,000 times per day. Women blink twice as often as men.

How Does the Nervous System Send Signals throughout the Body?

The *nervous system* uses billions of neurons to send electrochemical messages, also known as *neural impulses*, throughout the body. These messages control and direct many functions of the body. Neurons also receive information from internal and external receptors. These receptors interpret information so the body can respond either voluntarily (*consciously*) or involuntarily (*unconsciously*). Voluntary responses are controlled mostly by the brain. The two types of involuntary responses are autonomic responses and reflexes. These regulate the body's internal environment (for example, blood pressure) or cause a reaction that starts in the spinal cord.

The nervous system is made up of the central and peripheral nervous systems. The *central nervous system (CNS)* consists of the brain and spinal cord. The *peripheral nervous system (PNS)* consists of 12 pairs of cranial nerves and 31 pairs of spinal nerves.

Central Nervous System (CNS)

The *central nervous system (CNS)* is the command center of the body. The structures of the CNS respond to all neural messages in the body, monitor functions throughout the body, and help maintain homeostasis. The brain is the center of *cognition*, or mental functions such as thinking, reasoning, and remembering. The spinal cord connects the brain with the rest of the body.

The brain and spinal cord are covered with three layers of tissue known as *meninges*. The outer layer, called the *dura mater*, is a tough, protective membrane. The middle layer, the *arachnoid mater*, is a thin, transparent membrane resembling a loosely fitting sac. The arachnoid mater connects the dura mater with the innermost tissue layer, the *pia mater*. The pia mater is a thin membrane that sticks to the surface of the brain and the spinal cord. The pia mater has a rich supply of blood vessels that provide nutrients to nerve tissue. *Cerebrospinal fluid* fills the brain cavities and the central canal of the spinal column to cushion and protect these structures from injury.

Regions of the Brain

The brain is divided into four areas—the cerebrum, cerebellum, diencephalon, and brain stem (**Figure 9.10**). Each area plays an important role in the complex functions carried out by the brain.

- **Cerebrum**: the largest region of the brain, it is divided into left and right hemispheres. The right and left hemispheres are divided into four lobes: frontal, parietal, occipital, and temporal. The cerebrum is covered by the *cerebral cortex*, which contains gray matter arranged in folds and depressions. The cerebrum controls high-level cognitive functions such as language, reasoning, memory, and sensory integration (how the brain understands sensory information from the body and the environment).

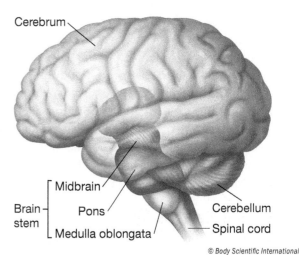
© Body Scientific International

Figure 9.10 Each area of the brain has special and complex functions.

- **Diencephalon**: found beneath the cerebrum, it has three glands: the thalamus, pineal gland, and hypothalamus. The *thalamus* plays a role in memory and sends messages such as pain from the sensory organs to the cerebrum. The *pineal gland* helps regulate the body's circadian rhythm, or 24-hour sleep-wake cycle. The *hypothalamus* monitors and controls involuntary body functions such as heart rate, blood pressure, temperature, and digestion.
- **Cerebellum**: located in the posterior part of the brain, it controls the body's sense of equilibrium (balance). It also coordinates the voluntary movement of muscles.
- **Brain stem**: connects the cerebrum with the spinal cord and has three parts: the midbrain, pons, and medulla oblongata. The *midbrain* is the passageway through which neural messages travel from the brain to the spinal cord. The *pons* connects the cerebellum to the rest of the brain and plays a role in breathing. The *medulla oblongata* connects the brain to the spinal cord and regulates heart rate, breathing, and blood pressure.

Spinal Cord

The *spinal cord* extends from the base of the brain to the lower back. It is inside the spinal column and is protected by vertebrae. It is made up of nerve tissue, and 31 pairs of spinal nerves branch off it and exit through either side of the spinal column. The spinal cord is divided into four regions, starting at the top of the cord and going to the bottom: the cervical region, thoracic region, lumbar region, and sacral region.

Neural messages travel up and down the spinal cord and make it possible for the brain and body to communicate. Sensory neurons in the CNS transmit messages to the brain and control basic body functions. Motor neurons transmit messages away from the brain, stimulating skeletal and smooth muscle to enable voluntary and involuntary movements. For example, if you touch something hot, neurons in the spinal cord will activate the speedy reflex needed to quickly move your hand before you are burned.

Peripheral Nervous System (PNS)

The *peripheral nervous system (PNS)* connects the CNS with the rest of the body. Cranial nerves transmit neural messages to and from the brain, and spinal nerves transmit neural messages to and from the spinal cord. The PNS is divided into the autonomic and somatic nervous systems (**Figure 9.11**).

Autonomic Nervous System (ANS)

The *autonomic nervous system (ANS)* controls involuntary, unconscious body functions. The two divisions of the ANS are the sympathetic and parasympathetic nervous systems, which you learned about in Chapter 7. The *sympathetic nervous system* controls the body's *fight-or-flight response*, which prepares the body for an emergency. Physical reactions to the fight-or-flight response include a racing heart and rapid breathing. The *parasympathetic nervous*

system controls the body's *rest-and-digest response*, which calms the body after the fight-or-flight response by decreasing heart rate and respirations.

Somatic Nervous System

The *somatic nervous system* controls voluntary body functions and stimulates skeletal muscle. This system also sends neural messages about pain.

What Is the Role of the Sensory System?

The *sensory system* is made up of sense organs, some of which are shared with other body systems. These sense organs include the eyes, ears, nose (also part of the respiratory system), tongue (also part of the gastrointestinal system), and skin (also part of the integumentary system). The structures of the sensory system transmit neural messages that make the senses of vision, hearing, smell, taste, and touch possible.

The Eye

The eye is the sense organ of vision. It has external and internal structures that receive and translate light into neural messages (**Figure 9.12**). External structures of the eye, including the eyelashes, eyebrows, lacrimal glands (which secrete tears), tear ducts, ciliary glands, and eye socket protect the eye and

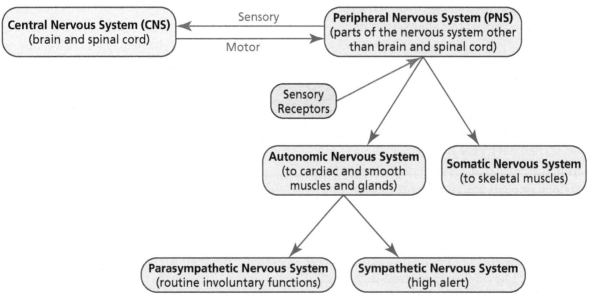

Goodheart-Willcox Publisher

Figure 9.11 The CNS and PNS work together to carry sensory and motor messages throughout the body.

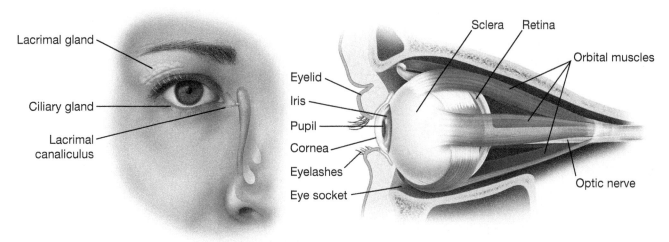

Figure 9.12 The external structures of the eye protect the eye, while the internal structures are responsible for vision.

prevent foreign substances from entering the eye. The orbital muscle moves the eye in the eye socket. The internal structures that cause vision include:

- The sclera (or *white of the eye*) protects the eye and maintains the eye's shape. The transparent, anterior portion of the sclera is the *cornea*, which protects the iris and the pupil.
- The *iris* is a colored, muscular layer of tissue. It surrounds the small, black *pupil*, which lets light into the eye. The light then passes through a *lens*, which is a flexible, clear, curved structure that focuses images on the retina at the back of the eye.
- The interior of the eye has two fluid-filled chambers: the anterior and posterior chambers. The anterior chamber contains *aqueous humor*, a clear, watery fluid that gives the eyeball its shape. The posterior chamber contains a clear, gel-like substance called the *vitreous humor*, which helps keep the retina in place.
- The *ciliary muscle* inside the eye regulates the shape and thickness of the lens, which allows the lens to focus light on the retina.
- The *retina* consists of special, light-sensitive receptor cells known as *rods* and *cones*. These cast images onto the retina to enable vision. The brain then interprets what is seen on the retina. The retina contains approximately 120 million rods, which are sensitive only to black and white and allow a person to see in dim light. Rods also provide peripheral (lateral) vision. The 6–7 million cones are sensitive to color and provide more acute vision.

- The *optic nerve* located at the back of the eye transmits neural messages from the retina to the brain.

The Ear

The ear has three divisions: the outer (external) ear, the middle ear (tympanic cavity), and the inner (internal) ear (**Figure 9.13**). All three sections of the ear are responsible for hearing, and the inner ear also plays a role in balance and equilibrium.

Sound enters the auditory canal and is translated into vibrations in the tympanic membrane, or *eardrum*. The middle ear is connected to the throat by the Eustachian tube. The Eustachian tube is closed except when a person swallows. It helps equalize pressure within the ear. The three *ossicles* in the eardrum, which are the smallest bones in the body, then transmit these vibrations from the eardrum to the fluid in the cochlea of the inner ear. Within the cochlea is the *organ of Corti*, which is the primary receptor for hearing. The organ of Corti contains four rows of hair cells that respond to sound vibrations. These cells transmit neural messages using the *cochlear nerve* and help a person determine the pitch and loudness of another person's voice. The cochlear nerve transmits neural messages to the auditory center of the brain, where sound is processed and interpreted.

The inner ear also contains structures and receptors to maintain equilibrium. At the base of the cochlea is the *vestibule*, which connects the cochlea to fluid-filled semicircular canals. Sensory information about equilibrium is transmitted from the vestibule

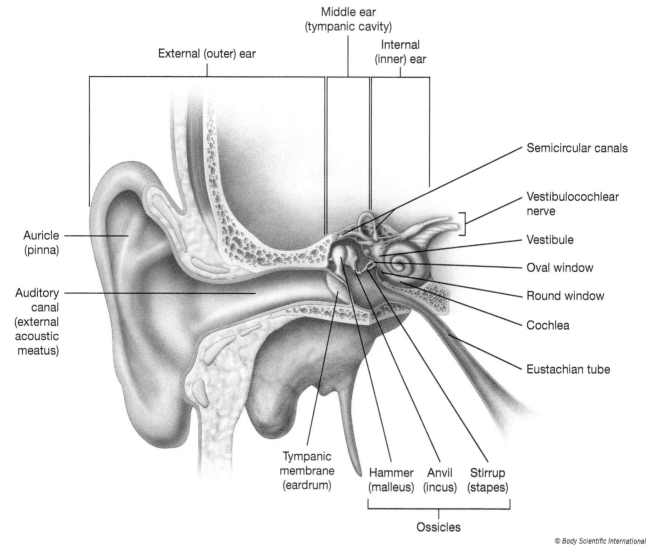

Figure 9.13 The structures of the ear are responsible for hearing. The inner ear plays a role in balance and equilibrium.

© Body Scientific International

by way of the *vestibular nerve* to the neurons that control eye movements, to the muscles that keep the body standing tall, and to the brain (so that the body's position can be adjusted). Together, the cochlear nerve and vestibular nerve form a cranial nerve called the *vestibulocochlear nerve*.

Other Sense Organs

The nose, tongue, and skin are also sense organs. Inside the nose are thousands of olfactory (smell) receptor cells containing *olfactory hairs*. When these hairs are stimulated by smell, neural messages are transmitted by way of the *olfactory nerve* (a cranial nerve) to the brain, where smell is processed.

The average adult tongue contains about 5,000 working taste buds. *Taste buds* are special receptors on the surface of the tongue. They sense

the flavor of food, as well as temperature. As you learned earlier in this chapter, the skin contains sensory receptors responsible for touch, pressure, temperature, pain, and itch.

How Do Hormones of the Endocrine System Regulate Body Functions?

The endocrine system is made up of **endocrine glands**, which are different from **exocrine glands**. *Endocrine glands* are located throughout the body (**Figure 9.14**) and secrete *hormones*, or chemical messengers that initiate and regulate specific body processes. Endocrine glands are ductless and secrete hormones directly into the bloodstream. *Exocrine glands* have ducts that transport substances to other organs or to the surface

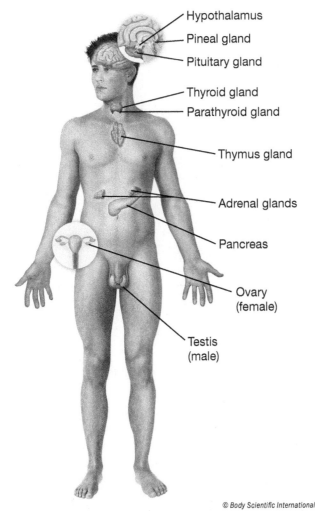

Hypothalamus
Pineal gland
Pituitary gland
Thyroid gland
Parathyroid gland
Thymus gland
Adrenal glands
Pancreas
Ovary (female)
Testis (male)

© Body Scientific International

Figure 9.14 Endocrine glands located throughout the body secrete hormones directly into the bloodstream.

of the skin. Sweat glands are an example of exocrine glands because sweat is secreted through ducts in the skin. The pancreas is different—it has both endocrine and exocrine functions.

The structures and functions of the endocrine system include:

- **Hypothalamus:** directly or indirectly controls all other endocrine glands. It is also part of the nervous system and coordinates responses and activities of these two body systems. Hormones secreted from the hypothalamus control body functions such as temperature regulation, thirst, hunger, sleep, mood, and sex drive. The hypothalamus also releases hormones that stimulate other glands to release specific hormones.
- **Pituitary gland:** divided into two lobes—the anterior pituitary and posterior pituitary. For example, the anterior pituitary releases the growth hormone (GH). The posterior pituitary

secretes *antidiuretic hormone (ADH),* which controls water absorption in the kidneys; and *oxytocin,* which stimulates uterine contractions during childbirth and helps with the release of milk in nursing mothers.

- **Pineal gland:** releases melatonin when the body is exposed to darkness. *Melatonin* is the hormone that regulates circadian rhythm, or the 24-hour sleep-wake cycle. When melatonin is released, you feel sleepy.
- **Thyroid gland:** wrapped around the front and sides of the windpipe, or *trachea,* the thyroid gland releases *thyroid hormones* that control metabolism, regulate body temperature, and increase the rate of protein production. The thyroid gland also releases *calcitonin,* which regulates the amount of calcium in the blood and helps the body maintain strong, stable bones.
- **Parathyroid glands:** two pairs of *parathyroid glands* are located on the back of the thyroid gland. Each parathyroid gland is smaller than a grain of rice. The parathyroid glands release *parathyroid hormone (PTH),* which helps balance levels of calcium in the blood and stimulates the activation of vitamin D.
- **Thymus:** releases *thymosin,* a hormone that helps with the development and maturation of immune cells. As a result, the thymus is part of the endocrine and immune systems. This gland shrinks in size as people age and is very small by the time people reach adulthood.
- **Adrenal glands:** sitting on top of the kidneys, each of the two adrenal glands have two layers. The outer layer, the *adrenal cortex,* releases cortisol (promotes the use of carbohydrates, fats, and proteins and increases the storage of blood glucose), cortisone (regulates blood glucose levels), and aldosterone (regulates blood pressure and fluid volume). The inner layer, the *adrenal medulla,* releases epinephrine (triggers the body's fight-or-flight response) and norepinephrine (narrows blood vessels and raises blood pressure). The adrenal glands also release some sex hormones.
- **Pancreas:** serves as an exocrine gland by secreting enzymes during digestion. Within the pancreas, islets of Langerhans release the hormones insulin and glucagon. *Insulin* lowers blood sugar levels, and *glucagon* stimulates the liver to increase blood sugar levels when needed.

- **Ovaries:** the ovaries secrete the majority of *estrogen* in the body. Estrogen regulates the female reproductive system and stimulates secondary sex characteristics, including the development of breasts and the growth of pubic and underarm hair. The ovaries also produce *progesterone*, which stimulates the growth of the mammary glands, regulates menstruation, and promotes the growth of the endometrium (the mucous membrane lining the inside of the uterus).
- **Testes:** release *testosterone*, which regulates secondary sex characteristics, including facial, underarm, and pubic hair growth; increased muscle mass; and a deeper voice. It is also essential for sperm maturation.

How Does the Cardiovascular System Pump Blood through the Body?

The main function of the cardiovascular system is to circulate (move) oxygen-rich blood throughout the body and to remove carbon dioxide and other waste products. To accomplish this task, the cardiovascular and respiratory systems work together to complete the exchange of oxygen and carbon dioxide.

The Heart

The *heart* is located in the chest, between the two lungs (**Figure 9.15**). It is composed of involuntary cardiac muscle, which contracts and relaxes in a rhythmic cycle. These contractions circulate blood through the heart to the rest of the body. The heart sits in a sac called the *pericardium* and is made up of three layers of muscle:

- **Epicardium:** serous, thin, watery layer
- **Myocardium:** located in the middle of the heart
- **Endocardium:** the innermost layer that lines the chambers of the heart

The heart is divided into right and left sides by the *septum*. Each side of the heart is further divided into an upper and lower chamber. The upper chambers are called *atria*, and the lower chambers are called *ventricles*. The lowest point of the heart is called the *apex*.

Blood Flow through the Heart

The heart is the engine that circulates blood through the body. Blood flows in one direction, through the

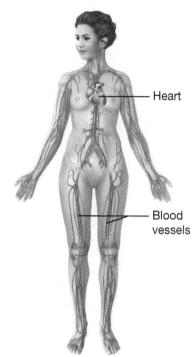

Heart

Blood vessels

© *Body Scientific International*

Figure 9.15 The heart contracts and relaxes in a rhythmic cycle to circulate blood through the body.

upper chambers of the heart to the lower chambers, and valves between the chambers prevent any blood from flowing backward. Once blood leaves the heart, it circulates throughout the body by way of the blood vessels (**Figure 9.16**).

Heart Rate and Blood Pressure

The heart's muscle fibers allow it to contract, relax, and pump blood through the heart. This action is regulated by the autonomic nervous system, which operates unconsciously. The heart's actions are also regulated by an electrical system that has sites throughout the heart muscle. The process by which the heart is electrically stimulated is *conduction*. During this process, electrical impulses in the atria and ventricles stimulate contractions needed for the heart to circulate blood. When the heart contracts, blood is forced through the arteries to the rest of the body. This is called *systole*. Between contractions, the heart relaxes (*diastole*) and fills with blood. Blood pressure measures the contraction (systolic) and then the relaxation (diastolic) of the heart. The normal range for an adult's blood pressure is 120/80 mmHg or below.

The normal pulse for adults is 60–100 beats per minute and depends on a person's health and physical activity. Pulse is most commonly felt and measured

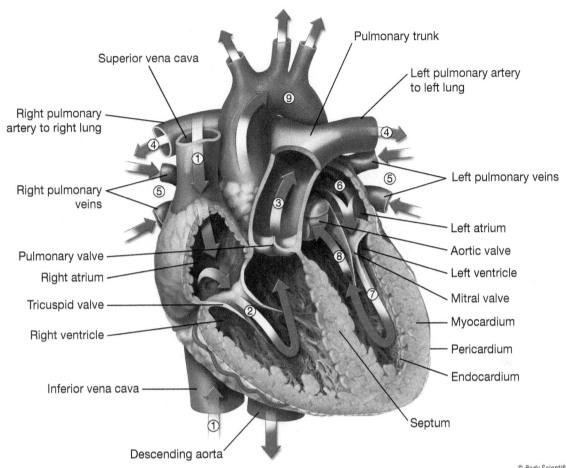

Superior vena cava

Pulmonary trunk

Left pulmonary artery
to left lung

Right pulmonary
artery to right lung

Right pulmonary
veins

Left pulmonary veins

Left atrium

Pulmonary valve

Aortic valve

Right atrium

Left ventricle

Tricuspid valve

Mitral valve

Right ventricle

Myocardium

Pericardium

Endocardium

Inferior vena cava

Septum

Descending aorta

© Body Scientific International

Figure 9.16 Follow the flow of blood through the heart using this diagram.

at the wrist, but is sometimes taken at the apex of the heart using a stethoscope. Pulse can also be taken at other points on the body. See Chapter 15 for a detailed discussion about measuring and recording blood pressure and pulse.

Blood Vessels

Blood vessels provide blood to the heart so that it can function properly. They also transport blood between the heart and the rest of the body. Many different blood vessels help to circulate blood throughout the body. Arteries, arterioles, and capillaries transport fully oxygenated blood from the heart to the body. Veins and venules carry oxygen-poor blood from the body back to the heart.

Blood

The average adult has between 10 and 15 pints of blood. *Blood* has two basic components: blood cells and plasma. **Plasma** is the liquid component of blood and makes up one-half of the blood's volume.

It is mostly water, but also transports hormones, protein, sugar, and waste products to or from the body tissues.

There are three types of blood cells—red blood cells (RBCs), white blood cells (WBCs), and platelets. Red blood cells (RBCs), or *erythrocytes*, are responsible for carrying oxygen throughout the body and removing carbon dioxide, a waste product. Hemoglobin molecules on red blood cells carry oxygen from the lungs to body organs and tissues and carry carbon dioxide from body organs and tissues to the lungs. White blood cells (WBCs), or *leukocytes*, defend the body against pathogens. Both red and white blood cells are created primarily in the bone marrow. Platelets, or *thrombocytes*, help the blood clot, or clump together to stop the bleeding, when there is an injury.

┌─── **THINK ABOUT THIS** ───
│ There are 60,000 miles of blood vessels in a human
│ body, enough to wrap around the Earth twice.

How Does the Respiratory System Supply the Body with Oxygen?

The respiratory system's primary function is breathing, or *respiration*. During respiration, oxygen is inhaled (*inspiration*) and carbon dioxide is exhaled (*expiration*). The process of respiration includes two important activities: ventilation and gas exchange.

Ventilation is the movement of oxygen-rich air into the lungs and the movement of carbon dioxide out of the lungs. Ventilation is measured by counting each inspiration and expiration. The normal ventilation rate for adults is 12–20 breaths per minute.

The respiratory and cardiovascular systems work together to complete the second activity, *gas exchange*. Gas exchange occurs in the alveoli of the lungs, where the gases oxygen and carbon dioxide are exchanged, or swapped. Inhaled oxygen moves through the alveoli and into capillaries so it can move to the body's cells, organs, and tissues by way of the blood vessels. Carbon dioxide moves from the capillaries into the alveoli so it can be breathed out into the environment.

The respiratory system is divided into two parts: the upper and lower respiratory tracts. The upper respiratory tract consists of the nose and nasal cavities, mouth, pharynx, and larynx. The lower respiratory tract consists of the trachea, bronchi, bronchioles, and two lungs, which contain alveoli (**Figure 9.17**).

Air enters the body through the nose and flows into the *nasal cavity*, the space behind the nose. Tiny hairs called *cilia* line the nasal cavity and filter pathogens from the air. The pharynx, or *throat*, is the passageway into the body for air, liquid, and food. The last organ in the upper respiratory tract is the semi-rigid larynx, or *voice box*. A large plate of thyroid cartilage known as the *Adam's apple* and the epiglottis are part of the larynx. The epiglottis opens to allow air to flow through the trachea (*windpipe*) into the lower respiratory tract. The epiglottis closes over the trachea when a person is eating or drinking to prevent foods and liquids from going into the trachea.

When air enters the trachea, it flows over *cilia* that trap foreign substances and sweep them up toward the larynx and pharynx. Midway down the chest, the trachea divides into the right and left bronchi. The bronchi are the passageways into the lungs. Air

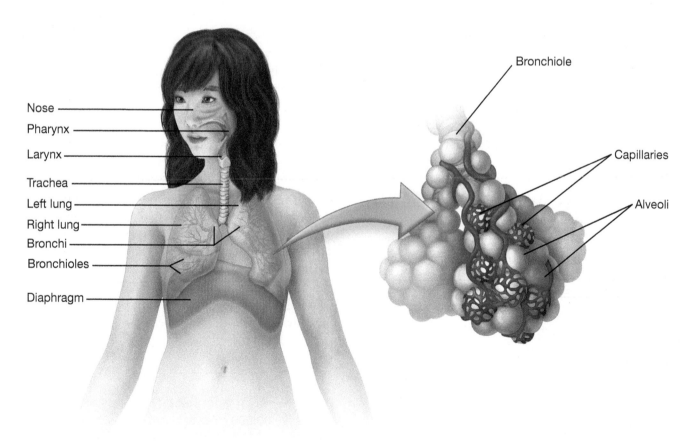

Nose
Pharynx
Larynx
Trachea
Left lung
Right lung
Bronchi
Bronchioles
Diaphragm

Bronchiole
Capillaries
Alveoli

© Body Scientific International

Figure 9.17 The respiratory system supplies oxygen to the body's cells and removes carbon dioxide.

flows into the bronchi, into smaller structures called *bronchioles*, and finally into the alveoli. *Alveoli* are tiny sacs in the lungs.

The lungs are the main organs of the respiratory system. There is a right and a left lung. The right lung sits a little higher in the thoracic cavity than the left because of the location of the liver. There are three lobes in the right lung (superior, middle, and inferior) and two lobes in the left lung (superior and inferior). The area between the two lungs is called the *mediastinum*. Several organs and structures are found in the mediastinum, including the heart.

The lungs are made of porous, spongy tissue. A *pleural membrane* covers the lungs. Fluid fills the pleural cavity in which the lungs are located to reduce friction during breathing. Each lung is cone-shaped and contains a network of blood, lymph vessels, and nerves. At the base of the lungs is the *diaphragm*, a muscle that contracts to help inflate the lungs.

How Do the Immune and Lymphatic Systems Keep You Healthy?

The *immune* and *lymphatic systems* protect the body against pathogens. The immune system does not have its own organs or vessels. Instead, it relies on organs from other body systems to fulfill its vital tasks. The lymphatic system also plays a major role in immunity and protection against pathogens. There are two different types of immunity:

- **Natural immunity**: is a type of immunity people have when they are born. Natural immunity is affected by a person's race, gender, genes, and cells (such as white blood cells).
- **Acquired immunity**: a type of immunity that people develop. This type of immunity can be active or passive. People develop *active immunity* by being exposed to a disease or through *immunization*. Immunization is a process in which a small or modified dose of a pathogen is usually injected to stimulate the production of antibodies. *Passive immunity* is short-term and passes from one body to another. For example, a fetus can develop passive immunity when a mother passes antibodies through the placenta.

Immune Cells

The immune system is activated when pathogens attack the body. A variety of cells are involved in responding to this attack. *T cells* are a type of white blood cell and include *cytotoxic cells*, which destroy cells that are harmful. White blood cells known as *B cells* transform into plasma and secrete antibodies for protection. When these antibodies are released into blood and lymph, they target foreign substances and destroy them.

Lymph and Lymph Vessels

Lymph is a colorless fluid that is found in the capillaries of the cardiovascular system and travels through lymph vessels. As it travels, lymph replaces harmful substances in the body with healthy white blood cells and plasma before returning to the cardiovascular system. The primary cell found in lymph is the *lymphocyte*, a type of white blood cell that is specialized to defend the body against pathogens. *Lymph vessels* include ducts that propel lymph through the body.

Lymph Organs

Organs of the lymphatic system include the lymph nodes, spleen, tonsils, and thymus (**Figure 9.18**). *Lymph nodes* are small organs located throughout the body. Some lymph nodes can be found in the armpit (*axilla*), for example. Lymph nodes contain lymphocytes that detect and destroy cells that are foreign to the body.

The *spleen* is the largest organ in the lymphatic system. It is filled with blood vessels and a reserve of blood. The spleen is an important part of destroying worn-out red blood cells, producing lymphocytes, storing platelets, and increasing blood volume in the body.

What Is the Gastrointestinal System's Role in Nutrition?

The *gastrointestinal system* has several functions related to the ingestion (eating and drinking), breakdown, absorption, and elimination of food and liquid. The structures and organs of the gastrointestinal system work together to absorb nutrients from the foods you eat and give you the energy you need to survive and be healthy (**Figure 9.19**).

Alimentary Canal

The gastrointestinal system includes the gastrointestinal tract (*GI tract*). Another name for the gastrointestinal tract is the **alimentary canal**. The alimentary canal leads from the mouth to the anus and connects many digestive organs. Many other organs assist the alimentary canal in achieving gastrointestinal functions.

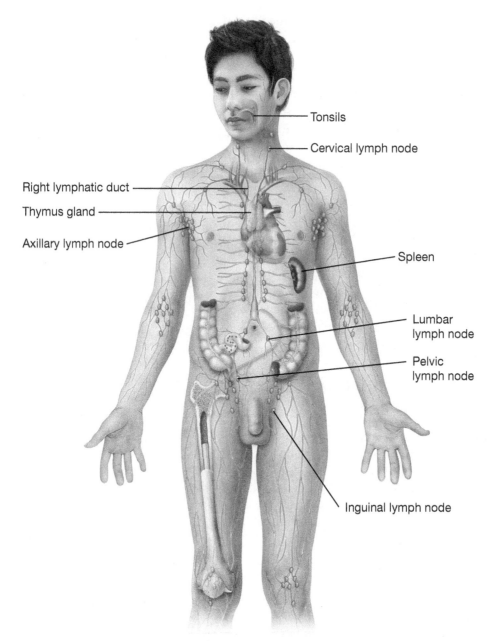

Tonsils

Cervical lymph node

Right lymphatic duct

Thymus gland

Axillary lymph node

Spleen

Lumbar lymph node

Pelvic lymph node

Inguinal lymph node

© Body Scientific International

Figure 9.18 The lymphatic organs work together to circulate and filter lymph.

The Mouth

Food and liquid enter the mouth through the lips, or *labia*. The mouth is lined with a mucous membrane that secretes *saliva* produced by the salivary glands. The lips and cheeks make up the front and the lateral walls of the mouth, and the hard and soft palates form the top, or *roof*, of the mouth. The *uvula*, a fingerlike projection found on the soft palate, hangs at the very back of the mouth to prevent liquid and food from entering nasal passages.

The *tongue* is an accessory organ that aids the teeth in chewing (*mastication*). The tongue uses muscular action to direct and move food in the mouth toward the pharynx. On the surface of the tongue are tiny bumps called *papillae* that contain taste buds. The underside of the tongue is made up of tiny blood vessels that aid in absorption. Because of these blood vessels, medications can be given under the tongue, or *sublingually*.

THINK ABOUT THIS

The tongue can identify five basic tastes: sweet, sour, bitter, salt, and umami (meaty or savory). All parts of the tongue can detect these tastes, but the sides of the tongue are more sensitive than the middle of the tongue, and the back of the tongue is most sensitive to bitter tastes.

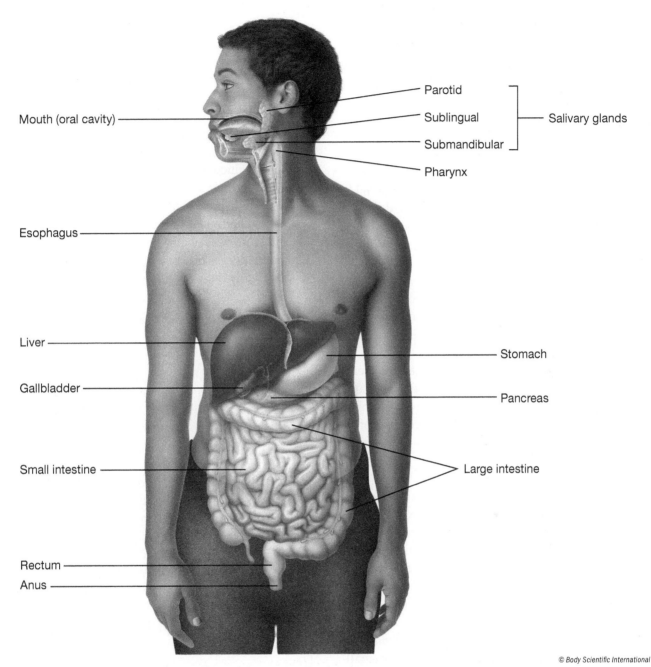

Mouth (oral cavity)

Parotid

Sublingual

Submandibular ⎤ Salivary glands

Pharynx

Esophagus

Liver

Stomach

Gallbladder

Pancreas

Small intestine

Large intestine

Rectum

Anus

© Body Scientific International

Figure 9.19 The organs of the digestive system include those that are part of the GI tract as well as accessory, or helper, organs that aid in digestion and nutrient absorption.

Each tooth is divided into two areas: the crown and the root. The outermost layer of the tooth is *enamel*. The root of each tooth is surrounded by bone and a layer of soft tissue called *gingiva* or *gums*.

Three pairs of *salivary glands* surround the oral cavity and are important in digestion. These glands produce 10,000 gallons of saliva over a person's lifetime. Saliva contains enzymes that aid in the chemical breakdown of food.

Pharynx and Esophagus

The pharynx, or *throat*, is the passageway to the mucus-lined, muscular esophagus. The *epiglottis* closes over the trachea to direct liquid and food to the esophagus. At the end of the esophagus is a **sphincter**, called the *cardiac sphincter*, that controls the flow and backflow of food and liquid traveling from the esophagus to the stomach.

Stomach

The *stomach* is made up of three layers of muscle that give it strength when it expands. These muscle layers also help mix food during digestion. The stomach is lined with a mucous membrane containing *rugae* (folds), which allow the stomach to expand when filled with food. This membrane also protects the lining of the stomach from harsh gastric (stomach) acid. When food mixes with gastric acid in the stomach, the mixture becomes *chyme*. Chyme enters the small intestine through a narrow passageway called the *pylorus*. The size of the pylorus is regulated by the pyloric sphincter.

Small Intestine

The *small intestine* is the longest section of the alimentary canal (between 17 and 20 feet long). The small intestine continues the process of digestion and helps the body absorb nutrients, water, and electrolytes (such as sodium) into the blood. Small, threadlike extensions called *villi* line the small intestine, absorbing nutrients as they help move chyme along the twisted path of the small intestine. The small intestine consists of three sections—the duodenum, jejunum, and ileum.

Large Intestine

The mucus-lined large intestine gets its name because it is much larger in diameter than the small intestine. There are six sections in the large intestine. The first section, the *cecum*, is connected to the ileum in the small intestine and receives unused food and waste. The *appendix*, which has no known function, hangs from the lower part of the cecum. The second, third, and fourth parts of the large intestine are the ascending, transverse, and descending colons. The *ascending, transverse*, and *descending colons* surround the small intestine. The *sigmoid colon* leads into the rectum, and the *rectum* stores waste (*feces*) until waste can be eliminated in a process called *defecation*.

Anus

The *anus* is the last structure of the alimentary canal. With help from the nervous system, voluntary and involuntary sphincters within the anus help regulate and control elimination—the process by which feces are removed from the body.

Accessory Organs

Three additional accessory organs within the gastrointestinal system aid digestion:

- **Pancreas:** produces insulin, glucagon, and enzymes that are secreted through the pancreatic duct into the small intestine to assist in digestion.
- **Liver:** responsible for making bile, which is needed to digest food and break down fat in the small intestine. The liver also stores nutrients, filters and removes waste products from the bloodstream, and changes carbohydrates into sugar (glucose).
- **Gallbladder:** a small, pear-shaped pouch that stores bile produced by the liver. When bile is needed, it travels to the duodenum in the small intestine by way of cystic and bile ducts. The gallbladder is not an essential organ and may be surgically removed, if necessary.

How Does the Urinary System Produce, Store, and Eliminate Urine from the Body?

The *urinary system* is responsible for filtering the blood and eliminating liquid waste from the body in the form of urine. This system determines which waste products need to be filtered from the blood and which can be reabsorbed. It also maintains the body's homeostasis by monitoring fluid levels and electrolytes in the body. Fluids and electrolytes will be discussed in more detail in Chapter 19.

The urinary system is made up of two kidneys, two ureters, the urinary bladder, and the urethra (**Figure 9.20**). The kidneys produce urine containing waste products that need to be *excreted*, or expelled from the body. The urinary bladder stores urine until it is excreted through the urethra. Gravity and peristalsis move urine through the urinary system.

Kidneys

The *kidneys* are two bean-shaped organs that weigh approximately 4–6 ounces each and are found in the abdominal cavity. Fat (*adipose*) and connective tissue line the kidneys to protect them and hold them in place. The kidney is made up of three regions: the renal cortex, renal medulla, and renal pelvis. The renal cortex is the outer layer of the kidney. It has microscopic *nephrons* that filter blood to remove waste products. Some waste products are reabsorbed by the body, while others pass to the renal medulla in the form of *urine*. Urine moves through the renal medulla to the renal pelvis, where it is expelled from the kidney by way of the ureters.

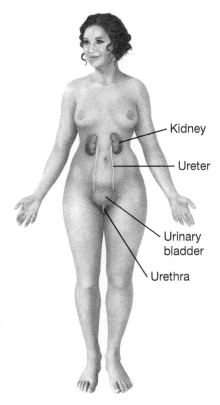

Kidney

Ureter

Urinary
bladder

Urethra

Urinary system

© Body Scientific International

Figure 9.20 The organs of the urinary system filter blood and eliminate (excrete) liquid waste (urine) from the body.

Ureters, Urinary Bladder, and Urethra

The two *ureters* are narrow tubes that transport urine from the renal pelvis to the urinary bladder. The hollow, muscular *urinary bladder* stores urine until it is expelled from the body. The urinary bladder can store up to 16 ounces of fluid before nerves in the bladder send a message to the brain that the bladder needs to be emptied. The *urethra* is the tube that passes urine out of the body. Two sphincters control the flow of urine out of the body. The first sphincter moves involuntarily, while the second (located at the end of the urethra) moves voluntarily. In both males and females, urine passes out of the body through an opening called the *meatus*.

How Do the Male and Female Reproductive Systems Differ?

There are several anatomical and physiological differences between the male and female reproductive systems; however, both systems are designed to achieve the same purpose—to produce children. The *male reproductive system* is designed to facilitate *conception*

(the union of a sperm and an ovum). To do this, the male reproductive system produces sufficient sperm to fertilize an ovum, or *egg*. The *female reproductive system* produces ova, supports the development of an embryo, and nourishes a baby through lactation after birth.

Male Reproductive System

The male reproductive system contains both external and internal organs and structures (**Figure 9.21**). The external organs are the scrotum and the penis. Internal organs help in the creation, storage, and transport of **sperm**. The sperm is the male reproductive cell that fertilizes a female's ovum.

External Male Reproductive Organs

The *scrotum* is a pouch covered by skin that hangs outside the body between the thighs. The scrotum contains the testes, or *testicles*, glands responsible for developing sperm.

Sperm form in small tubes within the testes. Sperm then move to the *epididymis*, a tube located outside the testes. Sperm continue to mature, and each sperm develops a tail called a *flagellum*, which help sperm move up the vagina.

The penis is located above the scrotum and is made up of three layers of spongy erectile tissue and sensory receptors. The penis is responsible for excreting both urine and sperm through the *glans penis*, the portion located at the distal end. In uncircumcised males, a fold of skin, called the foreskin or *prepuce*, covers the glans penis.

Internal Male Reproductive Organs

The internal male reproductive organs include the interior duct system, seminal vesicles, and prostate gland. The interior duct system moves sperm from the epididymis to the *vas deferens*. From there, sperm are transported to the pelvic cavity and to ejaculatory ducts within the *prostate gland*. The prostate gland opens into the urethra.

Seminal vesicles located in the pelvic cavity produce *semen*, the fluid that transports sperm during sexual intercourse. Semen empties into the ejaculatory duct until it is released during a process called *ejaculation*. The muscular prostate gland, located under the urinary bladder, secretes a thick fluid that lowers the acidity of semen and also aids in the release of semen during ejaculation.

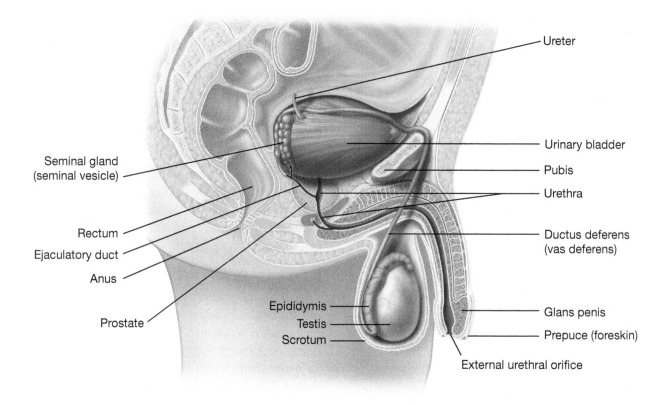

Seminal gland (seminal vesicle)

Rectum

Ejaculatory duct

Anus

Prostate

Epididymis

Testis

Scrotum

Ureter

Urinary bladder

Pubis

Urethra

Ductus deferens (vas deferens)

Glans penis

Prepuce (foreskin)

External urethral orifice

© Body Scientific International

Figure 9.21 The organs of the male reproductive system create and transport sperm.

Female Reproductive System

The female reproductive system also has both external and internal organs and structures. The external structures include the breasts, vulva, labia, and clitoris. Internal structures include the vagina, uterus, fallopian tubes, and ovaries.

External Female Reproductive Organs

The primary external female reproductive organs are the mammary glands, or *breasts*. Breasts change in size and function during puberty, during pregnancy, and after childbirth. On the outsides of the breasts are nipples surrounded by dark areas called *areolas*. Within the breasts are lobes, and each lobe contains lobules. Lobules produce breastmilk after childbirth. The milk produced by lobules is carried to the nipples via *lactiferous ducts*. Layers of fat (adipose) tissue surround the internal structures of the breast.

In females, the external genitalia is called the *vulva*. The vulva includes the *mons pubis*, where pubic hair grows (**Figure 9.22**). Two pairs of skin folds called the *labia* protect the vulva, vagina, and urethra from pathogens. Each outer fold of the labia is

a *labium majus* (collectively called the *labia majora*). Each inner fold is a *labium minus* (collectively called the *labia minora*). Between the labia minora is the *vestibule*, an area that contains the openings of the urethra (meatus) and vagina. Glands on the sides of the vaginal opening secrete mucus for lubrication. Also located at the anterior end of the vestibule is the *clitoris*, which is composed of erectile tissue.

Internal Female Reproductive Organs

The *vagina* is a flexible, tubelike structure with a mucous lining (**Figure 9.23**). The vagina conducts monthly menstrual flow, receives sperm during intercourse, and serves as the birth canal. The vagina extends into the body and is attached to the uterus at the cervix. The *uterus*, a hollow, muscular organ, is sometimes called the *womb*. The uterus has a mucous lining and a rich blood supply.

The two ovaries are filled with ova (*eggs*), the female sex cells. The ova grow inside fluid-filled sacs called *follicles*. Once a female reaches puberty, she starts ovulating, and ova are released into the *fallopian tubes*.

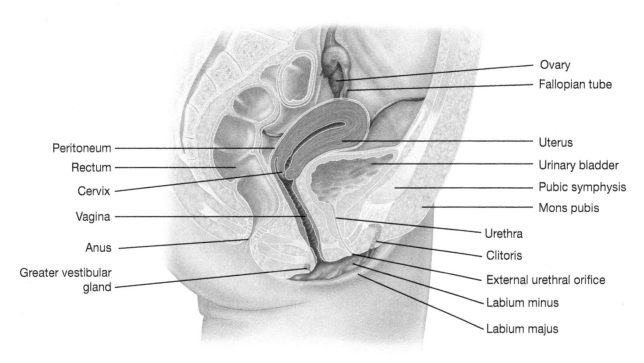

Figure 9.22 This side view of the female reproductive system shows both the external and internal female reproductive organs.

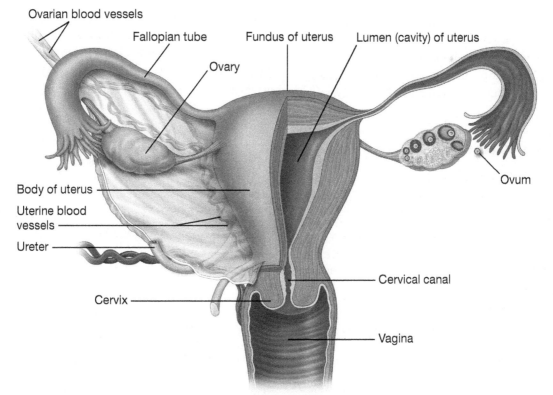

Figure 9.23 The internal organs of the female reproductive system create and transport ova. The uterus provides a home for a developing fetus for an average of 40 weeks.

Pharmacogenomics

John recently read a report online about a local company that was offering people the opportunity to learn about their DNA. The company was offering to analyze an individual's genome using a sample of saliva. The program, called "Getting to Know Your Genome," claimed it could help individuals be more aware of their genetic risks. It also claimed that individuals would learn how to choose the best medications and doses as part of a new science called *pharmacogenomics*.

Apply It

1. What benefits might John and his family have by participating in this program?
2. What disadvantages might John and his family have by participating in this program?

The fallopian tubes transport ova released from the ovaries during ovulation. If an ovum is not fertilized by a sperm, it will be removed from the uterus during *menstruation*, the monthly shedding of the uterine lining. If the ovum is fertilized, it will implant in the wall of the uterus. The uterus provides the "home" for a *fetus*, or unborn child. The uterus has enough elasticity to manage the growth of a fetus for an average of 40 weeks.

DNA and Reproduction

Deoxyribonucleic acid (DNA) plays an important role in reproduction. DNA molecules are found within the nucleus of every human cell. The complete set of DNA is known as the *genome*. The genome contains the instructions needed for an organism to reproduce, develop, and survive. It also contains the biological instructions that make each human unique. Each DNA sequence that contains these instructions is called a *gene*.

DNA molecules are tightly packaged and unwind only when DNA is reproduced. When DNA molecules are packaged, they are called *chromosomes*. The complete DNA genome has approximately 20,000 genes on 23 pairs of chromosomes. When reproduction occurs, humans inherit half of their DNA from their fathers and half from their mothers.

How Do Lifestyle Choices and Aging Affect Body Systems?

Not only are people responsible for forming opinions about their health and levels of wellness or illness, but they also make lifestyle choices that affect the body's health as they age. For instance, maintaining a healthy weight during adulthood and exercising regularly will

---

The Effects of Aging

Aging has many consequences on the human body. A resident's physical ability and movement can be greatly affected. A resident's appearance may also change, and there may be less interest in personal hygiene and eating. As people age, reading and oral communication may slow down. Residents may become frustrated with their slowness and memory changes. Attention to detail and the ability to organize information may lessen or deteriorate, leading to changes in daily habits, personal interests, and even the desire to drive. Some may avoid other older adults and believe they are less interesting. Residents may also lose their interest in interacting with others.

Changes that residents experience due to aging can have a significant impact and can greatly influence their lifestyles, needs, and desires. As a holistic nursing assistant, you must be sensitive to residents' responses to aging. You should also look for opportunities to promote residents' well-being and support their physical, emotional, and spiritual needs.

Apply It

1. Have you had experiences with older adults? If you have, what have you noticed about how older adults respond to their physical and mental changes?
2. If you were asked to care for an older adult, what could you do to help the adult improve his or her physical activity or lifestyle?
3. Now that you know the effects of aging, what can you do to slow down your aging process?

help prevent certain diseases and conditions, such as diabetes, that often come with age. Exercise also increases mobility and balance, which help people avoid the risk of falling.

Even if people follow the best health practices and make the best lifestyle choices, the body changes with age. These changes affect the structures and functions of individual cells and major body systems.

Changes to Cells, Tissues, and Organs

When cells age, they begin to function poorly or even abnormally. Cells also die as a part of normal body processes, usually to make room for new cells. Cells also die because they can only divide and multiply a limited number of times over a lifetime. If a cell cannot divide, it will grow larger and then die. Cells may also die if damaged by harmful substances such as sunlight, radiation, or certain medications.

Body tissues also change with age. For example, connective tissue becomes stiffer. This causes organs and airways to become more rigid, which makes it more difficult for the body to breathe and receive adequate nutrition. Tissue can also shrink (*atrophy*) or develop lumps called *nodules*.

Because of cell and tissue changes, organs also change and begin to function less effectively. Most body functions peak shortly before age 30 and then begin to gradually decline. As people age, their organs do not have the same ability to function as they once did. Overworking a weak organ can cause damage to the organ or even organ failure.

Over time, the most significant organ changes occur in the heart, lungs, and kidneys. Often, the aging of one organ also affects the functions of other organs. A person with rigid or narrow blood vessels may also experience breathing problems because the cardio-vascular and respiratory systems work together.

The Aging Body

All people age differently; however, the first signs of aging usually involve the skeletal and muscular systems. As people age, they begin to lose bone density, lose balance, and have problems with mobility. These signs may be followed by changes in the eyes and ears. **Figure 9.24** lists common changes in the aging body systems.

Body System Changes with Age

Body System	Signs of Aging
Integumentary system	• Skin tears more easily and bruises take longer to heal. • The ability to tolerate cold decreases. • Old-age spots appear on the skin. • Blood flow to the skin decreases. • Skin becomes dry. • Nerve endings become less sensitive to sensations such as pain. • Skin has a harder time converting sunlight to vitamin D, leading to a possible deficiency. • Hair thins and becomes gray or white. • Fingernails become rigid and may yellow or split. • Toenails change shape and thicken.
Skeletal system	• Bone loss occurs (called *osteoporosis*). • The face may sag, and eyes appear to shrink into the head due to decreases in bone and fat volume. • Deterioration to the vertebra at the top of the spine causes the head to tip forward. • Cartilage lining the joints thins and becomes less flexible, increasing likelihood of injury. • Lubricating fluid in the joints lessens, causing ligaments to lose flexibility.

(continued)

Goodheart-Willcox Publisher

Figure 9.24 The process of aging affects all of the body systems.

Body System	Signs of Aging
Muscular system	• Muscle tissue and strength starts decreasing at age 30. • The number and size of muscle fibers permanently decrease, making exercise more challenging. • Muscle is replaced by fatty or fibrous tissue, making muscles stiff. • Muscle is replaced by body fat. This changes the shape of the body as fat settles in the abdomen and buttocks.
Nervous system	• Chemical messages in the brain slow down. • Sensation may decrease. • Blood flow to the brain decreases. • The cerebellum may deteriorate, causing loss of balance. • By age 70, short-term memory, the learning of new material, and recall may be more difficult.
Sensory system	• The lens of the eye stiffens, making it harder to focus on close objects. • The lens becomes denser, and it is more difficult to see in dim light. • The lens yellows, changing the way colors are perceived. • Sensitivity to glare increases. • The eyes produce less fluid and tears, making them feel dry. • Tiny black specks (floaters) move across the field of vision. • Changes in ear structure and nerve cells cause age-related hearing loss. • Inner ear structures stiffen and deteriorate slightly, making a person unsteady. • Hearing worsens, making it harder to hear high- and low-pitched sounds.
Endocrine system	• The thyroid may shrink and function less effectively. • Metabolism of sugar and carbohydrates is less effective, possibly leading to type 2 diabetes. • Levels and activity of growth hormones decrease, affecting muscle mass. • Metabolism of fat, cholesterol, calcium, and vitamin D may change.
Cardiovascular system	• Heart muscle reduces in size, and blood vessels become stiff and less elastic. • Plaque accumulates on the insides of the arteries (*atherosclerosis*). • Arteries harden and lose their elasticity (*arteriosclerosis*), decreasing blood flow. • The amount of bone marrow decreases. • Blood cell production slows.
Immune and lymphatic systems	• The thymus slows down. • Cells are less able to destroy pathogens and other foreign substances, increasing the risk of infection; sometimes cells attack normal, healthy blood cells.
Respiratory system	• Alveoli, airways, and tissues lose elasticity and become more rigid. • The diaphragm weakens. • Pathogen-fighting cells fail, making it harder for the lungs to fight infection. • A person's cough weakens, making it harder to clear the lungs.

(continued)

Goodheart-Willcox Publisher

Figure 9.24 *(Continued)*

Body System	Signs of Aging
Gastrointestinal system	• Muscles in the esophagus weaken, sometimes causing problems with swallowing. • The stomach is less elastic and holds a smaller amount of food. • Less lactase (an enzyme needed to digest milk) is produced. • Food moves more slowly through the large intestine, increasing the possibility of blockage and constipation. • Liver enzymes function less effectively, making it harder to remove drugs and other substances from the body. • Taste buds lose sensitivity. • The sense of smell lessens. • Mouth dryness increases because less saliva is produced. • Dry mouth and loss of taste and smell reduce the ability to taste food and lessen appetite. • Teeth weaken and become brittle, and tooth enamel tends to wear away. • Gums may start to pull away from the teeth, causing the gumline to become exposed to bacteria and food.
Urinary system	• The number of kidney cells decreases, causing the kidneys to shrink in size. • Fewer nephrons filter the removal of waste products. • Bladder volume can shrink by one-half, causing more frequent urination. • Overactive bladder muscles may cause a feeling of needing to urinate, and muscles can weaken so the bladder is not completely emptied. • Weakened urinary sphincter muscles may cause leakage. • The prostate gland may enlarge, interfering with the passage of urine and full emptying of the bladder. • Older men may experience a longer start to their urine streams, have less force when urinating, and dribble at the end of urination.
Reproductive systems	• Estrogen levels decrease, causing the ovaries and uterus to become smaller and causing the tissues and lining of the vagina to become thinner, drier, and less flexible. • Breasts may become less firm and more fibrous and often will sag. • Male sex drive decreases. • Fewer sperm are produced. • Erectile dysfunction may occur due to changes in aging blood vessel circulation.

Goodheart-Willcox Publisher

Figure 9.24 *(Continued)*

SECTION 9.2 **Review and Assessment**

Key Terms Mini Glossary

alimentary canal a muscular tube of organs that starts in the mouth and leads down to the anus; a part of the gastrointestinal system; also called the *gastrointestinal (GI) tract*.

anatomy the study of the body's structure and parts.

appendicular skeleton the skeletal structure that enables the body to move; includes bones in the body's appendages (arms and legs).

autonomic nervous system (ANS) the part of the peripheral nervous system that controls involuntary, unconscious body functions.

axial skeleton the skeletal structure that provides stability for the body; includes bones in the body's trunk.

central nervous system (CNS) the part of the nervous system that consists of the brain and spinal cord.

deoxyribonucleic acid (DNA) a chemical compound that contains instructions for developing and directing the growth and activities of living organisms.

ducts tubes for conveying substances in the body.

endocrine glands ductless glands that secrete hormones directly into the bloodstream.

exocrine glands glands with ducts that transport hormones to other organs or to the surface of the skin.

gland a group of specialized cells that secrete substances.

ligaments fibrous cords of tissue that attach bone to bone and support organs.

peripheral nervous system (PNS) the part of the nervous system that consists of 12 pairs of cranial nerves and 31 pairs of spinal nerves.

physiology the study of how the body functions.

plasma the liquid component of blood; composed of water, hormones, protein, sugar, and waste products.

platelets flat, circular cells in the blood that assist in the clotting process.

receptors sensory nerve endings on or within a cell that react to various stimuli and produce an effect.

red blood cells the components of the blood that contain hemoglobin; responsible for oxygen and carbon dioxide exchange; also called *erythrocytes*.

somatic nervous system the part of the peripheral nervous system that controls voluntary body functions and the movement of skeletal muscle.

sperm the male reproductive cell; fertilizes the ovum during reproduction.

sphincter a circular muscle that can open or close; found in the heart and gastrointestinal system.

tendons bands of fibrous tissue that connect muscle to bone.

white blood cells components of the blood that fight infection and provide protection; also called *leukocytes*.

Apply the Key Terms

Complete the following sentences using the key terms in this section.

1. _____, or erythrocytes, are components of the blood that contain hemoglobin and are responsible for oxygen and carbon dioxide exchange.
2. The fibrous cords of tissue that attach bone to bone and support organs are called _____.
3. When a person studies the body's structure and parts they are learning _____.
4. _____ are ductless and secrete hormones directly into the bloodstream.
5. The skeletal structure that provides stability for the body and includes bones in the body's trunk is called the _____.

Know and Understand the Facts

1. Which organ is primarily responsible for breathing?
2. Which body systems are responsible for body movement?
3. Describe how the urinary system excretes waste.
4. List one lifestyle habit that can be changed to delay the aging of a body system.
5. Identify two organs that are affected by aging and explain how they change.

Analyze and Apply Concepts

1. Select one body system and describe the locations and functions of its organs.
2. Identify two body systems whose organs work together to achieve a particular function and describe that function.
3. Explain how the hormones of the endocrine system regulate body functions.

Think Critically

Read the following care situation. Then answer the questions that follow.

Seventy-five-year-old Mrs. V fell last week. She is now back at the healthcare facility with her right humerus, wrist, ankle, and two ribs fractured (broken). She still has bruises on her face and neck, and her balance is not good. Prior to the accident, she was having difficulty breathing and used a walker to ambulate. She also has a urinary catheter.

1. Which body systems were affected by Mrs. V's accident?
2. List three body functions that will be affected by Mrs. V's injuries.
3. How has and will her aging process influence her injuries and healing process?

9 Summary and Review

Key Points

Reviewing the key points for this chapter will help you practice more safely and competently as a holistic nursing assistant and will help you prepare for the certification competency examination.

- Holistic nursing assistants use medical terminology daily to make observations, understand and provide descriptions, and receive and give instructions about care.
- Specific terms refer to body cavities and body positions. There are also terms that refer to body directions and movements.
- Cells, membranes, and tissues are the foundation of life and have unique and specific functions.
- The body systems include the integumentary, skeletal, muscular, nervous, sensory, endocrine, cardiovascular, lymphatic and immune, gastrointestinal, respiratory, urinary, and reproductive systems. These body systems work independently and as a whole.
- People make lifestyle choices that affect their health as they grow older. While following best health practices helps the aging process, the body changes as a result of aging. Change occurs in the structures and functions of individual cells and major body systems.

Action Steps to Holistic Care

Review the information in this chapter. Complete the following activities.

1. As a nursing assistant, you will be expected to know many medical abbreviations and acronyms.

Using Figure 9.1 as a guide, create flash cards by writing the abbreviation or acronym on one side and the definition on the other. Then review these with a partner.

2. Research one body system and describe two facts about the system that were not discussed in this chapter.
3. With a partner, prepare a poster about the structure or function of a body system or organ. List the information that is most important to know when providing care.
4. Find two pictures in a magazine, in a newspaper, or online that best demonstrate the aging process. Explain why you selected these images.
5. Body systems often work together to achieve homeostasis. Identify two body systems that work together, explain their relationship, the contributions of each system, and the shared goal. Then prepare a report outlining your findings.

Building Math Skill

Juan is taking Mrs. G's blood pressure. When he charts her blood pressure, he knows that the systolic measure is the higher number and the diastolic is the lower number. The following is what he charted.

Mrs. G: 128/88 at 9 a.m.

Mrs. G: 150/96 at 6 p.m.

What is the difference in Mrs. G's blood pressure from her morning B/P to the one in the evening?

Preparing for the Certification Competency Examination

To prepare for the nursing assistant certification competency examination, you will need to know content found in this chapter. This content may be tested in the knowledge (written or oral) and skills (hands-on demonstration) portions of the exam. The following areas will be emphasized:

- medical terminology and abbreviations
- the structure of the body and body systems, including cells, tissues, and organs
- the functions and normal aging of the following body systems: integumentary, muscular, skeletal, respiratory, cardiovascular, nervous, sensory, lymphatic and immune, gastrointestinal, endocrine, urinary, and reproductive systems

These sample test questions are similar to ones you will find on the certification competency exam. See how well you can answer them. Be sure to select the *best* answer.

1. Which of the following is the smallest structural and functional unit of the human body?
   A. tissue
   B. membrane
   C. cell
   D. organ

2. What is the medical abbreviation for *activities of daily living*?
   A. ACLs
   B. ACDLs
   C. ADALs
   D. ADLs

(Continued)

3. A nursing assistant is asked to write the medical term meaning "disease of the nerves." Which of the following terms should he or she use?
   A. neuralgia
   B. neuropathy
   C. arthroscopy
   D. arthritis

4. What is a ligament?
   A. a fibrous cord of tissue that attaches bone to bone
   B. a fibrous cord of tissue that attaches muscle to bone
   C. a fibrous cord of tissue that attaches muscles to blood vessels
   D. a fibrous cord of tissue that attaches bone to nerves

5. You are taking care of Mr. M, an 85-year-old resident. He shares that his eyes feel very dry and itchy. Why might this be happening?
   A. aging of his skin and eyes
   B. drinking too much coffee
   C. using his walker too often
   D. aging of his lungs

6. The medical term *arthritis* is composed of a
   A. root word and prefix
   B. prefix and suffix
   C. root word and suffix
   D. root word and combining vowel

7. Which of the following is *not* a structure of the alimentary canal?
   A. oral cavity
   B. nasal cavity
   C. duodenum
   D. esophagus

8. A new nursing assistant is asked to have Mrs. A seated in her bed with the backrest of her bed at a 45° angle and her legs extended flat. Which position is this?
   A. supine
   B. Fowler's
   C. lateral
   D. prone

9. Which of the following is a change associated with the aging process?
   A. Skin becomes thick and calloused.
   B. Skin becomes less sensitive to pain.
   C. Skin becomes very hairy.
   D. Skin becomes very flexible.

10. Which structures filter blood and remove waste products from the body?
    A. rugae
    B. cilia
    C. nephrons
    D. gallbladder

11. Which of the following cells helps blood clot?
    A. fibrinogen
    B. red blood cell
    C. white blood cell
    D. platelet

12. Which of the following terms describes the front part of the body?
    A. ventral
    B. dorsal
    C. coronal
    D. proximal

13. Which word part is the central part of a medical term?
    A. suffix
    B. prefix
    C. acronym
    D. root word

14. Mrs. M has arthritis and cannot ambulate well. As a result, she has trouble having bowel movements. Which part of her gastrointestinal tract is primarily affected?
    A. large intestine
    B. gallbladder
    C. esophagus
    D. small intestine

15. Which of the following terms is used to describe the function of the human body?
    A. chemistry
    B. physiology
    C. biology
    D. anatomy

Did you have difficulty with any of the questions? If you did, review the chapter to find the correct answer(s).

10 Diseases, Conditions, and Pain

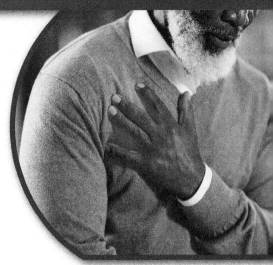

katleho Seisa/E+ via Getty Images

Welcome to the Chapter

As a nursing assistant, you will provide safe, quality care for residents who have various diseases and conditions. This chapter provides information about the relationship between wellness and illness. *Wellness* (a feeling of good health) and *illness* (a feeling of poor health) can occur at the same time. You will also learn the signs, symptoms, treatments, and care needed for common diseases and conditions. The body systems discussed in Chapter 9 provide the information needed for this discussion. You will also learn related medical terminology and abbreviations.

Diseases and conditions often cause pain. Understanding pain and knowing the best ways to observe and report it will provide you with the knowledge and skills you will need to help residents feel more comfortable.

What you learn in this chapter will help you develop your knowledge and skills to become a holistic nursing assistant. The topics discussed in the chapter are highlighted on the Providing Holistic Care Framework.

Chapter Outline

Section 10.1
Wellness, Illness, Diseases, and Conditions

Section 10.2
Pain Relief

Providing Holistic Care Framework

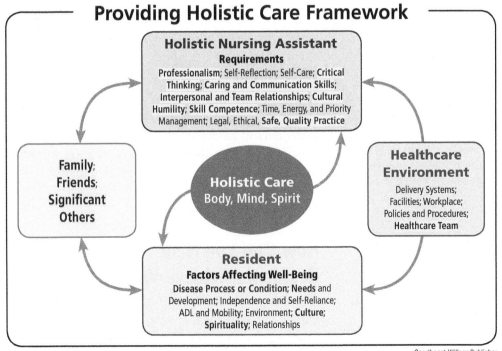

Holistic Nursing Assistant
Requirements
Professionalism; Self-Reflection; Self-Care; Critical Thinking; Caring and Communication Skills; Interpersonal and Team Relationships; Cultural Humility; Skill Competence; Time, Energy, and Priority Management; Legal, Ethical, Safe, Quality Practice

Holistic Care
Body, Mind, Spirit

Family; Friends; Significant Others

Healthcare Environment
Delivery Systems; Facilities; Workplace; Policies and Procedures; Healthcare Team

Resident
Factors Affecting Well-Being
Disease Process or Condition; Needs and Development; Independence and Self-Reliance; ADL and Mobility; Environment; Culture; Spirituality; Relationships

Goodheart-Willcox Publisher

Wellness, Illness, Diseases, and Conditions

Objectives

To achieve the objectives for this section, you must successfully:

- **identify** the differences among health, wellness, and illness.
- **explain** the difference between acute and chronic diseases and conditions.
- **identify** the signs and symptoms of common diseases and conditions for each body system.
- **describe** the treatments and care required for common diseases and conditions.
- **use** medical abbreviations and terminology related to the diseases and conditions discussed in this section.

Key Terms

Learn these key terms to better understand the information presented in the section.

acute disease	hemiplegia
analgesic	hypertension
anesthetic	illness
aneurysm	incontinence
aphasia	malignant
arrhythmias	metastasis
arteriosclerosis	necrosis
atherosclerosis	nodules
benign	pathology
biopsy	plaques
chronic disease	sclerosis
coma	sign
dialysis	symptom
disease	well-being
edema	wellness
health	

Questions to Consider

- Living with a disease or medical condition can be very challenging and difficult. Do you know someone who is living with a serious disease or condition? If so, what has this person told you about the experience?
- What changes has the person made to learn to live with the disease or condition and achieve some level of wellness? Have these changes been helpful?

What Is the Relationship between Wellness and Illness?

The relationship between *wellness* (a feeling of good health) and *illness* (a feeling of poor health) is not simple. Some healthcare providers show *wellness* on one end of a straight line and *illness* on the other end. This is not always a real picture. Even when people experience illness, parts of their bodies and minds can still be well. For example, when you catch a cold, you may have a cough and a runny nose but at the same time your heart is beating properly, your muscles and bones allow you to walk, and you may still have a good appetite.

Illness vs. Disease

Being ill, or having an illness, is not the same as having a disease. A *disease* occurs when an organ or body system is not working properly, causing specific symptoms that can be diagnosed by a licensed healthcare provider, such as a doctor. *Illness* is your personal interpretation of how you are feeling. You may feel dizzy even if nothing is wrong with any of your body systems. Anxiety or fear may be causing shallow, rapid breathing, which causes you to feel dizzy.

People often have different understandings about diseases they have. How they understand the disease and accept it will influence the way they react to it. People who understand the disease and are able to accept it will likely agree to, and follow, the needed treatment. If they have little or no understanding and acceptance, they may react with fear and confusion. A person with a disease who feels well will be more likely to manage the disease in a way that has a positive impact on his or her *health* (physical, mental, social, and spiritual condition).

Well-Being

The relationship between wellness and illness influences a person's sense of *well-being* (state of health). Every person has his or her own sense of well-being, which may not be affected by disease. This is important to remember as you care for others. No matter how ill a resident may be, some level of wellness is always possible (**Figure 10.1**).

How Can You Help Yourself and Residents Achieve Wellness?

Achieving wellness is a daily, 24-hour responsibility. Eating a healthy meal one day a week is not enough to achieve wellness. Achieving wellness requires

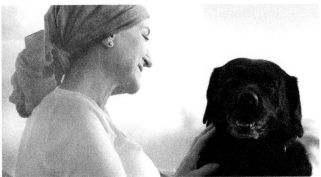

Figure 10.1 Even if a person has a serious disease, he or she can achieve some level of wellness.

self-awareness, commitment to wellness strategies, and ongoing change. Using wellness strategies will not only allow you to achieve your own wellness, but will also help you better care for others.

Wellness and Residents

Remember that, while you can support and promote residents' wellness and well-being, residents have the responsibility to take action and improve their own states of health, wellness, or illness. If you find that a facility or healthcare provider focuses more on residents' diseases and illnesses than on health and well-being, do not let that stop you from promoting wellness as you work with residents.

As a holistic nursing assistant, you can use your knowledge of residents' conditions to help them progress by finding time during your shift to informally provide information to residents while giving care. For example, you can show a resident the importance of exercising hands and feet when assisting with daily hygiene. You can remind residents of important safety precautions while helping them ambulate. Paying attention to possible opportunities can be very beneficial.

Use a positive approach and attitude when you care for residents. Your support can make a difference in residents' wellness and can help residents choose to feel better about themselves and their situations. Your support and encouragement can help residents see themselves as worthwhile.

Encourage residents to be as independent as possible. When appropriate, ask residents to be more involved in their daily hygiene, such as bathing or brushing their teeth. You can also encourage increased activity and ambulation (walking) as residents are able. These activities will help residents establish a routine and help them become more independent. Being independent can be comforting to some residents.

Try to increase residents' social interactions and activities. If a resident has not been out of his or her room, and is able, encourage the resident to visit the dining room or participate in a facility activity. Participating in social activities is a strategy for achieving wellness. Sometimes a simple invitation or suggestion can make a difference. Forming supportive, positive relationships with residents can help you have a greater influence on residents' wellness.

Wellness and the Holistic Nursing Assistant

It is important to remember that you must also be aware of your *own* health and well-being. Becoming more aware starts with how you see illness, wellness, and health. As you decide what *illness*, *wellness*, and *health* mean to you, you will be better able to personalize your care for others. Start by being alert, present, and nonjudgmental. Including behaviors and actions in your daily life that help maintain your health and well-being will help you succeed. The following questions will help you establish your own level of health and well-being:

- What are your eating habits? Do you regularly choose healthy foods? Do you snack on candy or skip meals? Do you eat in front of the television, or do you sit down at a table and eat your meal slowly?
- How often do you exercise and participate in physical activities? Do you maintain a healthy weight and exercise at least 150 minutes each week?
- Do you choose not to use tobacco products and drugs, and do you keep your alcohol consumption to a minimum?
- Do you get between 7 and 9 hours of sleep each night?
- Have you found strategies (methods) to manage stress effectively?
- Do you participate regularly in social activities? Are you part of a group that enjoys playing sports or going to the movies?
- Do you have a strong support group of family and friends?
- Do you think about your personal safety and that of others? Do you avoid driving when you are tired? Do you refuse to text and drive at the same time?
- Do you attempt to prevent and control the spread of disease? Do you wash your hands or use hand sanitizer before meals? Do you cover your mouth when you cough or sneeze?
- How happy do you feel every day? Do you wake up and look forward to your day? Do you appreciate nature and the environment around you?

Think about your answers to these questions. Do you feel you have achieved the best health and well-being possible, or is there room for improvement? What strategies can you use to maintain your own health and wellness?

What Is the Difference between a Disease and a Condition?

As you learned earlier in this chapter, a *disease* occurs when an organ or body system functions incorrectly and particular signs and symptoms appear. In contrast, the term *condition* is a particular physical or mental state of health or illness. For example, a person might say, "I have a heart condition," which means the person's heart may not be functioning properly. The person's disease may be coronary artery disease due to a buildup of plaque in the arteries.

Diseases and conditions can be acute or chronic. An *acute disease* is short-term and usually starts suddenly. A *chronic disease* is long-term or recurring. With treatment, an acute disease will go away or will not recur (come back) for a long time. For a disease or condition to be considered chronic, it must last for at least three months. Most chronic diseases and conditions, however, can last a lifetime.

Living with any chronic disease or condition can be frightening and frustrating. A chronic disease often requires constant attention. Many people with chronic diseases or conditions go through periods of sadness, discouragement, hopelessness, anger, and depression.

Classifying Diseases by Cause

Diseases are classified to show similarities and differences. This type of classification is also a way to study the trends, causes, and effects of certain diseases in particular populations. The following classifications are by causes of disease:

- **Genetic or congenital disorder**: caused by a person's genes or by an event at birth. Examples include Down syndrome, sickle cell anemia, and cerebral palsy (**Figure 10.2**).
- **Infectious disease**: also called *pathogenic disease*; caused by microorganisms such as bacteria or viruses. Examples include hepatitis (caused by a virus) or tuberculosis (caused by bacteria).
- **Degenerative disease**: a result of cell breakdown over time, which causes changes in tissues and organs. Examples include arthritis and Parkinson's disease.

- **Nutritional disease**: a deficiency or excess in a person's diet. An example is rickets, which is caused by vitamin deficiency.
- **Cancer**: caused by the production of abnormal or excess body cells. Examples include melanoma, breast cancer, and leukemia.

Classifying Diseases and Conditions by Body System

Another method for classifying diseases and conditions is by the affected body system. Conditions are categorized using the body system or organ that is affected. For example, a person may have a skin or lung condition. Each disease is related to a particular ***pathology***, or changes that occur in the body's tissues and organs as a result of the disease. Pathology includes a disease's signs and symptoms. A ***sign*** is objective, or factual, information about a disease or condition. A ***symptom*** is subjective information about a disease or condition based on a person's feelings or opinions. Each disease has unique signs, symptoms, treatments, and specific plans for care.

In this chapter, you will learn about the diseases and conditions you will encounter most often when you begin working as a nursing assistant. For many of these diseases and conditions, treatments include prescribed medications. If a resident is taking prescribed medications, be sure to observe the resident closely. If the resident changes his or her normal patterns—physically, mentally, or emotionally—he or she may be experiencing a side or adverse effect from the medication or an allergy or sensitivity to its chemical or natural ingredients. These observations need to be reported

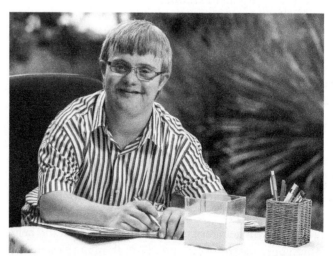

karelnoppe/Shutterstock.com

Figure 10.2 Down syndrome is an example of a genetic disease.

to the licensed nursing staff immediately so that action can be taken. Also, always confirm with the licensed nursing staff that the care you give follows facility policy, the doctor's orders, and the plan of care.

Which Diseases and Conditions Affect the Integumentary System?

Several common diseases and conditions that affect the integumentary system (skin, hair, and nails). Among others, these include keratosis, psoriasis, shingles, and decubitus ulcers.

Keratosis

Keratosis is a condition in which there is too much *keratin* (a skin protein) in the skin. Two forms of keratosis are keratosis pilaris and seborrheic keratosis.

Keratosis pilaris is a skin condition that cannot be prevented or cured. It is identified by patches of thick, dry skin; painless rough patches; and tiny bumps. Treatment usually consists of moisturizers, and in some cases, prescription creams to improve the skin's appearance.

Seborrheic keratosis, identified by round or oval-shaped growths, is noncancerous, and may develop with age or from increased exposure to the sun. The growths start as small, rough patches that develop into thick, wart-like growths. They look waxy; are slightly raised; and are usually brown in color, but can also be yellow, white, or black. A growth should be surgically removed if it looks suspicious or is causing physical discomfort or emotional distress.

Psoriasis

Psoriasis is a condition with an unknown cause that is identified by the excessive growth of new skin cells on the top layer of the skin. This condition typically

affects the knees, elbows, and scalp. Thick, red patches called *plaques* develop due to swollen blood vessels below the skin. Plaques are often covered with loose, silver-colored scales that may be itchy and painful (**Figure 10.3**).

Treatments for psoriasis are primarily topical (applied to the surface of the skin) over-the-counter or prescription ointments, creams, and shampoos. Other treatments include oral and injectable medications and light therapies. Sunlight is also helpful for treating psoriasis, although sunscreen should be worn and sun exposure should be limited to 20 minutes daily, three days a week.

When caring for residents with psoriasis, lotions or creams keep the skin moist and avoid itchiness. However, use these less frequently in warm weather, as the combination of sweat and lotion can make psoriasis worse. Regular baths using lukewarm water can help avoid dry skin. Pat, rather than rub, the skin with a dry towel after bathing. Wrap the affected skin in a bandage or plastic wrap and wash gently in the morning to reduce scaling.

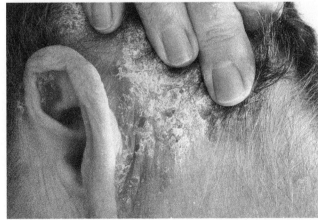

Lipowski Milan/Shutterstock.com

Figure 10.3 Psoriasis causes plaques, which are often covered with silver-colored scales.

Shingles

Shingles, or *herpes zoster*, is a painful skin rash caused by the varicella-zoster virus. The varicella-zoster virus also causes chickenpox. Everyone is at risk for shingles; however, shingles is more common among people who are over 50 years of age or who have weakened immune systems (due to stress or taking certain medications, for example). A vaccine exists for shingles, which lowers a person's chance for getting the virus. If a vaccinated person gets shingles, the person will have less pain and a rash that clears more quickly. Shingles itself is not contagious, although exposure to shingles blisters can cause chickenpox in people who have never had chickenpox or received its vaccine.

Shingles symptoms typically develop in stages. The first stage starts with a headache and the person may have light sensitivity and flu-like symptoms. The next stage includes tingling, itching, or pain in the area where a rash may appear. For some people, no rash appears; others have a mild rash; and yet others have a noticeable rash with fluid-filled blisters that crust over in two to four weeks and may leave scars (**Figure 10.4**). Shingles is treated with antiviral medications and **analgesics** (pain medications).

Decubitus Ulcers

A decubitus ulcer is sometimes called a *bedsore*, *pressure ulcer*, or *pressure injury*. It is a skin condition caused by continuous pressure on the skin and on bony areas (or *projections*) that restricts or prevents

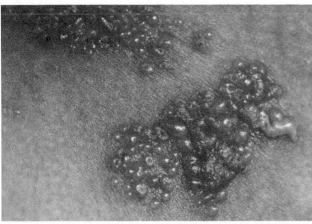

santol/Shutterstock.com

Figure 10.4 Shingles rashes often contain fluid-filled blisters, which may be painful. Check the resident's pain levels and alert the licensed nursing staff if pain relief is needed.

blood flow. Continuous pressure can result from resident immobility (inability to move) or from rubbing on the skin. Items that rub the skin may include bed covers, clothing, wrinkled or wadded-up sheets, tubing on or around the body, and even food crumbs in the bedding. Fragile skin is particularly at risk for decubitus ulcers. Other risk factors for this condition are inability to feel pain, muscle spasms, poor nutrition, extreme weight loss, and **incontinence** (lack of bowel or bladder control).

Stages of Decubitus Ulcers

The severity of decubitus ulcers is identified using four stages (**Figure 10.5**):

- **Stage 1**: the skin is not open, but appears red, blue, or purple depending on the resident's skin tone.
- **Stage 2**: the decubitus ulcer is still considered superficial, or *shallow*, but the skin is now open. A blister filled with fluid, an abrasion, or a shallow sore that looks like a crater (hole) can be seen. The surrounding area may be irritated and red. As soon as the skin is broken, there is risk for *cellulitis*, or infection of the skin and connective tissue.
- **Stage 3**: the ulcer is much deeper than in stage 2 and may extend into underlying connective tissue. The sore looks more like a crater and may ooze, bleed, or contain pus.
- **Stage 4**: the damage is deep and may reach muscles, tendons, ligaments, joints, and bone. The ulcer will bleed, and skin and tissue **necrosis** (death) may occur. At this stage, there is risk not only of bone and joint infections, but also of system-wide infection leading to *sepsis* (a life-threatening infection in the bloodstream) and organ failure.

Sometimes a decubitus ulcer is considered *unstageable*. This happens when the ulcer is covered by a mass of dead tissue or contains dry scabs. In these situations, it is difficult to see the depth of the ulcer, and therefore, its stage cannot be identified.

Pressure Points

Certain areas of the body are more likely to develop decubitus ulcers. These susceptible areas are known as *pressure points*. Pressure points can be found where skin covers the bony areas of the body (**Figure 10.6**).

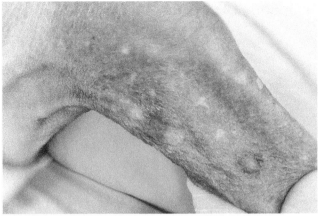

A—Stage 1

Arthit Premprayot/Shutterstock.com

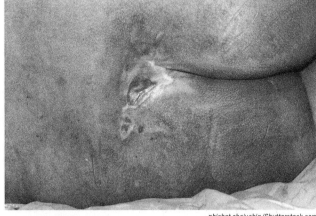

B—Stage 2

phichet chaiyabin/Shutterstock.com

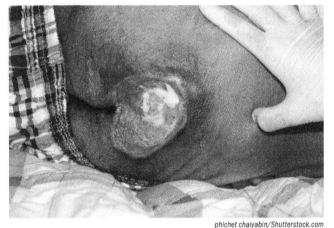

C—Stage 3

phichet chaiyabin/Shutterstock.com

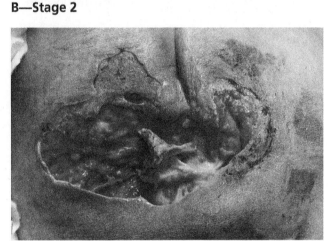

D—Stage 4

Elena Kitch/Shutterstock.com

Figure 10.5 The stages of a decubitus ulcer are shown here.

Prevention, Treatment, and Care for Decubitus Ulcers

Good skin care prevents the formation of decubitus ulcers. You will learn more about skin care in Chapter 18, but basic guidelines follow:

- Keep pressure points dry and clean.
- Ulcers must be kept clean, and dressings should be applied when needed.
- Wet or creased dressings and bandages should be changed regularly.

Regularly repositioning the resident, ambulation, and range-of-motion exercises, as directed, also help prevent decubitus ulcers. (See Chapter 14 for more information.) If a resident is immobile, the resident's position in bed or in a chair should be changed at least every two hours on a schedule, and support devices for positioning should be used. Bed linens should be smooth and free from crumbs.

If a resident develops a decubitus ulcer, good nutrition will promote wound healing. Also assist

with pain relief, as appropriate. Observe and report on the resident's skin condition, as needed. Immediately report any new redness or ulcers. Remember that residents who have a healed decubitus ulcer are at higher risk of developing the same ulcer again.

How Do Diseases and Conditions Influence Skeletal System Function?

Diseases of the skeletal system may affect a resident's mobility, cause joint pain, and increase the risk for broken bones. Common skeletal diseases and conditions include osteoporosis, arthritis, and fractures.

Osteoporosis

Osteoporosis is a condition in which the bones are *porous*, or full of holes. This occurs when the body makes too little bone or starts losing bone density, or *mass*. Loss of bone density makes the bones brittle,

Pressure Points for Decubitus Ulcers

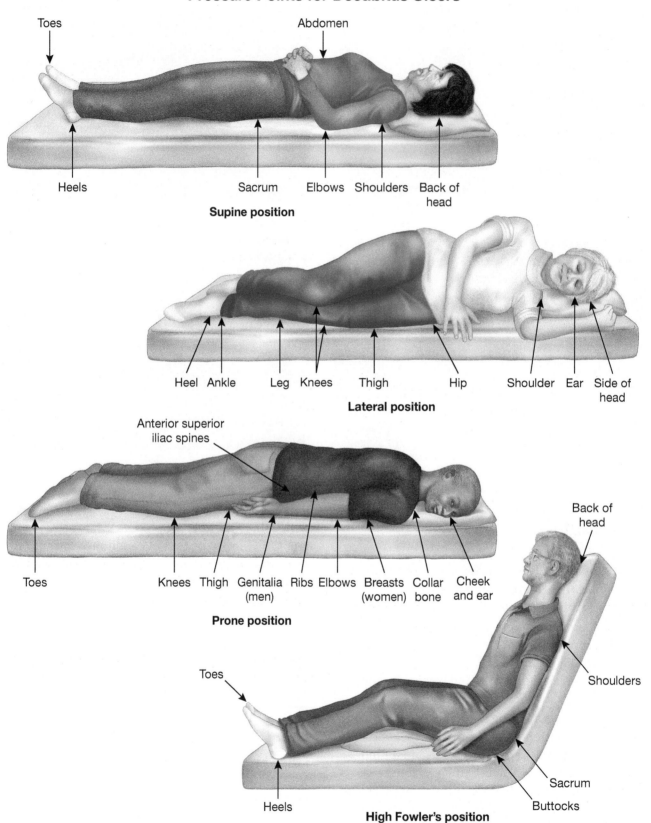

Figure 10.6 Decubitus ulcers are more likely to develop at pressure points. Bed linens may create pressure points on the toes or abdomen if the resident is lying in supine position, for example.

© Body Scientific International

increasing the risk of fracture, particularly in the hip, spine, and wrist. Symptoms such as back pain usually do not occur until the bones begin to weaken. If osteoporosis affects the vertebrae, the resident will lose height and may become stooped or hunched (**Figure 10.7**).

Older people and women are most at risk. Racial or ethnic background, too much alcohol or tobacco use, certain medical conditions or medications, and a family history of osteoporosis can also increase the risk.

Lifestyle changes are usually recommended to treat osteoporosis. These may include smoking cessation (quitting), increased physical activity, and a balanced diet. Prescription medications are available to both prevent and treat the disease. If a resident has osteoporosis, pay extra attention to how the resident is moved, positioned, and assisted with ambulation. The resident may need gentle assistance. In addition, fall-prevention strategies must be in place.

Arthritis

Arthritis describes a variety of chronic diseases and conditions in which joints are inflamed, swollen, tender, and red. While the risk of arthritis does increase with age, about two-thirds of people with arthritis are younger than 65. Arthritis is more common among women than men and affects all racial and ethnic groups.

Common symptoms of arthritis include pain, aching, stiffness, and swelling in or around joints, leading to decreased range of motion (**Figure 10.8**). The joints

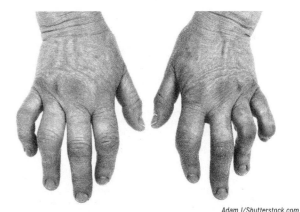

Adam J/Shutterstock.com

Figure 10.8 One sign of arthritis is inflammation of the joints.

most commonly affected by arthritis are in the hands, lower back, hips, knees, and feet. Symptoms may appear suddenly or develop gradually.

Good lifestyle habits are the best treatment for arthritis. A healthy diet and exercise help maintain a normal weight, so that extra weight does not press on inflamed, sore joints. While exercise can be painful and tiring, it is very important for maintaining range of motion. Rest periods can help when residents get tired. Mobility aids can assist with stability, balance, and gait.

You can help residents who have arthritis become more comfortable by using positioning, giving a warm bath, and maintaining a restful environment. These actions will lead to better and more restful sleep and will help the resident conserve energy.

Pain is another factor in treating arthritis. As a nursing assistant, you can assist the licensed nursing staff by providing routine information about pain levels. Also, support residents with nonmedical pain-relief approaches such as warm and cold applications (see Chapter 18), as ordered by the doctor.

Fractures

Broken bones, or *fractures*, are common skeletal system conditions. There are different types of fractures (**Figure 10.9**). Fractures can occur throughout life, but are more frequent for children and older adults, due to falls. Certain medications, lack of proper nutrition or activity, and osteoporosis can also lead to fractures, particularly in the hip. Women over 65 years of age have the highest risk of hip fractures. Some hip

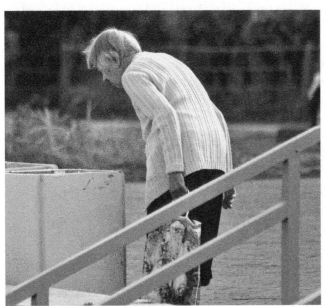

Michkasova Elena/Shutterstock.com

Figure 10.7 A resident with osteoporosis may appear stooped or hunched.

> **THINK ABOUT THIS**
>
> Bone is so strong that one cubic inch of bone can withstand 19,000 pounds or more, roughly the weight of five standard pickup trucks.

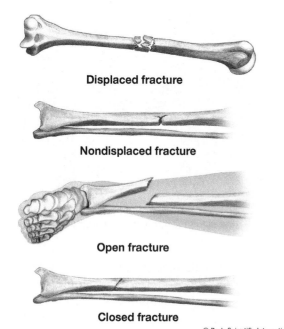

Displaced fracture

Nondisplaced fracture

Open fracture

Closed fracture

© Body Scientific International

Figure 10.9 There are four different types of bone fractures.

fractures are repaired surgically; in other cases, the hip is replaced with a prosthesis (artificial device).

After a fracture occurs, a bone needs to be set, or positioned into its proper place, using a process called *reduction*. No surgery is required for a closed reduction; in a closed reduction, a cast is used to immobilize (keep from moving) the fractured bone. Sometimes bones need to be pinned together, which requires surgery through open reduction. In open reduction, rods, screws, or plates are used to properly position the bone before a cast is applied. Casts are often made from fiberglass or plaster, and some are removable.

Cast Care

When a cast is applied, it needs to be kept dry to prevent a bad smell and skin irritation. Skin care will be needed at the edges of the cast. When caring for a resident with a cast, cover the cast with plastic and do not let water get under the cast during bathing. Keep the cast from becoming soiled if the resident uses a bedpan or urinal. Sometimes sprinkling baking soda or rubbing a fabric softener wipe on the outside of the cast can help reduce any odor. Remind residents never to push items such as hangers or pencils under the cast if the skin is itching. This can damage the skin and dislocate the cast.

Observing the Cast

Observation of a resident with a cast is extremely important. Casts must never restrict blood flow. Signs of restricted blood flow include numbness,

tingling, cold skin in the area outside the cast, and pale or bluish-colored skin (called *cyanosis*). Infection under a cast may cause the skin around the cast to be unusually warm, or odor or drainage may come out from under the cast. The resident may also have chills or a fever. Immediately report any of these signs to the licensed nursing staff.

Supportive devices such as pillows, trochanter rolls, and footboards can be used to provide proper positioning and comfort for a resident in a cast. See Chapter 14 for more information on the use of these devices.

Which Common Diseases Are Associated with the Muscular System?

There are several common muscular system diseases. Two will be discussed in this section: muscular dystrophy (MD) and amyotrophic lateral sclerosis (ALS).

Muscular Dystrophy (MD)

Muscular dystrophy (MD) is a group of diseases that cause progressive weakness and loss of muscle mass due to atrophy. In MD, abnormal genes interfere with the production of proteins needed to maintain healthy muscle tissue. There are different types of MD. Each type is caused by a unique genetic mutation (change), which is usually inherited. About one-half of MD cases are *Duchenne MD*, which typically affects young boys. There is no cure for MD.

Some types of MD are mild, progress slowly, and occur in adulthood. The main sign of MD is progressive muscle weakness. Some residents with MD will lose the ability to walk. In milder forms of MD, muscles often cannot relax following contraction, and facial and neck muscles are the first to be affected. Muscle weakness can affect breathing, and residents with MD may need breathing assistance, such as a *ventilator* (a machine that forces air in and out of the lungs). MD can reduce the efficiency of the heart muscle and can also cause difficulty swallowing (*dysphagia*).

Amyotrophic Lateral Sclerosis (ALS)

Amyotrophic lateral sclerosis (ALS) is a slow decline and deterioration of motor neurons in the brain and spinal cord. In ALS, motor neurons in the spinal cord break down, which leads to scarring or **sclerosis** (hardening) of the muscles they control. As a result, muscles waste away, or *atrophy*. When motor neurons die, the

THINK ABOUT THIS

Humans do not grow new muscle fibers; instead, existing muscles just grow thicker. This is important to know when thinking about diseases that cause muscle atrophy, or weakening.

brain's ability to start and control muscle movement is lost. Because voluntary muscle action is affected, a resident with ALS may lose the ability to speak, eat, move, and breathe.

The onset of ALS is gradual and often occurs between the ages of 40 and 70. On average, people with ALS survive 5–10 years after diagnosis. Initial symptoms may vary; one person may experience trouble speaking, and another may have a hard time picking something up. Because ALS affects only motor neurons, the senses of sight, touch, hearing, taste, and smell, as well as the muscles of the eyes and bladder, are generally not affected.

Caring for Residents with Muscular Diseases

There are a variety of ways a holistic nursing assistant can provide care for residents with progressive muscular diseases or conditions. Each of these should be guided by the resident's plan of care. For example, residents may need encouragement and assistance with ambulation, range-of-motion exercises, ADLs, and skin care. Be patient and supportive. They may also need canes, walkers, or wheelchairs to maintain mobility and independence. Elevating the head of the bed may ease shortness of breath and provide comfort if the resident has breathing issues. Good nutrition is important. Assistance with eating such as the resident sitting up straight, putting the chin on the chest when swallowing, and concentrating while eating may also help. Monitor daily fluid intake to make sure the resident gets 2,500 mL, unless **contraindicated** (advised against) because of difficulty swallowing. Also be aware of any changes in elimination patterns. Any observed changes in a resident's status should be reported to the licensed nursing staff immediately.

How Is the Nervous System Affected by Disease?

Common nervous system diseases include multiple sclerosis (MS), Parkinson's disease, and neuropathy. Injuries to the spinal cord, discussed in Chapter 21, also affect the function of this body system.

Multiple Sclerosis (MS)

Multiple sclerosis (MS) is a condition in which the immune system attacks *myelin,* the protective material that surrounds nerve fibers in the brain and spinal cord. Eventually, nerves themselves may become damaged, and nerve signals to the body may slow or be blocked (**Figure 10.10**). There are treatments for this disease, but there is no cure.

There are several different types of MS. The first symptoms of MS usually appear between the ages of 20 and 50. Women are more likely to be diagnosed with MS than men. Early MS signs and symptoms that are common among the types of MS include fatigue (exhaustion); muscle stiffness, weakness, or spasms; tingling; numbness in the face, body, arms, or legs; trouble walking; blurred vision; difficulty processing thoughts; pain; and depression.

The type of MS determines the severity of the disease and the effectiveness of treatment. Treatment may include medications to ease symptoms and manage stress. Rehabilitation may be used to promote strength and balance and reduce fatigue. People who have difficulty speaking or swallowing may also receive occupational therapy.

Parkinson's Disease

Parkinson's disease progresses gradually and causes neurons in the brain to slowly break down or die. Neurons in the brain are responsible for producing

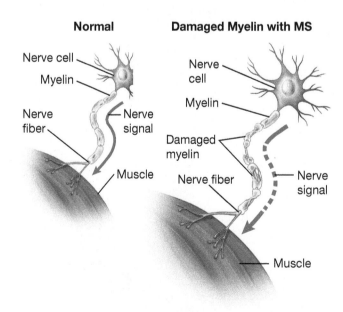

© Body Scientific International

Figure 10.10 Damage to myelin slows and interrupts the transmission of neural messages.

dopamine, an important chemical messenger. Decreased dopamine levels cause abnormal brain activity that leads to the signs and symptoms of Parkinson's disease.

Risk factors for Parkinson's disease include gender (men have a higher risk than women); age (often begins toward the middle or end of a person's life); heredity; the environment, such as exposure to certain toxins; and changes in the brain that include certain signs specific to Parkinson's disease.

Symptoms of Parkinson's disease usually begin on one side of the body. This side will always have the worst symptoms, even if symptoms eventually appear on the other side. **Figure 10.11** shows some of the typical symptoms of Parkinson's disease. Another common symptom is a movement called *pill rolling*, where the person rubs the tip of the thumb and the forefinger back and forth; tremors in the head, hands,

and fingers (when relaxed); and stooped posture and balance problems. Speech may become soft, quick, slurred, and monotone (flat-sounding). Difficulty processing thoughts, frequent waking during the night, fatigue, difficulty swallowing, accumulation of saliva in the mouth (causing drooling), depression, anxiety, constipation, and loss of bladder control may also occur.

A treatment plan of care for Parkinson's disease may include prescription medications to help improve movement and walking, reduce tremors, and treat depression. Physical therapy, speech-language therapy, exercise, and a healthy diet may be helpful. Surgery to regulate certain parts of the brain and improve symptoms may be advised for certain residents.

Neuropathy

A *neuropathy* is a disease that can affect three types of nerves:

- **Sensory nerves:** causes tingling, pain, and numbness.
- **Motor nerves:** there is weakness in the feet and hands.
- **Autonomic nerves:** there may be problems with internal organs, which can increase heart rate and lower blood pressure.

Neuropathy can involve a single nerve (*mononeuropathy*) or many nerves (*polyneuropathy*). About one-third of all neuropathies are *idiopathic*, which means the cause is unknown.

Peripheral neuropathy is one of the most common types of neuropathy in which nerves carrying messages to the body are damaged or diseased. It can be a side effect of many medications. Diabetes, vitamin deficiencies, some cancers, chronic kidney disease, and inflammatory conditions can also cause peripheral neuropathy. Injury, infection, or pressure from a tumor or broken bone lying next to or on a nerve can cause neuropathy.

Treating neuropathy may include over-the-counter and prescription pain medications, as well as topical medications such as an **anesthetic** (a medication that produces a loss of sensation). Mechanical aids, including braces or specially fitted shoes, help with muscle weakness to better support walking and reduce pain.

Caring for Residents with Neurological Diseases

As a holistic nursing assistant, there are several ways to provide care for residents with neurological

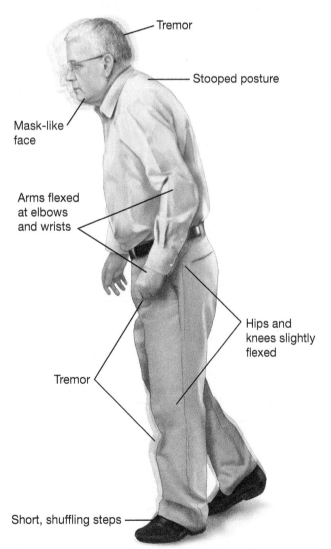

Tremor

Stooped posture

Mask-like face

Arms flexed at elbows and wrists

Hips and knees slightly flexed

Tremor

Short, shuffling steps

© Body Scientific International

Figure 10.11 There are several observable symptoms of Parkinson's disease.

diseases and conditions. The most important is to be patient and supportive. Help promote regular activity, as appropriate, and support residents who use canes or walkers. Make sure fall-prevention measures are in place. Communicate clearly, slowly, and in simple terms if the resident has cognitive challenges. Encourage residents to drink plenty of fluids to prevent constipation and assist with eating, as needed. Observe for signs of pain or depression and report any emotional or behavioral changes to the licensed nursing staff.

How Does Disease Alter Sense Organ Function?

Common sensory system diseases and conditions are cataracts, glaucoma, macular degeneration, otitis media, and Ménière's disease. Care for vision and hearing impairment or loss are discussed in detail in Chapter 21.

Cataracts

A *cataract* is a condition in which a slow buildup of protein on the lens of the eye causes clouding (**Figure 10.12**). This buildup makes it harder for light to pass through the lens, affecting sight. Vision becomes blurry as the cataract grows. The lens may become yellow or brown, which makes reading difficult, images less sharp, and colors dull. Cataracts may cause sensitivity to light and glare and the person may see halos (rings) around lights.

Cataracts can occur in one or both eyes. They are not harmful to the eye, are not contagious, and do not spread from eye to eye. Most cataracts form

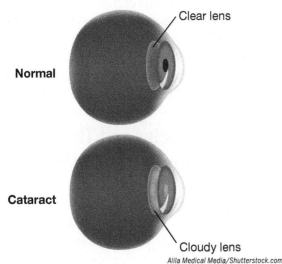

Normal

Clear lens

Cataract

Cloudy lens

Alila Medical Media/Shutterstock.com

Figure 10.12 A cataract causes clouding of the lens.

due to aging, but cataracts can also develop as a result of other diseases, such as diabetes, long-term use of steroid medications, eye injury, or congenital disorders. Risk factors for cataracts include smoking and alcohol use, family history, and prolonged exposure to the sun.

People with cataracts may benefit from changing eyeglass or contact lens prescriptions, using anti-glare sunglasses and magnifying lenses, using brighter lamps, and limiting night driving. When vision loss interferes with daily activities, such as driving or reading, surgery to replace the eye's lens with an artificial lens is recommended.

Glaucoma

Glaucoma is an incurable condition that may result in vision loss and blindness. Fluid builds up at the open angle of the eye (where the cornea and iris meet), creating pressure that can damage the optic nerve. The amount of intraocular pressure (pressure within the eye) that the optic nerve can tolerate is different for each person.

People over the age of 60, African-Americans over the age of 40, people with a family history of glaucoma, and those with high blood pressure are at risk. Glaucoma can occur in one or both eyes. Without treatment, side vision (*peripheral* vision) is lost. Glaucoma can also cause tunnel vision (narrowing of vision) and blindness.

Glaucoma can be treated using prescription oral medications and eye drops that lower eye pressure or cause the eye to make less fluid. Other treatments may include surgery to increase fluid drainage. Early diagnosis is important to prevent vision loss. Lost vision cannot be restored.

Macular Degeneration

Macular degeneration is an incurable eye disease caused by the deterioration of the *macula*, the central portion of the retina. As macular degeneration progresses, people experience wavy or blurred vision. Central vision may be completely lost over time and may leave people legally blind (**Figure 10.13**). Peripheral vision is not affected.

There are two types of macular degeneration—wet and dry. *Dry macular degeneration* is more common

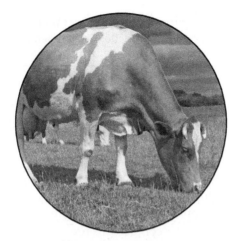

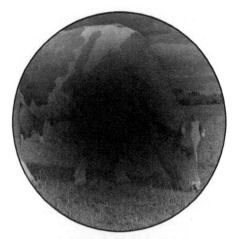

How a scene appears with normal vision

How a scene appears with vision affected by macular degeneration

smereka/Shutterstock.com; concept adapted from Lighthouse International

Figure 10.13 In macular degeneration, central vision deteriorates most quickly.

and is characterized by yellow deposits called *drusen*. When drusen are small and scattered, they may not affect vision. When they become large and grow close together, *wet macular degeneration* can develop and cause more severe vision loss. Wet macular degeneration is caused by the growth of abnormal blood vessels underneath the macula.

The biggest risk factor for macular degeneration is age. *Age-related macular degeneration (AMD)* refers to macular degeneration that develops over the age of 60. Other risk factors are genetics, race (Caucasians are more likely to develop the disease than other races), smoking, and cardiovascular disease.

Good nutrition, including foods with vitamins K and C, is important for preventing macular degeneration. Exercising regularly, avoiding smoking, and protecting the eyes from sunlight are also prevention strategies. Wet AMD may be treated with the use of a laser to lower intraocular pressure, chemical injections, or prescription medications.

Otitis Media

Otitis media, commonly called an *ear infection*, is the most common cause of earaches. The infection is located in the middle ear. Infection is usually due to a cold, influenza, or other respiratory infection. Infection can also be caused by allergies, smoke, fumes, and other environmental toxins. Although otitis media usually affects infants and children, it can also affect adults. Otitis media can happen suddenly and causes ear pain or an earache, drainage of fluid from the ear, and reduced hearing. The eardrum becomes red and appears to be bulging.

Ménière's Disease

Ménière's disease affects the inner ear. This condition causes sudden episodes of spinning (called *vertigo*), hearing loss, ringing in the ear (*tinnitus*), and pressure in the ear. Ménière's disease usually begins between the ages of 20 and 50. A combination of factors may cause Ménière's disease, including allergies, viral infection, improper fluid drainage or blockage in the inner ear, migraines, or a genetic predisposition (tendency to suffer from a condition).

Ménière's disease is chronic and does not have a cure; however, medications, rehabilitation to improve balance, hearing aids, and sometimes surgery can help reduce the severity and frequency of vertigo episodes. Vertigo episodes can occur weeks or years apart, and symptoms may improve or disappear entirely between episodes. In most cases, Ménière's disease affects only one ear.

Vertigo may cause residents to lose their balance easily, resulting in a high risk of falling. Sudden movements and bright lights should be avoided during an episode, and residents should rest after an episode before returning to normal activities.

How Do Diabetes and Thyroid Disease Affect the Endocrine System?

Diabetes mellitus and thyroid disease (hyperthyroidism and hypothyroidism) are common diseases of the endocrine system. Although these diseases are caused by changes in the endocrine system, they impact the whole body.

Diabetes Mellitus

Diabetes mellitus, commonly referred to as *diabetes,* is a disease in which the body's ability to produce or respond to insulin is damaged. This causes abnormal *metabolism* (chemical reactions in the body that maintain cells and the organism) of carbohydrates and elevates glucose (*sugar*) levels in the blood and urine.

There are four types of diabetes: type 1 diabetes, type 2 diabetes, prediabetes, and gestational diabetes. *Gestational diabetes* occurs during pregnancy and often goes away after the baby is born. Type 1 diabetes typically begins during childhood or adolescence. In *type 1 diabetes,* the immune system destroys the cells that produce insulin, causing *hyperglycemia* (high blood sugar levels) as glucose builds up in the bloodstream. Type 2 diabetes more commonly appears after age 40. Type 2 diabetes develops when cells become resistant to insulin and the pancreas is unable to make enough insulin to overcome this resistance.

Risk Factors, Signs, and Symptoms of Type 2 Diabetes

Age, weight (being overweight increases the risk), lack of exercise, family history, race, high blood pressure, and abnormal cholesterol and triglyceride levels are all risk factors for type 2 diabetes. Some people with type 2 diabetes have such mild symptoms that they go unnoticed for a time. The signs and symptoms include:

- increased thirst
- frequent urination
- extreme hunger
- unexplained weight loss
- tingling pain or numbness in the hands and feet
- ketones in the urine (ketones are by-products of muscle and fat breakdown that develop due to insufficient insulin)
- fatigue and irritability
- blurred vision
- slow-healing sores and frequent infections

Diabetes is often diagnosed using a blood test called *glycated hemoglobin (A1C),* which measures the percentage of blood glucose attached to *hemoglobin* (oxygen-carrying molecules in red blood cells). When glucose levels are high, more glucose attaches to hemoglobin. Other tests, such as random and fasting blood sugar, determine the amount of glucose in the blood under different conditions; the normal range of blood sugar is 70–100 mg/dl.

Caring for Residents with Diabetes

Diabetes cannot be cured. Symptoms can be managed when blood glucose levels are carefully and continuously monitored using glucometers or continuous glucose monitors to make sure levels stay within the target (**Figure 10.14**). Oral medications to stimulate the production of insulin may be used, as are insulin replacement injections or pumps (dispense prescribed amounts of insulin). Urine may be tested to determine the presence of ketones.

Diet and exercise are particularly important for managing diabetes. Meals should be healthy and eaten on a regular schedule. Residents with diabetes should not skip meals or eat partial meals. Carefully document what a resident has eaten during a meal and report any changes to the licensed nursing staff. Assist residents with diabetes to complete the

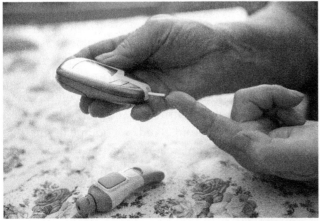

urbans/Shutterstock.com

A

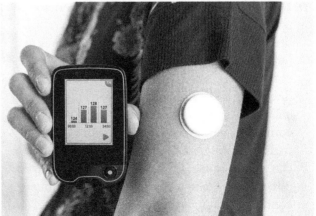

Click and Photo/Shutterstock.com

B

Figure 10.14 Glucometers (A) and continuous glucose monitors (B) help people check their glucose levels. Glucose levels may be checked between four and eight times a day or several times a week.

exercise and activities prescribed by the doctor. Exercise lowers blood glucose levels and increases sensitivity to insulin.

Foot care is very important for residents who have diabetes. Feet should be washed daily in lukewarm water, dried gently (particularly between the toes), and moisturized. Do not cut the toenails of residents with diabetes, unless permitted. These residents usually need professional foot care. Look for blisters, cuts, sores, redness, or swelling that may lead to gangrene. Dental and gum care are also important. Observe the resident for red or swollen gums. Stress management is also important. Stress can prevent insulin from working properly and cause blood glucose levels to rise.

Possible Complications

Long-term complications are possible if blood glucose levels are poorly managed. These can include dry skin conditions, hearing loss, heart disease, cerebrovascular accidents (strokes), kidney damage, retinopathy (eye damage), peripheral neuropathy, and severely limited blood circulation (gangrene) to the lower limbs. Gangrene can lead to amputation of the toes and feet.

Even if residents with diabetes carefully manage their blood glucose levels, they must be observed closely for three possible conditions:

- **Hyperglycemia**: high blood sugar. Blood glucose levels can become too high if residents overeat, have an illness, or do not take enough of their prescribed medications. Signs and symptoms include excessive thirst, a dry mouth, fatigue, nausea, and blurred vision. Hyperglycemia is commonly treated by adjusting a resident's meal plan, prescribed medications, physical activity, or exercise.
- **Diabetic ketoacidosis**: buildup of ketones in the urine. When the body lacks adequate insulin, it breaks down fat for energy, causing ketones to build up in the blood. Diabetic ketoacidosis most commonly occurs in type 1 diabetes and may occur due to illness or missed doses of insulin. Signs and symptoms include loss of appetite, weakness, confusion, vomiting, fever, stomach pain, and fruity-smelling breath. Diabetic ketoacidosis can lead to **coma** (a state of deep and prolonged unconsciousness) and death and is a serious condition that may require emergency care.
- **Hypoglycemia**: low blood sugar. Blood glucose levels sometimes drop too low if a resident does not have enough calories at a meal, skips a meal,

significantly increases physical activity, drinks large amounts of alcohol, or takes too much of a prescribed medication. Signs and symptoms include sweating, shakiness, weakness, hunger, dizziness, headache, blurred vision, heart palpitations, irritability, slurred speech, drowsiness, confusion, fainting, and seizures. Hypoglycemia can be reversed if a resident consumes a quick source of sugar, such as fruit juice, regular soda, or glucose tablets. A glucagon emergency injection kit consisting of a syringe and glucagon that can be injected into the arm, thigh, or buttocks may be prescribed by a doctor.

Signs of hyperglycemia, diabetic ketoacidosis, or hypoglycemia must be reported immediately to the licensed nursing staff.

Thyroid Disease

Thyroid disease is usually caused by too much or too little thyroid hormone. *Hyperthyroidism* and *hypothyroidism* are the two types of thyroid disease you will most commonly come across when working as a holistic nursing assistant.

Hyperthyroidism

Hyperthyroidism refers to excess production of the thyroid hormone. Hyperthyroidism can be caused by Graves' disease, in which the immune system attacks the thyroid gland and the thyroid reacts by making too much thyroid hormone. Other common causes of hyperthyroidism include **nodules** (lumps of body tissue) that develop in the thyroid gland and increase the secretion of thyroid hormone.

People with hyperthyroidism often experience nervousness, tremors, agitation, *tachycardia* (rapid heartbeat), heart palpitations (pounding heartbeat), heat intolerance, mental fogginess and poor concentration, and menstrual changes (reduced flow). Signs and symptoms of Graves' disease include protruding eyeballs, red or swollen eyes, tearing or discomfort in one or both eyes, light sensitivity, and blurry or double vision. When the thyroid gland or a nodule in the thyroid enlarges, it can create a growth called a *goiter*.

Hyperthyroidism is treated by slowing down or stopping excess thyroid hormone production. Some common treatments prescribed are radioactive iodine treatments, a year of antithyroid medications, or sometimes surgery.

Hypothyroidism

Hypothyroidism occurs when the thyroid gland does not produce enough thyroid hormone or the thyroid gland has been surgically removed. The most common cause of hypothyroidism is an autoimmune disorder called *Hashimoto's thyroiditis*. In Hashimoto's thyroiditis, the body produces antibodies that attack and destroy the thyroid gland, and the thyroid gland becomes inflamed. Symptoms commonly seen include feeling cold, sluggishness, depression, menstrual changes (excessive flow or prolonged cycle), mental fogginess and poor concentration, a bloated feeling, weight gain, and high cholesterol levels.

Hypothyroidism is treated with lifelong thyroid hormone replacement using prescription medications. Side effects of these medications might include nervousness or even chest pain. Some medications, such as antidepressants, can interfere with thyroid hormone replacement.

When caring for a resident with thyroid disease, observe the resident for any signs or symptoms of changes or side effects from medications. Also, be sensitive to and watch for any emotional issues, such as mood changes or depression. Report any changes to the licensed nursing staff.

How Does Disease Affect the Cardiovascular System?

Common cardiovascular system diseases include coronary artery disease, angina, myocardial infarction, and congestive heart failure. (You learned about angina and myocardial infarction in Chapter 5.) Cerebrovascular accidents (CVAs), or *strokes*, and peripheral vascular disease are also common.

Coronary Artery Disease

Coronary artery disease occurs when there is damage, injury, or disease in the inner layers of coronary arteries. These arteries supply the heart with blood, oxygen, and nutrients. When these are damaged, plaque and other waste products form at the site, resulting in a condition called *atherosclerosis* (**Figure 10.15**).

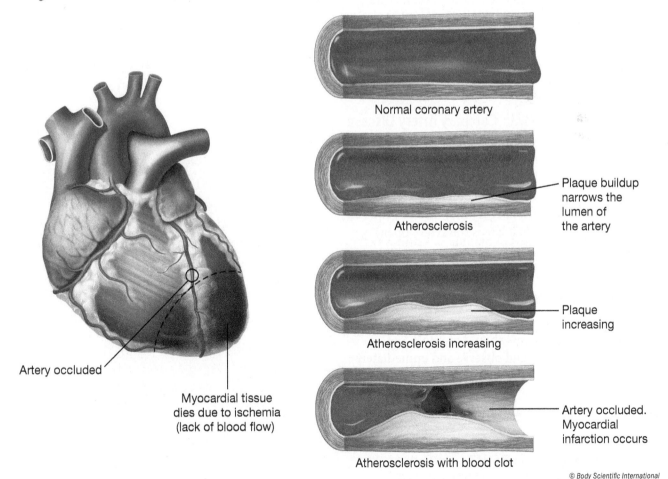

Artery occluded

Myocardial tissue dies due to ischemia (lack of blood flow)

Normal coronary artery

Atherosclerosis — Plaque buildup narrows the lumen of the artery

Atherosclerosis increasing — Plaque increasing

Atherosclerosis with blood clot — Artery occluded. Myocardial infarction occurs

© Body Scientific International

Figure 10.15 Atherosclerosis narrows the arteries, restricting blood flow. When blood flow is mostly or completely restricted, myocardial infarction can result, as shown here.

Plaque hardens and narrows the arteries, allowing less blood to flow to the heart. This may cause chest pain, shortness of breath, or even a heart attack, if the arteries become completely blocked.

Symptoms are not usually felt until there is a major blockage. Risk factors include aging, gender (men are more likely to get it), family history, smoking, high blood pressure, high LDL (low-density lipoprotein, or bad cholesterol) levels, being overweight or obese, lack of physical activity, and excessive, unrelieved stress.

Congestive Heart Failure

Congestive heart failure occurs when the heart does not have the oxygen and nutrients it needs to pump blood effectively. This weakens the heart's pumping power, causing blood to move through the heart at a slower-than-normal rate and pressure in the heart to increase. Congestive heart failure can be the result of coronary artery disease.

Congestive heart failure can affect the kidneys and cause *edema*, or retention of fluid, in the arms, legs, ankles, feet, and lungs. Fluid buildup in the lungs may cause shortness of breath and sometimes a dry, hacking cough or wheezing. Fluid buildup can also cause swelling in the ankles and legs, bloating in the abdomen, and weight gain. Dizziness, fatigue, rapid heartbeats, and *arrhythmias* (abnormal heart rhythms) are also possible.

Caring for Residents with Coronary Artery Disease

Aspirin may be prescribed to reduce blood clotting. Other prescription medications may be used to widen blood vessels, relax blood vessels to improve blood flow, slow heart rate, decrease blood pressure, or lower blood cholesterol. Surgery may also be required to insert stents (a coil that keeps the artery open) or to bypass a blocked artery.

Lifestyle changes are typically part of the plan of care for coronary artery disease. These lifestyle changes may include smoking cessation, healthful eating, weight loss, regular exercise, and stress reduction. Holistic nursing assistants should promote and support these changes and observe and immediately report any changes in residents, including changes in blood pressure, pulse, respiration, and mental or emotional behaviors or attitudes.

THINK ABOUT THIS

The brain does not have any pain receptors, and therefore, cannot feel pain.

Cerebrovascular Accident (CVA)

A *cerebrovascular accident* (*CVA*) or *stroke* occurs when a blood vessel in the brain becomes blocked due to atherosclerosis or *arteriosclerosis* (hardening of the arteries) or bleeding due to a ruptured *aneurysm* (a distended or weak area in a blood vessel). Risk factors include smoking, diabetes, high cholesterol, and *hypertension* (high blood pressure).

There are three types of strokes:

- **Ischemic stroke:** most common; occurs due to blocked arteries that keep blood from flowing to the brain (**Figure 10.16**).
- **Hemorrhagic stroke:** occurs when an artery in the brain leaks blood or ruptures due to an aneurysm. The bleeding causes damaging pressure on brain cells.
- **Transient ischemic attack (TIA):** also called a *ministroke*, because it only lasts for a short amount of time, a TIA is caused by a blocked artery in the brain. Some people have a TIA and do not even know it.

Signs and Symptoms of Stroke

The signs and symptoms of a stroke include a sudden, severe headache that feels different from other headaches. A person who is having a stroke may

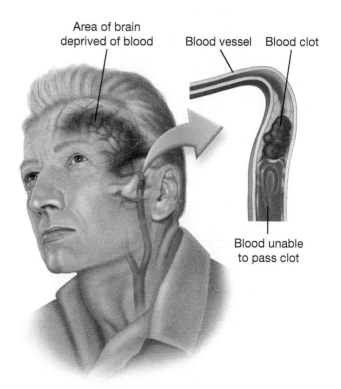

Area of brain deprived of blood

Blood vessel   Blood clot

Blood unable to pass clot

© Body Scientific International

Figure 10.16 Ischemic strokes result from blocked arteries in the brain.

also have numbness; tingling; weakness (causing drooping of the face and mouth); loss of movement in the face, arm, or leg; or *hemiplegia* (loss of movement on one whole side of the body). These symptoms may make it difficult for a person to walk. Trouble seeing, slurred speech, *aphasia* (inability to understand and use words), confusion, dizziness, and difficulty understanding simple statements may also occur.

Time is critical for treating strokes. The longer a person goes without treatment, the greater the damage from the stroke will be.

Care After a Stroke

One of the most important concerns about care after a stroke is the damage the stroke may leave. Damage from a stroke can significantly affect people physically, mentally, and emotionally. Holistic nursing assistants can help residents who have suffered a stroke by assisting with ambulation and making sure fall-prevention measures are in place. Residents may also require help dressing or eating. If bladder control is lost, change residents quickly to prevent skin irritation. Paralysis may also lead to vision problems. Be sure residents are familiar with the room and do not try to get up on their own.

It is important to be patient and respectful with residents who have had a stroke. Residents will be very frustrated if they can no longer do what they were able to do prior to the stroke. This is especially true if residents have aphasia. When caring for these residents, speak slowly and listen carefully. Also encourage residents' families to provide support during recovery. Show residents' families proper and supportive ways they can help.

Peripheral Vascular Disease (PVD)

Peripheral vascular disease (PVD), or *peripheral artery disease*, occurs when there is damage to the blood vessels that supply blood to the extremities (legs, feet, arms, or hands) and other body parts. Damage usually occurs due to atherosclerosis and arteriosclerosis. Plaque buildup and hardening of the blood vessels can progress until arteries become narrow or blocked. Other causes include the presence of a blood clot, inflammation of the arteries (*arteritis*), infection, or injury. Blood vessels in the legs are most often affected, but blood vessels in the arms and kidneys may also become narrow and blocked.

PVD Symptoms

The first signs of PVD begin slowly. A person may feel discomfort such as fatigue or cramping in the in one or both calves, thighs, or hips while walking. Other signs and symptoms are numbness, tingling, or weakness in the legs; burning or aching pain in the feet or toes, even at rest; cold feet; loss of hair on the legs; and skin that becomes pale and bluish in color. When symptoms are more severe, pain is present even during rest at night. If left untreated, gangrene can develop in the affected limb, and tissues may die and decay. This can lead to amputation (surgery to remove the limb).

PVD Treatment

Treatment for PVD depends on the underlying cause of the disease. One of the greatest risk factors for PVD is smoking, particularly if a person also has diabetes. Helpful strategies for the treatment of PVD include smoking cessation, a healthful diet, physical activity, and efforts to lower blood pressure and cholesterol. A holistic nursing assistant can provide care for residents with PVD by helping them find comfortable positions and observing for any changes in the skin (sores that do not heal) or complaints of new sensations or pain in the legs. If these changes and complaints occur, they need to be reported to the licensed nursing staff immediately.

Treatment may also include prescription medications that dilate (open) the blood vessels, prevent blood clots, relieve pain, and lower blood pressure and cholesterol. Surgery to widen the arteries, insert stents, remove plaque, or bypass the blockage may be helpful, but is usually performed only if medication does not work.

How Does Disease Affect Respiratory System Structures?

The *common cold* is a viral infection of the respiratory system and affects the nose and throat. Because most people have experienced a cold in their lifetimes, this section will focus on other common respiratory diseases: asthma, chronic obstructive pulmonary disease (COPD), pneumonia, and tuberculosis.

THINK ABOUT THIS

The medical term for sneezing is *sternutation*. One sneeze can spray about 100,000 germs about 3–5 feet.

Asthma

Asthma is a chronic lung disease in which the airways swell, narrow, and become inflamed. Inflammation causes mucus to develop, which narrows the airways even more and reduces airflow to the lungs. Asthma may cause periods of wheezing, which sounds like high-pitched whistling during expiration. Other symptoms may include a tight chest, shortness of breath, and coughing, usually at night or early in the morning. For some people, symptoms are mild and go away with or without treatment. For others, symptoms get worse, and attacks or *flares* may occur.

Asthma attacks are usually caused by particular substances or circumstances. Triggers (causes) are typically specific to the individual. A trigger can be dust, animal fur, mold, pollen, cigarette smoke, a new chemical used in the home, a certain food, exercise, a newly prescribed medication, or an upper respiratory infection. There is no cure for asthma. Treatment focuses on managing asthma symptoms.

Asthma symptoms may be managed using oral medications or an *inhaler* or *nebulizer* to breathe medication into the lungs. Quick-relief or *rescue inhalers* relax tight muscles in the airways during a flare. If a rescue inhaler does not provide relief, this becomes a medical emergency. A nebulizer is a machine that provides a fine mist of liquid medicine that goes directly into the lungs. These are long-term medications taken daily and are not considered quick relief for asthma symptoms.

When caring for residents who use inhalers and nebulizers, be sure you understand the purpose of the inhaler or nebulizer and check with the licensed nursing staff to be sure there is a quick-relief inhaler nearby. Also, encourage residents with asthma to avoid their triggers while still making sure they are getting the physical activity they need.

Chronic Obstructive Pulmonary Disease (COPD)

Chronic obstructive pulmonary disease (COPD) is also known as *chronic obstructive airway disease* or *chronic obstructive lung disease*. In COPD, thick, inflamed airways filled with mucus reduce the amount of airflow into the body. When people have COPD, they usually have two conditions—chronic bronchitis and emphysema (**Figure 10.17**). The severity of these conditions will vary for each person.

Chronic Bronchitis

Bronchitis is a condition in which the bronchial passages become inflamed. Irritated membranes in the bronchial passages swell and narrow the airways to the lungs. Bronchitis can be acute or chronic.

When people have acute bronchitis, they experience a persistent, hacking cough, mucus in their airways, and a feeling of breathlessness. Acute bronchitis is most often the result of a viral infection and typically lasts one to three weeks. Treatments for acute bronchitis usually include cough suppressants, over-the-counter medications to relieve fever and body aches, rest, and fluids.

Chronic bronchitis lasts three months or longer, becomes more serious over time, and requires ongoing medical treatment. Repeated episodes of acute bronchitis, which weaken the airways, may result in chronic bronchitis. Smoking and secondhand smoke may also cause chronic bronchitis.

Emphysema

Emphysema causes damage to the walls of air sacs (*alveoli*) in the lungs, which reduces the amount of gas exchange that can occur. Because the alveoli do not work properly, carbon dioxide becomes trapped during exhalation, leaving no room for fresh oxygen during inhalation. People with emphysema experience a gradual increase in shortness of breath, even at rest. Heart problems may also result from this disease.

Signs and Symptoms of COPD

COPD is the third-leading cause of death in the United States. Symptoms of COPD appear slowly and worsen over time, limiting activities of daily living. Symptoms of COPD include a persistent cough that produces large amounts of mucus, a tight-feeling chest, shortness of breath (usually with physical activity), and wheezing. Severe symptoms—such as difficulty catching one's breath, tachycardia (rapid heart rate), edema, mental confusion, and weight loss—vary depending on the amount of lung damage. There is no cure for COPD; lung damage is irreversible.

Caring for Residents with COPD

The goals for treating COPD are to relieve symptoms, slow disease progression, improve tolerance to activity, and prevent complications. *Bronchodilators*, inhaled medications that relax muscles around the airways, help improve breathing. Long-acting bronchodilators are used daily, while short-acting bronchodilators are

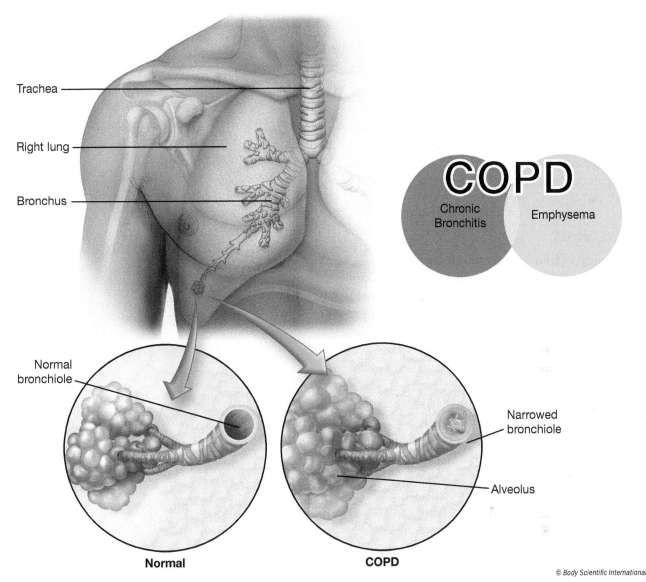

Trachea

Right lung

Bronchus

Normal bronchiole

Normal

COPD

Chronic Bronchitis

Emphysema

Narrowed bronchiole

Alveolus

COPD

© *Body Scientific International*

Figure 10.17 COPD includes chronic bronchitis and emphysema.

used only when needed. Residents who have severe COPD may also need oxygen therapy delivered by nasal cannulas. Residents with COPD should receive an annual flu shot and pneumonia vaccine to prevent complications. Surgery may benefit those with severe COPD or emphysema.

Living with COPD can be frustrating, scary, and can cause stress and depression. Residents with COPD should quit smoking, avoid secondhand smoke, and remove irritants in their environment. Holistic nursing assistants can assist by listening and providing support and resources, as directed.

As a holistic nursing assistant, you can help residents with daily activities and slow down activities to help ease breathing. Residents who are short of breath will also need to have personal items within easy reach,

have assistive devices, and receive help eating. If residents are on oxygen therapy, good hygiene around the nose and mouth is very important. Maintaining good hygiene is also important, as there may be large amounts of coughed-up mucus. Always observe residents for worsening symptoms, such as trouble breathing, gasping, or changes in attitude or emotions. Immediately report this to the licensed nursing staff if these occur.

Pneumonia

Bacterial pneumonia is an infection of the lungs that causes inflammation and fluid buildup. Risk factors for bacterial pneumonia include an age over 65, asthma, diabetes, heart disease, smoking, surgery, poor nutrition, and alcohol consumption. Common signs and symptoms are high fevers; chills and sweating; greenish, yellow, or bloody mucus; dyspnea (difficulty breathing); sharp, stabbing pain in the lungs; fatigue; little appetite; cyanosis in the lips and fingernails; and confusion. Prevention strategies are regular hand hygiene, good nutrition and exercise, sufficient sleep, isolation from those who are sick, and vaccines. Effective treatments include antibiotics (until the bacteria are destroyed), medications for fever and pain, rest, plenty of fluids, a humidifier to loosen mucus, smoking cessation, oxygen therapy, and IV fluids.

Tuberculosis

Tuberculosis (TB) is a bacterial infection that is spread through droplets in the air (from coughing and sneezing). TB primarily attacks the lungs, but can also damage the kidneys, spine, and brain. Risk factors include a weakened immune system and travel to areas where TB is common. TB may be latent (inactive) or active. In latent TB, bacteria are in the body, but no symptoms are present. Active TB causes painful coughing that lasts more than three weeks, coughing up blood, fatigue, fever, night sweats and chills, loss of appetite, unintentional weight loss, back pain, and blood in the urine. Residents with TB take antibiotics for at least six to nine months and must take all of the medication prescribed. Active TB can spread; therefore, infection control precautions (such as covering the mouth with a tissue and putting dirty tissues in a sealed bag) are necessary.

How Are the Immune and Lymphatic Systems Affected by Disease?

The primary function of the immune system is to defend the body against infection. As you learned in Chapter 9, there are two different types of immunity. *Natural immunity* is the immunity with which people are born. *Acquired immunity* is immunity to specific bacteria or viruses. Both types give the body the ability to protect itself.

Autoimmune Disorders

When a person has an *autoimmune disorder*, the body produces antibodies that attack the body's own tissues instead of fighting infection. There is no known cause of autoimmune disorders, although a person's genes, along with infection and other environmental factors, play a role. There are more than 80 known autoimmune

disorders, and these disorders tend to run in families. Women (particularly African-American, Hispanic, and Native American women) are at higher risk for some autoimmune disorders.

Treatments for autoimmune disorders generally focus on using medications and other approaches to reduce immune system activity. No cure has been discovered.

Several diseases and conditions, including rheumatoid arthritis and multiple sclerosis (MS), are thought to be affected by the autoimmune response. Another autoimmune disorder is *systemic lupus erythematosus* (commonly called *lupus* or *SLE*). People who have lupus develop autoimmune antibodies that attack multiple body tissues. While lupus is different for each person, it typically affects the joints, lungs, blood cells, nerves, kidneys, and skin. *Ulcerative colitis* and *Crohn's disease* are autoimmune inflammatory bowel diseases (IBDs). These diseases cause antibodies to attack the lining of the intestines, resulting in abdominal pain, diarrhea, rectal bleeding, fever, and weight loss. Another autoimmune disorder called *vasculitis* results in the immune system attacking and damaging blood vessels.

HIV/AIDS

Human immunodeficiency virus (HIV) weakens the immune system and causes people to become sick with infections that would not normally affect them. *Acquired immunodeficiency syndrome (AIDS)* is considered the most advanced stage of HIV.

HIV is not transmitted by simple casual contact, such as kissing or sharing drinking glasses. HIV is most commonly spread by:

- vaginal or anal intercourse without a condom with someone who has HIV/AIDS
- sharing needles or syringes with someone who has HIV/AIDS
- deep puncture with a needle or surgical instrument contaminated with HIV
- HIV-infected blood, semen, or vaginal secretions that get into open wounds or sores
- birth or breast-feeding when the mother is infected with HIV/AIDS

HIV/AIDS Signs, Symptoms, and Diagnosis

HIV symptoms vary depending on the stage of the virus. In the first stage of HIV infection, people may have a fever, headache, diarrhea, sore throat, swollen lymph glands (in the neck), muscle aches and joint pain, and red rashes that do not itch. These symptoms will usually last for a few weeks. At this time, the virus is highly infectious.

The second stage of HIV is called *clinical latent infection* (or *chronic HIV*). There are no specific signs or symptoms of this stage; however, some people continue to have swollen lymph glands. At this stage, untreated HIV will continue to attack and destroy the immune system, leaving a person susceptible to other serious infections. This stage can last for a long time and usually does not progress if the person is taking medication.

HIV may progress to the third and final stage, which is AIDS. The signs and symptoms of AIDS are:

- constant tiredness
- headaches and dizziness
- swollen lymph glands in the neck or groin
- a fever that lasts more than 10 days
- night sweats
- unexplained weight loss of 10 or more pounds
- purplish spots on the skin or mouth
- shortness of breath
- a persistent, deep, dry cough
- severe, chronic diarrhea
- yeast infection in the mouth (thrush), throat, or vagina
- unexplained bruises or bleeding from a body opening
- frequent or unusual skin rashes
- severe numbness or pain in the hands or feet, loss of muscle control and reflexes, paralysis, or loss of muscular strength
- confusion, personality changes, or decreased mental abilities

People with AIDS who do not take medications will only survive about three years, or less if they get a serious infection. There is currently no cure for HIV/AIDS, but there are treatments.

The current treatment for HIV/AIDS is a combination of medications (called a *cocktail*) that helps control the growth of the virus, keeping HIV from progressing into AIDS. Cocktails may not be available to everyone, can be expensive, and may have serious and uncomfortable side effects. They may only work for some people and only for limited periods of time.

Protection against HIV/AIDS is very important. The surest way to prevent HIV/AIDS is to abstain from sexual intercourse and from sharing needles. If people choose to have sex, they should practice safe or safer sex (for example, using condoms for protection) to reduce the risk of exchanging blood, semen, or vaginal fluids.

Caring for Residents with HIV

As a holistic nursing assistant, you should use consistent hand hygiene and put on gloves if touching infected fluids or waste. It is also important to prevent skin puncture; pay attention to any potential sharp instruments that have potentially been exposed to body fluids or left in the linens. If present, these instruments must be removed carefully.

Encourage mobility if the resident is weak and frail, and maintain skin integrity through frequent positioning and by keeping the skin clean and dry. Mobility can also be improved through range-of-motion exercises and gentle massage, if ordered.

Be aware of potential side effects from medications and observe and report to the licensed nursing staff any physical, behavioral, or emotional changes. Good nutrition, fluids, exercise, rest, and stress management are important for helping residents maintain a healthy lifestyle.

How Does Disease Influence Gastrointestinal System Function?

The gastrointestinal (GI) system uses its essential functions of ingestion, digestion, absorption, and elimination to transform foods eaten into energy that is needed to survive and thrive. Any change or interruption in this process may result in a gastrointestinal disease or condition. Common gastrointestinal system diseases and conditions are gastroesophageal reflux disease (GERD), peptic ulcers, gallbladder disease, and diverticulitis.

Gastroesophageal Reflux Disease (GERD)

Gastroesophageal reflux disease (GERD) is commonly called *acid reflux* and is caused by the flow of acidic stomach contents back into the esophagus. This backflow occurs when the cardiac sphincter between the esophagus and the stomach is weak or relaxes when it should not. GERD may also be caused by a *hiatal hernia* (the stomach bulges through the diaphragm). Severe coughing, vomiting, or straining are possible causes of a hiatal hernia.

The primary symptom of GERD is *heartburn*, which is also called *indigestion*. Heartburn feels like a burning pain in the middle of the chest. Along with the burning sensation, there may be an acidic taste. Food may also move up the throat and into the mouth. Heartburn is usually worse after eating, lying down, or bending over.

Other symptoms of GERD include a chronic cough, laryngitis, and nausea. A serious complication is *esophagitis*, or damaging inflammation in the esophagus that may lead to esophageal bleeding and ulcers. Easing the symptoms of heartburn is an important step in treating GERD. Simply standing up may reduce heartburn, and taking over-the-counter antacids will neutralize acid in the stomach.

Heartburn is often triggered by eating chocolate, peppermint, coffee, fried or fatty foods, citrus fruits and juices, tomato products, pepper, and alcohol, so avoiding these may bring relief. Dietary changes can be challenging, particularly if these foods are favorites or are an important part of a resident's culture. Controlling portions and eating at least two to three hours before going to bed can also decrease GERD. Elevating the head of the bed or sleeping on wedges will lessen reflux. Do not use pillows for these positions, as they may increase pressure on the stomach. If feeding a resident, position the head of the bed at 75–90 degrees and leave the head of the bed elevated for one to two hours after eating. Encouraging weight loss for overweight residents can provide relief.

Nicotine relaxes the sphincter responsible for GERD, so smoking cessation can be helpful. Some residents take prescription medications to reduce the secretion and amount of acid in the stomach. Surgery may be necessary to treat very severe GERD.

Peptic Ulcers

Peptic ulcers are sores or sometimes holes in the lining of the GI tract. They may form in the stomach, duodenum of the small intestine, or esophagus (**Figure 10.18**). A bacterial infection caused by *Helicobacter pylori* (*H. pylori*) is present in most people who have duodenal and gastric ulcers and may be the primary cause of ulcers. Ulcers are more likely to develop in older adults, as older adults may take medications that irritate the GI tract.

Peptic ulcers cause a dull abdominal pain that becomes more intense when the stomach is empty. Bloating, burping, acid reflux, weight loss (because it hurts to eat), and nausea or vomiting are other symptoms. Symptoms that require immediate treatment are continuing, sudden sharp pain in the abdominal area; black or bloody stools; and bloody vomit that looks like coffee grounds. These signs can mean the ulcer has worn through the stomach lining or that a blood vessel has broken.

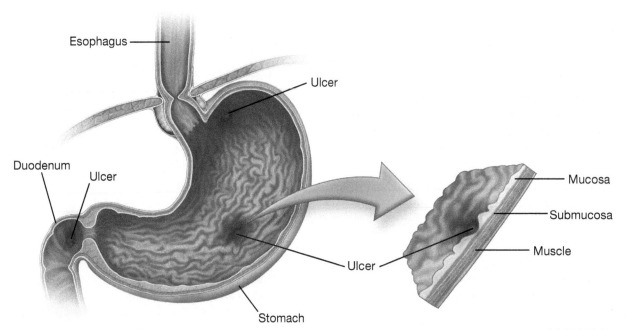

© Body Scientific International

Figure 10.18 Peptic ulcers are sores or sometimes holes in the lining of the GI tract.

Antacids and prescription medications may be used to decrease stomach acids. If *H. pylori* is present, antibiotics are given to kill the bacteria. Ulcers must be monitored to make sure they do not get worse. If an ulcer does not heal, if there is bleeding, or if there is a tear in the GI lining, the next step may be blood transfusions or surgery.

While ulcer-related symptoms may lessen quickly with treatment, prescribed medications must be taken, and smoking, alcohol, and foods that trigger symptoms must be avoided. Managing stress also helps improve or eliminate symptoms. As a holistic nursing assistant, observe and report any side effects that may be caused by treatment. These side effects include headaches, dizziness, and diarrhea.

Gallbladder Disease

Gallbladder disease occurs when *gallstones* (a hardened mixture of cholesterol and other substances found in bile) form in the gallbladder (**Figure 10.19**). Gallstones can form if the gallbladder does not empty normally. People who are overweight are at greater risk for gallstone formation.

Gallbladder disease sometimes causes mild pain in the upper right part of the abdomen, and pain may spread to the right upper back or shoulder blade. If a bile duct is blocked the person may experience pain, as well as fever and chills. The person's skin and the whites of the eyes can become yellow, or *jaundiced*. This symptom could mean that gallstones are in the bile duct or that there is an infection in the gallbladder. This is an emergency.

To prevent or reduce the risk of gallstones, residents should not skip meals, should maintain a healthy weight, and should lose weight slowly if needed. Prescription medications may be used to dissolve gallstones. Surgical removal of the gallbladder (called a *cholecystectomy*) is required if gallstones become large and if attacks recur frequently. Removing the gallbladder does not affect important body functions.

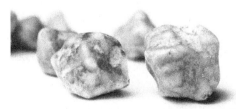

Roblan/Shutterstock.com

Figure 10.19 Gallstones form in various shapes and sizes.

If caring for residents who have had a cholecystectomy, be aware that they may experience diarrhea for a short period while their bodies become accustomed to changes in digestion.

Diverticulitis

Diverticulitis occurs when pouches in the wall of the colon, called *diverticula*, become inflamed or infected. Low fiber in the intestine can create pressure, which causes diverticula to become inflamed in weak spots in the intestinal wall. This causes intense pain in the lower left abdomen that worsens during activity, fever and chills, bloating and gas, nausea and vomiting, and diarrhea or constipation.

As a holistic nursing assistant, you should follow the resident's plan of care to help prevent diverticulitis. Residents should be encouraged to maintain a high-fiber diet with whole grains and fresh fruit and vegetables. These foods will help digested food pass through the intestines quickly, thus reducing pressure. Exercise also helps promote normal bowel function. During a mild diverticulitis attack, low heat on the abdomen, if prescribed, can be comforting. Guiding a resident through relaxation techniques, such as deep breathing, may also be helpful. Prescription medications, including antibiotics, are given if there is an infection. At first, solid food should be replaced with liquids to allow the intestine to heal. Severe attacks may require IV antibiotics and possible surgery.

How Is the Urinary System Affected by Disease?

Urinary tract infections (UTIs), kidney stones, and acute kidney failure are urinary system diseases and conditions discussed in this section. You will learn about a urinary condition called *incontinence* in Chapter 20.

Urinary Tract Infection (UTI)

A *urinary tract infection (UTI)* is an infection in any part of the urinary system, such as in the urinary bladder (*cystitis*) or the urethra (*urethritis*). UTIs typically develop when pathogens enter the body through the urethra and begin to grow. The body usually defends against these bacterial invasions, but sometimes the defense fails, resulting in an infection.

Common causes of UTIs include the transfer of bacteria from the anus, sexual activity, certain types of birth control, menopause, kidney stones, an enlarged prostate, the presence of a urinary catheter, or a surgical procedure. Women are at greater risk for UTIs due to their anatomy, because the female urethra is located very close to the anus.

Signs and symptoms of UTIs depend on the infection's location. In general, there is a strong and persistent urge to urinate and a burning sensation when urinating. Only very small amounts of urine may be excreted, and urine may appear cloudy and have a strong smell. Blood may also be present in the urine, causing urine to look red, bright pink, or cocoa colored. People who have UTIs may also be confused and disoriented, and women may experience pain in the pelvic area. UTIs in the kidneys may cause upper back and side pain, fever, and chills. There may also be discharge from the urethra. If left untreated, UTIs may lead to serious complications, such as multiple and more serious infections, urethral narrowing (called a *stricture*), and kidney damage.

Antibiotics are typically used to treat UTIs, and several different antibiotics may be used. An analgesic may be prescribed if the resident is experiencing pain. Pay attention to residents' levels of pain and report that information to the licensed nursing staff. Sometimes it is helpful to apply heat to the resident's abdomen using a warm, dry compress or a heating pad, if ordered. Keep residents hydrated and avoid irritating fluids such as coffee, soft drinks, and citrus juices. If a resident has a urinary catheter, provide thorough catheter care to prevent UTIs (see Chapter 20). Provide excellent hygiene for residents by giving daily perineal care (see Chapter 19), ensuring cleanliness after elimination, and keeping dressings, briefs, and other linens near the urethra dry and clean.

Kidney Stones

Kidney stones (*renal lithiasis*) are small, hard deposits that form in the kidneys. There is no single cause for kidney stones. Dehydration, obesity, gout, family or personal history, gastrointestinal diseases, side effects of some medications, and diets high in protein, salt, and sugar are possible causes of kidney stones.

A person can have a kidney stone and not be aware of it. This is because symptoms may not occur until the stone starts to move. Signs and symptoms of moving kidney stones include:

- pain that comes in waves, changes in intensity, is located in the side and back below the ribs, and spreads to the lower abdomen and groin
- pink, red, or brown urine that is foul-smelling
- a persistent need to urinate, urination of small amounts, and pain during urination
- fever and chills, if an infection is present
- nausea and vomiting

The focus of treatment is on passing the kidney stone, which can be very painful. Drinking a lot of water (between 2 and 3 quarts) until urine is clear, pain medications, and sometimes using prescription medications that relax the muscles in the ureter may help pass a kidney stone. Larger kidney stones may be broken up using sound waves, a scope, or surgery. Prescription medications may help prevent future kidney stones from forming.

Encourage residents who have a history of kidney stones to drink plenty of fluids. Foods with a lot of salt, animal protein, beets, spinach, sweet potatoes, nuts, chocolate, and soy products may cause kidney stones and should be avoided. If you are caring for a resident who is passing a kidney stone, follow the instructions given by the licensed nursing staff.

Renal Failure

Renal failure, or *kidney failure*, occurs when the kidneys are unable to filter waste products from the blood. As a result, dangerous levels of waste products build up in the body, creating an imbalance in the body's chemical balance.

Renal failure can develop over a long period of time or in a few hours, depending on the cause. Failure that develops quickly, or *acute renal failure*, is an emergency. If not treated, it can be irreversible and fatal. A person can also have chronic kidney disease, or *chronic renal failure*, in which there is a gradual loss of kidney function.

Usually, renal failure is the result of some other disease, such as hypertension, diabetes mellitus, or PVD. Other causes are urinary blockage, infections, allergic reactions, medications, blood loss, severe burns, and cancer.

Signs and symptoms of renal failure are decreased urine output, edema, shortness of breath, chest pain, muscle weakness, drowsiness and fatigue, confusion, and nausea. Advanced stages of renal failure or *end-stage renal disease (ESRD)* can lead to seizures or a coma (a state of deep and prolonged unconsciousness). Complete loss of kidney function leads to death.

Renal failure may require hospitalization. Treatment goals are established to balance fluids, and prescription medications may be used to control high potassium levels due to lack of kidney filtering. High potassium levels can cause arrhythmias and muscle weakness. A diet that limits potassium, salt, protein, calcium, and phosphorus (a mineral found in milk, cheese, and nuts) may be recommended. Temporary **dialysis** (removal of waste products from the body) may be needed to get rid of wastes, toxins, and excess fluids from the blood. The resident may receive *hemodialysis* (through a machine that filters the blood) or *peritoneal dialysis* (through a catheter inserted into the abdominal cavity that delivers a solution that absorbs waste and excess fluids) when in ESRD. A kidney transplant may be needed if dialysis does not work.

Diet is extremely important for treating renal failure, and low-potassium foods are an essential component. Low-potassium foods include apples, cabbage, green beans, and strawberries. A diet that limits salt and phosphorus is also a requirement to help reverse renal failure. Phosphorus is a mineral found in milk, cheese, and nuts. Limiting protein and calcium intake may also be recommended.

Which Diseases Are Associated with the Reproductive Systems?

A common reproductive system disease for males is benign prostatic hypertrophy (BPH). Reproductive system diseases for females include vaginitis and uterine prolapse. A discussion of sexually transmitted infections (STIs) is included in Appendix C.

Benign Prostatic Hypertrophy (BPH)

Benign prostatic hypertrophy (BPH), also called *benign prostatic hyperplasia*, is an enlarged prostate gland. This is a common occurrence for men as they age and their hormones change and cells grow. When the prostate gets bigger than normal, it can partially block the urethra (**Figure 10.20**). This can cause problems with urination.

The signs and symptoms of BPH include:
- trouble starting the urine stream and difficulty stopping it, which causes "dribbling"
- a weak urine stream

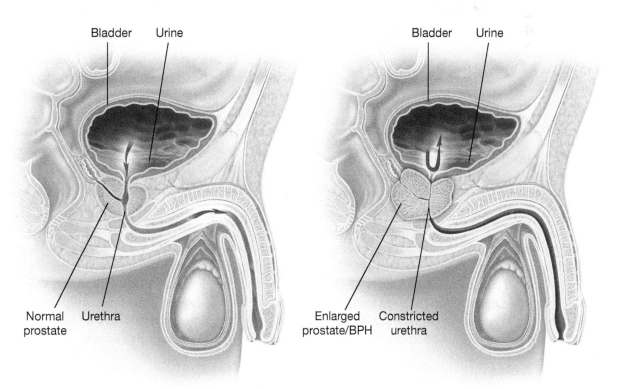

© Body Scientific International

Figure 10.20 BPH can block the male urethra if the prostate grows too large.

- the feeling that the bladder is not completely empty after urination
- extreme difficulty urinating when the bladder is nearly blocked, which can cause a backup of urine (called *urinary retention*), infections, and kidney damage

Medications may be prescribed, and lifestyle and physical strategies may be recommended to control symptoms. If symptoms are severe, surgery may be performed to remove part of the prostate gland.

Difficulty urinating may cause a resident to become anxious and fearful. This anxiety may cause the resident to be tense, making it even more difficult to urinate. Encourage residents to relax and stay calm. You can also help residents *double urinate*, or urinate as much as possible, relax for a moment, and then urinate again. Avoiding caffeine and alcohol will help lessen the need to urinate. As a holistic nursing assistant, you can help residents maintain good body hygiene and skin care and provide special briefs if there is dribbling. Be respectful and do not call these briefs *diapers*.

Vaginitis

Vaginitis is an infection or inflammation of the vagina. The source of the infection might be bacteria, a virus, or yeast. Vaginitis can be caused by a *yeast infection*, or an overgrowth of the yeast normally found in the vagina. Vaginitis may also result when there are more bacteria than usual in the vagina. It can also be caused by sexual contact; poor hygiene; lower levels of hormones, which make the vagina dry; or allergic reactions to detergents, fabric softeners, soaps, or vaginal sprays.

A healthy vagina may have clear or slightly cloudy discharge. Vaginitis may cause changes in the color, smell, and texture of this discharge. For example, a yeast infection may cause vaginal discharge to look like cottage cheese. Vaginal discharge may also have a fishy smell if the infection is bacterial. Irritation, itching, or burning during urination may also occur.

Medications and topical creams may be prescribed to treat vaginitis. Cold compresses may also help. Avoid irritants to the vagina and abstain from sex until the infection is completely gone. To prevent vaginitis, encourage residents to maintain good hygiene and avoid using sprays or perfumed soaps. For immobile residents, providing daily perineal care is essential. (See Chapter 18 for the perineal care procedure.) Vaginal irrigation (*douching*) is not recommended, as it can disrupt the normal organisms in the vagina and increase the risk of another infection. Nylon clothing or tight pants that hold in heat and moisture will further the problem of vaginitis. Yogurt with active cultures may help reduce infection.

Uterine Prolapse

Uterine prolapse occurs when the muscles and ligaments of the pelvic floor stretch, weaken, and provide inadequate support for the uterus. The uterus can then slip down into the vagina or even protrude out of the vagina (**Figure 10.21**).

Uterine prolapse can vary in its severity and can happen to women of any age. It can be caused by damage to tissues during pregnancy and childbirth, large babies, loss of muscle tone, loss of estrogen during menopause, or continuous straining during elimination. Additional risk factors include age, obesity, heavy lifting, excessive coughing, and genetic predisposition.

Mild uterine prolapse usually goes unnoticed. The signs and symptoms of moderate-to-severe prolapse include tissue protruding from the vagina, urine leakage or retention (held in the body), trouble having a bowel movement, a pulling feeling in the pelvis, and low back pain.

Encourage residents with uterine prolapse to drink plenty of fluids, eat high-fiber foods (if appropriate), avoid straining during elimination, and to avoid coughing, if possible. Remind residents to use good body mechanics when lifting and maintain a proper weight (if needed) to decrease pressure. Sometimes a *vaginal pessary*, a device that fits inside the vagina and holds the uterus in place, may be ordered. Surgery is usually required to repair a severe prolapse.

How Does Cancer Affect the Body?

The effects of cancer provide a good example of how the body systems are all connected. Cancer can begin at a site in one body system and then spread to other systems. If it spreads, it affects not only the structure and function of the system where it started, but also the structure and function of other systems.

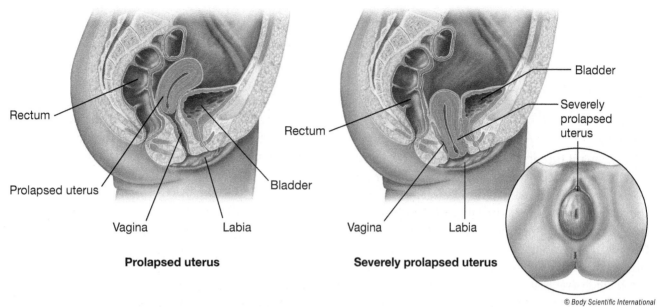

© Body Scientific International

Figure 10.21 A prolapsed uterus can slip into or protrude from the vagina.

Cancer occurs when cells grow abnormally and out of control, crowding out normal cells. Some cancers grow quickly, while others are slow-growing. There are many types of cancer, and cancer cell growth can start in any location of the body.

Cancer cells spread to other locations in the body through a process called *metastasis*. When metastasis occurs, cells from the original site of cancer (for example, the intestine) spread to other parts of the body (for example, the bones). Once cancer metastasizes, it is much harder to treat. The most common cancers are breast, lung, prostate, intestine and rectum, urinary bladder, skin, thyroid, and pancreatic cancer.

In many cancers, a lump called a *tumor* forms; if it is *malignant*, it is cancerous. If a tumor is *benign*, it does not contain cancer cells. A tumor might also be a *lipoma*, which consists of fat cells. Some cancers, such as blood cancer, do not form tumors. Blood cancer occurs within blood cells.

Cancer is classified using stages 1–4, with stage 1 meaning the cancer has not likely spread from its original site. As the stage numbers increase, the cancer is spreading further from its original site. Stage 4 is the most advanced stage of cancer. Some people will completely recover from cancer, some will live with cancer for many years in remission (which can mean all signs of cancer are gone), and others will die of cancer.

Cancer Risk Factors, Signs and Symptoms, and Diagnosis

Living a healthy lifestyle, not smoking, and avoiding toxic substances such as secondhand smoke will reduce the risk of developing cancer. Risk factors for cancer include age, family history of cancer, and exposure to sunlight without protection.

The signs and symptoms of cancer are different depending on the type and location of the cancer. For example, breast cancer often causes a lump to form in the breast, while a lesion on the skin may be a sign of melanoma. Some general signs and symptoms of cancer include:

- weight loss of 10 or more pounds with no reason
- consistent fatigue and fever
- pain that does not go away
- changes in the color or texture of the skin
- sores that do not heal
- changes in elimination
- unusual bleeding or discharge
- lumps
- trouble swallowing
- ongoing hoarseness and coughing

X-rays, blood tests, or a *biopsy* (the removal of a small piece of tissue for testing) are usually performed to diagnose cancer.

Cancer Treatments

Common treatment approaches for cancer usually include some combination of surgery, chemotherapy agents (toxic drugs), or radiation. The treatment method used depends on the type of cancer, its stage, and individual response.

Surgery

If a malignant tumor is present, the goal of surgery is to remove the entire tumor and its edges and be sure no cancerous cells remain. During surgery, sometimes the surgeon also removes surrounding tissue to prevent possible spread. Sometimes chemotherapy is given before surgery to shrink a tumor. If a resident has had surgery, he or she will need post-surgical care, which can include dressing changes, proper positioning, and careful monitoring of blood pressure.

Chemotherapy

Chemotherapy consists of a group of drugs that target cancer cells. Some chemotherapy drugs destroy cancer cells, some keep cancer from spreading, or others shrink tumors before surgery. Chemotherapy may be administered (given) by injection, an IV, topically, or orally. Chemotherapy is usually administered in timed cycles. Common side effects of chemotherapy include fatigue, dry mouth, sores in the mouth, easy bruising, appetite and weight changes, nausea and vomiting, constipation or diarrhea, hair loss, and changes in mood and concentration. These side effects usually go away soon after treatment, but some may take longer.

Radiation

Radiation is used to kill or slow the growth of cancer cells. A radiation treatment consists of high-energy waves directed at cancer cells. Side effects of radiation are different for each person, are associated with the location of radiation therapy, and can be mild or severe. Early side effects generally include nausea, fatigue, and skin problems. If radiation is administered (given) to the scalp, hair loss may be a side effect. Eating problems may result if treatment is administered to the head, face, or throat. Resulting eating problems usually do not last long.

Caring for Residents with Cancer

When people receive a diagnosis of cancer, their lives may no longer be the same. People will experience many changes in their self and body images, work schedules, family lives, and daily routines.

Providing Emotional Support

Many residents may become frightened and anxious after a cancer diagnosis, worrying about what will happen next and how long they will live. This can be overwhelming. There are many decisions to make and much to think about—not only for the present, but also for the future. A holistic nursing assistant must be sensitive to and aware of a resident's feelings about and approaches to cancer diagnosis and treatment. Supportive care and attention to residents' needs are fundamental. Being positive and adding humor, when appropriate, can be helpful.

Responding to Chemotherapy Side Effects

If a resident is having chemotherapy, he or she may have a catheter, port, and attached pump to control the delivery of medications (**Figure 10.22**). Skin care and observation for possible infection are very important. Attention to a resident's response to

---

HEALTHCARE SCENARIO

Effects of Exercise on Cancer

The National Cancer Institute recently reported the results from a large-scale study. The study found that greater levels of exercise—such as walking, running, or swimming—can result in a lower risk of developing 13 different types of cancer, including intestine, breast, and endometrial cancers. It is believed that exercise lowers the risk of cancer growth due to changes in cells' chemical reactions.

Apply It

1. How can you best use this research when caring for residents with cancer?
2. What challenges or barriers might you or others come across when using this research?

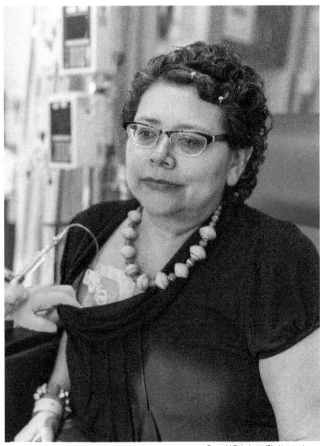

Emerald Raindrops/Shutterstock.com

Figure 10.22 Chemotherapy is delivered via a catheter and port.

chemotherapy and its side effects requires good observation and reporting.

- If a resident feels fatigued, be sure he or she rests after treatment and takes short naps during the day. If ordered and appropriate, a short walk can boost energy. Practice fall-prevention strategies.
- If a resident feels nauseous, small, frequent meals can help, as can apples, juice, tea, and flat ginger ale. Sometimes drinking fluids slowly before and after meals, but not during, can also help. Avoid strong-smelling foods, sweets, and fried fatty foods. Food may taste metallic; using plastic utensils may help.
- If a resident is experiencing hair loss, use a soft-bristle brush during hair care and mild, moisturizing shampoo and conditioners. The resident should wear a wig only if the scalp is clean and free from irritation or sores. Be sure the wig is clean.

- If a resident seems to have mental fog after treatment (sometimes called *chemo brain*), provide daily activities, talk with the resident, and focus on one thing or task at a time.
- Sun sensitivity is another side effect. Residents should go outside when the sun is the weakest (before 10 a.m. and after 4 p.m.). Sunscreen, clothing that covers the skin, and a wide-brimmed hat should be worn.

Report any unusual side effects to the licensed nursing staff.

Responding to Radiation Side Effects

Side effects of radiation may include skin that looks sunburned, is swollen or blistered, or becomes dry, flaky, and itchy. When caring for residents, be gentle during skin care and use mild soap and lukewarm water. Apply ointment or lotion as ordered but do not use hot or cold compresses, tape, or bandages unless instructed.

Use sun precautions even after the radiation has ended. Radiation therapy to certain parts of the body can have side effects that influence eating and cause nausea. Follow the same care discussed for residents experiencing nausea after chemotherapy. If radiation is administered to the head and neck, residents may experience mouth sores, lack of or thick saliva, and trouble swallowing. Take special care during oral hygiene (see Chapter 18). Diarrhea is another side effect. A doctor may prescribe medications and change the diet to ensure there is adequate nutrition. Be sure to keep the resident's skin and bed linens clean and dry.

End-of-Life Care

End-of-life experience is different for each person. For some, poor quality of life and the spread of cancer lead to a decision to end treatment. Holistic care is most important at this time. Some people choose to receive end-of-life care at home, others stay in long-term care settings, and others who are close to death may choose to use hospice services. Guidelines for providing end-of-life care can be found in Chapter 22.

SECTION 10.1 **Review and Assessment**

Key Terms Mini Glossary

acute disease a short-term disease or condition that usually starts suddenly.

analgesic a type of pain medication that does not cause loss of consciousness.

anesthetic a medication that produces a loss of sensation.

aneurysm a distended and weak area in the wall of an artery supplying blood to the brain.

aphasia a condition in which a resident cannot understand or use words.

arrhythmias abnormal heart rhythms.

arteriosclerosis a condition in which arteries thicken, harden, and lose elasticity.

atherosclerosis a condition in which arteries narrow due to plaque buildup.

benign not cancerous.

biopsy the removal of a small piece of tissue from a tumor using a special needle; the sample is tested for cancer cells.

chronic disease a long-term or recurring disease or condition.

coma a state of deep and prolonged unconsciousness.

dialysis the process of removing waste products and excess fluid from the body.

disease a condition in which an organ or body system functions incorrectly and exhibits particular signs and symptoms.

edema the retention of fluid in body tissues.

health the condition of a person's physical, mental, social, and spiritual self.

hemiplegia a condition of paralysis on one side of the body.

hypertension high blood pressure.

incontinence a lack of bowel or bladder control.

illness a feeling of poor health; not always caused by a disease.

malignant cancerous.

metastasis the spread of cancer cells to other locations in the body.

necrosis the death of body tissue.

nodules small, round lumps of body tissue; can be felt by touch.

pathology a collection of changes to the body's tissues or organs; can trigger a disease or can be caused by a disease.

plaques superficial, solid, elevated lesions.

sclerosis the thickening or hardening of a body part.

sign a piece of objective or factual information about a disease or condition.

symptom a piece of subjective information about a disease or condition; is based on a person's feelings or opinions.

well-being the state of a person's health; influenced by balancing one's diet, exercise, relationships, financial resources, work, education, and leisure.

wellness a feeling of good health

Apply the Key Terms

Think about the definitions of the following key terms. Describe one difference between each pair of key terms.

1. analgesic and anesthetic
2. illness and well-being
3. arteriosclerosis and atherosclerosis
4. arrhythmia and hypertension
5. edema and sclerosis

Know and Understand the Facts

1. What is the difference between an acute and chronic disease?
2. List two risk factors for one of the diseases discussed in this chapter.
3. What is hypertension, and how does it affect the body?
4. Explain the difference between atherosclerosis and arteriosclerosis.
5. Describe what happens when a resident has a hemorrhagic stroke.

Analyze and Apply Concepts

1. Discuss the typical treatment for a resident with diabetes mellitus.

2. Describe one way in which you can help a resident develop a sense of wellness or well-being.

Think Critically

Read the following care situation. Then answer the questions that follow.

Mrs. M was diagnosed with type 2 diabetes 15 years ago. She is 25 pounds overweight and has maintained her diabetic management plan for several years. Last month, she had a stroke. Mrs. M is now in a skilled nursing facility because she has left-sided weakness and is having trouble with her speech. The doctor feels that her diabetes is not stable, so he has prescribed insulin injections.

1. Which signs and symptoms should you watch for to determine if Mrs. M becomes hypoglycemic or hyperglycemic?
2. How are hypoglycemia and hyperglycemia treated?
3. Describe three important approaches to use when caring for Mrs. M.

Pain Relief

Objectives

To achieve the objectives for this section, you must successfully:

- **describe** types of pain and the pain cycle.
- **explain** reactions to pain and pain's impact on people's lives.
- **use** scales and measures to determine pain levels.
- **discuss** different ways to relieve pain and provide comfort.

Key Terms

Learn these key terms to better understand the information presented in the section.

acute pain	integrative medicine (IM)
addictive	nonpharmacological
chronic pain	pain scales
conventional medicine	stoic

Questions to Consider

- Think about the last time you felt physical pain. Did you hurt yourself, or was the pain from an illness?
- What was your initial reaction to pain? How long did the pain last? What did you do to lessen the pain?

What Is Pain?

Pain is an uncomfortable feeling or sensation that can be recognized by each of us. Sometimes pain occurs suddenly and goes away quickly. Pain may also start slowly and last for a long time.

Pain can be mild, moderate, or severe. When asked, people often describe their pain in different ways. Some might say their pain is sharp, dull, aching, throbbing, stabbing, crushing, or stinging. Pain can start as a sharp feeling and become achy, or it can begin as a dull pain and become crushing.

Many factors influence the development and severity of pain. Pain's cause, such as arthritis, a cut, or an abrasion, influences its sensation and severity. Other factors, such as the person's experience, cultural and ethnic influences, and the length of time pain is experienced, must also be considered when understanding pain.

Pain is felt, or *perceived*, when pain receptors in the nervous system are stimulated. Pain receptors send a signal to the spinal cord, which responds by causing a reflex action signaling motor nerves to act on the sensation of pain (**Figure 10.23**). The spinal cord also carries the pain message to the brain, which

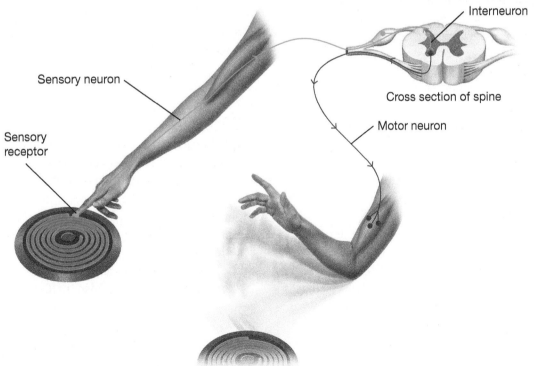

© *Body Scientific International*

Figure 10.23 Sensory receptors in the finger transmit pain messages to the spinal cord and brain to alert the person to remove her finger from the hot stove.

alerts the person that he or she is having pain. It also causes particular reactions, such as increased heart rate or sweating. This process happens very quickly so the body can take immediate action.

Acute and Chronic Pain

When pain is sudden and goes away quickly with treatment (within six months), it is acute. *Acute pain* may be the result of an injury, such as a broken bone, surgery, or even childbirth. When pain persists over time, it is chronic. *Chronic pain* may be the result of a past injury, disease, or condition. Some examples of chronic pain are low back pain, recurring headaches, or joint pain from arthritis.

Acute pain is felt (often intensely), begins to subside (lessen), and typically goes away quickly with or without treatment. Because chronic pain is usually from a disease, a person may have continuing pain from degenerative diseases, such as arthritis. People with chronic pain tend to react differently to pain they've had for a long time. For those with chronic pain, even the slightest touch can feel severe.

Cycle of Chronic Pain

Chronic pain occurs over and over again and feels endless to those experiencing it. This is why people with chronic pain experience the *cycle of chronic pain*. A repeating cycle of pain can lead to decreased activity, low interest in daily living, and decreased feelings of happiness and joy. Both physical reactions and psychological (emotional) responses are part of the cycle of chronic pain.

For example, a resident with chronic, painful muscle spasms in his lower back feels pain when he moves because movement causes immediate muscle tension or spasms. Muscle spasms lead to less blood flow, inflamed muscles, reduced mobility, muscle weakness, and decreased activity. When the resident moves and feels severe pain, he avoids further activity to reduce his pain.

The psychological or emotional aspect of the cycle of chronic pain includes fear, anxiety, and a stress response to pain. The resident who has muscle spasms in his lower back may become depressed due to his physical pain. Depression may lead to even more inactivity, because the resident may have little desire to do anything. If the resident uses pain medications for a long time, he may feel confused, very tired, and will lack energy. This will likely result in choosing to move even less (**Figure 10.24**).

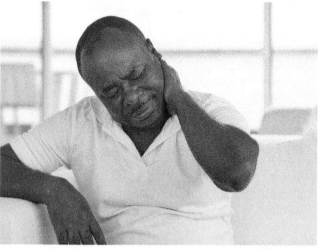

lunopark/Shutterstock.com

Figure 10.24 Chronic pain can have a major impact on residents' lives.

It is easy to imagine how the cycle of chronic pain affects people's lives. More time is spent focusing on the pain, and less on living life. Limited mobility leads to painful muscle tightening and atrophy, decreasing a person's motivation to be active. There is little joy, happiness, and desire. These experiences lead to frustration, sadness, depression, grief, and anger about a life that feels lost. It is not surprising that people who are in chronic pain have very little interest in ADLs and resist requests to exercise, be active, or socialize. While this is the cycle of chronic pain, not all people who have chronic pain experience it in this way. A great deal depends on how a person individually perceives pain.

The Pain Experience

Each person is the best judge of his or her own pain. One's experience and interpretation of pain can either strengthen or weaken the ability and willingness to withstand pain. A person who has a weakened capacity for pain may describe even the smallest pain as severe. For some, the threshold is high; these people are not particularly sensitive to pain. Others have a low threshold for pain; these people feel pain to a greater degree and feel stressed and emotionally exhausted.

The experience of pain also influences how people respond to pain medications. For some people, the need for medications to relieve pain is great. These people expect that, if medication is taken, the pain will go away. This may not always happen, however. A medication may not relieve the pain or may not be the right strength.

If medications are taken too often or for too long a period, they may become less effective, and the body may require larger amounts to reach the same relief. Some people are *stoic* (detached from feeling) and feel that they can withstand pain without the help of medication. This is based on the person's pain threshold.

It is always hard to judge others when it comes to perceived pain. The balance is a person's desire to control pain, the relief felt from pain medication, and efforts to avoid developing resistance to or overuse of pain medication.

What Is the Best Way to Observe and Report Pain?

When working as a holistic nursing assistant, you will need to help determine the level and intensity of a resident's pain so you can report it properly. This is important because it helps licensed nursing staff members make sure the most appropriate and effective pain medication is provided. This knowledge can also help holistic nursing assistants take *nonpharmacological* (not medication-based) actions, based on the plan of care, to help comfort and ease pain.

If pain is severe, the doctor might write an order for a prescription opioid. *Opioids* are a strong and powerful pain medication. They can be very helpful after surgery, or if a resident has pain from cancer. They are not usually helpful for chronic pain because they may be *addictive* (produce a psychological and physical inability to control or stop taking a medication). Research has shown that one in four people who take opioids for a long time become addicted, and some may even overdose. This happens because over time the body gets used to opioids and the same level of pain relief may not happen. To get that same relief, more is taken.

Opioids can have serious side effects if they are not given correctly:

- breathing problems and a slow heart rate
- confusion, dizziness, and mental disturbances, such as moodiness or outbursts of temper
- constipation
- drowsiness
- nausea and vomiting

Opioid medication must be stopped slowly, especially if the medication has been taken for a long time. The body needs to adjust. Otherwise *withdrawal symptoms* such as sweating, goosebumps, vomiting, anxiety, insomnia, and muscle pain may occur.

Awareness of Pain

The first step in determining others' pain is to be aware of your beliefs, attitudes, and feelings about pain. For example, if you have a high threshold for pain and come from a culture that is stoic, you might not be as sensitive to and aware of others' pain.

The next step is to understand how people express their pain. Many residents can describe their pain in detail. Others may just say, "I hurt." Many times, a resident's facial expressions and gestures are key signs of pain. For example, a resident who keeps her eyes closed and tenses the muscles in her jaw may be in pain. Other gestures that show pain include keeping the hands closed around the body or rubbing the part of the body that hurts.

CULTURE CUES
Expressions of Pain

A resident's feelings about disease, pain, and the use of pain medications are often learned through tradition and family values. Some residents are very expressive about pain, while stoic residents may feel they should bear pain silently, perhaps even smiling through the pain. Residents may have learned growing up that pain should be ignored and that it is just part of life. As a result of their experiences, they will be affected by pain differently. Some residents may need a great deal of pain relief, and others will not ask for or even require it.

A resident's willingness to report pain may also be influenced by his or her cultural background. Bearing pain means suffering pain well, a quality valued by some. Not everyone in every culture conforms to a set of expected behaviors or beliefs; however, being mindful and sensitive to how others respond to and express pain is important when giving care.

Apply It

1. What assumptions or values do you have about pain based on your culture and family values?
2. How have your assumptions or values affected your response to pain?
3. In your opinion, what two actions can you take as a holistic nursing assistant to demonstrate you are aware of a resident's pain?

Pain Scales

When providing holistic care, you must always be objective in how you observe and report the resident's subjective perceptions and feelings about pain. This is particularly important when discussing pain. Pain is sometimes considered the fifth vital sign (along with blood pressure, pulse, respiration, and temperature). Objectively reporting the resident's subjective feelings of pain can help the licensed nursing staff assess a resident's condition. *Pain scales*, or devices used to measure the perception of the severity of pain, can help you do this (**Figure 10.25**). Check to see which scales your healthcare facility uses. Pain scales can help residents describe the intensity of pain using numbers from 0 (no pain) to 10 (severe pain).

A pain scale that uses expressive cartoon faces to show different levels of pain can be helpful when working with those who do not speak English well. The resident selects the face that best describes the intensity of pain on a range from *does not hurt* to *hurts a whole lot*.

Pain scales also exist for residents who cannot communicate verbally. These pain scales require that you observe residents for certain expressions and gestures classified as pain indicators. For example, you would look at a resident's face and determine, based on expressions, where the resident falls and how much pain the resident is experiencing. These scales may also determine the resident's level of activity—from lying quietly to thrashing about in the bed—and whether the resident is crying, moaning, or whimpering. Careful listening and observation help a holistic nursing assistant find out the real story behind a resident's pain.

Pain Relief

Depending on the pain and its severity, pain may be relieved using over-the-counter medications or prescribed pain medications. Physical therapy and pain-relief therapy can also help.

Integrative medicine may also be used for pain relief. *Integrative medicine (IM)* is alternative approaches that are used along with, or in place of, *conventional medicine* (symptoms and diseases are treated using prescription medications, clinical procedures, radiation, or surgery). IM approaches can be used to relieve pain. Some IM approaches used for pain relief include:

- acupuncture or acupressure
- relaxation techniques, such as deep breathing
- meditation
- massage therapy
- biofeedback (the use of a device to practice relaxation techniques)
- hypnotherapy
- yoga
- tai chi or qigong

IM approaches must be reviewed by a doctor before they are used to make sure they do not interfere with pain-relief goals or the disease process. They must also be performed by providers who have required training and credentials.

Some IM approaches are more effective when combined with other methods. For example, some prescribed medications are more effective when combined with massage or meditation. Residents might need to try various methods to maintain maximum pain relief. A pain-relief action plan or a consultation

PAIN MEASUREMENT SCALE

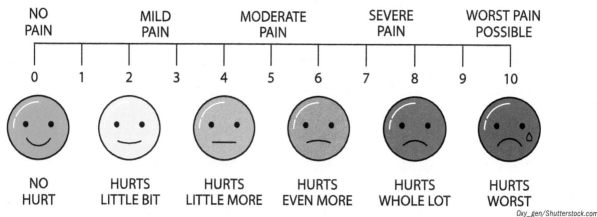

Oxy_gen/Shutterstock.com

Figure 10.25 Pain scales may use numbers and faces to help residents identify their levels of pain.

with a pain-relief specialist can be helpful. To assist in pain relief, a holistic nursing assistant can:

- be sensitive to and aware of a resident's pain during care
- help residents relax before, during, and after procedures by encouraging them to use deep breathing during times of pain
- provide comfortable positioning
- encourage residents to listen to favorite music before, during, and after procedures to stay calm
- talk with residents about their memories of peaceful and calm experiences

- use distraction by providing reading materials, favorite television shows, or opportunities to talk with family and friends
- provide a gentle massage, which is particularly helpful during bathing
- apply warm and cold packs and compresses, if ordered
- use pleasing aromas in the room, if acceptable

If you have residents who have difficulty talking about pain, you might ask them to write about their pain and discuss their thoughts with family members, a doctor, or the licensed nursing staff.

SECTION 10.2 **Review and Assessment**

Key Terms Mini Glossary

acute pain an intense discomfort, often the result of trauma, that goes away within six months with treatment.

addictive causing a psychological and physical inability to control or stop taking a medication.

chronic pain a persistent, uncomfortable feeling that does not go away over time.

conventional medicine symptoms and diseases are treated using prescription medications, clinical procedures, radiation, or surgery; also called *Western medicine* or *allopathic medicine.*

integrative medicine (IM) alternative approaches that are used along with, or in place of, conventional medicine

nonpharmacological without the use of medication.

pain scales devices used to measure a person's perception of the severity of pain.

stoic detached from emotion or feeling.

Apply the Key Terms

Identify the key term used in each sentence.

1. Licensed nursing staff used a pain scale to measure the perception of the resident's severity of pain.
2. Using prescription medications is an example of conventional medicine.
3. Meditation is considered an integrative medicine approach.
4. Chronic pain can be persistent, uncomfortable, and does not go away over time.
5. When residents are detached and show no emotion or feeling they are stoic.

Know and Understand the Facts

1. Describe the two types of pain.
2. What is the difference between acute and chronic pain?
3. Identify two nonpharmacological or IM approaches to pain relief.
4. Describe the cycle of chronic pain.

Analyze and Apply Concepts

1. List three ways in which pain can impact people's lives.
2. How might the chronic pain cycle affect a resident's pain experience?
3. List two reasons why residents might react to pain differently.
4. Explain why and how pain scales are used.

5. A nursing assistant is providing morning care for a resident. The resident states that she has pain in her right wrist and arm. What three actions can the nursing assistant take to assist with pain relief?

Think Critically

Read the following care situation. Then answer the questions that follow.

You are caring for Mrs. G in an assisted living center. Mrs. G has advanced rheumatoid arthritis that affects many of her joints. She also has COPD. Your assignment is to help Mrs. G with bathing and ambulation. Mrs. G is 82 years old and has been at the center for six months. She is quite thin and frail. She uses a walker for ambulation and seems very independent. When you walk into Mrs. G's room, she tells you that today she has quite a bit of pain in her hips and would rather stay in bed and not bathe.

1. How should you respond to Mrs. G using what you know about arthritis and COPD?
2. How can you best determine Mrs. G's pain intensity and level so you can inform the licensed nursing staff?
3. What do you need to know about Mrs. G's diseases to help with pain relief?
4. What nonpharmacological approaches might you use with Mrs. G?
5. Identify two ways you can provide safe, quality, holistic nursing care.

Key Points

Reviewing the key points for this chapter will help you practice more safely and competently as a holistic nursing assistant and will help you prepare for the certification competency examination.

- There is a relationship between wellness and illness. A person can experience both wellness and illness at the same time. Even when a person is ill, parts of his or her body and mind can still have some level of wellness.
- Diseases and conditions can be acute or chronic. An acute disease or condition lasts a short amount of time and happens suddenly. Chronic diseases or conditions last for at least three months and are often lifetime challenges.
- A holistic nursing assistant must be knowledgeable about common diseases and conditions and their causes, signs and symptoms, general treatments, and ways to provide care.
- Pain is an uncomfortable feeling or sensation. Pain that is sudden and goes away relatively quickly with treatment is acute. When pain does not go away over time, it is chronic.
- Pain can be severe, moderate, or mild, and the perception of pain is individual. Diseases or conditions, individual and familial experiences with pain, cultural and ethnic influences, and how long pain is experienced all influence a person's perception and expression of pain.
- Pain scales help determine levels of pain and intensity and provide important information for the licensed nursing staff.
- Nonpharmacological actions such as deep breathing and massage can help comfort and ease pain.

Action Steps to Holistic Care

Review the information in this chapter. Complete the following activities.

1. Select a disease or condition not discussed in this chapter. Conduct research and prepare a short paper or digital presentation that summarizes the causes, signs and symptoms, and three ways to best provide care.
2. Find two pictures in a magazine, in a newspaper, or online that best demonstrate various levels and intensities of pain. Describe each image and discuss how it represents pain.
3. Select one cultural, ethnic, or religious group and research values or traditions they might have surrounding pain. Describe these values or traditions and identify two approaches to best provide care.

Building Math Skill

Lorraine has been taking care of Mr. V for several days. He has lung cancer and has quite a bit of pain. When she goes into his room he complains of pain in his back. Lorraine uses the pain scale to ask him how bad the pain is. He says, "8." The licensed nursing staff member then comes in and gives Mr. V. his pain medication When Lorraine checks on him after an hour, he says his pain is now a "3". Four hours later, Mr. V's call light goes on and Lorraine goes into his room. Mr. V. is moving about in his bed and is crying. He says his pain is now a "10."

1. What is the difference in Mr. V's pain level before his pain medication and after it has taken effect?
2. What is the difference in Mr. V's pain level from when the medication is working to when it wears off?

Preparing for the Certification Competency Examination

To prepare for the nursing assistant certification competency examination, you will need to know content found in this chapter. This content may be tested in the knowledge (written or oral) and skills (hands-on demonstration) portions of the exam. The following areas will be emphasized:

- common health problems involving the body systems
- signs and symptoms of common health problems, types of pain, and factors that lead to discomfort and pain
- expressions and gestures that indicate discomfort and pain
- scales and measures for determining level of pain
- nonpharmacological measures that nursing assistants can use to enhance comfort

The sample test questions are similar to ones you will find on the certification competency exam. See how well you can answer them. Be sure to select the *best* answer.

1. Which of the following is the best strategy for people to achieve long-lasting health and wellness?
   A. talking with their friends about the medications they take
   B. visiting the doctor only when they are ill
   C. taking responsibility for their own care
   D. reading a chapter in a book about wellness

2. Which of the following describes pain that goes away rather quickly?
   A. chronic
   B. mild
   C. acute
   D. sharp

3. Mrs. D has had psoriasis for several years. How would you expect her skin to look?
   A. very dry, thick, or scaly and itchy
   B. with rough patches and thick, wart-like growths
   C. dry with rough patches and tiny bumps
   D. thick with red patches or plaques

4. Mr. K is admitted to the emergency department with severely low blood sugar. What is this condition called?
   A. hypotension
   B. hypoglycemia
   C. hyperglycemia
   D. hypertension

5. When a resident is diagnosed with arthritis, this is considered a(n)
   A. degenerative disease
   B. infectious disease
   C. nutritional disease
   D. environmental disease

6. Mr. F has coronary artery disease. He is complaining of shortness of breath. This is called
   A. angina
   B. lupus
   C. aphasia
   D. dyspnea

7. A nursing assistant wants to help Mrs. B be more comfortable and get some relief from her back and hip pain. Which of the following actions would *not* be helpful?
   A. using the pain scale to report the level of pain
   B. making Mrs. B walk around the room to exercise her back and hip
   C. helping Mrs. B deep-breathe and think about a pleasant experience
   D. using distraction by suggesting a favorite TV program to watch

8. A nursing assistant is caring for a resident who has had a stroke. The resident is having trouble speaking. What is this symptom called?
   A. GERD
   B. hemiplegia
   C. metastasis
   D. aphasia

9. Today, Mr. O is seeing Dr. Smith to tell her about his unexplained weight loss of 15 pounds, consistent fatigue, and trouble swallowing. Which of the following conditions might Mr. O have?
   A. cancer
   B. COPD
   C. renal failure
   D. GERD

10. Mrs. Q has a superficial decubitus ulcer on her hip. The ulcer has only one blister filled with fluid, and the surrounding area is irritated and red. What stage is the decubitus ulcer?
    A. stage 4
    B. stage 2
    C. stage 1
    D. stage 3

11. Ms. N has COPD. Her primary symptoms are most likely
    A. mental confusion
    B. nausea and vomiting
    C. coughing and mucus
    D. chest pain

12. Research has shown that bacterial infection can cause
    A. GERD
    B. gastritis
    C. diverticulitis
    D. peptic ulcer

13. Which of the following is another name for GERD?
    A. acid reflux
    B. angina
    C. stroke
    D. heart attack

14. What is one way to prevent a resident from contracting a UTI?
    A. provide good catheter and perineal care
    B. make sure you use warm compresses on the urethra
    C. be sure the resident takes daily medications
    D. keep the linens free from crumbs and wrinkles

15. Your best friend has asthma. She usually is able to control her flares, but today she is short of breath and is having trouble breathing. What should she do first?
    A. use her quick-relief inhaler
    B. call 9-1-1
    C. call her doctor
    D. use her nebulizer

Did you have difficulty with any of the questions? If you did, review the chapter to find the correct answer(s).

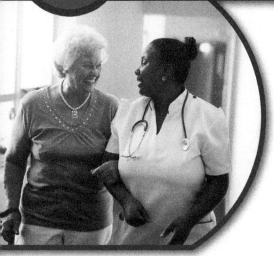

Jacob Lund/Shutterstock.com

Welcome to the Chapter

In this chapter, you will learn how to use verbal and nonverbal communication to positively influence your interpersonal relationships with others. You will also develop listening skills and learn to overcome communication barriers. As a holistic nursing assistant, you will help licensed nursing staff communicate important information about residents' health. Learning to communicate holistically will help you establish positive, caring relationships with residents. In this chapter, you will also learn to recognize how anxiety, fear, anger, and conflict affect communication and interpersonal relationships and how you can respond effectively to these emotions and situations.

What you learn in this chapter will help you develop your knowledge and skills to become a holistic nursing assistant. The topics discussed in the chapter are highlighted on the Providing Holistic Care Framework.

Chapter Outline

Section 11.1
Holistic Communication

Section 11.2
Caring Skills
and Interpersonal
Relationships

Section 11.3
Anxiety, Fear, Anger,
and Conflict

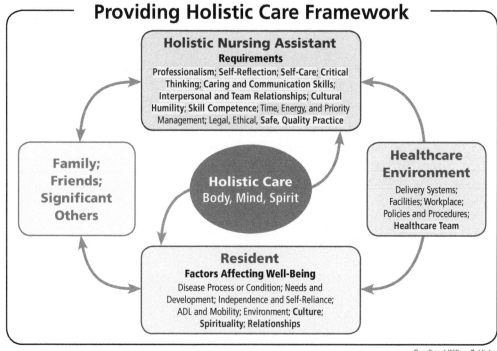

Providing Holistic Care Framework

Holistic Nursing Assistant
Requirements
Professionalism; Self-Reflection; Self-Care; Critical Thinking; Caring and Communication Skills; Interpersonal and Team Relationships; Cultural Humility; Skill Competence; Time, Energy, and Priority Management; Legal, Ethical, Safe, Quality Practice

Family; Friends; Significant Others

Holistic Care
Body, Mind, Spirit

Healthcare Environment
Delivery Systems; Facilities; Workplace; Policies and Procedures; Healthcare Team

Resident
Factors Affecting Well-Being
Disease Process or Condition; Needs and Development; Independence and Self-Reliance; ADL and Mobility; Environment; Culture; Spirituality; Relationships

Goodheart-Willcox Publisher

Holistic Communication

Objectives

To achieve the objectives for this section, you must successfully:

- **explain** the basic principles of holistic communication.
- **describe** verbal and nonverbal communication and active listening.
- **identify** barriers to holistic communication.
- **demonstrate** holistic communication strategies.

Key Terms

Learn these key terms to better understand the information presented in the section.

active listening
body language
clarification
closed-ended question
communication barriers
defense mechanisms

health literacy
interpreter
jargon
labeling
open-ended question
prejudice

Questions to Consider

- Do you enjoy talking with others?
- Do you think you are an effective communicator? What special qualities and characteristics do you have that help you communicate effectively with others?
- What can you do to improve your communication skills?

Humans have been communicating with one another since the beginning of time. Even before people began to speak and write, they used cave paintings, rock carvings (*petroglyphs*), and rock paintings (*pictographs*) to communicate. We have come a long way since those very early days.

Today, people communicate with one another in many ways. In addition to face-to-face communication and talking on the telephone, smartphones, tablets, and laptops give people the ability to communicate electronically using e-mail, text messaging, video chatting, and social media. Healthcare facilities also use e-mail, video conferencing, and social media to communicate with staff, advertise services, and provide education.

What Is Holistic Communication?

A large part of your responsibility as a nursing assistant will be communicating effectively. *Communication* is the way people exchange information with one another.

People send and receive messages—both verbal and nonverbal—with the goal of communicating thoughts, needs, and feelings.

When communication is holistic, it considers all aspects of a resident's body, mind, and spirit. *Holistic communication* is more than just talking. It is being fully present and fully focused on a conversation with another person. Holistic communication promotes healing and well-being and keeps lines of communication open to achieve a caring environment. Successful holistic communicators are accurate, honest, timely, and nonjudgmental. Holistic communication helps nursing assistants and residents develop trusting, respectful relationships, which are very important to delivering safe, quality care.

Components of Communication

As a holistic nursing assistant, you will communicate verbally with residents, residents' families, and members of the healthcare team. You will give residents instructions, talk with residents and their families, share information about resident care with the healthcare team, and discuss procedures with the licensed nursing staff. These are only a few examples of how you will communicate verbally during your shift. The ability to communicate effectively, being sure your message is heard and understood, is necessary for delivering safe, quality care. To communicate a message effectively, you must understand the four basic components (parts) of communication (**Figure 11.1**):

1. **The sender:** begins the conversation and decides what the message is and the best way to share it.
2. **Mode of communication:** chosen by the sender, the message can be sent by speaking, listening, using gestures or body language, and writing. The mode of communication should always fit the situation and be clear.
3. **Recipient (receiver):** the message is received when the recipient listens carefully to the spoken words, including the tone and pitch of the sender's voice, and observes the sender's body language.
4. **Feedback:** the response from the recipient that confirms that the sender and recipient have the same, or similar, understanding of the message.

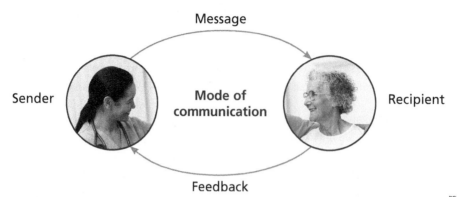

Figure 11.1 The four components of communication are the sender, mode of communication, recipient, and feedback.

ESB Professional/Shutterstock.com

Verbal and Nonverbal Communication

As you learned in Chapter 2, *verbal communication* occurs when people use spoken words to express themselves. *Nonverbal communication* does not use words, but instead includes pointing your finger, shaking your head, making facial expressions, or using body gestures. Body posture also reflects your feelings. For example, standing with your back straight indicates confidence, while slumped shoulders can convey a lack of confidence or interest.

Body language is a type of nonverbal communication that uses gestures (such as nodding your head or shrugging your shoulders) and body movements. Messages sent using body language can be clear or require interpretation. Unfortunately, people are not always aware of their body language. A person might communicate an opinion verbally, but communicate a differing opinion with his or her body language. Even when body language accurately communicates thoughts or feelings, others may not interpret the body language in the way it was meant.

Other types of nonverbal communication include making eye contact, moving the eyebrows and forehead, using touch, and recognizing zones of personal space. In the United States, comfortable zones of personal space are expressed in the following ways:

- *Intimate space* (1.5 feet or less) might be shared with family, very close friends, and pets.
- *Personal space* (1.5–4 feet) is used for friends and acquaintances.
- *Social space* (4–12 feet) is often seen in business settings or when meeting new people.
- *Public space* (12 feet or more) is observed when speaking in front of a group of strangers.

In your role as a nursing assistant, you will often enter residents' personal space to give care. When entering a resident's intimate space, remember to be courteous and respectful. Ask permission to touch the resident prior to each procedure. If doing a procedure that involves an intimate body part, move slowly and explain what you are doing. Avoid standing over a resident if you can, as this can make him feel uncomfortable. When possible, remain at the resident's eye level when you are working or talking (**Figure 11.2**). If you use your hands to deliver care, make sure your hands are warm. If you need to use gloves or a mask, explain why.

Observation

To communicate holistically, you must use your senses of sight, smell, touch, and hearing. Using your senses will strengthen your observations, improve the care you give, and make your interactions more meaningful. One way to use your senses is to observe changes in residents. For example, observing a resident's facial expressions can let you know if the resident is in pain. You may use your sense of smell to identify a foul odor, which can help identify a possible new condition.

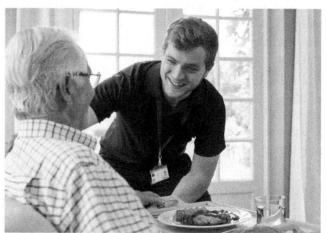

Monkey Business Images/Shutterstock.com

Figure 11.2 Talking with residents at eye level will help them feel more comfortable.

Personal Space

Different cultures have different views about personal space. For example, in public places in Japan, personal space is limited, and people push up against each other when standing and walking. In Italy, the personal space between strangers is an arm's length, but personal space is much closer with friends and family, and people often hug and kiss in public. In Egypt, gender plays an important role in personal space. If two people of the same sex are talking, personal space will be very close; however, if two people of the opposite sex are talking, they will usually stand an arm's length apart or more. In the United States, people value personal space and tend to be most comfortable 2–3 feet from another person during conversation. Pay attention to your residents' cultures and adjust your actions and care accordingly.

Apply It

1. Describe any experiences you have had with your own personal space and different cultures.
2. How do you think the views of personal space in different cultures will affect the care you give as a holistic nursing assistant?

Your sense of touch can help others feel cared about and also allow you to feel changes in skin temperature. You will learn more about observation and reporting in Chapter 13.

What Communication Devices Are Used in Healthcare?

In healthcare facilities, urgent needs and information are often communicated using a pager or paging system, landline telephone, or cell phone provided by the facility. E-mail is also used, but only for information unrelated to the resident and care. For example, e-mail might be used to communicate announcements, scheduling, or meeting invitations and reminders.

Telephones in healthcare facilities provide a way to share and gather information. Typically, landline telephones are located at a nurse's station, and answering the telephone is an important part of a nursing assistant's daily responsibilities.

The same legal requirements and confidentiality required for face-to-face and written communication also affect information shared over the telephone. If you share important information about a resident over the telephone, you should write this information down and verify by restating the information back to the caller. If you believe taking the information is outside your legal scope of practice, let the caller know and find a member of the licensed nursing staff.

The following guidelines will help you communicate properly using the telephone. Remember to always follow facility guidelines.

- Answer the telephone promptly. Greet callers in a friendly, professional manner. Identify yourself and your unit.

- If you are making a call, state your first or preferred name and title when your call is answered. Let the person know immediately why you are calling (**Figure 11.3**).
- Speak clearly, confidently, and using a moderate volume and speed. Listen carefully and ask questions, if needed. If you are taking a message, ask the caller to spell his or her name and any unfamiliar words and include the date and time of the call.
- If a doctor calls to communicate medical orders, let the doctor know receiving this information is outside your scope of practice. You may ask the doctor to hold while you get a licensed nursing staff member or ask if the doctor would like his or her call returned.

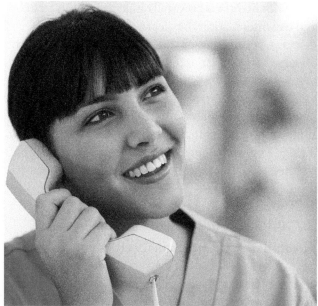

wavebreakmedia/Shutterstock.com

Figure 11.3 When calling, immediately identify yourself and the reason for the call.

- If you need to place a caller on hold, ask for the caller's permission before doing so.
- Never use jargon or medical abbreviations.
- Listen to the other person carefully to determine the best way to assist him or her.
- Take notes while listening, wait for the other person to finish speaking, repeat key points, and ask questions to clarify the person's statements.
- Finish the call in a friendly, professional way.

In many healthcare facilities, telephones are located in resident rooms. Facilities may also provide secure cell phones that nursing assistants and licensed nursing staff members can use during their shifts. These phones are sometimes connected to the call lights in resident rooms, allowing the nursing assistant to answer a call light using the phone.

What Are Barriers to Effective Holistic Communication?

Communication barriers are actions, behaviors, or situations that interfere with or block effective holistic communication. For example, language can be a communication barrier. You can avoid this barrier by using words that others will understand. You may need to adjust these words if a resident speaks another language or does not have a good understanding of English. If a resident speaks a different language, be sure to ask for an *interpreter* who can translate for you. If there are no interpreters available, use pictures to communicate your message.

Health literacy is how well residents fully understand and use information they learn about their health, diseases, conditions, or treatments. A person's health literacy can be a barrier to communication. Poor health literacy can result when people ignore what they are told, misinterpret messages, or lack the information or understanding to follow instructions or report abnormal symptoms. Factors that may influence health literacy include English reading and writing skills, beliefs about wellness and illness, and knowledge about healthcare topics and systems.

Jargon and Slang

Jargon and slang are informal words, phrases, and language used by a specific group of people or culture. The use of jargon or slang is another barrier to effective holistic communication. The words in jargon and slang may be unfamiliar to residents and can complicate a conversation or cause misunderstanding. People from different generations, cultures, or geographical areas may have their own unique jargon or slang. Examples of slang include the word *selfie* and *lol* (short for "laugh out loud").

Some jargon is specific to healthcare and is acceptable to use with other healthcare staff members. Examples of healthcare jargon include medical abbreviations, such as *BP* for "blood pressure"; *NPO*, which means "nothing by mouth"; or *vitals*, which is short for "vital signs." Do not use healthcare jargon with residents. Instead, use words that everyone you work with and care for will understand. If you must use a word that may cause confusion, explain what the word means.

Stereotypes and Labels

Another barrier to communication is *stereotyping*, which you learned about in Chapter 7. Some people use stereotypes to make negative and discriminatory behaviors against others acceptable. To avoid this communication barrier, always be aware of any biases you have against groups or types of people. It is important to treat everyone with respect.

Labeling, or negatively describing someone in one word or a phrase, is also a barrier to communication. Labeling can cause *prejudice*, or an opinion or feeling that is formed without facts and often leads to an unfair feeling of dislike for a person because of race, sex, or religion. Prejudice can prevent people from examining whether there is truth to a label. Labeling is also hurtful to the person who is labeled. For example, saying that someone who talks a lot has a "big mouth" may make that person not want to share an important opinion. If you call someone lazy and laugh, the other person may feel hurt.

Words can hurt others. Think about the words you use. Do not use labels as part of your day-to-day communication. The role of the nursing assistant is to assist others in their daily lives, not to make their lives more difficult.

Advice

It is not the nursing assistant's role or responsibility to give advice or opinions to residents, family members of residents, or healthcare staff. If nursing assistants give advice instead of listening, they may ignore what a resident really wants to communicate, and this will result in a poor quality of care. Giving personal advice crosses professional boundaries. Giving medical advice about a resident's disease, condition, or treatment plan is outside the scope of practice for a nursing assistant and can be dangerous. Refer any medical questions to the licensed nursing staff. If you are asked a question you cannot answer, be polite and explain that you will let the licensed nursing staff know about the concern.

Cultural Barriers

It is important for caregivers to be aware of other people's cultures. If you do not know a resident's culture or beliefs, you may do something hurtful to the resident. Take time to learn about residents' cultural beliefs. Where are residents from? Do they speak English? Do they have cultural beliefs that influence how they communicate (for example, not making eye contact with others)? As a holistic nursing assistant, always look for any special attention or changes in care that residents may need because of cultural beliefs.

Hearing Impairments

The tone of your voice and the rate at which you speak may present a challenge when you communicate with residents who have hearing impairments (difficulties). When caring for a resident who has a hearing impairment, always approach the resident from the front. When talking, always face the resident, use good eye contact, and avoid mumbling (**Figure 11.4**). You may need to speak slower or louder for those who cannot hear well, but you do not need to yell. Use short sentences and simple words. Remember that high-pitched tones may be difficult to hear, even if a resident uses a hearing aid. Always make sure that residents' hearing aids are turned on and that the batteries are working.

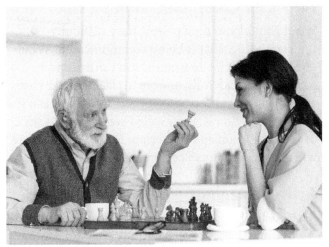

LightField Studios/Shutterstock.com

Figure 11.4 Always make eye contact when communicating with a resident who has a hearing impairment.

Some residents and their families may rely on *sign language* to communicate. In these situations, an American Sign Language (ASL) interpreter may be needed. An ASL interpreter may be very helpful when important instructions or information need to be communicated. Check with the licensed nursing staff to learn how you can find this resource.

Vision Impairments

Eyesight tends to worsen as people age, so many residents will have vision impairments, and some may wear eyeglasses. The holistic nursing assistant's responsibility is to make sure that eyeglasses are clean and fit well. If eyeglasses are not clean, use a soft cloth to clean them. If there are any problems with the eyeglasses or if a resident refuses to wear his or her eyeglasses, tell the licensed nursing staff.

To avoid startling residents, knock on the door before entering a resident's room and always announce who you are. This is very important for all residents, but is even more important for those with vision impairments who may have difficulty seeing you without eyeglasses. When entering a resident's room, you could say, "Good morning, Mrs. O. I'm Tammy, your nursing assistant. I'm here to help you get dressed."

Speech Impairments

Speech impairments may make it harder for residents to communicate with you. For example, *aphasia* is one speech impairment you may experience when caring for residents. Aphasia may be caused by a stroke, brain tumor, brain injury, infection, or dementia.

There are different types of aphasia. In one type, residents know what they want to say, but have difficulty communicating. In another type, residents struggle to find the right words to speak or write. At its most severe, aphasia causes difficulty speaking and understanding words.

When working with residents who have speech impairments, check for understanding. Speak slowly and calmly in simple sentences. Give residents the time they need to talk, and do not finish residents' sentences or correct errors. Gesturing or pointing to objects can also help with explanations.

Cognitive Challenges

People with cognitive challenges such as dementia (progressive, permanent cognitive disorders that get worse over time) may forget events, have trouble learning, be unable to process and understand information, and behave inappropriately. These challenges are the result of changes in the brain.

These changes result in memory loss, confusion about time and dates, disorientation, and trouble finding the right words or being a part of a conversation. Holistic nursing assistants should approach residents with dementia in a calm, professional manner and should use proper body language to show respect and interest. As a nursing assistant, you may smile and gently touch or hug a resident, when appropriate. Always keep an even tone of voice, as loud noises can cause an aggressive response. Maintain eye contact and calmly explain why you are there and what is needed. Keep instructions simple and break them down into steps and wait between questions for answers. When needed, use questions, such as, "Would you like to wear this sweater today?" Use simple words, such as "Roll to the right" or "Stand up," followed with praise.

Defense Mechanisms

Some of the most serious barriers to communication are *defense mechanisms*. Defense mechanisms are unconscious behaviors that enable people to ignore or forget situations or thoughts that cause fear, anxiety, and stress. Defense mechanisms are a form of stress management. For example, a person may deny that he or she has an illness such as diabetes to decrease feelings of fear or anxiety.

Defense mechanisms can prevent people from being honest about and sharing their feelings. There are many defense mechanisms, and only some of them interfere with communication. Common defense mechanisms that may create communication barriers include the following:

- **Denial**: rejecting the truth about one's feelings, experiences, or facts. An example of denial is a resident insisting he feels fine when he does not. The resident is using the defense mechanism to convince himself and others that he is fine.
- **Repression**: refusing to remember a traumatic or painful situation. An example might be forgetting a terrifying childhood event.
- **Regression**: returning to childlike behaviors when fearful, anxious, or angry. A resident who has a temper tantrum may be exhibiting signs of regression.
- **Displacement**: transferring a bad or negative feeling, such as anger, away from the source and onto someone or something else. For example,

you might be angry with your friend, but hold the anger in until you get home and express your anger at a family member.
- **Projection**: believing that others feel a certain way when, in fact, the feelings are yours. For example, you might say, "I know my teacher dislikes me," when the real truth is that you dislike your teacher.
- **Reaction formation**: feeling one way inside, but outwardly expressing the feeling in an opposite way. For example, you may not like a person, but still go out of your way to be nice to her.
- **Intellectualizing**: focusing on facts, logic, and reasoning instead of a stressful feeling or uncomfortable emotion. For example, a resident recently diagnosed with a terminal illness may focus on learning everything about the disease and possible treatments instead of dealing with his or her feelings about the diagnosis.
- **Rationalization**: using logic to excuse unacceptable behaviors and feelings. Often, people use this defense mechanism after they have done something they regret. An example would be stealing money from a friend and then making it sound acceptable by saying, "She owed me money anyway."

We all use defense mechanisms. When defense mechanisms are overused, however, they are no longer protective and can become harmful. It is important to recognize when defense mechanisms are being used, either by yourself or by others. Recognizing defense mechanisms is a good first step in making sure defense mechanisms do not become barriers to communication.

How Can Communication Be Improved?

What should you do if people have difficulty understanding what is being communicated? When you are in difficult communication situations, be patient, listen carefully, and try to clarify (make clear) and reflect what is being communicated. You can use a communication strategy called *active listening*, which uses clarification and reflection. Proper questioning will also help improve communication.

Active Listening

Active listening promotes understanding and successful communication. Active listening involves showing interest in the person speaking and what is being said. Pay attention and use good eye contact. Eye contact helps the speaker feel that what he or she is saying is important and that the message has been received. Eye contact also shows you are willing to take the time to pay attention. Sitting down, leaning toward the speaker, and nodding your head also show you are actively listening (**Figure 11.5**).

Clarification involves restating what you believe was said to make sure you heard the message correctly. To ask for clarification, you might say to the speaker, "I want to be sure I understand. What I heard you say was…"

Reflection is an approach in which you listen, identify feelings a resident is expressing nonverbally, and ask a question to bring those feelings forward. For example, you might ask, "Are you feeling frustrated about not being able to walk as well as you did yesterday?" The goal of reflection is to identify a resident's feelings so they can be expressed and discussed. Often, just stating the feeling will relieve a resident's tension and frustration and lead to increased comfort and well-being.

Questioning

Questions are helpful communication tools. The most effective questions are *open-ended questions* that lead to more than a one-word answer. Open-ended questions help you get the information you need to provide safe, quality holistic care.

An example of an open-ended question is "How well did you sleep last night?" As the resident considers the answer to this question, he or she may also think of other details to share and tell you that, "Although I slept for about seven hours, I had a hard time falling asleep and had some strange dreams." This answer begins a conversation with the nursing assistant. The

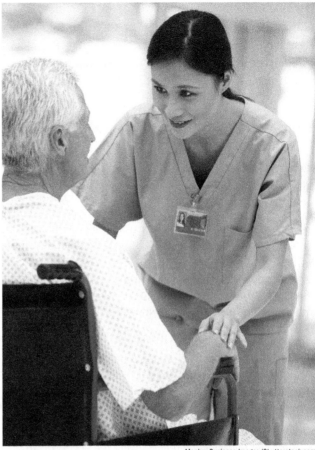

Monkey Business Images/Shutterstock.com

Figure 11.5 This nursing assistant is demonstrating that she is actively listening.

nursing assistant can explore the length and quality of the resident's sleep by asking more open-ended questions.

A more specific or *closed-ended question* often does not produce detailed answers. A closed-ended question, such as "Did you sleep well last night?"

BECOMING A HOLISTIC NURSING ASSISTANT

Holistic Communication

The more personalized your interactions with residents are, the more comfortable residents will feel. Including the following holistic communication guidelines into your daily practice will help you develop strong relationships with those in your care:

- Always face residents when speaking.
- Do not hesitate to ask residents if you are unsure about what they want and need.
- If you want to move personal items, ask first.
- Before you leave a resident's room, let the resident know when you plan to return.

- Ask if the resident wants the curtains or door open or closed when you leave the room.
- For residents with vision impairments or mobility issues, be sure needed items are within reach and can be found easily.

Apply It

1. Why are these guidelines important to holistic communication?
2. What situations may prevent you from using these guidelines? Explain your answer.

may result in a one-word answer of "yes" or "no." If an open-ended question had been asked, the answer might have been more detailed.

When using questioning, avoid "why" questions since these types of questions may be difficult to answer.

"Why" questions can make people feel defensive. An example of a "why" question that might make a resident feel defensive could be "Why did you ring your call light? I was just in your room 10 minutes ago."

SECTION 11.1 **Review and Assessment**

Key Terms Mini Glossary

active listening the process of showing interest in what a person is saying; includes paying attention, making eye contact, clarifying, summarizing and reflecting on what a person has said.

body language gestures, posture, and movements that communicate a person's thoughts and feelings.

clarification the process of restating what you believe was said to make sure you heard the message correctly.

closed-ended question a question that requires only a one-word answer, such as yes or no.

communication barriers any actions, behaviors, or situations that block or interfere with a person's ability to successfully send and receive communication messages.

defense mechanisms unconscious behaviors that enable people to ignore or forget situations or thoughts that cause fear, anxiety, and stress.

health literacy a person's ability to understand fully and use information about health, diseases, conditions, or treatments.

interpreter a person who translates written or spoken words into another language.

jargon words, phrases, and language used by a specific group of people or culture.

labeling describing someone using a specific word or phrase.

open-ended question a question that requires more than a one-word answer.

prejudice an opinion or feeling that is formed without facts and that often leads to unfair feelings of dislike for a person or group because of race, sex, or religion.

Apply the Key Terms

Complete the following sentences using the key terms in this section.

1. "Did you sleep well last night?" is an example of a(n) _____.
2. Mr. F speaks only Spanish. To make sure he understands instructions about his treatment, he should have a(n) _____.
3. When a resident gestures that she is okay, she is using _____.
4. The RN is paying attention, making eye contact, summarizing, and clarifying what the resident is saying. She is using _____.
5. A nursing assistant just told a resident that he would be NPO for a procedure. The resident looks confused because he does not understand the _____ used by the nursing assistant.

Know and Understand the Facts

1. What is holistic communication?
2. Explain the four basic components of communication.
3. Describe the difference between verbal and nonverbal communication.
4. List three barriers to communication.

Analyze and Apply Concepts

1. Provide two examples of defense mechanisms and explain the influence of the two defense mechanisms on holistic communication.

2. Explain how active listening and questioning can promote holistic communication.
3. You are a nursing assistant working in a long-term care facility. Write a care situation in which holistic communication is used effectively between yourself and a resident. Identify the communication approaches used and how they affect the conversation.

Think Critically

Read the following care situation. Then answer the questions that follow.

Harry has just started his job as a nursing assistant and is caring for Mrs. N. Mrs. N had a stroke three months ago, which paralyzed the left side of her face. As a result, she is unable to speak clearly. Mrs. N also has a hearing impairment. Harry brings lunch to Mrs. N, puts it on the overbed table, and quietly tells Mrs. N that lunch is ready. He then walks out of her room.

When Harry returns later to pick up Mrs. N's tray, he notices that nothing has been eaten. He says to Mrs. N, "Why didn't you eat anything? Well, if you don't want to eat, you don't have to." While Harry is talking, Mrs. N mumbles and points to her bathroom.

1. What are the communication barriers in this situation?
2. How could Harry make sure he is aware of Mrs. N's hearing and speaking problems?
3. What should Harry do differently in this situation?

SECTION 11.2 Caring Skills and Interpersonal Relationships

Objectives

To achieve the objectives for this section, you must successfully:

- **explain** the four types of interpersonal relationships.
- **describe** behaviors and attitudes that demonstrate caring.
- **discuss** how caring relationships are established.

Key Terms

Learn these key terms to better understand the information presented in the section.

caring
giving of self
interpersonal relationships
intimate relationships

Questions to Consider

- Have you ever met someone for the first time and immediately felt like that person's friend? Or, maybe you disliked a person you just met? Why do you think you responded to these people in this way?
- Many times, your first impressions of people help you determine the relationships you build. Building relationships is even more important when you are asked to care for someone. Think of a time you were asked to care for a person or a pet. How did you feel? Was giving care difficult, or did you enjoy it? Why?

What Are Interpersonal Relationships?

Interpersonal relationships develop between two or more people who have similar interests or goals. These relationships are built and maintained when people's needs and desires are met. There are four types of interpersonal relationships: family relationships, friendships, intimate relationships, and professional relationships.

Family Relationships

Family relationships are based on interactions between parents, siblings, and extended family members. Families form their own patterns of communication, which are typically based on culture, habit, and familiarity. These are often the strongest interpersonal relationships in a person's life.

Friendships

Friendships are also strong interpersonal relationships that are usually built on similar likes and dislikes. As time passes, more personal information is shared, and trust develops. The relationship continues to build and often, private information and secrets are shared. Both friendships and family relationships usually offer protection, support, and acceptance for those involved.

Intimate Relationships

Intimate relationships develop from romantic feelings and love. These relationships are close, romantic, and sometimes sexual. If this type of relationship is to thrive, those in the relationship must pay attention to each other's emotions and feelings.

Professional Relationships

Professional relationships are developed and maintained in professional, or work, settings. As a nursing assistant, you will develop professional relationships with coworkers, residents, and residents' family members (**Figure 11.6**). Interpersonal relationships in professional settings do not have the same strength as family relationships and friendships and do not always extend outside the workplace.

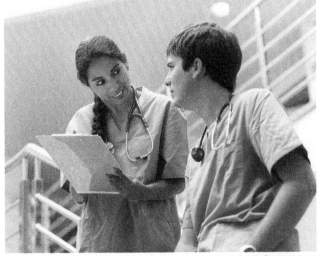

wavebreakmedia/Shutterstock.com

Figure 11.6 Professional relationships are those you have with your coworkers.

Intimate relationships are not appropriate in professional settings.

Although professional relationships may not be as deep or long-lasting as other relationships, they require the same level of attention and effective communication. Developing professional relationships can improve care and health outcomes. For example, the way you approach, communicate, listen, and respond can impact a resident's willingness to agree to your requests. It can also influence whether or not a resident follows his or her treatment plan. Residents may even feel better about themselves as a result of your relationships with them.

How Are Professional Relationships Built and Maintained?

You can use several important approaches and skills to build and maintain professional relationships. Professional relationships are at their strongest when you follow these approaches:

- Be present. Be responsive and focus on others.
- Respect others' views and opinions. Actively listen, ask open-ended questions, and show interest in what others have to say.
- Be helpful. Take the time needed to give residents and staff the assistance they need, even when you are busy.
- Be fair. Avoid stereotypes and labels.
- Be trustworthy and reliable. Others should be able to count on you at all times.
- Be appreciative, positive, and optimistic. Offer positive feedback and comments when appropriate.
- Be a team player. Provide support and help when needed, even if you are busy or tired.
- Manage anger and conflict in an appropriate manner.

Your ability to build and maintain professional relationships may be influenced by your personal experiences and feelings. Perhaps you are caring for a resident whose comments or behaviors remind you of someone you do not like. It is possible that you will transfer that feeling of dislike onto the resident. This can negatively affect your relationship with that resident and your ability to provide holistic care.

Feelings that transferred because of association can also be good. For example, a resident may like a nursing assistant because he reminds the resident of a close friend or family member.

Feelings that are transferred are often unconscious. If you find yourself being short or angry with a resident without cause, stop and think about your feelings. Or, you may find yourself being too friendly. Ask yourself why. If you experience a resident being too friendly or directing anger toward you, do not take these feelings personally. Rather, recognize and be aware of what is happening. Then focus on effective communication skills and the way you can best deliver care. Use your active listening and questioning skills to help divert residents' feelings to their recovery, treatment, and family members. If you are unable or have difficulty redirecting either your own feelings, or the feelings of a resident, let a member of the licensed nursing staff know. Sometimes a change of assignment helps.

What Are Caring Skills?

As a holistic nursing assistant, you will be asked to care for people who are ill. How do you feel about having this responsibility? Maybe you have already had this experience with a family member or friend.

When people hear the word *caring*, they may already have an idea of what the word means. In healthcare, the term **caring** means providing assistance and comfort to positively affect the health and well-being of a resident. Caring may also involve giving of yourself, showing empathy and patience, being reliable and resourceful, and seeking information.

Giving of Self

To care for others, you must be ***giving of self***. A person who is giving of self makes himself or herself available and open to others. To be giving of self, nursing assistants must understand that residents' needs come first. Nursing assistants who are giving of self impact both the physical and emotional well-being of residents. These caregivers are positive and earn the trust and respect of others. This quality is important. Residents who do not trust or respect their caregivers may not cooperate, making it harder to provide care.

Empathy

Caring and being giving of self also require *empathy*, or understanding another person's feelings and emotions. Empathy is different than sympathy. Sympathy is a feeling of concern for others with a hope that they become happier or better off. Empathy goes beyond sympathy. It is a more active response where you are "feeling with" another.

An example of empathy might be telling a resident, "I understand you may be frightened about your upcoming procedure." If appropriate, you could even hold a sad-looking resident's hand as an expression of caring and empathy. A good way to hold a resident's hand is to rest the resident's hand on top of yours (**Figure 11.7**).

A person who tends to be empathetic usually demonstrates several qualities. These include caring deeply about others, being a good active listener, and quickly sensing how others feel.

Patience and Reliability

Holistic nursing assistants who exhibit caring behaviors are *patient* and are willing to understand. They are *reliable*, never take shortcuts, and know their responsibilities. These behaviors demonstrate caring and competence. They show that nursing assistants understand their roles, take the time to make sure they are accurate, and are consistent in their practice.

Information Seeking

Another way to show that you care is to take the time to learn more about residents. You can use the information you learn to help residents experience their past joys and present desires (**Figure 11.8**).

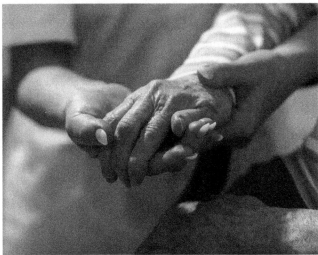

thodonal88/Shutterstock.com

Figure 11.7 Holding a resident's hand shows caring and empathy. However, it is best to hold a resident's hand in such a way that the resident can remove his or her hand if desired.

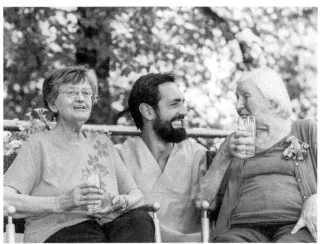

Kzenon/Shutterstock.com

Figure 11.8 Learning more about residents will help you form good relationships when delivering care.

Suppose a resident has shared with you that she once enjoyed running with her dog, but can't now because she is in a wheelchair. She is depressed because she misses the companionship of her dog. By connecting with a volunteer animal therapy program, you might be able to help this resident. Animal therapy organizations bring therapy dogs into healthcare facilities and allow residents to spend time with the animals. Just seeing a dog could improve this resident's spirits and well-being.

Resourcefulness

People who are *resourceful* think and act quickly to overcome challenges or solve problems. Caring can be demonstrated with simple, resourceful actions.

Think about a resident with Alzheimer's disease who always sits quietly in the activity room of a long-term care facility. When nursing staff members try to talk with the resident and ask questions, the resident never responds with more than one word. A nursing assistant speaks with the resident's daughter, who says that her father loves big band music. The next day, the nursing assistant gives the resident a pair of headphones and plays big band music for him. The resident sits up in his wheelchair, sings, taps his feet, and moves his hands in a rhythmic way. As a result, the resident is more open to answering questions. More importantly, the resident and those around him experience joy. Something as simple as music and a nursing assistant's care can make a big difference in a resident's life.

SECTION 11.2 **Review and Assessment**

Key Terms Mini Glossary

caring providing assistance and comfort to affect the health and well-being of a resident positively.

giving of self the quality of putting a resident's health and wellness needs before one's own needs as a caregiver.

interpersonal relationships relationships between two or more people who share similar interests or goals; meet physical and emotional needs.

intimate relationships relationships between two people who have romantic feelings of love for each other.

Apply the Key Terms

An incorrect key term is used in each of the following statements. Identify the incorrect key term and then replace it with the correct term.

1. The quality of putting a resident's health and wellness needs before your own is called caring.
2. An intimate relationship is between two or more people who share similar interests or goals.
3. Providing assistance and comfort to residents that positively affect health and well-being is giving of self.
4. When two people have romantic feelings of love for each other, they have an interpersonal relationship.

Know and Understand the Facts

1. Identify and define the four types of interpersonal relationships.
2. List five strategies for building and maintaining strong professional relationships.
3. What does it mean to be *giving of self*?
4. Identify two skills that demonstrate caring.

Analyze and Apply Concepts

1. Explain how to handle a situation in which a resident tells you he or she does not like the nursing assistant who gave care yesterday.
2. Identify two qualities or behaviors you can demonstrate to help form effective professional relationships.

3. Give two examples of situations in which a nursing assistant can demonstrate caring behaviors or actions.

Think Critically

Read the following care situation. Then answer the questions that follow.

Jennifer, a nursing assistant, has been caring for Mr. H, a war veteran, for several weeks. Both of Mr. H's legs were amputated at the knee as a result of an explosion during his tour of duty. Mr. H has always been pleasant and cooperative, and he and Jennifer have developed a good relationship. Today, Mr. H received bad news, but Jennifer was not aware of the news. When Jennifer entered Mr. H's room to help him with morning care, Mr. H threw an object from his nightstand at her. Jennifer was shocked at his behavior. She asked him what was wrong. Mr. H was crying and was embarrassed to have anyone see him cry, so he yelled, "Leave me alone!"

1. What feeling is Mr. H displaying, and is it directed toward Jennifer?
2. What should Jennifer do next to maintain her strong interpersonal relationship with Mr. H?
3. What attitudes and behaviors can Jennifer demonstrate to show she cares about Mr. H?

Anxiety, Fear, Anger, and Conflict

Objectives

To achieve the objectives for this section, you must successfully:

- **identify** the causes of anxiety, fear, anger, and conflict.
- **describe** the behaviors and feelings related to anxiety, fear, anger, and conflict.
- **explain** ways a holistic nursing assistant can ease anxiety, fear, anger, and conflict.

Key Terms

Learn these key terms to better understand the information presented in the section.

anger	conflict
assertive	fear
collaboration	phobias
compromise	

Questions to Consider

- Think about a time you felt anxious, fearful, or angry. What caused these feelings, and what did you do about them? If you acted on these feelings, did you feel better or worse as a result?
- Now think about a time you had a conflict with a friend or family member. What caused the conflict? How did you and your friend or family member feel? Were you able to settle the conflict? If you were, how did you do it?

What Is Anxiety and How Can It Be Managed?

As you learned in Chapter 2, *anxiety* is a feeling of worry, uneasiness, or nervousness. Anxiety is common. Mild, brief anxiety may occur when you look forward to an event that has not yet happened. For example, a student may have anxiety before taking an important test. Anxious feelings may produce physical reactions. Before the test, a student might feel his heart pounding, notice his foot shaking, or start chewing on his lips or fingernails. People handle anxiety differently. Some people deal with it by crying, expressing anger, or shutting down emotionally. Others do not know why they are feeling anxious and may recognize the cause of anxiety only after it has passed.

Anxiety disorders are different from experiencing mild or brief anxiety caused by a stressful event. Anxiety disorders include **phobias** (unsupported, exaggerated fears), panic, post-traumatic stress disorder (PTSD), and obsessive-compulsive disorder (OCD). An estimated 40 million adults in the United States ages 18 and older are affected by an anxiety disorder. That is about 18 percent of the US population. Anxiety disorders usually last at least six months and can continue for a lifetime. They may get worse if left untreated.

Anxious Residents

Anxiety is something you may observe in residents. To recognize anxiety, watch for heavy, short breaths and complaints about heart palpitations or chest pain. If the chest pain is described as severe, notify the licensed nursing staff immediately. You might also observe unusual shakiness, dizziness, sweating, muscle aches, dry mouth, and fluctuations (changes) in behavior and mood. Some residents will tell you they feel anxious. Others might experience the physical symptoms of anxiety, but be unaware of the cause and not tell you.

If a resident shows physical symptoms of anxiety, let licensed nursing staff know so they can follow up. If a resident is feeling anxious, encourage the resident to talk with you about his or her feelings. Use good eye contact and be present during the conversation. You might ask if a resident would like some water, since dry mouth is often a result of anxiety. If a resident is not sure what is causing his or her feelings, know that just your calm, positive presence can help (**Figure 11.9**).

You can tell anxiety is subsiding, or *lessening*, when physical symptoms start to disappear. If you observe that the resident's anxiety is intense or long lasting, let the licensed nursing staff know. Some residents may need medication to relieve their symptoms. The goal of your care is to ease anxious feelings and to keep these feelings from getting out of control.

THINK ABOUT THIS

According to the National Institutes of Mental Health, women are more than twice as likely as men to experience anxiety disorders in their lifetimes.

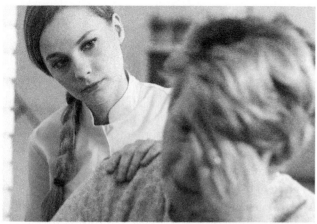

Photographee.eu/Shutterstock.com

Figure 11.9 One way to help ease resident anxiety is to just be present. Sometimes a caring touch can help residents be calm.

Anxiety as a Caregiver

Working in healthcare may put you in many situations that can cause anxiety. For example, thinking about performing a procedure for the first time or caring for a resident in isolation may cause anxiety. As a nursing assistant, you will need to handle your feelings appropriately. If you do feel anxious while giving care, the following suggestions may help you overcome those feelings:

- Know what causes you to feel anxious and what physical symptoms are typical for you. Recognizing your own patterns of anxiety will help you become aware of and manage them.
- If you start to feel anxious, take slow, deep breaths. This will have a calming effect.
- If you feel your anxiety is getting in the way of providing safe care, take a brief break.
- Talk about your feelings and anxiety with a coworker.
- Never feel embarrassed about your anxiety. Everyone has been anxious at one time or another.

What Is Fear and How Can It Be Overcome?

Some people describe *fear* as a paralyzing feeling. You may describe fear as feeling scared, feeling emotionally out of control, or being overwhelmed. Fear is different from anxiety. While anxiety occurs in response to an *anticipated* event, fear is an unpleasant emotion or feeling that occurs in response to an *identified* threat or the presence of danger.

Fear is a personal experience. Some fears may develop from terrifying and real experiences, while other fears may develop from the possibility or threat of a frightening experience. Reactions to fear may range from a low level of fear to fear that overpowers you, leaving you feeling weak, tired, and out of control. Common fears include fears of flying, public speaking, heights, the dark, failure, or rejection.

Fearful Residents

Depending on your point of view and experience, you can view fear as either positive or negative. Positive fear can serve as a healthy warning sign and motivate you to do or be better. Fear can also be immobilizing. Some people react to fear in an aggressive manner. They may scream, yell, or lash out physically (**Figure 11.10**). Others may shut down emotionally and not be able to face their fear.

Fear has physical effects due to the actions of the *sympathetic nervous system (SNS)*, which causes the *fight-or-flight response*. When people are fearful, they may become short of breath and sometimes sweat. The heart may race, and people may become shaky or nervous. Depending on their level of fear and the threats they are facing, people may run and scream or stand strong and physically fight.

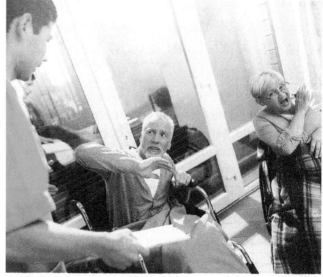

VGstockstudio/Shutterstock.com

Figure 11.10 Fear may cause residents to become angry. When this happens, it is important to remain calm, try to identify the cause of the fear or anger, and do not take their reactions personally.

Fear cannot be overcome unless a person commits to reducing or eliminating his or her fear. As a nursing assistant, you may find that some residents ignore their fear. Residents may bottle the fear up inside, and all you see may be anger, self-pity, or sadness, which are feelings that often accompany fear. Holistic communication and caring, even in the form of an empathetic response of understanding, can help identify and relieve a resident's fear.

Fear as a Caregiver

Fear can sometimes be hard to recognize in yourself. You can practice identifying your fears in writing or out loud. Once you have identified your fears, you must learn ways to manage them. Taking deep breaths when you feel fearful may help. You might also ask yourself why you are feeling afraid. This will help you understand how the fear started. You may set goals to begin overcoming your fears. For example, you might set a goal to find someone with whom to share your feelings. Some people find that professional help can assist in overcoming fears. If people do not deal with their fears, the fears may prevent them from helping others.

What Strategies Can Be Used to Manage Anger?

Anger is a powerful feeling that develops from frustration, displeasure, or a threat (**Figure 11.11**). Anger can be very damaging to one's self and others. Everyone has experienced anger and its many degrees of intensity. *Frustration* is a mild form of anger; *rage* is an extreme form. Many situations or experiences can cause anger.

Anger causes physical reactions. Typically, when you are angry, your heart rate increases, you may frown, your eyes narrow, your body heats up, your breathing may change, and your feelings turn into behaviors. Some people erupt in anger and yell, scream, or pound on something. Others have the same physical reactions, but instead of showing their anger outwardly, they turn anger inward. This can cause serious internal physical symptoms and depression.

Angry Residents

Some residents believe they have lost control over their own lives, and this causes them to feel frustrated or helpless. Residents may not know how to talk

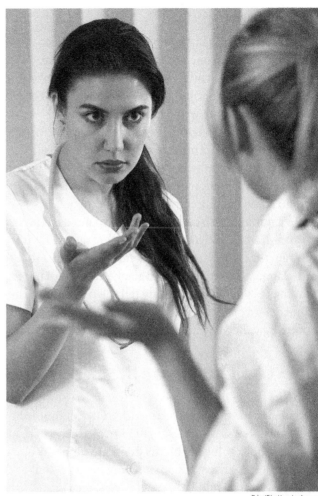
Edw/Shutterstock.com

Figure 11.11 Anger can be a powerful emotion. It is important not to let anger keep you from acting professionally.

about their feelings and instead keep them inside. As their feelings increase, residents may become angry. The following are strategies you can use to help calm angry residents:

- Use active listening.
- Do not personally respond to the anger.
- Ask questions to clarify why the resident is angry.
- Speak in a soft tone at a low volume level. This will help defuse, or reduce, the anger.
- Never raise your voice or yell. Some residents just need to voice their anger.

Calming residents is very important, particularly if anger is getting out of hand or if residents are at risk of hurting themselves or others. If residents ask you to leave them alone, do that, but tell residents you will return in a certain amount of time. Always respect residents' wishes and be sure to keep residents safe. If residents do ask you to leave them alone, report this situation to the licensed nursing staff.

Anger as a Caregiver

Managing anger is not always easy. As a nursing assistant, you will need to recognize what situations can and will make you angry and learn to control your anger. It is unprofessional to show your anger or to gossip about people with whom you are angry.

As a nursing assistant, you must manage your anger and deal with it appropriately. If you feel yourself getting angry, try to remove yourself from the situation that is causing your anger. Walk away, take a break, and do some deep breathing to calm down.

As a nursing assistant, you may also need to speak up and share if someone is making you angry. If you can remain calm, you can respond to situations that cause anger. For example, if someone calls you a name that makes you angry, politely tell the person that the name hurts your feelings and that you would appreciate not being called by that name again.

How Can Conflict Be Resolved?

Conflict is any disagreement between two or more people. It can be as simple as a difference of opinion or as complex as a war. Conflict is not always bad and may help solve problems or create new ways of completing tasks. A conflict may be centered on facts, values, beliefs, expectations, feelings, or behaviors. Conflicts may be *external*, or exist between people or groups. Conflicts may also be *internal*. For example, a person may struggle to make an important decision. Conflict must *never* be ignored. If conflict is not resolved, it will continue and grow in intensity.

A conflict may cause feelings of anxiety, fear, and some level of anger. These feelings must be handled before any problem-solving can occur to resolve the conflict (**Figure 11.12**). Each of us has a different style when dealing with and resolving conflict. Conflict-management styles range from avoiding conflict altogether to directly dealing with conflict. Many times, *compromise* (in which there is a give and take between people) can help reduce a conflict situation. *Collaboration* (in which people work together to resolve conflict in a way that satisfies everyone) is considered the most inclusive and positive approach to managing conflict. Conflict resolution is important, and it is always possible to

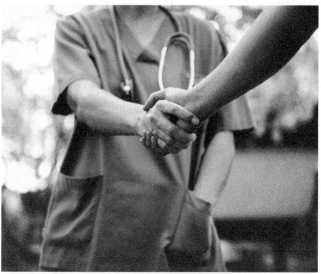

Studio4dich/Shutterstock.com

Figure 11.12 Conflict resolution is important, and it is always possible to resolve disagreements in a productive manner.

Conflict Management

In last night's news broadcast, a local journalist reported on a conflict between a local community agency and a group of citizens in the community. The citizens requested that the agency provide community outreach services for the large population of older adults. The citizens were asking for special resources for people with dementia and for family caregivers.

The reporter stated that, early that morning, citizens from the community were outside the agency distributing information. Agency officials responded to the citizens' request with a public letter. The officials stated that they did not see how or why they should take responsibility for providing these services. The officials also said they did not have the financial resources to support the requested resources.

Apply It

1. What is the source of the conflict described in this scenario?
2. Did either side take any actions that increased the conflict? Explain.
3. What action could the agency take next?
4. How would you suggest that the agency and community members resolve this conflict?

resolve disagreements in a productive manner. If you do not respond to conflict, the situation can get out of control.

Conflict management has two parts—first, you must manage feelings and second, you must solve the problem.

To manage feelings:
- cool down any angry feelings
- stay in the present and focus on the situation
- avoid assigning any blame

To begin problem solving:
- attack the problem, not the person with whom you have the conflict
- focus on the issue
- don't make assumptions
- be *assertive* (bold and clear) when expressing your feelings and requests
- use active listening
- seek a solution by finding common interests and agreement

SECTION 11.3 **Review and Assessment**

Key Terms Mini Glossary

anger a strong feeling or emotion that develops from frustration, displeasure, or a threat.
assertive bold and clear.

collaboration the process by which people work together to resolve conflict in a way that satisfies everyone.
compromise the process by which two sides of a conflict give and take to find the best resolution.

conflict a disagreement between two or more people.
fear an unpleasant feeling or emotion resulting from the threat or presence of danger.
phobias unsupported, exaggerated fears that sometimes interfere with daily life.

Apply the Key Terms

Write a sentence using each key term properly.
1. collaboration
2. compromise
3. conflict
4. fear
5. phobia

Know and Understand the Facts
1. What is the difference between fear and anxiety?
2. Identify one way in which a holistic nursing assistant can help relieve a resident's fear.
3. Describe three physical responses to anger.
4. Identify three strategies to calm angry residents.
5. What is the difference between compromise and collaboration?

Analyze and Apply Concepts
1. List two ways to deal with anxiety.
2. A resident is yelling at another resident and pounding his fists on his wheelchair. What can a nursing assistant do to help calm this resident?

3. Identify three strategies a holistic nursing assistant can use to resolve conflict.

Think Critically
Read the following care situation. Then answer the questions that follow.

Janet is a nursing assistant caring for Mrs. K, an 88-year-old woman, today. Mrs. K was admitted to a local long-term care facility yesterday afternoon. In the morning, Janet knocks on Mrs. K's door and introduces herself. Mrs. K looks frightened and pulls the bed covers up to her eyes. Janet asks if Mrs. K would like to get ready for breakfast. Mrs. K shakes her head. Janet asks her again about eating breakfast and says, "Would you like to eat in your room today?" Mrs. K continues to shake her head and keeps her covers pulled up to her neck.

1. What feelings might Mrs. K be expressing?
2. What might be the reason for Mrs. K's feelings?
3. What would you advise Janet do or say to help Mrs. K feel more comfortable?

Key Points

Reviewing the key points for this chapter will help you practice more safely and competently as a holistic nursing assistant and will help you prepare for the certification competency exam.

- Holistic communication is important when giving safe, quality care.
- Cultural differences, labeling, jargon, and stereotyping may cause communication barriers. Defense mechanisms are unconscious ways of diminishing stress and anxiety.
- To build and maintain strong interpersonal relationships, you must be self-aware, respectful, helpful, fair, trustworthy, appreciative, a team player, and able to manage anger and conflict.
- Caring means providing assistance and comfort to positively affect the health and well-being of residents.
- Feelings of anxiety, fear, and anger, as well as conflict, will be a part of your work as a holistic nursing assistant. Allowing residents to share their feelings and emotions is one way to respond.

Action Steps to Holistic Care

Review the information in this chapter. Complete the following activities.

1. Working with a partner, select one barrier to holistic communication discussed in the chapter. Create a skit that shows the communication barrier in action, with one of you acting as a resident and the other as a holistic nursing assistant. Be sure to include a way to respond to this barrier, using holistic communication.

2. Select one defense mechanism you learned about in this chapter. Prepare a short paper or digital presentation that describes the defense mechanism, how it is demonstrated, why a person would use this defense mechanism, and how to best respond to the defense mechanism.

3. With a partner, select one of the following: anxiety, fear, anger, or conflict. Prepare a poster that best shows your selection. Include a definition of your selection and two action steps to decrease it.

4. Find pictures in a magazine, in a newspaper, or online that best demonstrate three types of nonverbal communication you use.

Building Math Skill

Mrs. B's family just left after visiting with her for several hours. After they left, Mrs. B started crying. When you asked her what happened, she would not say. Rather, she became so upset that you checked her B/P, pulse, and respirations because she was not able to catch her breath. Since you have cared for her over several days, you found that the readings were much higher than her normal. Her respirations were 28 and her pulse was 110 beats per minute. Normally they are 18 breaths per minute and 80 beats per minute. Later, when you report the change to the licensed nursing staff you share the differences in the readings. What did you say?

Preparing for the Certification Competency Examination

To prepare for the nursing assistant certification competency examination, you will need to know content found in this chapter. This content may be tested in the knowledge (written or oral) and skills (hands-on demonstration) portions of the exam. The following areas will be emphasized:

- verbal and nonverbal communication
- barriers to communication
- care that supports communication and behavior in a positive, nonthreatening way
- effective communication with residents, families, and the healthcare team
- dynamics of interpersonal relationships
- caring skills

These sample test questions are similar to ones you will find on the certification competency exam. See how well you can answer them. Be sure to select the *best* answer.

1. When residents pat you on the arm, how are they communicating?
   A. verbally
   B. using slang or jargon
   C. nonverbally
   D. using active listening

2. Which of the following is the best way to communicate with a resident who is hearing impaired?
   A. yell loudly until the resident responds
   B. use short sentences and simple words
   C. stand behind the resident while you talk
   D. increase the tone of your voice

3. Which of the following is the most effective way to be sure a resident understands your explanation of a new treatment?
   A. have the resident write it down
   B. have the resident read the procedure
   C. have the resident repeat back what he or she heard
   D. have the resident ask you questions

4. A nursing assistant wants to be sure she is expressing herself in a caring way. Which of the following qualities would best show this skill?
   A. projection
   B. gossip
   C. privacy
   D. respect

5. Mrs. L shares with her nursing assistant that she is afraid of dying. How should the nursing assistant best respond?
   A. He should say, "If you pray, you will not be so afraid."
   B. He should ask Mrs. L open-ended questions and listen quietly.
   C. He should tell Mrs. L that she is not going anywhere soon.
   D. He should tell Mrs. L that he will ask for medications to help calm her down.

6. When the same message is sent using both verbal and nonverbal communication, the message is considered which of the following?
   A. effective
   B. assertive
   C. caring
   D. empathetic

7. How do nursing assistants show they are actively listening?
   A. by interrupting as much as possible
   B. by starting to make the bed
   C. by using good eye contact and responding appropriately
   D. by using laughter

8. What are the four components of communication?
   A. listener, receiver, communicator, and observer
   B. sender, mode of communication, recipient, and feedback
   C. observer, method of communication, receiver, and participant
   D. sender, observer, strategy, and feedback

9. Which of the following describes a health-literate resident?
   A. is not able to read books and information about his or her health conditions and diseases
   B. is able to understand what is shared with him or her about his or her disease or condition
   C. is able to search the Internet for information about specific diseases
   D. is not able to follow instructions about his treatments.

10. Mr. P is angry about how ill he feels today. What would be the best way to communicate with him?
    A. yell at him and tell him to settle down immediately
    B. call his daughter and tell her that she needs to visit him
    C. ignore Mr. P and get him water to help him calm down
    D. help him share his feelings and give him time to calm down

11. Two nursing assistants have worked well together for several years. They like each other and believe they have an excellent professional relationship. Which of the following best describes why they have this relationship?
    A. They are respectful and appreciative of each other.
    B. They have created an intimate way of talking to each other.
    C. They have formed an excellent friendship.
    D. They both like their nurse supervisor.

12. This morning, Mrs. W told you that she feels so much better today and is sure she will be going home by the end of the week. You both know she has terminal cancer and is in her final days. What defense mechanism is she using?
    A. repression
    B. denial
    C. regression
    D. displacement

13. A new nursing assistant is not yet comfortable in her position. She walks with a stooped posture and keeps her arms crossed over her chest when talking with staff. What behavior is she using to express her discomfort?
    A. tone of voice
    B. slang
    C. body language
    D. stereotyping

14. The *first* action someone should take to resolve a conflict between two people is which of the following?
    A. give the two people a resource on conflict
    B. focus on the issues that are causing the conflict
    C. collaborate with all the people involved
    D. manage the feelings the people have

15. What communication barrier is present when a nursing assistant says to a resident, "I need your vitals, stat"?
    A. jargon
    B. labeling
    C. stereotyping
    D. empathy

Did you have difficulty with any of the questions? If you did, review the chapter to find the correct answer(s).

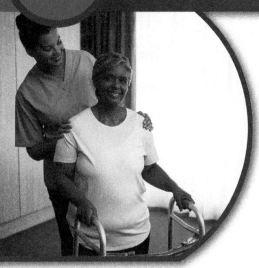

wavebreakmedia/Shutterstock.com

Welcome to the Chapter

Nursing assistants provide care to diverse residents who come from all races, ethnicities, and cultures. It is important to be aware of and sensitive to other cultures, as well as your own culture. This sensitivity leads to a deeper appreciation and understanding between people. It also helps build an open-minded relationship and stronger partnership with others. This is an important part of delivering safe, quality care.

What you learn in this chapter will help you develop your knowledge and skills to become a holistic nursing assistant. The topics discussed in the chapter are highlighted on the Providing Holistic Care Framework.

Chapter Outline

Section 12.1
Diverse Cultures

Section 12.2
Cultural Humility
and Cross-Cultural
Communication

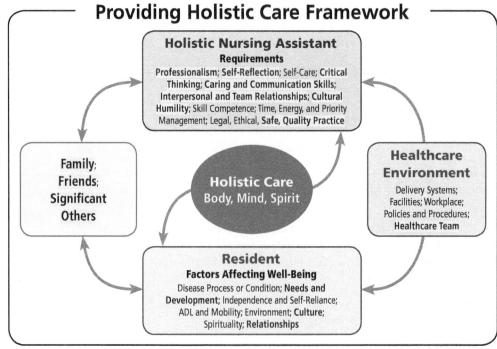

Providing Holistic Care Framework

Holistic Nursing Assistant
Requirements
Professionalism; Self-Reflection; Self-Care; Critical Thinking; Caring and Communication Skills; Interpersonal and Team Relationships; Cultural Humility; Skill Competence; Time, Energy, and Priority Management; Legal, Ethical, Safe, Quality Practice

**Family;
Friends;
Significant
Others**

Holistic Care
Body, Mind, Spirit

**Healthcare
Environment**
Delivery Systems;
Facilities; Workplace;
Policies and Procedures;
Healthcare Team

Resident
Factors Affecting Well-Being
Disease Process or Condition; Needs and Development; Independence and Self-Reliance; ADL and Mobility; Environment; Culture; Spirituality; Relationships

Goodheart-Willcox Publisher

SECTION 12.1 Diverse Cultures

Objectives

To achieve the objectives for this section, you must successfully:

- **describe** the differences among race, ethnicity, and culture.
- **identify** the challenges related to appreciating and working within diverse cultures, groups, and populations.

Key Terms

Learn these key terms to better understand the information presented in the section.

beliefs
customs
diversity
ethnicity
ethnocentrism

race
racism
rituals
traditions
trait

Questions to Consider

- Have you ever communicated or worked with people who have different beliefs or who come from cultural groups different from your own? These people may have dressed differently or spoken a language other than yours.
- What did you do when you interacted with these people? How did you react?
- When you interacted with these people, did you ever not know what to say or do? What feelings did that cause? How did you deal with your feelings?

What Is Diversity?

In healthcare, you will meet, care for, and work with many different people. While people all have the same basic needs, they all also come from a variety of family backgrounds, places, ethnic groups, generations, religions, orientations, and belief systems. This is *diversity*, or the presence of differences among people (**Figure 12.1**). There are many types of diversity, including racial and ethnic diversity, family diversity, religious diversity, geographic diversity, generational diversity, and sexual diversity, among others.

Racial and Ethnic Diversity

To be comfortable with diversity, you must understand the terms related to this topic. Two terms you will hear often that relate to diversity are *race* and *ethnicity*. **Race** is a person's genetic makeup and cannot be changed. Race can be identified using a person's physical characteristics, or *traits*. People of the same race may share certain traits, including skin, hair, or eye color.

Ethnicity describes the ethnic group a person belongs to and is different from race. Ethnicity is a group's identification with shared social, cultural, and traditional practices. For example, an Italian family that follows traditional Italian practices would be ethnically Italian. Another example is a person who has the racial characteristics of a Hispanic but may not identify with his or her Hispanic ethnicity, or social, cultural, and traditional practices.

As you have learned, *culture* is a set of learned behaviors and is passed down through generations. People of the same culture have shared *traditions* (behaviors that have special meanings), *beliefs* (ideas accepted to be true), and languages. They also have shared *rituals* (actions always done in the same way), eating habits, dress, and *customs* (established practices and beliefs). For example, Hispanic or Latino cultures often value family, both immediate and extended. In many Asian cultures, older adults play major roles in making decisions that affect the entire family.

The US Census Bureau recognizes the following races in the United States: Caucasian, African-American, American Indian or Alaska Native, Asian, Native Hawaiian or other Pacific Islander, and Hispanic or Latino. Today, most of the US population is made up of Caucasians, although the African-American and Hispanic populations are growing quickly.

Family Diversity

Diversity exists among families. Some families are considered *traditional* and include a mother, a father, and a child or children. Other families are made up

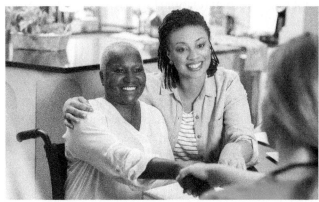

asiseeit/E+ via Getty Images

Figure 12.1 Diversity refers to the many differences among people. In healthcare, communicating and giving care require knowledge of diversity and respect for others' differences.

of a single parent, who is either male or female, and a child or children. In *blended families*, divorced parents marry other people and may have children from both marriages. Some families have two parents of the same sex. Additionally, some families adopt or foster children. An *intergenerational family* is one in which several generations live in the same house. Interracial families have family members from different races.

Religious Diversity

Successful holistic nursing assistants should have a general familiarity with diverse religions. A *religion* is defined by a specific set of spiritual beliefs about supreme beings, a particular philosophy of life, a code of ethics, and a set of rituals. In some religions, a supreme being is seen as responsible for all healing. The most common religion in the United States is Christianity, which a little over 70 percent of people follow and which primarily includes Protestantism and Catholicism. Nearly 6 percent of people in the United States follow other religions, such as Judaism, Buddhism, and Islam. The final 23 percent of people in the United States do not identify themselves as having a religion. These people may consider themselves atheists (people who deny or disbelieve the existence of a supreme being), agnostics (people who believe they cannot know if any supreme being exists), or they do not have a formal relationship with a religion.

Geographic Diversity

The places where people live, or people's geographic locations, must also be considered when discussing diversity. Various regions of the United States have different cultural practices. For example, people who grow up on the East Coast of the United States have a different experience from those who grow up in the Southwest. Regional accents vary, people may be familiar with different types of food, and people may call items such as clothing or furniture by different names (for example, a *sofa*, *couch*, or *divan*). People may even be used to different types of transportation because of their geographic locations. People who live in the city may use public transportation, while people in rural areas rely on personal vehicles.

Generational Diversity

You learned about the different generations in Chapter 7. In today's society, there are five diverse generations: the silent generation, baby boomers, Generation X, millennials, and Generation Z. Remember that it is important not to believe stereotypes about particular generations. Rather, you should recognize generational diversity and value the qualities of each generation. The better you understand the differences between generations, the easier it will be for you to understand the members of these generations and build rapport through improved communication.

Sexual Diversity

As a holistic nursing assistant, you will take care of or work with people with different sexual orientations and gender identities. *Sexual orientation* describes a person's emotional, romantic, and sexual attraction to males or females. A person's sexual orientation may be:

- heterosexual (attracted to members of the opposite sex)
- homosexual (attracted to members of the same sex)
- bisexual (attracted to members of both sexes)
- asexual (lacking sexual attraction for other people)

Gender identity refers to a person's sense of being a man or a woman and the expression of that sense. For example, a person may feel that his or her assigned sex (male or female) is the same as his or her gender identity. Another person may feel that his or her assigned sex is incorrect and instead identify with the opposite gender. This person's assigned sex may be male, but she may have a female gender identity. People with this type of gender identity are *transgender*. Transgender people may identify with different sexual orientations.

Some people have *differences or disorders of sexual development (DSDs)*, also called *intersex*. People with DSDs are born with variations in their biological structures—that is, their sexual anatomy is not in alignment with the female or male sex. For example, a female may be born without a vaginal opening. A male may be born with a scrotum that looks like labia. A person may have male anatomy on the outside, but have typical internal female anatomy, or have a mix of XX and XY chromosomes. In some cases, a DSD is recognized at birth. In other cases, it is not identified until puberty or not identified at all.

Other types of diversity include diversity in people's mental and physical abilities, differences in levels of education, and varied political beliefs. As a holistic nursing assistant, you will likely care for many, if not all, of the diverse cultures, groups, and populations discussed. Each resident, no matter his or her background, always deserves safe, quality care.

What Are Challenges to Appreciating Diversity?

Appreciating diverse cultures requires you to first develop an awareness about your *own* cultural values and beliefs. This will allow you to determine how your cultural perspectives, values, and beliefs differ from those of your residents and coworkers (**Figure 12.2**). This awareness can help you overcome challenges in establishing relationships and providing care. Making the conscious choice to accept and appreciate diversity will also help you avoid potential challenges and communication barriers.

Challenges to appreciating diversity include ethnocentrism, biases, prejudices, racism, and stereotypes.

- *Ethnocentrism*: involves judging another culture based on the beliefs and standards of one's own culture.
- **Bias**: is an unfair belief that some people, objects, or situations are better than others. Ethnocentrism can create a bias.

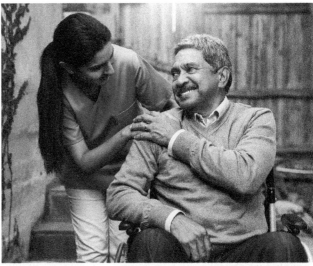

PeopleImages/E+ via Getty Images

Figure 12.2 When you better understand your own background and culture, you will be more able to communicate with people from different backgrounds and cultures.

- **Prejudice**: is an opinion or feeling that is formed without facts. Prejudice develops when a person is biased. It often leads to unfair feelings of dislike for a person or group based on race, sex, or religion. For example, a family member may have had an experience with a person from another culture that caused him to form a negative opinion about that culture as a whole. This may also cause him to form prejudices against people from that culture.
- *Racism*: is a form of prejudice. It is the belief that one's own race is superior.

CULTURE CUES

Valuing Diversity

The following guidelines will help you recognize and appreciate diversity as a holistic nursing assistant:

- Treat people respectfully by paying attention to the way *they* wish to be treated, not the way *you* wish them to be treated.
- Question your own assumptions and the assumptions of others. This will help you avoid limiting your opportunities to understand another person.
- Offer to assist others whose backgrounds and experiences are different from your own.
- When asking someone to explain a point of view or an opinion that is different from your own, let the person know that you are asking because you want to understand, not because you want the person to justify the opinion.
- Do not joke about or make fun of people's differences. When you see another person joking this way, be direct and ask him or her to stop.

- Welcome ideas that are different from your own.
- Look at issues from another person's point of view before making decisions.
- Continually monitor your thoughts and language for any assumptions or stereotypes you might have.
- Always use facility policies and procedures. Healthcare facilities often have resources, including staff members who have expertise in diversity.

Apply It

1. Which of these guidelines do you follow as part of your typical interactions with others?
2. Which of these guidelines do you not often follow? Which guidelines would you like to include in your interactions with others? Explain.
3. How can you include the guidelines you do not often follow in your interactions with others?

- **Stereotyping**: is also a form of prejudice. It is a simple and general way to communicate a usually negative opinion about a group of people. A stereotype, for example, might be that all old people are cranky or that all people who are overweight are sloppy.

Challenges to appreciating diversity can interfere with your ability to be culturally aware, sensitive, and respectful. Overcoming these challenges, should they occur, is important to delivering safe, quality care.

SECTION 12.1 **Review and Assessment**

Key Terms Mini Glossary

beliefs ideas that a person or group of people accepts to be true.

customs established practices and beliefs that are followed by a group of people over multiple generations.

diversity the presence of differences among people.

ethnicity identification with common social, cultural, and traditional practices that are shared within a group.

ethnocentrism an outlook in which one judges another culture based on the beliefs and standards of one's own culture.

race a set of inherited physical characteristics, such as skin, eye, and hair color.

racism intolerance, discrimination, or prejudice based on race.

rituals actions that are always done in the same way, often for religious purposes or as part of a ceremony.

traditions behaviors or practices that have special meanings or symbolism and that are handed down from one generation to another.

trait a distinctive physical quality or characteristic.

Apply the Key Terms

Think about the definitions of the following key terms. Describe one difference between each pair of key terms.

1. ethnicity and race
2. ethnocentrism and traditions
3. traits and customs
4. rituals and racism
5. diversity and beliefs

Know and Understand the Facts

1. In your own words, explain the meaning of diversity.
2. Explain the difference between *race*, *ethnicity*, and *culture*.
3. Identify and describe two types of diversity.
4. Give one example of ethnocentrism.
5. Describe what someone does when he or she stereotypes.

Analyze and Apply Concepts

1. How might the family, religious, or generational diversity among residents impact the way you give care?
2. Discuss two challenges that can interfere with a person's ability to appreciate diversity.
3. A nursing assistant has been asked to care for a resident who comes from a different generation than she, has lived in a different geographic area, and has a different cultural background. What three guidelines can she use when caring for the resident that shows she values diversity?

Think Critically

Read the following care situation. Then answer the questions that follow.

Mrs. P is a 75-year-old woman whose admission forms show that she is Jewish and follows Judaism's religious traditions and customs. Mrs. P had a broken hip and now needs therapy after hip-replacement surgery. After talking with her second husband and his children, Mrs. P has decided that her rehabilitation will be most successful if she spends a few weeks in a specialized facility that offers daily therapy. She will stay in the specialized facility until she is able to safely walk at home. When Aamir, a nursing assistant, meets Mrs. P and her husband, he realizes they both have heavy accents and are difficult to understand. Aamir has worked with a similar resident in the past, and it was not a good experience. Aamir found that resident to be demanding and stubborn.

1. Which types of diversity are present in this situation?
2. What challenges to appreciating diversity might arise in this situation?
3. What actions could Aamir take to prevent any challenges to appreciating diversity?

Objectives

To achieve the objectives for this section, you must successfully:

- **recognize** that routines and procedures may need to be changed due to cultural and religious traditions and customs.
- **include** the practice of cultural humility when giving care.
- **demonstrate** cross-cultural communication when giving holistic care.

Key Terms

Learn these key terms to better understand the information presented in the section.

cross-cultural   cultural humility
  communication   kinship

Questions to Consider

- How do your values, traditions, and customs make you different from others?
- Have people ever shared with you that they see you as different? How did that make you feel?
- Have others tried to understand your differences? If so, how did they show that they understood? What have you done in the past to show that you understand others' differences?

What Is Cultural Humility?

It is important to understand that people interpret their own cultures and beliefs uniquely. No two people or families are exactly the same, even if they share a common religion or culture. People within a culture or religion may interpret, practice, or feel comfortable following traditions in different ways. Therefore, it is never fully possible to understand another culture and all of the people in it.

Because of this, it is important that holistic nursing assistants practice cultural humility. *Cultural humility* acknowledges that it is impossible to learn and know everything about another person's culture. Instead, cultural humility recognizes that there are differences among all people and focuses on the importance of evaluating one's own culture to understand its limitations, barriers, and gaps in knowledge. Cultural humility tries to achieve a sense of equality by encouraging people to be respectful of one another, be open to new ideas, and understand

that each person should be treated as an individual. Therefore, cultural humility has a positive effect on care.

A person who practices cultural humility is positively curious about how other people see the world and live. This positive and respectful curiosity leads a person to be open-minded and present when observing and asking questions of others.

Respecting the beliefs and traditions of those in your care is a very important part of your role and responsibility as a holistic nursing assistant. As you provide care with cultural humility, you may discover differences in the ways your residents approach their health, the procedures they agree to follow, and the medications they are willing to take. Individuals may have special family traditions, communication styles, dietary preferences and restrictions, religious customs, and levels of modesty (regard for decency of behavior, dress, and exposure of body parts to others) that impact the care you give.

Perspectives on Illness and Disease

Each person has his or her own understanding and feelings about illness and disease. These may have been formed from childhood and are often based on the family's culture and tradition about illness and disease, from experiences with loved ones who either struggled with or accepted their illnesses and diseases, or from the their own experiences. Religious and spiritual beliefs may also play a role. It is important to realize that each person presents his or her unique perspective differently. Perspectives can range from the resident being terrified and fearful to being accepting and willing to do whatever is necessary to move to a healthier state.

To increase your awareness about resident's perspectives, it is often best to ask them about their experiences. You can focus on how they feel about being ill or having a particular disease, or who they cared for and how that affected them, or how their family views someone who is ill or has a specific disease. This will give you a much better understanding about how to approach residents when you perform a procedure, how they might respond to having diagnostic tests, or how they act and what questions they ask when a doctor visits.

Family Dynamics

As a holistic nursing assistant, you will come in close contact with residents' family members. Family members communicate and relate to each other in many different ways. In some cultures, a particularly strong emphasis is placed on the family and everyone is included in decision making. Family members may also be heavily involved in caregiving. There is often *kinship* (feelings of closeness) between members of an extended family or community. A resident may be close with a support group or with people in his or her neighborhood. Sometimes these relationships are as important as relationships with family and friends. Because these relationships are so important, they should be acknowledged and respected.

Communication Styles

A nursing assistant's ability to communicate effectively with residents may be influenced by residents' cultural and communication practices. In some cultures, self-control is valued to the extent that people are unwilling to acknowledge strong emotions or pain. This may make it difficult for residents to share how they are feeling. Other cultures have great respect for authority figures, such as doctors. As a result, residents may smile and nod out of respect, even if they are feeling confused or embarrassed. This reaction may be misleading. It may lead to the assumption that everything is all right with the resident, when everything is not.

Dietary Preferences and Restrictions

People's diets are often influenced by their cultural or religious practices. For example, many Buddhists abstain from consuming alcohol, and some are vegetarians. Jewish individuals may follow a *kosher* diet and eat only foods that meet the requirements of Jewish dietary laws. Muslim residents may not eat pork or any foods prepared with any form of alcohol. Some religions require the consumption of particular foods during ceremonial times (**Figure 12.3**). Other religions do not allow the use of alcohol, tobacco, tea, or coffee. As a holistic nursing assistant, you must be aware of any medical and religious dietary restrictions your residents have and assist with accommodating any special requests, as appropriate.

Religious Customs

Residents' religions may affect the care they require even in ways beyond dietary restrictions. For example, residents' religious beliefs may prevent them from taking certain medications, receiving blood transfusions (replacing lost blood with a donor's blood), donating or receiving organs, or allowing life support. Residents may also require specific arrangements to practice their religious beliefs. Religious beliefs may impact a resident's daily schedule as the resident includes prayer, meditation, or other religious practices as activities during his or her day.

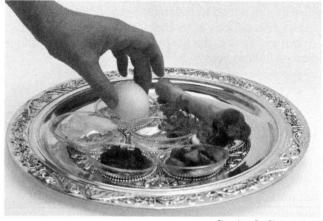

ChameleonsEye/Shutterstock.com

Figure 12.3 One example of a religious ceremony involving food is the Jewish Passover. This arrangement of food, known as the Seder plate, has symbolic meaning.

As a holistic nursing assistant, you may be asked to make sure residents have what they need to follow their religious practices. For example, Muslims may require supplies and equipment for washing prior to prayer, a clean sheet to place on the floor, and assistance kneeling to get into prayer position facing the city of Mecca. Jewish residents may observe the *Sabbath*, which begins on Friday at sundown and lasts until sundown on Saturday. During the Sabbath, a Jewish person who practices his or her religion may not write, bathe, or use electricity (for example, turn on or off lights). You may need to assist these residents with any activities they are not able to do. For example, you may need to turn lights in the resident's room on or off during Sabbath.

Levels of Modesty

Nursing assistants see residents in their most vulnerable moments. As a holistic nursing assistant, you should provide extra care and consideration for residents whose cultural practices or religious beliefs require modesty. In an effort to maintain their modesty, some residents prefer to receive treatment from someone of the same gender. Some women may also keep their hair covered.

How Can a Nursing Assistant Integrate Cross-Cultural Communication into Care?

When holistic nursing assistants practice cultural humility, they have the ability to use *cross-cultural communication*. Cross-cultural communication uses practices and approaches that promote and improve relationships with people from different cultures. This includes awareness and sensitivity; learning about another culture's values, traditions, and customs; and understanding differences in how members of the culture communicate. The following guidelines are part of cross-cultural communication:

- Be present, make eye contact, and use active listening skills.
- Pay attention to your body language. Be mindful of your gestures and avoid using your arms and hands when talking, as this may seem intimidating.
- Smile and be open to hearing what is said.
- Enter a resident's personal space only when appropriate.
- Use plain language when speaking. Avoid words that have two meanings or similar sounding words (such as *pair* and *pear*).
- Avoid slang, jargon, and humor. Residents are not likely to understand them.
- Use short, simple sentences. Keep questions and answers brief.
- Speak slowly to give residents time to understand what you are saying.
- Ask the resident to repeat back what he or she heard.
- If the resident does not repeat back what you said, ask the resident if he or she has any questions.
- Ask questions so you can respect traditional practices.

BECOMING A HOLISTIC NURSING ASSISTANT
Cultural Humility and Cross-Cultural Communication

The following list includes qualities of holistic nursing assistants who practice cultural humility and use cross-cultural communication skills. Read through this list and determine whether you have each quality.

- I have a good understanding of my own cultural and ethnic identity.
- I use self-reflection and avoid making assumptions or believing stereotypes.
- I respect others and do not try to make others accept my values and beliefs.
- I work hard at understanding differing perspectives.
- I know that a person's skill in the English language has nothing to do with his or her level of intelligence or literacy.

- I ask questions and seek training when I am uncertain about a cultural group or religion.
- I always use cross-cultural communication skills when working with residents, their families, and staff from different cultures or religions.

Apply It

1. Which of the qualities in this list do you already have?
2. Consider which qualities you do not have and identify ways you can develop your knowledge and skills so you can use them in the future.

- Summarize what you have said, if you can. Repeat the same message, with patience, so the resident has more time to understand what was said.
- Use other forms of communication to support oral communication (**Figure 12.4**).
- Attempt to learn key words in other languages.
- Provide written resources in a resident's native language.
- Ask the licensed nursing staff for an interpreter, when appropriate and necessary.

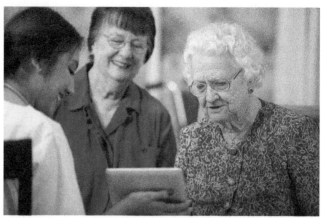
fstop123/Signature collection via Getty Images
Figure 12.4 If the resident is struggling to understand what you are saying, sometimes showing her an image or written word may help understanding.

SECTION 12.2 **Review and Assessment**

Key Terms Mini Glossary

cross-cultural communication the use of practices and approaches that promote and improve relationships between people from different cultures.

cultural humility awareness and understanding of one's own culture, as well as the cultures of others; includes knowledge of personal limitations, barriers, and gaps in knowledge and provides the openness needed to be sensitive to and respectful of other cultures.

kinship a feeling of being close or of having an association or connection.

Apply the Key Terms

Identify the key term used in each sentence.

1. A nursing assistant practices cultural humility when she is aware of her own personal limitations and barriers and gaps in her knowledge about other cultures.
2. Mr. T has kinship with the community he lives in because he is very close with his neighbors. They visit with him every weekend.
3. Last week, the health care facility provided training in cross-cultural communication to help new staff learn practices and approaches that promote and improve relationships between people from different cultures.

Know and Understand the Facts

1. Identify two ways a nursing assistant can show cultural humility.
2. Give two examples of specific religious customs holistic nursing assistants must be aware of when providing care.
3. Describe two examples of family traditions that represent cultural diversity.
4. What is cross-cultural communication?

Analyze and Apply Concepts

1. Identify one area in which you can improve your practice of cultural humility.
2. How can cultural dietary preferences and restrictions affect care?
3. Name four cross-cultural communication skills.

Think Critically

Read the following care situation. Then answer the questions that follow.

Tiana, a nursing assistant, has been asked to care for Mrs. E who was recently admitted to a long-term care facility. Mrs. E spends the majority of her time with her family. Mrs. E speaks little English. Tiana has been assigned to perform morning care. As Tiana enters the room, Mrs. E's daughter is feeding her something she brought from home.

1. What is the first action Tiana should take when she enters the room to show cultural humility?
2. What cultural knowledge will be important for Tiana to know to provide safe, quality care?
3. Which cross-cultural communication skills could help Tiana care for Mrs. E?

Key Points

Reviewing the key points for this chapter will help you practice more safely and competently as a holistic nursing assistant and will help you prepare for the certification competency examination.

- People of a variety of races and ethnicities live in the United States. Learning to appreciate others' differences, or diversity, will enable you to provide safe, quality care.
- Nursing assistants give care to residents from diverse family structures, religious beliefs, geographic locations, and generations.
- Ethnocentrism, bias, prejudice, stereotypes, and racism prevent a nursing assistant from appreciating diversity.
- Cultural humility recognizes that there are differences among all people and focuses on the assessment of one's own culture to understand its limitations, barriers, and gaps in knowledge.
- Cross-cultural communication is based on being aware and sensitive; building knowledge about another culture's values, traditions, customs; and understanding how members of a culture communicate both verbally and nonverbally.

Action Steps to Holistic Care

Review the information in this chapter. Complete the following activities.

1. Select one challenge to appreciating diversity. Prepare a short paper or digital presentation that provides more detail than is found in this chapter.
2. Write a short paper that explains the concept of cultural humility. Discuss why cultural humility is an important quality for holistic nursing assistants to practice. Also identify the qualities a person who practices cultural humility must have. Finally, explore an area such as family traditions, modesty, or religious customs, that might impact the care you will give as a holistic nursing assistant and explain how you could use cultural humility to respond to any challenges or differences.
3. With a partner, prepare a poster that shows three cross-cultural communication skills. Identify how these skills will lead to more effective resident interaction.
4. Research one cultural or religious group in the United States. Write a brief report describing three traditions or customs that would be important for a holistic nursing assistant to know.

Building Math Skill

There are 30 residents on your unit. Twelve residents are Hispanic. What percent of the total unit population do the Hispanic residents represent?

Preparing for the Certification Competency Examination

To prepare for the nursing assistant certification competency examination, you will need to know content found in this chapter. This content may be tested in the knowledge (written or oral) and skills (hands-on demonstration) portions of the exam. The following areas will be emphasized:

- influence of cultural attitudes
- the nursing assistant's role in respecting and accommodating cultural differences
- recognizing cultural and religious beliefs that require specific diets

These sample test questions are similar to ones you will find on the certification competency exam. See how well you can answer them. Be sure to select the *best* answer.

1. When a person evaluates another culture based on the beliefs and standards of his or her own culture, this is called
   A. bias
   B. prejudice
   C. stereotyping
   D. ethnocentrism

2. A nursing assistant is caring for an older woman who practices her culture's traditions. Which of the following would *not* be a cultural or religious practice to be aware of?
   A. The woman may have cultural dietary restrictions.
   B. The woman may be very modest and want to be covered.
   C. The woman may want the nursing assistant to assist her with meals.
   D. The woman may have many family members visiting at the same time.

(Continued)

3. Which of the following *best* describes the difference between race and racism?
   A. Race is a group of people who share many physical characteristics. Racism is the belief that one's race is superior.
   B. Race is intolerance or discrimination. Racism is the belief that one's race is inferior.
   C. Race is a group of people who have family traditions. Racism is the belief that one's race is built on values.
   D. Race is related to geographic area. Racism is the belief that one's race is superior.

4. The difference between a ritual and a tradition is that a tradition is
   A. a religious ceremony
   B. a practice that requires dietary restrictions
   C. handed down from one generation to another
   D. a practice that involves only current family members

5. A new nursing assistant is caring for a Muslim resident. What should the nursing assistant know about practicing cultural humility when giving care?
   A. In Islam, food is used to honor the dying.
   B. She should treat each resident as an individual.
   C. She does not need to worry about any dietary customs.
   D. All Muslim people usually act the same way.

6. Which of the following is true of ethnicity?
   A. It is based on the racial roots, customs, and rituals as a group sees them and practices them.
   B. It is based on a group's decision about how they will practice their rituals and traditions.
   C. It is based on a group's identification with common social, cultural, and traditional practices.
   D. It is based on a cultural group's perception of their likes and dislikes and how they are practiced.

7. Nursing assistants who demonstrate cultural humility always
   A. use journaling to describe their experiences
   B. use team meetings to discuss conflicts
   C. use meditation to deal with stress
   D. use self-evaluation to understand their own culture

8. Which of the following actions demonstrates cross-cultural communication skills?
   A. being present and using active listening skills
   B. providing clean linen during morning care
   C. providing comfortable chairs
   D. keeping the curtains closed during a procedure

9. What is a blended family?
   A. a family that is made up of several generations
   B. a family of members from difference races
   C. a family that consists of remarried parents and their children
   D. a family that includes two single people

10. What is a stereotype?
    A. an opinion that is not based on facts
    B. a simple, general, and usually negative opinion about a group of people
    C. a judgment about another culture based on the beliefs and standards of one's own culture
    D. an unfair belief that some people, objects, or situations are better than others

11. If a nursing assistant is being prejudiced, she is
    A. being rude and mean to another person
    B. paying special attention to another person
    C. forming an opinion before getting the facts
    D. creating rumors and spreading them

12. Mrs. H, a 45-year-old woman, is Jewish and observes her religion's traditions and customs. What is the most important thing to know about her dietary needs?
    A. She will likely not have a midday snack.
    B. She will likely need a diet free from fats and carbohydrates.
    C. She will likely ask for a meal that has no spices or salts.
    D. She will likely need a meal that is kosher.

13. A nursing assistant is taking care of Mrs. A, an older Asian woman. Mrs. A doesn't ask for much, and the nursing assistant provides her limited care because she always seems so happy. Is this nursing assistant practicing cultural humility?
    A. yes, because he likes taking care of her
    B. no, because he provides only limited care
    C. yes, because he doesn't bother her with a lot of daily care
    D. no, because he may not really know what she needs

14. A nursing assistant who asks questions to learn about a resident's cultural values, traditions, and customs is using
    A. cultural sensitivity
    B. cross-cultural communication
    C. transpersonal communication
    D. cultural awareness

15. What is sexual orientation?
    A. one's attraction to males or females
    B. one's personal identity of being male or female
    C. one's romantic engagement
    D. one's personal expression

Did you have difficulty with any of the questions? If you did, review the chapter to find the correct answer(s).

Welcome to the Chapter

This chapter provides information about the holistic nursing assistant's role in planning, organizing, and documenting care. Some tools used to organize care include plans of care and care conferences. In this chapter, you will also learn how to use objective and subjective observation when reporting and documenting important information about the care you give. Reading and completing assignment sheets, participating in rounds, and filling out change-of-shift reports are other skills you will learn. You will also need to know how to properly and accurately document care in an electronic health record (EHR), electronic medical record (EMR), or paper record.

What you learn in this chapter will help you develop your knowledge and skills to become a holistic nursing assistant. The topics discussed in the chapter are highlighted on the Providing Holistic Care Framework.

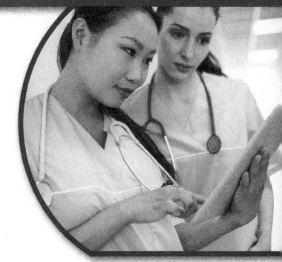

wavebreakmedia/Shutterstock.com

Chapter Outline

Section 13.1
Planning and Organizing Care

Section 13.2
Observing and Reporting Care

Section 13.3
Documentation

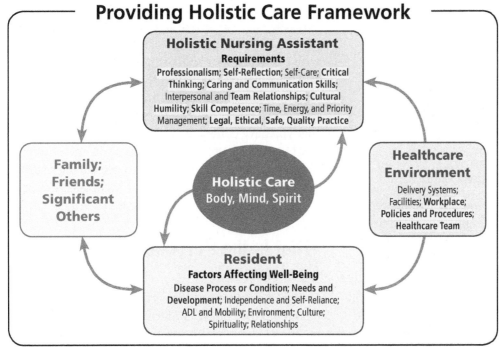

Providing Holistic Care Framework

Holistic Nursing Assistant
Requirements
Professionalism; Self-Reflection; Self-Care; Critical Thinking; Caring and Communication Skills; Interpersonal and Team Relationships; Cultural Humility; Skill Competence; Time, Energy, and Priority Management; Legal, Ethical, Safe, Quality Practice

Family; Friends; Significant Others

Holistic Care
Body, Mind, Spirit

Healthcare Environment
Delivery Systems; Facilities; Workplace; Policies and Procedures; Healthcare Team

Resident
Factors Affecting Well-Being
Disease Process or Condition; Needs and Development; Independence and Self-Reliance; ADL and Mobility; Environment; Culture; Spirituality; Relationships

Goodheart-Willcox Publisher

Planning and Organizing Care

Objectives

To achieve the objectives for this section, you must successfully:

- **identify** the purposes and key components of plans of care, care conferences, rounds, and change-of-shift reports.
- **explain** how nursing assistants participate in care planning, care conferences, rounds, and change-of-shift reports.
- **describe** how to read and use assignment sheets to organize and deliver care.

Key Terms

Learn these key terms to better understand the information presented in the section.

care conferences   nursing orders
change-of-shift report   rounds

Questions to Consider

- Have you ever planned or organized an activity and had others depend on you for the activity to be successful? The activity might have been a party or event.
- When planning the activity, what did you do to make sure you accomplished your responsibilities?
- What type of planning was involved for the activity? Did you have to ask others to help? What did you learn from this experience?

What Is a Plan of Care?

As you learned in Chapter 6, a *plan of care* is a written document that licensed nursing staff develop for each resident (**Figure 13.1**). The plan of care is developed from a thorough assessment and provides guidance for delivering personalized, consistent care to residents. In some facilities, plans of care are called *service plans*.

Plan of Care Organization

Plans of care may be different in each healthcare facility; however, they are generally organized using the steps of the nursing process. The plan also includes other important information needed to deliver care (for example, doctors' orders). Plans of care are usually made up of important medical information, including:

- medical diagnoses (identify diseases or medical conditions)
- ordered medications and treatments

- nursing diagnoses (identify potential or actual health problems that can be improved through nursing care, such as poor nutrition or difficulty ambulating)
- nursing goals (the desired changes or outcomes in a resident's condition, such as promoting independence; may be called *critical* or *clinical pathways* in some facilities)
- *nursing orders* (instructions for achieving care goals, such as help a resident ambulate at least twice per shift)

Plan of Care Evaluation

Evaluation is ongoing and is used to track and update the progress that is made toward achieving a goal. Plans of care are evaluated and updated routinely, and when any changes occur. The information provided by nursing assistants helps licensed nursing staff members determine if nursing actions should be stopped, continued, or adjusted. Evaluation is also used to assess the overall effectiveness of the nursing plan of care. Any updates or changes in care are documented by the licensed nursing staff and then communicated to staff members across all shifts to be sure there is consistency in the care given.

Plans of Care and the Nursing Assistant

Although nursing assistants do not create plans of care, they have an important role in the care planning process. Because nursing assistants work closely with residents, they share important observations and information that affect the plan of care. When you are a nursing assistant, members of the licensed nursing staff may ask you for specific information that you have collected. This information may be used to write the plan of care. An updated, written plan of care is usually available to use during a shift. This plan of care may be in the form of a *Kardex* or part of an electronic medical record (EMR).

What Is the Purpose of a Care Conference?

Care conferences, or *plan of care conferences*, are held regularly. These conferences bring together all members of the healthcare team who deliver care to a particular resident. Nursing staff members, social

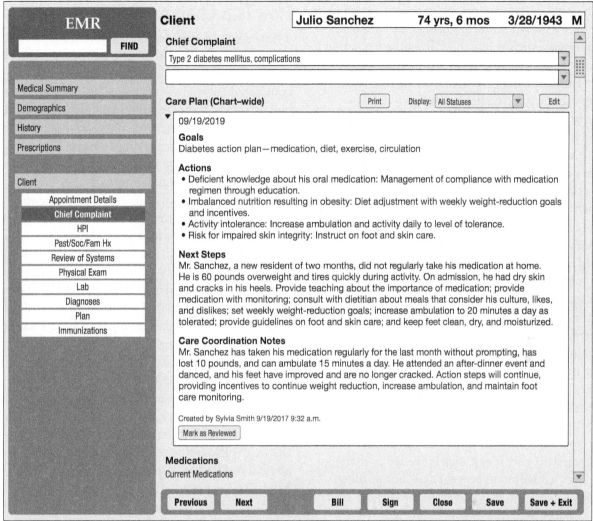

Figure 13.1 This is a sample of an electronic plan of care.

workers, dietitians, and rehabilitation and therapy staff members all participate in care conferences and discuss the plan of care. The resident and a family representative may also attend. It is a resident's right to participate in care planning and care conferences.

The purpose of the conference is to review progress and make needed changes to the plan of care, if necessary. Plans for continuing care, progress being made, problems or challenges in providing care, and changes in treatments are discussed. Questions may come up about how well a resident is eating and drinking, if a resident's weight has changed, whether or not the resident participates in activities, or if the resident needs personal items. These are questions the nursing assistant, who most often provides direct care, can typically answer. If a nursing assistant has been caring for a resident regularly, he or she may also share information on the resident's progress.

What Are Rounds?

Rounds or *rounding* are opportunities to physically monitor and discuss the status of a resident's condition or disease. *Nursing rounds* are conducted by the licensed nursing staff. These rounds typically occur right outside or in a resident's room, either at the beginning or end of a shift. Their purpose is to check on the resident's condition and any special needs. Rounds are used to provide staff members with information about their assigned residents. When nursing rounds are performed at the end of a shift, they can take the place of change-of-shift reporting.

Hourly or more regular rounding may also be performed. Hourly rounds improve safety, encourage more effective delivery of care, and increase resident satisfaction. Hourly rounding involves checking on residents at regular times during a shift to determine levels of comfort, safety, and environmental needs. Frequent and consistent monitoring helps prevent harmful events, such as possible falls or the formation of decubitus ulcers due to immobility. Rounds also provide information to licensed nursing staff members about pain medication needs.

Hourly rounds also help nursing staff members respond more quickly and effectively to resident needs. This can also prevent residents from having to always use call lights to make requests. Rounding information may be written on a facility-tracking document or entered directly into the electronic medical record (EMR).

When you work as a nursing assistant, you may be included in rounds or delegated to perform rounds on assigned residents during your shift. During rounding, you may be asked to observe a resident's condition, check on the effectiveness or outcome of treatment, or ask a resident about his or her pain levels after taking medication. If you are included in rounds, provide specific, factual information about those in your care. Conduct rounds as you are directed by the licensed nursing staff. If any follow-up care is needed, you are responsible for providing that care as directed. Follow-up care may include informing the licensed nursing staff that pain medication is needed or changing the resident's position to prevent a decubitus ulcer.

How Is a Change-of-Shift Report Used?

The *change-of-shift report* is a verbal report that provides important information about residents from one shift to the next. Change-of-shift reports are completed approximately 15–30 minutes prior to the end of a shift. These reports may be communicated from the outgoing nurse in charge to the incoming nurse in charge, from nursing assistant to nursing assistant, or the entire incoming nursing staff may attend the outgoing nurse's report.

During a change-of-shift report, nursing staff members share accurate information about resident status. Detailed plans for future care are discussed based on reports from the outgoing nursing staff. Nursing staff members must share any safety concerns (such as fall risks) and information about changes in a resident's condition or disease (such as changes in vital signs). Nursing staff members should also discuss future plans, including any tests that may affect care during the next shift and restrictions in eating or ambulation (**Figure 13.2**).

Nursing assistants may be present when the change-of-shift report is shared and may provide the nurse in charge with information about residents in their care. Providing detailed, accurate information about a resident's status is very important. It can be helpful to keep notes about the care you give during a shift so you do not forget important items.

CULTURE CUES
Cultural Beliefs About Healthcare

Cultural traditions and practices help form beliefs about healthcare, health, illness, and disease. These beliefs influence when a person seeks care and treatment, and who a person is willing to see for healthcare needs. Beliefs about healthcare also affect healthcare choices, responses to specific treatments, and willingness to make the changes needed to achieve health and well-being.

For example, if a resident has been diagnosed with cardiovascular disease, she will likely need to change her dietary habits, take medications, and exercise regularly. If these requirements interfere with her healthcare beliefs and cultural traditions and practices, she will be less likely to follow the plan of care. The resident may refuse to change her diet because it does not include traditional foods she eats.

Another resident may believe that only herbal remedies work and refuse to take medications prescribed by

his doctor. If the resident does this, his disease or condition may be greatly affected, causing serious consequences. As a nursing assistant, you must pay attention to cultural practices and help, as appropriate, to balance residents' cultures with their treatment needs. This is an important part of planning and organizing effective care delivery.

Apply It

1. Select one disease or condition and describe how cultural traditions or practices might influence treatment or care. Explain why you picked the disease or condition.
2. Identify three specific cultural traditions or practices that could impact the progress or treatment of a disease. Explain how these cultural traditions or practices might be effectively included in the treatments or care being given.

During the change-of-shift report, listen carefully and take notes, particularly about information related to your assignments and the residents in your care. Ask questions if the previous shift's change-of-shift report is unclear.

What Is an Assignment Sheet?

Assignment sheets are used in healthcare facilities to identify which residents a nursing assistant will be caring for and what specific care is required. These sheets provide detailed information about specific residents and will help you plan and organize your shift (**Figure 13.3**). Review your assignment sheet and ask the licensed nursing staff any questions you may have. This review is very important if you are

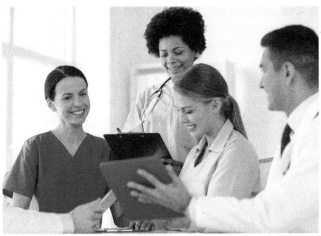

Syda Productions/Shutterstock.com

Figure 13.2 The information shared during a change-of-shift report is important. Nursing staff members should be alert and listen carefully during the report.

RM	RESIDENT	BATH	ACTIVITY	TRTMT	FLUIDS	ADDED INSTR
2	John S	☑ Bed ☐ Tub ☐ Shower ☐ Shampoo ☑ Shave ☐ Nails	☑ Bed ☐ Brp/Help ☐ Amb/Help ☐ Amb ☐ Walker ☐ Whlchr ☐ Crutches	☐ Enema ☐ BM ☐ Void ☐ Incont. ☑ Bed Sore ☐ Eggcrate ☐ Handrolls	☐ Encourage ☐ Limit to _____ ☐ Sips/W ☐ I & O ☐ Dist/W ☑ Catheter	*Catheter and Skin Care*
3	Don L	☐ Bed ☐ Tub ☑ Shower ☐ Shampoo ☐ Shave ☐ Nails	☐ Bed ☐ Brp/Help ☐ Amb/Help ☑ Amb ☐ Walker ☐ Whlchr ☐ Crutches	☐ Enema ☐ BM ☐ Void ☐ Incont. ☐ Bed Sore ☐ Eggcrate ☐ Handrolls	☐ Encourage ☐ Limit to _____ ☐ Sips/W ☐ I & O ☐ Dist/W ☐ Catheter	*Warm Compress*
4	Ruth Z	☐ Bed ☐ Tub ☑ Shower ☑ Shampoo ☐ Shave ☐ Nails	☐ Bed ☐ Brp/Help ☐ Amb/Help ☐ Amb ☑ Walker ☐ Whlchr ☐ Crutches	☐ Enema ☐ BM ☐ Void ☐ Incont. ☐ Bed Sore ☐ Eggcrate ☐ Handrolls	☐ Encourage ☐ Limit to _____ ☐ Sips/W ☑ I & O ☐ Dist/W ☐ Catheter	
5A	Lillian B	☐ Bed ☐ Tub ☑ Shower ☐ Shampoo ☐ Shave ☐ Nails	☐ Bed ☑ Brp/Help ☐ Amb/Help ☐ Amb ☐ Walker ☐ Whlchr ☐ Crutches	☑ Enema ☐ BM ☐ Void ☐ Incont. ☐ Bed Sore ☐ Eggcrate ☐ Handrolls	☐ Encourage ☐ Limit to _____ ☐ Sips/W ☑ I & O ☐ Dist/W ☐ Catheter	*Foot Care*
5B	Jane D	☐ Bed ☑ Tub ☐ Shower ☐ Shampoo ☐ Shave ☐ Nails	☐ Bed ☐ Brp/Help ☐ Amb/Help ☐ Amb ☐ Walker ☑ Whlchr ☐ Crutches	☐ Enema ☐ BM ☐ Void ☐ Incont. ☐ Bed Sore ☑ Eggcrate ☐ Handrolls	☑ Encourage ☐ Limit to _____ ☐ Sips/W ☐ I & O ☐ Dist/W ☐ Catheter	

Goodheart-Willcox Publisher

Figure 13.3 This is a sample assignment sheet. Using this sheet will help you be organized and keep track of important information.

caring for unfamiliar residents or if there have been changes in a resident's condition or progress. Also review any treatments you have not done recently.

During your shift, you may add information to the assignment sheet. For example, you may record a resident's response to treatment so you remember to report it to the licensed nursing staff.

Use assignment sheets to plan your shift and prioritize tasks. For example, if you have to give two complete bed baths and a shower, you may give the shower first since bed baths take much longer. You might also take care of urgent needs first before performing any treatments or procedures that take longer. Assignment sheets are planning tools for your shift that will help you be organized, efficient, and effective.

SECTION 13.1 **Review and Assessment**

Key Terms Mini Glossary

care conferences routinely scheduled meetings that bring together all members of the healthcare staff who deliver care to a particular resident; during the meeting, the resident's plan of care is discussed.

change-of-shift report a verbal report that transfers essential information about residents from one shift to the next.

nursing orders instructions outlining the actions that should be taken to achieve stated goals of care; written by the RN.

rounds opportunities to monitor and discuss the status of a resident's condition or disease; conducted inside or right outside the resident's room.

Apply the Key Terms

Think about the definitions of the following key terms. Describe one difference between each pair of key terms.

1. nursing orders and care conference
2. change-of-shift report and rounds
3. rounds and nursing orders
4. care conference and change-of-shift report

Know and Understand the Facts

1. Describe the purpose of a plan of care.
2. What is the purpose of a care conference?
3. Why are change-of-shift reports important?
4. Explain the process used to share critical information during rounds.

Analyze and Apply Concepts

1. Discuss the role of nursing assistants during care conferences.
2. What types of information can a nursing assistant provide during change-of-shift reports?
3. What might a nursing assistant be asked or delegated to observe during rounds?
4. Describe how nursing assistants use assignment sheets to plan, prioritize, and organize care.

Think Critically

Read the following care situation. Then answer the questions that follow.

Sima has been caring for Mrs. F for the past week. She has enjoyed this assignment and is very comfortable with the care she is providing. Sima has become so used to caring for Mrs. F that she no longer spends any time observing, asking Mrs. F questions about how she feels, or making notes on her assignment sheet. When the nurse in charge asks for change-of-shift report information today, Sima says that nothing has changed.

1. Do you think Sima is properly caring for Mrs. F? Explain your answer.
2. Is Sima's answer appropriate? Why or why not?
3. When you are caring for someone for a long period of time, how can you be sure you are observing and recording important and necessary information?

Observing and Reporting Care

Objectives

To achieve the objectives for this section, you must successfully:

- **explain** the difference between objective and subjective observation.
- **describe** the process used to provide accurate, complete, and timely reports.

Key Terms

Learn these key terms to better understand the information presented in the section.

critical observation	objective observations
deformity	subjective observations
numbness	tingling

Questions to Consider

- How observant do you think you are?
- How well can you describe an event or situation after it has happened? Are you able to use specific details, or do you remember only generalities?
- What might you do to be more observant?

Holistic nursing assistants must be sensitive to and aware of changes in a resident's daily routine, behavior, communication, appearance, general mood, and physical health. Always expect that changes in a resident's condition will occur as the resident's condition may improve or worsen. Regularly observe residents to help identify changes. A good time to do this is during routine care. It is also important to practice observation skills when you have been asked to observe a resident for specific changes (for example, a change in breathing patterns or wound drainage).

What Are Objective and Subjective Observations?

Observation is one of the most important responsibilities of a nursing assistant. Nursing assistants must observe residents while providing care, looking for physical changes, expressions of emotion, responses to treatment, and the progress of the resident's disease or condition. These observations may be either objective or subjective. ***Objective observations*** are based on facts. ***Subjective observations*** are based on feelings or opinions.

Objective Observations

The primary purpose of objective observation is to focus only on facts that are based on sight, hearing, touch, and smell. The measurement of a resident's oxygen status, vital signs, wound drainage, and urinary output are objective observations (**Figure 13.4**). Objective observations are never opinions or based on a personal bias.

For example, if a resident tells you about a rash she has, an objective observation would state that the resident has a red, bumpy irritation on the upper arm. You would describe only what you saw by observing the rash objectively. You would not say, "the resident has a rash" because that would be a personal opinion. If a resident had a bruise on his leg, you would describe its location, how large it is, the color of the bruise, if it was inflamed or swollen, the temperature of it to the touch, and if there was drainage coming from the bruise.

Subjective Observations

Subjective observations are ideas, thoughts, or opinions. While subjective observations are helpful and important observations, they are not facts. If residents provide subjective information, the residents' exact words must be shared with the licensed nursing staff.

As an example of subjective observation, a resident may complain of pain. To make an objective observation, you would need to see physical evidence of pain. This physical evidence might include the holding or rubbing of the painful body part, discoloration on the body part that hurts, or movement of the resident away from you when you touch that body part.

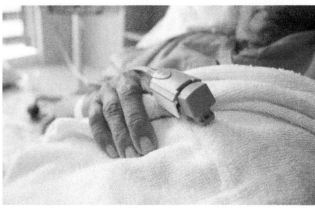

Piyada Jaiaree/Shutterstock.com

Figure 13.4 A specific measurement, such as oxygen status, is an example of an objective observation.

Without physical evidence, there is no way to know if pain is an objective fact or not. To report the pain subjectively, you might say, "The resident states that his pain feels like a dull ache and never lets up. In the morning, it feels worse than in the evening."

Another example is a resident who shares that he did not sleep well last night. The objective observation is the resident's eyes are swollen and the lids are red-rimmed. The subjective observation is his exact words. You can make a subjective observation more detailed by asking questions such as, "What happened during the night that kept you awake?" The resident might say, "I was worried about my son. He is going on a business trip today by car, and because of the weather the roads are dangerous." The subjective observation you provide would again use the exact words stated by the resident.

Critical Observation

To be successful and provide safe, quality care, holistic nursing assistants need to develop strong observational skills. *Critical observation* occurs when both objective and subjective observation are reported and recorded

appropriately. Part of critical observation is knowing when you should share your observation with the licensed nursing staff. Some observations, such as those related to routine care or treatments, can wait until the change-of-shift report. Other observations, such as complaints of pain or changes in vital signs, are critical and must be reported immediately. Failing to do so may cause you to incorrectly remember important details. If you do not remember specific events or details, always tell the licensed nursing staff that you cannot recall the specifics.

How Does Accurate Reporting Make a Difference in Care?

The healthcare team communicates observations and other important information by accurately reporting care. Accurate reporting makes certain that residents' conditions are always being effectively monitored so licensed nursing staff members can promptly respond to any issues or concerns. The best way to report information is through face-to-face communication.

Always use your notes to give a specific, accurate report. Report only those details you saw or actions you did yourself. Give the report to the licensed nurse at the change of shift and whenever you leave the unit during your shift. If the observation is cause for concern, share it as soon as possible. Always tell the licensed nursing staff immediately if there is a change in a resident's condition. You should always report any changes related to:

- the resident's ability to respond
- mobility
- complaints of sudden, severe pain
- a sore or reddened area on the skin or swelling
- complaints of a sudden change in vision
- complaints of pain or difficulty breathing
- abnormal respirations
- complaints or signs of difficulty swallowing
- vomiting
- bleeding
- vital signs outside the normal ranges

- joint pain, tenderness, or *deformity* (distortion)
- complaints of *numbness* (lack of feeling) or *tingling* (a sensation like sharp points digging into the skin)
- lightheadedness or dizziness

Whenever you are reporting, use the following steps:

1. Give the resident's name, room number, and bed number.
2. Include the time you made your observation or gave specific care.
3. Provide objective observations, such as what you saw, heard, smelled, or felt.
4. Provide only those subjective observations that were communicated to you by the resident (for example, any reported feelings of pain).
5. Identify any possible or requested resident needs.

Always be prepared to give a report during the change of shift, when there are immediate issues, and whenever you are requested to do so by the licensed nursing staff.

SECTION 13.2 **Review and Assessment**

Key Terms Mini Glossary

critical observation the appropriate use of both objective and subjective observation.

deformity the distortion of a body part.

numbness an inability to feel sensations due to changes in nerve function.

objective observations descriptions of the facts about a situation.

subjective observations descriptions based on feelings or opinions about a situation.

tingling a sensation that feels like sharp points digging into the skin due to changes in nerve function.

Apply the Key Terms

An incorrect key term is used in each of the following statements. Identify the incorrect key term and then replace it with the correct term.

1. The nursing assistant reported that the resident was not able to feel sensations due to changes in her nerve function. She was describing tingling.
2. Objective observation is based on feelings or opinions about a situation.
3. Numbness is a sensation that feels like sharp points digging into the skin.
4. Reporting blood pressure is a subjective observation.
5. Deformity is the appropriate use of both objective and subjective observation.

Know and Understand the Facts

1. What is an objective observation?
2. What is a subjective observation?
3. When is it appropriate to give an immediate report to the licensed nursing staff?

Analyze and Apply Concepts

1. What are two examples of critical observations?
2. List three guidelines you can use to improve your observation skills as a holistic nursing assistant.
3. A nursing assistant is leaving the unit on break. List the five steps he should take when reporting to the licensed nursing staff.

Think Critically

Read the following care situation. Then answer the questions that follow.

Jim, the nurse in charge, asked nursing assistant Jaylene to check on Mr. L and see if his pain had gone away. Jim gave Mr. L medication about a half hour ago for leg pain. When Jaylene got to Mr. L's room, she asked him how he was doing, but Mr. L was holding his leg and crying quietly.

1. How should Jaylene describe what she sees? What type of observation is this?
2. What should Jaylene do next? Explain your answer.
3. What type of report should Jaylene give Jim and when?

Objectives

To achieve the objectives for this section, you must successfully:

- **describe** the different types of records and their purposes.
- **describe** why documentation is important when providing care.
- **explain** the documentation scope of practice for nursing assistants.
- **apply** guidelines for accurate and timely documentation.

Key Terms

Learn these key terms to better understand the information presented in the section.

12-hour clock
24-hour clock
addendum
amendments
consultations

electronic health
  record (EHR)
electronic medical
  record (EMR)
manually

Questions to Consider

- Think about the last time you wrote something. Maybe you were writing for a school assignment or for a job. Did you plan ahead what you wanted to write, or did you just start writing?
- When you write, what steps do you take to be sure you communicate your thoughts effectively?

What Types of Records Are Used in Healthcare?

When you begin working in healthcare, using and maintaining records will be an important responsibility. Some records are electronic; others are physical forms and must be filled in *manually*, or by hand. For example, nursing assistants in some facilities record vital signs on a form; in other facilities, they enter this information into the resident's EMR (**Figure 13.5**).

Information about residents is kept on the unit in which residents reside and is readily available. When residents are discharged or expire, their records are sent to a department that stores and maintains the facility's health records. Because records are legal documents, their life spans are regulated by accreditation agency recommendations, federal and state retention laws and regulations, legal requirements,

and in some facilities, the needs of ongoing medical research and education. All healthcare facilities have policies and procedures regarding the maintenance, retention, and destruction of records and documents.

Two primary types of records are used in healthcare facilities:

- records that support and document care
- records that make sure all functions in a facility are organized and operate smoothly and efficiently

Records that support and document care include electronic health records (EHRs); electronic medical records (EMRs); paper records (sometimes

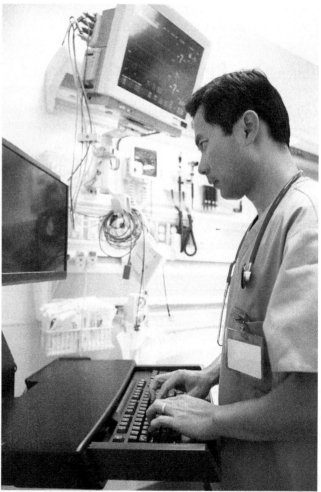

MBI/Shutterstock.com

Figure 13.5 Nursing assistants can enter information into a resident's EMR using digital devices.

called *charts*); admission, transfer, and discharge records; medication administration records (MARs); and plans of care. As a nursing assistant, you will be responsible for viewing, using, and adding to these health records. Careful, accurate documentation is an important part of providing effective, holistic care.

Some records used in healthcare facilities are not related to care. These include employment forms, policies and procedures (see Chapter 6), supply order forms, and incident reports (see Chapter 4). Some forms may be used by many healthcare staff members, while others may be specific to particular healthcare functions.

Electronic Health Record (EHR)

An *electronic health record (EHR)* is a digital record that contains all of a person's health information, including medical history and healthcare experiences. An EHR can include doctors' visits; hospital stays; surgical or medical procedures; annual physical examinations; referrals; and *consultations* (meetings) with other doctors, social workers, or therapists.

EHRs make information available instantly and they have all medical and healthcare information from every provider who has given care. One benefit of the EHR is that the information it contains can be shared across healthcare providers and facilities, making it possible for the information to travel with the person. Another benefit is that EHRs are environmentally friendly and eliminate the large amount of paper used with manual recordkeeping.

EHRs store specific healthcare data, and information such as age, medical history, diagnoses, medications, allergies, progress notes, immunization dates, laboratory test results, X-ray images, and insurance and billing data. This information can come from a variety of healthcare facilities. The goal of the EHR is to contain, in one place (such as with the person's primary care provider), all medical and health records. The use of an EHR makes coordinated, individual-centered care possible; eliminates duplication; and allows a smooth transition from one healthcare facility to another.

For example, when a pharmacist enters medication details into the EHR, this information becomes available to all healthcare providers. As a result, healthcare providers can see all drugs and dosages that have been ordered. When an EHR system is fully functional, a patient can go to his or her own EHR to view personal information, laboratory and X-ray results, special screening outcomes (for example, from a mammogram), and summaries of notes made by specialists.

Electronic Medical Record (EMR)

An *electronic medical record (EMR)* is a component of an EHR. An EMR typically uses the same technology as an EHR. However, instead of containing the *entire* health record, it includes information about a person's *single stay* in a facility (such as a hospital or an individual trip to the doctor's office).

The EMR contains administrative and clinical information about the person. Administrative information includes age, gender, insurance coverage, and other data such as religious preference. Clinical information includes all medical and health information, such as history, diagnosis, progress, laboratory test results, and consultations with specialists. EMRs track information over time, identify due dates for screenings or checkups, and provide information about and changes in treatment progress and response (**Figure 13.6**). They can also help monitor the quality of care given.

How Should Health Records Be Handled?

Information documented in an EHR should concern only the person receiving care, and confidentiality must be maintained. As you learned in Chapter 3, *confidentiality* requires that healthcare providers consider any information communicated by a resident to be private.

According to HIPAA, people can expect that their diagnoses, test results, and private information will be recorded accurately and kept confidential when they visit a healthcare facility. *Health information* is considered any paper, oral, or electronic record shared with a healthcare provider, insurer, or similar individual that can be used to identify a resident. Healthcare facilities often have detailed security measures to protect health information. If healthcare providers share information inappropriately, this can be considered an *invasion of privacy* and have legal consequences.

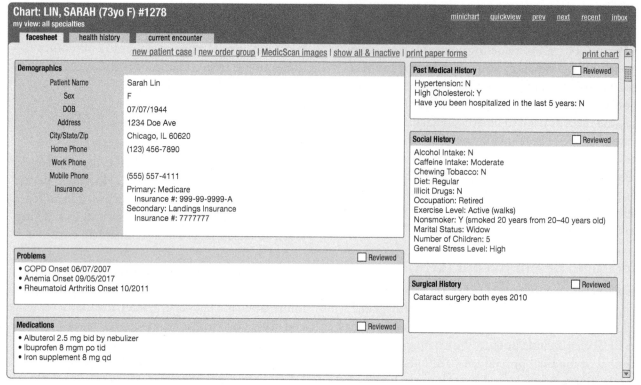

Chart: LIN, SARAH (73yo F) #1278
my view: all specialties

minichart   quickview   prev   next   recent   inbox

facesheet   health history   current encounter

new patient case | new order group | MedicScan images | show all & inactive | print paper forms   print chart

Demographics

Patient Name	Sarah Lin
Sex	F
DOB	07/07/1944
Address	1234 Doe Ave
City/State/Zip	Chicago, IL 60620
Home Phone	(123) 456-7890
Work Phone	
Mobile Phone	(555) 557-4111
Insurance	Primary: Medicare Insurance #: 999-99-9999-A Secondary: Landings Insurance Insurance #: 7777777

Past Medical History   ☐ Reviewed

Hypertension: N
High Cholesterol: Y
Have you been hospitalized in the last 5 years: N

Social History   ☐ Reviewed

Alcohol Intake: N
Caffeine Intake: Moderate
Chewing Tobacco: N
Diet: Regular
Illicit Drugs: N
Occupation: Retired
Exercise Level: Active (walks)
Nonsmoker: Y (smoked 20 years from 20–40 years old)
Marital Status: Widow
Number of Children: 5
General Stress Level: High

Problems   ☐ Reviewed

• COPD Onset 06/07/2007
• Anemia Onset 09/05/2017
• Rheumatoid Arthritis Onset 10/2011

Surgical History   ☐ Reviewed

Cataract surgery both eyes 2010

Medications   ☐ Reviewed

• Albuterol 2.5 mg bid by nebulizer
• Ibuprofen 8 mgm po tid
• Iron supplement 8 mg qd

Goodheart-Willcox Publisher

Figure 13.6 This is an example of an EMR.

Follow these guidelines to make sure residents' personal information is kept private and confidential:

- Maintain privacy and confidentiality at all times.
- Never use a personal device to take a photo or video of residents or their families.
- Do not identify residents by name outside the unit and facility.
- Do not post or publish information online that may lead to resident identification.
- Do not access records out of curiosity.
- Log off a computer once you are done using it (**Figure 13.7**).
- Choose a strong password and do not share it with others.
- Promptly report any identified breaches (violations) of confidentiality or privacy.
- Follow the facility's policies about using employer-owned electronic devices and personal devices in the workplace.
- Remember that violating confidentiality and privacy may result in discipline.

In addition to maintaining confidentiality, HIPAA also provides the right (with a few exceptions) for people to inspect, review, and receive copies of their health records. Residents must complete a formal request to review these records and receive them physically or electronically. Residents can also name personal representatives, such as family members, to access their records. They may also let other caregivers receive copies. Sometimes healthcare

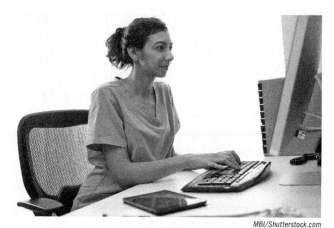

MBI/Shutterstock.com

Figure 13.7 When using a computer to open electronic records, always log off the computer once you are done.

facilities use secure, online health portals to give people access to their health information. Copies of health records cannot be denied, even if a person has not yet paid for healthcare services. If mailing records, some facilities may request a fee.

What Guidelines Should Be Followed When Documenting Care?

All care that is given to a resident needs to be documented (or *charted*). This information is used to make decisions about a resident's status and progress, necessary changes in treatment, medications, and care. Nursing assistants enter information into resident records and complete forms with specific information (such as vital signs or fluid intake and output measurements) within their scope of practice.

When working as a nursing assistant, never document something if it was not done. Never document for someone else, even if members of the licensed nursing staff ask you to document for them. If this situation occurs, report it to the nurse manager. Remember, documentation is always a description of what *you* have done.

Many healthcare facilities use electronic records, but if the facility uses paper records (charts), document in blue or black ink, write legibly, so that others can easily read what you have written. Draw a line through any blank spaces so that additional information cannot be written on the record. When you have finished documenting care, sign your full name and include your title.

If you are using electronic records, you will be given special training and a username for the electronic record system. After completing an entry in an electronic record, you should sign your full name using a digital signature and include your title.

Whether you are using electronic or paper records, follow these guidelines when documenting care:

- Check that you are documenting in the correct resident's record.
- Read any notes you have already written before you document. This will make sure the information written describes current care given.
- Identify the date and time that you are making the entry. Depending on the facility's preference, you may use a 12- or 24-hour clock. The *12-hour clock* splits each day into two 12-hour periods: the 12 hours from midnight

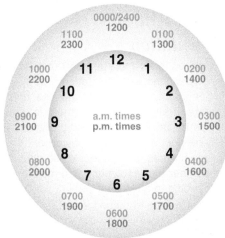

Goodheart-Willcox Publisher

Figure 13.8 If you are using a 12-hour clock, note if the time is a.m. or p.m. If you use a 24-hour clock, you will only need to identify the time.

to noon (called *a.m. hours*) and the 12 hours from noon to midnight (called *p.m. hours*). The *24-hour clock* divides the day into 24 hours, from midnight to midnight and numbered from 0 to 24 (**Figure 13.8**).

- Think and document in the order that you delivered care. For example, if you gave a bed bath before you helped a resident walk, document in that order.
- Document only what you observed, heard, and did and how the resident responded. Include objective and subjective observations. Use quotation marks when documenting subjective information, such as the resident saying, "I feel depressed today."
- Always document any response or behavior that is not typical for a resident.
- Use simple, descriptive terms, but avoid words such as *normal*, *good*, or *adequate*.
- Use abbreviations commonly accepted by the facility in which you work.
- Never remove pages from a paper record or delete an entry or section from an electronic record.

How Are Documenting Errors Corrected?

If an error has been made during documentation, it must be corrected quickly. The only person who can change, or *amend*, a record is the person who wrote

BECOMING A HOLISTIC NURSING ASSISTANT

Documentation

Documentation is an important part of providing safe, quality holistic care. Documentation provides ongoing information about the progress, changes, and status of residents. It also makes sure there is constant communication between shifts and provides information that may be needed or required by other healthcare staff and insurance companies. When documenting care, remember that documentation must always:

- be specific to a resident
- be kept private and confidential
- be yours (not someone else's)
- be timely (not done at the end of the shift)
- be accurate (if you are not sure how to spell a word, look it up)
- be written in the order care was given

- contain only what was observed or performed
- contain simple, descriptive terms and accepted abbreviations
- be corrected immediately and according to procedure if an error occurs (by the person who made the error)
- have a signature, title, date, and time of entry

Remember that if you do not document something, it is not considered done.

Apply It

1. Do you think any of these guidelines might be a challenge for you to put into action? Why or why not?
2. Describe how you can overcome any challenges you may have documenting care.

the original entry. Documentation corrections are legally called **amendments**. The following guidelines can guide you in correcting errors for both paper and electronic records. Always check your facility's guidelines for amending a health record.

- Make sure there really is an error before you continue. If the error is not your error, talk with the person who entered the incorrect information and encourage him or her to amend the problem. If the error is yours, take steps to correct it.
- If correcting a paper record, do not erase or use any correction liquid or tape. Instead, draw a single line through the incorrect information and make sure the original entry remains legible (clear). The new entry should be placed above or next to the error. Initial or sign and date the correction. The original and corrected entry should always be readable (**Figure 13.9**).

- If correcting an electronic record, add an **addendum** to the original electronic document that provides the corrected information. *Do not* delete the original information or rewrite it. Make sure the new entry is clearly identified as an addendum on the document.
- If you failed to enter information during documentation, add a late entry with the missing information and details.
- Once you correct an error or enter missing information, you must *authenticate* the information, or prove that it is real. To do this, digitally or manually sign the entry with your full name and title. Also include the date.
- Make sure the original document is retrievable (can be accessed in the future). Remember that health records are legal documents that must be stored and accessible at all times.

Each healthcare facility has its own policies and procedures about how to handle errors. Ask questions if you are uncertain about how to amend a record.

Did not want to ambulate after morning care. Stated, "I have a terrible headache and want to take a nap." VS taken. T—100.2, P—82, R—18, BP—116/86. When asked, pain level was a 5. Observed a red, bumpy irritation on her ~~left upper arm~~. left lower arm. Reported VS, headache, pain level, and skin irritation to the charge nurse.

9/17/20XX SCR

Figure 13.9 To correct a manual record, draw a line through the incorrect information, initial and date. Add the correct information on top of or beside the incorrect entry.

SECTION **13.3** **Review and Assessment**

Key Terms Mini Glossary

12-hour clock a method of indicating time that splits the day into two 12-hour periods: the 12 hours from midnight to noon (called *a.m. hours*) and the 12 hours from noon to midnight (called *p.m. hours*); each hour is numbered consecutively and labeled as *a.m.* or *p.m.*

24-hour clock a method of indicating time that divides the day into 24 hours, from midnight to midnight and numbered from 0 to 24; does not use *a.m.* or *p.m.* designations; also called *military time.*

addendum a type of amendment in which an item is added to a health record to correct an error.

amendments corrections to a health record.

consultations meetings with a healthcare expert; the expert gives advice or information.

electronic health record (EHR) an electronic record that includes information about a person's entire medical history and all healthcare experiences.

electronic medical record (EMR) a component of an EHR that includes administrative and clinical information about a single stay in a healthcare facility.

manually by hand.

Apply the Key Terms

Complete the following sentences using the key terms in this section.

1. A(n) _____ is a component of an EHR that includes administrative and clinical information about a single stay in a healthcare facility.
2. When documenting care, a nursing assistant writes that he ambulated the resident at 1:00 p.m. He is using a(n) _____ clock.
3. A nursing assistant needs to correct a health record. This is called a(n) _____.
4. A(n) _____ clock was used to document that a resident received a bed bath at 0930.
5. A(n) _____ is added to a health record to correct an error.

Know and Understand the Facts

1. Describe the difference between an EHR and EMR.
2. Explain why documentation is an important part of providing care.
3. Describe two ways to make sure documentation is accurate.
4. What is the difference between an amendment and an addendum?

Analyze and Apply Concepts

1. List three actions a holistic nursing assistant can take to maintain confidentiality and privacy when using electronic records.
2. Why is it important to never document for another nursing assistant or healthcare provider?

3. Describe how you would correct an error in a paper record.
4. Describe how you would correct an error in an electronic record.
5. How would you document 10 o'clock in the evening using a 12-hour clock and a 24-hour clock?

Think Critically

Read the following care situation. Then answer the questions that follow.

Mrs. E was admitted to a healthcare facility yesterday. Jack, a nursing assistant, is responsible for her care today. Mrs. E will need a complete bed bath, will need her vital signs taken every three hours, and will need to be turned and positioned every two hours. During Jack's shift, Mrs. E complains of nausea, and a member of the licensed nursing staff gives her medication. Jack stops providing care because Mrs. E wants to take a nap after her medication. After about an hour, Mrs. E says she feels much better, so Jack begins her care again and finishes the bed bath. He turns her every two hours and measures her vital signs as requested.

1. What specific information should Jack be documenting during his shift? Where should he be documenting this information?
2. If Jack makes an error documenting his care in Mrs. E's EMR, what should he do to correct the error? What should he do if he makes an error in a paper record?

Key Points

Reviewing the key points for this chapter will help you practice more safely and competently as a holistic nursing assistant and will help you prepare for the certification competency examination.

- A written plan of care provides the necessary direction and guidance for delivering personalized, holistic care. Care conferences are used to review a resident's progress and make updates to the plan of care, if necessary.
- Rounds are regularly performed to monitor residents' conditions or diseases.
- Change-of-shift reports share important information between shifts.
- Assignment sheets identify which residents each nursing assistant will be caring for during a shift.
- It is important that nursing assistants regularly observe residents for changes in daily routine, behavior, communication, appearance, general mood, and physical health.
- An electronic health record (EHR) provides information about a person's entire health history. An electronic medical record (EMR) provides information related to a single visit in a healthcare facility.
- Documentation must be timely, accurate, and to the point. Nursing assistants are responsible for documenting in resident records and recording information on forms.
- A health record is a legal document and must be accurate and maintained properly. If care is not documented, it is not considered done.
- Any documentation errors must be corrected quickly. The only person who can correct, or amend, a record is the person who made the original entry.

Action Steps to Holistic Care

Review the information in this chapter. Complete the following activities.

1. Create a poster or digital presentation that explains what a plan of care is and why it is important. Discuss how and why care plans are created, who uses them, the information that is typically included, and how they are organized and evaluated. Then think about how a nursing assistant might use a plan of care or contribute to its development.
2. With a partner, prepare a poster with information about the use of assignment sheets. Illustrate what is important about using the sheet and how the sheet can help organize care and manage time.
3. Research current scientific information about rounding and resident care. Provide a brief report that describes three current facts about rounding not covered in this chapter.

Building Math Skill

The unit you work on recently changed from using a 12-hour clock to a 24-hour clock. You usually document three times during your evening shift: right after vital signs are taken, after dinner, and before you leave. Convert these times to a 24-hour clock

4:00 p.m.
7:00 p.m.
10:00 p.m.

Preparing for the Certification Competency Examination

To prepare for the nursing assistant certification competency examination, you will need to know content found in this chapter. This content may be tested in the knowledge (written or oral) and skills (hands-on demonstration) portions of the exam. The following areas will be emphasized:

- observation and reporting of condition changes
- objective and subjective observations
- documentation
- confidentiality
- communication guidelines

These sample test questions are similar to ones you will find on the certification competency exam. See how well you can answer them. Be sure to select the *best* answer.

1. What is the purpose of a care conference?
   A. to discuss daily assignments
   B. to discuss admissions
   C. to discuss transfers
   D. to plan and change care as needed

2. If your facility uses a 24-hour clock, and you are performing care at 1:15 p.m., what time should you write on the documentation?
   A. 1315
   B. 0115
   C. 1115
   D. 1305

3. The purpose of a plan of care is to
   A. provide doctors with a way to review care
   B. provide the healthcare team with a plan so they can respond to different orders
   C. provide the necessary directions for delivering individualized, holistic care
   D. provide the resident and family with a set of teaching instructions

4. A nursing assistant was asked by the nurse in charge to perform rounds. The nurse is specifically asking the nursing assistant to
   A. monitor residents' conditions or diseases
   B. clean residents' rooms to ensure a safe and secure environment
   C. provide proper nutritional snacks when requested
   D. offer residents a way to be involved in activities

5. Why are change-of-shift reports important?
   A. They give staff a chance to talk with each other about shift issues and problems.
   B. They are a time to relax and get to know staff from other shifts.
   C. They are a time to communicate important resident information from one shift to the next.
   D. They provide time for nursing staff to document and talk with doctors.

6. Ms. C, a new resident, shares with you that her heart is beating fast. What should you document about what she said?
   A. The resident is having a lot of pain.
   B. The resident stated that "her heart is beating fast."
   C. The resident seems to be uncomfortable.
   D. The resident feels like her heart is beating fast.

7. Objective observation uses
   A. only facts
   B. opinions and beliefs
   C. opinions and facts
   D. your own beliefs

8. A nursing assistant used both objective and subjective observation to report on Mr. K's care. Which of the following is a subjective observation?
   A. Mr. K's urine appeared cloudy.
   B. Mr. K said he felt very nauseous.
   C. Mr. K felt warm to the touch.
   D. Mr. K's face was red and splotchy.

9. In which of the following records do nursing assistants do the majority of documentation?
   A. progress notes
   B. the plan of care
   C. the health record
   D. the assignment sheet

10. What positive outcome can be achieved by rounding?
    A. seeing family members more often
    B. taking a few minutes to rest
    C. monitoring the number of visitors
    D. monitoring possible fall risks

11. Which of the following is the best example of an objective observation?
    A. The resident was complaining of a lot of pain.
    B. The resident's blood pressure was 165/110, and her hands were shaking.
    C. The resident stated that "she had a lot of pain."
    D. The resident seemed anxious.

12. When a new nursing assistant transferred to your unit, he needed training on giving a change-of-shift report. Which skill or step is the most important?
    A. being sure to provide as much information as possible
    B. reporting only those things he saw or did himself
    C. waiting to report until he has all the information
    D. providing a report that includes the family and roommate

13. An electronic medical record (EMR) is an electronic document that
    A. is left at the bedside for ease of reading
    B. has health information from multiple providers
    C. has information about a specific person's single stay
    D. is left in the medical records department so it is safe and secure

14. A nursing assistant realizes he has made an error in an EMR. What should he do to correct the error?
    A. ask his supervisor to fix it before the shift ends
    B. check facility policy for the correct procedure
    C. cross the information out digitally and enter new information
    D. wait until the next shift

15. Which of the following helps make sure important information is continuously shared about resident care and progress?
    A. plan of care
    B. incident report
    C. the 24-hour clock
    D. the nursing process

Did you have difficulty with any of the questions? If you did, review the chapter to find the correct answer(s).

14 Mobility

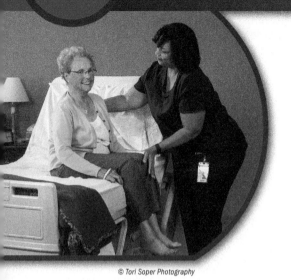

© Tori Soper Photography

Chapter Outline

Section 14.1
Positioning, Turning, Transferring, and Lifting

Section 14.2
Ambulation and Assistive Ambulatory Devices

Section 14.3
Rehabilitation and Restorative Care

Welcome to the Chapter

As a nursing assistant, you will be responsible for promoting, supporting, and assisting with mobility. Maintaining mobility is important for resident well-being. In this chapter, you will learn about the importance of ambulation and about ways to help residents who use assistive ambulatory devices such as canes, walkers, and wheelchairs. You will also learn the importance of rehabilitation and restorative care, ways to assist residents with range of motion, and guidelines for helping residents maintain as much independence and self-reliance as possible.

The information and procedures presented in this chapter will help you build the knowledge and skills needed to become a holistic nursing assistant. Check with your instructor to ensure that these procedures are within your state's regulations for nursing assistant practice. The topics discussed in the chapter are highlighted on the Providing Holistic Care Framework.

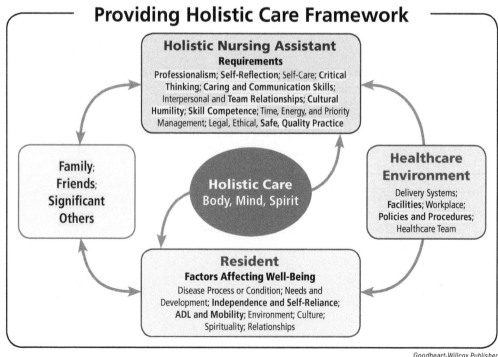

Goodheart-Willcox Publisher

Positioning, Turning, Transferring, and Lifting

Objectives

To achieve the objectives for this section, you must successfully:

- **explain** the importance of proper body alignment, positioning, and safe handling techniques.
- **identify** different body positions.
- **demonstrate** the procedures for positioning, turning, transferring, and lifting residents.

Key Terms

Learn these key terms to better understand the information presented in the section.

ankylosis
body alignment
contracture
foot drop

orthostatic hypotension
syncope
trochanter rolls

Questions to Consider

- Have you ever stayed in one position for too long? Maybe you had to lie in bed for a long time because of an illness or sat for hours working on a computer.
- How did you feel after staying in one position for too long? Did you feel aches and pains in particular body parts? If so, what did you do to relieve these aches and pains?

Nursing assistants are responsible for monitoring and changing resident positions to prevent the effects of immobility. The nursing assistant's responsibility may include positioning a resident in bed, moving a resident up in bed, turning a resident, helping (transferring) a resident into a wheelchair, or lifting a resident. Residents must maintain proper body alignment during these procedures.

Why Is Body Alignment Important?

Body alignment is the best placement of all body parts to allow the bones and muscles to be used efficiently. It is important for maintaining correct posture. When you are standing with good body alignment, your shoulder blades should be back, your chest should be forward, the top of your head should align (line up) with the ceiling, and your knees should be straight. When a resident is lying in bed, the spine should not be crooked or twisted, and the arms and legs should be comfortably positioned. Proper body alignment reduces stress on joints and skin.

How Should Residents Be Positioned, Turned, Transferred, and Lifted?

There are many benefits of positioning, turning, transferring, and lifting residents. Repositioning increases comfort and helps residents relax. It can also restore (bring back) body function such as helping improve the respiratory function and stimulating circulation, which prevents the possible formation of blood clots in the legs. When residents are not actively moving, muscles can atrophy (waste away) and develop *contracture* (shortening) and *ankylosis* (stiffening). Residents with *foot drop* (a condition in which the feet and toes drag) are unable to lift the front part of one or both feet due to muscle weakness or paralysis. Proper positioning and support in bed are very important for this condition. Finally, repositioning relieves pressure and strain on the skin, helping to prevent the formation of a decubitus ulcer.

Using Equipment and Devices

Different types of equipment and devices are used for positioning, support, and to reduce friction:

- pillows of various sizes to help protect the skin; prop up a limb; or support the head, a limb, or the back for comfort
- folded or rolled towels and blankets to prop up and support the resident and maintain proper body alignment
- *trochanter rolls*, made from rolled towels or blankets, that span from the top of the pelvic bone to the mid thigh to prevent external (outer) rotation of the hips
- a *draw sheet* (also called a *pull sheet*, *turning sheet*, or *lift sheet*) that is folded in half, placed on the middle of the bed, and used by the nursing assistant to turn the resident
- cotton padding to protect the skin and bony areas
- a *footboard*, which is a flat panel placed at the end of the bed to prevent foot drop
- a *hip abduction wedge*, which is usually made of stiff foam rubber material cut into a wedge and is used to separate the legs
- a *bed board*, which is a wide board placed under the mattress that provides additional support

If you have questions about a particular device, ask the licensed nursing staff, because some equipment and devices may be contraindicated in some residents. Some equipment and devices can be used or interpreted as restraints, which can violate resident rights and cause harm (for example, smothering from a pillow or possible entrapment).

Understanding Body Positions

Doctors usually prescribe a specific schedule for placing residents, particularly bedridden residents, into different positions, sometimes every hour. Even if there is no doctor's order, residents should be moved or repositioned every two hours. Residents should be rotated through at least four body positions during a shift, unless a particular position is contraindicated. Supportive devices such as pillows, towels, blankets, padding, trochanter rolls, and footboards may be used to maintain alignment. Position changes and the types of positions used should be recorded to make sure a correct schedule is maintained.

Fowler's Position

In Fowler's position, the resident is seated in bed, and the head of the bed is raised to a 45° angle (**Figure 14.1**). In *high Fowler's position*, the bed is raised to a 60–90° angle. The resident's knees may be elevated with a pillow under the knees and a pillow may also be used to support the resident's head.

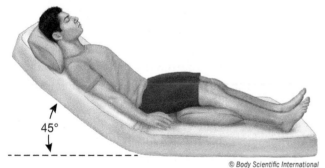

© Body Scientific International

Figure 14.1 In Fowler's position, the head of the bed is elevated to 45°.

Semi-Fowler's Position

In semi-Fowler's position, the resident is seated in bed, and the head of the bed is raised to a 30° angle (**Figure 14.2**). Support the resident's head and knees with pillows. You may need to use a foot support (such as a footboard) to prevent foot drop, if ordered by the appropriate healthcare provider.

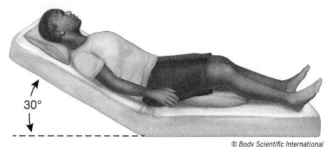

© Body Scientific International

Figure 14.2 In semi-Fowler's position, the head of the bed is elevated to 30°.

Supine Position

When placed in supine position, the resident is lying face up, flat on the back (**Figure 14.3**). The bed is flat, and both of the resident's arms and legs are extended. Support the resident's head with a pillow. The resident's arms, hands, back, and knees may also need to be supported with a pillow, or rolled towels or blankets. Use a footboard, if ordered, to prevent foot drop. You may need to place a trochanter roll to prevent the resident's hips from rotating outward. If needed, use padding to protect pressure points on the resident's elbows, knees, and tailbone.

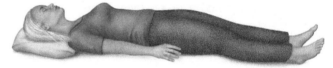

© Body Scientific International

Figure 14.3 In supine position, the resident lies flat on her back.

Trendelenburg Position

Trendelenburg position is a special supine position often used for residents who need certain medical or surgical procedures. The resident's legs are raised above the head and may be extended or bent (**Figure 14.4**).

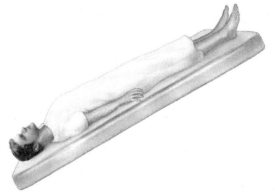

© Body Scientific International

Figure 14.4 In Trendelenburg position, the resident lies on his back. The legs are raised above the head.

Prone Position

In prone position, the resident is lying facedown, flat on the abdomen (**Figure 14.5**). The resident's legs are extended, and the head is turned to one side. The arms are extended down at the sides or bent upward at the elbows. You may need to support the resident's head and abdomen with pillows. To reduce pressure on the toes, place a pillow under the resident's lower legs or allow the resident's feet to hang off the bed.

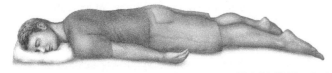

© Body Scientific International

Figure 14.5 In prone position, the resident lies facedown.

Lateral Position

The resident is lying on the left side (called *left lateral*) or the right side (called *right lateral*) in lateral position (**Figure 14.6**). Support the resident's head with a pillow. The resident's lower arm should be flexed. The resident's upper leg and hip should be bent at the knee to relieve pressure on the back. You may need to place a pillow against the resident's back to maintain the position. If needed, place a small pillow under the arm and between the resident's knees for protection and alignment.

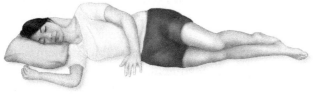

© Body Scientific International

Figure 14.6 In lateral position, the resident lies on one side.

Sims' Position

Sims' position is a partly left lateral and partly prone position (**Figure 14.7**). Support the resident's head and shoulder with a pillow. The resident's left leg and arm should be extended, and the right leg and arm

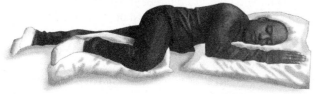

© Body Scientific International

Figure 14.7 In Sims' position, the resident lies partly prone and partly lateral.

should be flexed. The resident's left arm should rest behind him or her. The flexed right leg, hand, and arm should be supported with pillows.

Safety Guidelines for Positioning

Maintaining safe resident-handling at all times is very important when positioning or repositioning residents. Always practice safety by using proper body mechanics and asking for assistance if the resident is frail, overweight, or has drainage tubes or an IV. General safety guidelines include the following:

- Maintain a wide, stable base with your feet.
- Position the bed at the correct height (waist level when providing care, hip level when moving a resident).
- Try to keep your work directly in front of you and avoid rotating your spine.
- Keep the resident close to your body to keep from reaching.
- Always observe the skin before and after changing a resident's position. Give skin care to pressure points. Protect the resident from tubing that may rub the skin.
- Provide the most support to the heaviest part of the resident's body. Avoid placing one body part directly on top of another.
- Move the resident carefully and smoothly. Avoid *shearing*, or abrasion, of the skin.
- Always check that the bed linens are clean, dry, and smooth. Be sure that folds in the linens or food crumbs do not rub the skin and increase the risk of decubitus ulcers.
- Pay attention to any complaints of dizziness, shortness of breath, rapid heartbeat, chest or head pain, changes in ability or strength, or pain when bearing weight during positioning. If the resident makes one of these complaints, stop the procedure, maintain resident safety, and let the licensed nursing staff know immediately.

Preparing for Positioning

When preparing for any resident-handling activity, you should follow specific guidelines:

1. Observe the resident and determine what supplies or equipment (such as body lifts or gait belts) may be needed to maintain safety.
2. Know how positioning equipment works and understand the procedure for using it.

CULTURE CUES
Understanding Directions

As a holistic nursing assistant, you should always explain what you are doing when positioning or moving residents. Residents who do not speak your language may have a hard time understanding what is expected of them. You may need to ask for an interpreter or a family member to help explain the procedure. Understanding may be difficult even when an interpreter is used or when English is the resident's second language. Move and speak slowly. Ask questions along the way to be sure you are understood. Showing residents what you want them to do can be helpful.

Language skills and cultural differences may interfere with communication as you ask residents to turn, sit up, or move from the bed to a chair. Be observant and watch residents' nonverbal communication, as many cultures believe that people should be polite and show respect to authority figures (such as healthcare providers). Residents may follow your directions even if they do not understand, are uncomfortable, or do not really want to do what is being asked. Residents may frown as they are moved, and their bodies may become stiff due to pain. If this occurs, stop changing the resident's position. There may be other ways to change the position (for example, by finding a more comfortable position or supporting the body with additional pillows, towels, blankets, or padding to relieve pressure). Always work to maintain safety and prevent incorrect twisting or turning, which can increase risk for skin rubs, irritation, bruising, or falls.

Apply It

1. What two actions can a holistic nursing assistant take to make sure residents understand what is expected of them?
2. What precautions (safe actions) can be taken to prevent possible bodily harm or pain, maintain skin integrity, and reduce safety risks during a position change?

3. Gather the appropriate supplies and equipment and other staff members, if needed.
4. Organize the physical environment and equipment for safe completion of the procedure. Lock the wheels of the bed or wheelchair, raise or lower the bed or stretcher to the correct height, remove clutter, and check if any equipment needs to be charged.
5. If other staff members are needed for the procedure, make sure they know what to do.
6. Position yourself using the principles of body mechanics.

7. Tell residents what actions you expect from them. Show residents what to do and then help them during the procedure. Ask residents to assist as much as they safely can and to the level of their ability. Be sure to ask if residents are in pain. If a resident is in pain, let the licensed nursing staff know before changing a position.
8. Some residents (for example, residents who are paralyzed) may not be able to tell you if they are uncomfortable. You must pay special attention to these residents to prevent possible problems due to poor body alignment.

Procedure

Positioning in Bed

Rationale
Proper positioning in a bed provides good body alignment, helps maintain skin integrity, prevents decubitus ulcer formation, and promotes comfort and relaxation.

Preparation
1. Ask the licensed nursing staff if there are doctor's orders for the procedure, if there are any specific instructions listed in the plan of care, and if the resident can be moved into the positions required for this procedure.
2. Practice safety by asking for assistance from a coworker.
3. Wash your hands or use hand sanitizer before entering the room.
4. Knock before entering the room.
5. Introduce yourself using your first or preferred name and title. Explain that you work with the licensed nursing staff and will be providing care.
6. Greet the resident and ask the resident to state his full name, if able. Then check the resident's identification bracelet.
7. Use Mr., Mrs., or Ms. and the resident's last name when conversing.

8. Explain the procedure in simple terms, even if the resident is not able to communicate or is disoriented. Ask permission to perform the procedure.

9. Bring the necessary equipment into the room. Place the following items in an easy-to-reach place:
   - pillows of various sizes, if available and needed
   - folded or rolled towels and blankets
   - trochanter rolls
   - draw sheet
   - padding for skin and possible pressure points
   - bed board
   - footboard, if used to prevent foot drop
   - hip abduction wedge

   If you are unsure how to use a positioning device, check with the licensed nursing staff.

   Best Practice: An immobile resident, whether in bed or seated in a chair, should be repositioned at least every two hours. Some residents may need to be repositioned more often. Follow the plan of care.

The Procedure

10. Provide privacy by closing the curtains, using a screen, or closing the door to the room.

11. Lock the bed wheels and then raise the bed to hip level.

   Best Practice: Wear disposable gloves only if required for infection prevention and control.

12. Maintain safety during the procedure. If there are side rails, raise and lock the rails on the opposite side of the bed from where you will be working. Lower the rail on the side where you are working.

13. While the position may be prescribed by the plan of care, there may be times when residents can be asked about their personal comfort preferences. Be sure any tubing, such as IVs or urinary drainage bags, are not moved or pulled out of place or kinked during or after positioning.

14. If moving an immobile resident up in bed, place pillows under the head and against the headboard for safety. The resident should be in a supine position. Ask another nursing assistant to help you with this procedure and stand on the opposite side of the bed from the other nursing assistant. Grasp each side of the draw sheet, and together (on the count of three), gently slide the resident up in the bed. Use proper body mechanics by standing straight and facing the bed with your knees slightly bent and your feet pivoted (turned) toward the head of the bed.

15. If moving a resident with some mobility up in bed, place pillows under the head and against the headboard for safety. Put one arm under the resident's shoulders and the other arm under the resident's hips. Ask the resident to bend his knees, brace his feet firmly against the mattress, and place both hands on the mattress alongside his legs. On the count of three, ask the resident to push toward the head of the bed with his hands and feet. At the same time, slide the resident while still supporting his shoulders and hips. Use proper body mechanics by bending your knees, bending your body from the hips, pivoting toward the head of the bed, and shifting your weight from foot to foot as the resident moves.

16. Place pillows; soft, rolled towels; trochanter rolls; or blankets under the appropriate body areas, such as the head, shoulders, and small of the back; arms and elbows; thighs (tucking under to prevent external hip rotation); and ankles, calves, and knees (to raise the heels off the bed).

17. Do not raise the resident's ankles without first supporting the knees and calves.

18. If the knees are flexed, support them with a small pillow or blanket roll.

19. If appropriate, place a small pillow or blanket roll at the feet to prevent foot drop. (Use a footboard only if approved.)

20. Position the resident so the body is properly aligned. Then straighten the bed linens.

   Best Practice: Pay attention to all possible pressure points on the resident's body. Provide support and padding for these areas, as needed.

21. Raise the head of the bed to a level appropriate for the position.

22. Recheck that any tubing is in place. If you have any concerns, ask a licensed nursing staff member to check that the IV or other tubing is working properly. If the resident has a urinary drainage bag, be sure it is positioned below the bladder.

23. Check to be sure the bed wheels are locked, and lower the bed.

24. Follow the plan of care to determine if the side rails should be raised or lowered.

25. Remove, clean, and store equipment in the proper location. Remove soiled linens and discard disposable equipment.

Follow-Up

26. Wash your hands to ensure infection control.

27. Make sure the resident is comfortable and place the call light and personal items within reach.

(continued)

Positioning in Bed *(continued)*

28. Conduct a safety check before leaving the room. The room should be clean and free from clutter or spills.
29. Wash your hands or use hand sanitizer before leaving the room.

Reporting and Documentation

30. Report any specific observations, complications, or unusual responses to the licensed nursing staff. Document this information, along with the care provided, in the chart or EMR.

Turning a Resident in Bed

Turning a resident is an important part of positioning. Some positions, such as the lateral position, require turning the resident. You may also need to turn a resident during care (for example, when giving a bed bath or making an occupied bed). A draw sheet can assist you with turning residents, especially residents who have limited mobility.

Procedure

Turning a Resident in Bed

Rationale
When a resident must remain in bed, turning can help prevent skin breakdown, promote comfort, and prepare residents for care procedures (such as bathing and bed making).

Preparation
1. Ask the licensed nursing staff if there are doctor's orders for the procedure, if there are any specific instructions listed in the plan of care, and if the resident can be moved into the positions required for this procedure.
2. Practice safety by asking for assistance from a coworker.
3. Wash your hands or use hand sanitizer before entering the room.
4. Knock before entering the room.
5. Introduce yourself using your first or preferred name and title. Explain that you work with the licensed nursing staff and will be providing care.
6. Greet the resident and ask the resident to state her full name, if able. Then check the resident's identification bracelet.
7. Use Mr., Mrs., or Ms. and the resident's last name when conversing.
8. Explain the procedure in simple terms, even if the resident is not able to communicate or is disoriented. Ask permission to perform the procedure.
9. Bring the necessary equipment into the room. Place the following items in an easy-to-reach place:
   - pillows of various sizes, if available and needed
   - folded or rolled towels and blankets
   - trochanter rolls
   - draw sheet

   - padding for skin and bony areas
   - hip abduction wedge, if needed

   If you are unsure how to use a positioning device, check with the licensed nursing staff.

   Best Practice: An immobile resident, whether in bed or seated in a chair, should be repositioned or turned at least every two hours. Some residents may need to be repositioned or turned more often. Follow the plan of care instructions.

The Procedure
10. Provide privacy by closing the curtains, using a screen, or closing the door to the room.
11. Ask the resident if she has any concerns about turning.
12. Lock the bed wheels and then raise the bed to hip level.

    Best Practice: Wear disposable gloves only if required for infection prevention and control.

13. Maintain safety during the procedure. If there are side rails, raise and lock the rails on the opposite side of the bed from where you will be working. Lower the rail on the side where you are working.
14. Be sure any tubing, such as an IV or urinary drainage bags, are not moved or pulled out of place or kinked during or after positioning.
15. Place the resident's head pillow up against the headboard of the bed to protect the resident's head.
16. Ask the resident to assist as much as possible.

    Best Practice: Pay attention to how close the resident will be to the side rail after being turned.

17. If using a draw sheet to turn the resident toward you, reach over the resident and untuck the side of the draw sheet farthest from you so you can grasp it. The draw sheet may already be on the bed. If the draw sheet is not on the bed, place the draw sheet on the bed below the resident's shoulders and hips.
18. Ask or assist the resident to bend her knees.
19. Cross the resident's arms over her chest.
20. Cross the resident's leg farthest from you over the leg nearest to you.
21. Reach over the resident and support her behind the shoulders with one hand and behind the hip with the other.
22. Using proper body mechanics, roll the resident gently and smoothly toward you. If there is a draw sheet, you can use that to help roll the resident.
23. Bend the resident's upper knee and hip forward slightly into a comfortable position.
24. Place a pillow against the resident's back for support and place a pillow under the resident's top leg, behind the legs, and under the top arm for comfort.
25. Reposition the head pillow under the resident's head and check the neck for proper alignment.

> **Best Practice:** Provide padding to cushion pressure points and to support the natural curves of the body, if needed.

26. Raise the side rail, if used, on the side where you worked. Move to the opposite side of the bed (behind the resident) and lower the side rail. Place your hands under the resident's shoulders and hip.
27. Move the shoulder and hips, if needed, for comfort while the resident lies against a pillow.

> **Best Practice:** When positioning the resident, push instead of pulling. Pushing is much safer than pulling.

28. To turn a resident away from you, start by repeating steps 10–15.
29. Ask or assist the resident to bend her knees.
30. Cross the resident's arms over her chest.
31. Cross the resident's leg nearest to you over the leg farthest from you.
32. Place one hand under the resident's shoulders and the other hand under the resident's hip.
33. Using proper body mechanics, roll the resident gently and smoothly away from you. If there is a draw sheet, untuck it, or place a draw sheet on the bed to help roll the resident.
34. Bend the resident's upper knee and hip forward slightly into a comfortable position.
35. Reposition the head pillow under the resident's head and check the neck for proper alignment.

36. Place a pillow behind the resident's back to help maintain a side-lying position.
37. Move the shoulder and hips, if needed, for comfort while the resident lies against the pillow.
38. Use pillows to make further body position changes and straighten out the resident's clothing, bed linens, and any tubes (**Figure 14.8**).

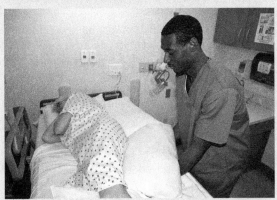

Figure 14.8   *Image courtesy of Wards Forest Media, LLC*

> **Best Practice:** Provide padding to cushion pressure points and to support the natural curves of the body, if needed.

39. Recheck that any tubing is secure and in place. If you have any concerns, ask a licensed nursing staff member to check that the IV or other tubing is working properly. If the resident has a urinary drainage bag, be sure it is positioned below the bladder.
40. Check to be sure the bed wheels are locked, and lower the bed.
41. Follow the plan of care to determine if the side rails should be raised or lowered.
42. Straighten the resident's clothing and bed linens.
43. Remove, clean, and store equipment in the proper location. Remove soiled linens and discard disposable equipment.

Follow-Up

44. Wash your hands to ensure infection control.
45. Make sure the resident is comfortable and place the call light and personal items within reach.
46. Conduct a safety check before leaving the room. The room should be clean and free from clutter or spills.
47. Wash your hands or use hand sanitizer before leaving the room.

Reporting and Documentation

48. Report any specific observations, complications, or unusual responses to the licensed nursing staff. Document this information, along with the care provided, in the chart or EMR.

Procedure

Logrolling

Rationale

Logrolling is a useful way to safely turn and move bedridden residents. During logrolling, the resident's body is kept in straight alignment (like a log). Logrolling is typically used for a resident who has had a spinal injury or who must be turned in one movement, without twisting. Two healthcare staff members are required to complete the logrolling procedure.

Preparation

1. Ask the licensed nursing staff if there are doctor's orders for the procedure, if there are any specific instructions listed in the plan of care, and if the resident can be moved into the positions required for this procedure.
2. Practice safety by asking for assistance from a coworker.
3. Wash your hands or use hand sanitizer before entering the room.
4. Knock before entering the room.
5. Introduce yourself using your first or preferred name and title. Explain that you work with the licensed nursing staff and will be providing care.
6. Greet the resident and ask the resident to state his full name, if able. Then check the resident's identification bracelet.
7. Use Mr., Mrs., or Ms. and the resident's last name when conversing.
8. Explain the procedure in simple terms, even if the resident is not able to communicate or is disoriented. Ask permission to perform the procedure.
9. Bring the necessary equipment into the room. Place the following items in an easy-to-reach place:
   • pillows of various sizes, if available and needed
   • folded or rolled towels and blankets
   • draw sheet

The Procedure

10. Provide privacy by closing the curtains, using a screen, or closing the door to the room.
11. Lock the bed wheels and then raise the bed to hip level.
12. Maintain safety during the procedure. If there are side rails, raise and lock the rails on the opposite side of the bed from where you will be working. Lower the rail on the side where you are working.
13. Be sure any tubing, such as IVs or urinary drainage bags, are not moved or pulled out of place or kinked during or after positioning.

> **Best Practice:** Wear disposable gloves only if required for infection prevention and control.

14. Make sure the bed is in the flat position and the resident is in the supine position. If allowed, remove the pillow beneath the resident's head.
15. Stand next to the bed on the side opposite of the way you will turn the resident.
16. Position one of your legs in front of the other and slightly bend your front knee.
17. Move the resident's entire body to the side of the bed nearest to you. Use the draw sheet, if necessary.
18. Place the resident's arms across his chest. Place a pillow lengthwise between the resident's legs to protect the knees.
19. Raise the side rail, if used, on the side where you worked. Move to the other side of the bed and lower the side rail.
20. Stand near the resident's shoulders and chest. A coworker should stand on the same side of the bed near the resident's hips and thighs.
21. Stand with your feet apart and with one foot in front of the other.
22. Ask the resident to hold his body rigid (stiff).
23. On the count of three, you and your coworker should roll the resident toward you in a single movement (**Figure 14.9A**). Use the draw sheet, if necessary or if instructed (**Figure 14.9B**). Keep the resident's head, spine, and legs aligned.

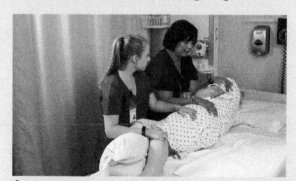

A

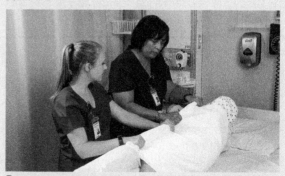

B
Figure 14.9

© Tori Soper Photography

24. Reposition the pillow under the resident's head and straighten the bed linens.
25. Position the resident to maintain good body alignment in a lateral position. Use pillows as instructed by the charge nurse or the plan of care.
26. Straighten the resident's clothing, bed linens, and any tubes.
27. Recheck that any tubing is in place. If you have any concerns, ask a licensed nursing staff member to check that the IV or other tubing is working properly. If the resident has a urinary drainage bag, be sure it is positioned below the bladder.
28. Check to be sure the bed wheels are locked and lower the bed.
29. Follow the plan of care to determine if the side rails should be raised or lowered.
30. Straighten the resident's clothing and bed linens.
31. Place any soiled linens in the appropriate laundry hamper.

Follow-Up
32. Wash your hands to ensure infection control.
33. Make sure the resident is comfortable and place the call light and personal items within reach.
34. Conduct a safety check before leaving the room. The room should be clean and free from clutter or spills.
35. Wash your hands or use hand sanitizer before leaving the room.

Reporting and Documentation
36. Report any specific observations, complications, or unusual responses to the licensed nursing staff. Document this information, along with the care provided, in the chart or EMR.

Dangling

In addition to positioning and turning residents, nursing assistants also help residents get out of bed. *Dangling*, or sitting at the edge of the bed, is an important first step to take before a resident moves out of bed to sit or stand. Dangling helps residents become comfortable in a seated position and is very important if residents have been bedridden for a period of time. Sitting before standing lowers the risk of **orthostatic hypotension**, a condition in which blood pressure falls when a resident stands. If orthostatic hypotension does occur, a resident may feel lightheaded or dizzy after standing up, feel weak, experience **syncope** (fainting), and become a fall risk.

Procedure

Dangling at the Edge of the Bed

Rationale
Helping a resident dangle, or sit, at the edge of the bed before getting up promotes safety. It reduces the risk of falling from possible dizziness or fainting.

Preparation
1. Ask the licensed nursing staff if there are doctor's orders for the procedure, if there are any specific instructions listed in the plan of care, and if the resident can be moved into the positions required for this procedure.
2. Wash your hands or use hand sanitizer before entering the room.
3. Knock before entering the room.
4. Introduce yourself using your first or preferred name and title. Explain that you work with the licensed nursing staff and will be providing care.
5. Greet the resident and ask the resident to state her full name, if able. Then check the resident's identification bracelet.
6. Use Mr., Mrs., or Ms. and the resident's last name when conversing.
7. Explain the procedure in simple terms, even if the resident is not able to communicate or is disoriented. Ask permission to perform the procedure.
8. Place the resident's robe and shoes nearby, if needed.
9. Clear the area of furniture and equipment to provide space to move.

The Procedure
10. Provide privacy by closing the curtains, using a screen, or closing the door to the room.
11. Lock the bed wheels and then raise the bed to hip level.

(continued)

Dangling at the Edge of the Bed (continued)

12. Maintain safety during the procedure. If there are side rails, raise and lock the rails on the opposite side of the bed from where you will be working. Lower the rail on the side where you are working.
13. Fanfold the linens to the foot of the bed.
14. Ask the resident to move to the edge of the bed, or assist the resident, if necessary.
15. Raise the head of the bed slowly so the resident is in a sitting position. Raising the head slowly will help prevent the resident from becoming dizzy or feeling discomfort.
16. Face the resident and stand at the side of the bed with your feet spread apart and your knees slightly bent to protect your back.
17. Slip one arm behind the resident's shoulders and grasp the far shoulder.
18. Slip your other arm under the resident's knees and rest your hand on the side of the resident's thigh (**Figure 14.10**).

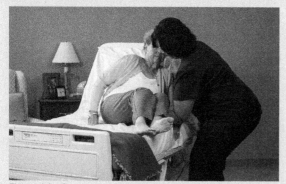

Figure 14.10   © Tori Soper Photography

19. In a single, smooth, pivoting movement, slide the resident's legs over the side of the bed and move her head and shoulders upward so that the resident sits on the edge of the bed (**Figure 14.11**).

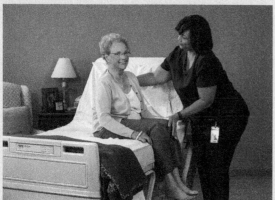

Figure 14.11   © Tori Soper Photography

20. Instruct the resident to hold on to the side of the mattress for support, if needed.
21. Stand in front of the seated resident to block her in case of a fall forward.
22. Do not leave the resident. Provide support, if necessary.
23. Observe the resident's condition during dangling. Ask how the resident is feeling (for example, dizzy or lightheaded). Check the resident's pulse and respirations. Check for any difficulty breathing and note if the skin is pale or bluish in color (called *cyanosis*).

> **Best Practice:** A resident may feel dizzy for the first few minutes of dangling, but this feeling should pass. If it doesn't, return the resident to a lying position with the head raised and immediately notify the licensed nursing staff.

24. If the resident is getting out of bed, make sure the resident is stable and feels well enough to continue the procedure.
25. To return the resident to a lying position after dangling, reverse this procedure and position the resident using proper body alignment.

Follow-Up

26. Wash your hands to ensure infection control.
27. Make sure the resident is comfortable and place the call light and personal items within reach.
28. Conduct a safety check before leaving the room. The room should be clean and free from clutter or spills.
29. Wash your hands or use hand sanitizer before leaving the room.

Reporting and Documentation

30. Report any specific observations, complications, or unusual responses to the licensed nursing staff. Document this information, along with the care provided, in the chart or EMR.

Transferring a Resident

Transferring residents from their beds to a chair, wheelchair, or stretcher (and back again) is another procedure that requires concentration and safety awareness. Transfers are performed when residents need assistance moving from their beds to sit in a chair or wheelchair (**Figure 14.12**). In addition to a transfer from a bed to a chair, transfers may also be required for toileting. When transferring a resident to another part of the facility, a wheelchair or stretcher is used. A wheelchair is also used when transferring a resident to a car or accessible vehicle.

Transfer sheets, slides, roll boards, and wooden or plastic slide or transfer boards are typically used for transfers between beds and stretchers. A *gait belt* (or *transfer belt*) can be used to transfer residents who may be too weak to support himself or herself. The use of the gait belt will help prevent falls. The gait belt also decreases the risk of the nursing assistant suffering a back injury. A gait belt should never be used to lift a resident and is contraindicated for residents who have had abdominal surgery. A gait belt should be used as directed in the plan of care and should never be used to lift a resident by the waist.

Lifts may be used for residents who are extremely overweight, cannot bend their bodies, or are unable to bear weight on their feet. Lifts can be mechanical or electronic (**Figure 14.13**). Facilities have policies about when and how to use a lift.

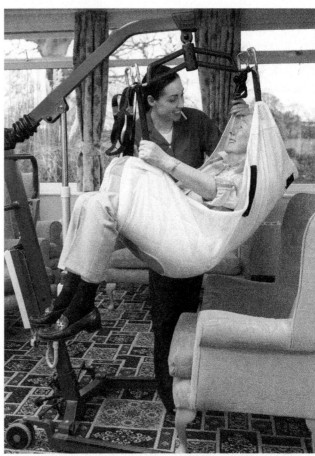

SolStock/iStock/Getty Images Plus via Getty Images

Figure 14.13 Lifts help transfer residents who are overweight, who cannot bend, or who cannot put any weight on their feet.

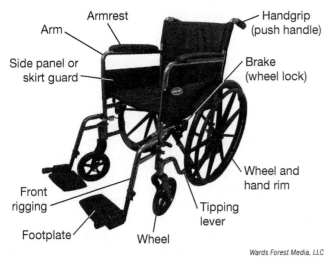

Wards Forest Media, LLC

Figure 14.12 Knowing the parts of a wheelchair can help you better provide wheelchair transport.

Procedure

Transferring a Resident from a Bed to a Chair or Wheelchair

Rationale
Transferring a resident in one smooth or pivoting motion lessens fatigue and promotes safety.

Preparation
1. Ask the licensed nursing staff if there are doctor's orders for the procedure, if there are any specific instructions listed in the plan of care, and if the resident can be moved into the positions required for this procedure.
2. Wash your hands or use hand sanitizer before entering the room.

(continued)

Transferring a Resident from a Bed to a Chair or Wheelchair (continued)

3. Knock before entering the room.
4. Introduce yourself using your first or preferred name and title. Explain that you work with the licensed nursing staff and will be providing care.
5. Greet the resident and ask the resident to state his full name, if able. Then check the resident's identification bracelet.
6. Use Mr., Mrs., or Ms. and the resident's last name when conversing.
7. Explain the procedure in simple terms, even if the resident is not able to communicate or is disoriented. Ask permission to perform the procedure.
8. Bring the necessary equipment into the room. Place the following items in an easy-to-reach place:
   • chair or wheelchair
   • a gait belt (in good condition and functional)
   • bath blanket
   • a robe and slippers or shoes
   • a pillow, if needed

The Procedure

9. Provide privacy by closing the curtains, using a screen, or closing the door to the room.
10. Lock the bed wheels and then lower the bed to its lowest appropriate position.
11. Maintain safety during the procedure. If there are side rails, raise and lock the rails on the opposite side of the bed from where you will be working. Lower the rail on the side where you are working.
12. Be sure any tubing, such as an IV or urinary drainage bags, are not moved or pulled out of place or kinked during or after positioning.
13. Position the chair or wheelchair next to the bed. If the resident has a weak side, position the chair or wheelchair so the resident can transfer using his stronger side.
14. For safety, stabilize the chair so that it cannot move. If transferring the resident into a wheelchair, lock the wheels of the wheelchair. Remove or swing footplates outward. Be sure the front swivel wheels of the wheelchair are facing forward.
15. Assist the resident to a seated position at the edge of the bed. Help the resident put on nonslip, properly fitting shoes and then place the resident's feet on the floor.
16. Apply a gait belt around the resident's waist over his clothing, per plan of care. The buckle of the gait belt should be in the front. Thread the belt through the teeth of the buckle and through the belt's two loops to lock it.
17. Check that the gait belt is snug, but that there is still enough room to place your fingers under the belt.
18. Stand in front of the resident with your feet about 12 inches apart.

19. Place one of your feet between the resident's feet and place your other foot outside one of the resident's feet. This will allow you to lock a sliding resident's knee with your knees.
20. Place your feet so that you have room to pivot them toward the chair.
21. Face the resident and hold onto the gait belt using an underhand grasp above each hip bone for greater safety.
22. Instruct the resident to push up, but not to put his arms on your shoulders or around your neck.
23. Signal the resident that it is time to stand. Using the gait belt, assist the resident into a standing position. Lift the resident using your arm and leg muscles. Bend your knees and keep your back straight. Do not twist your body.
24. Continue to hold on to the gait belt while the resident gains his balance. Stand knee to knee or toe to toe with the resident, to maintain stability of the resident's legs. Have the resident stand erect with his head up and back straight. Suggest that the resident shift his weight from one foot to the other to become comfortable standing before starting the transfer.
25. Face the chair or wheelchair and move your feet toward it as the resident follows, taking baby steps.
26. Once the resident is standing in front of the chair or wheelchair, ask if the resident feels the chair or wheelchair on the back of his legs.
27. Instruct the resident to put his hands on the armrests.
28. Assist the resident into a seated position using proper body mechanics.
29. Position the resident properly. The back and buttocks should be supported by the back of the chair or wheelchair. If there are footrests, place the resident's feet on them. There should be some space between the backs of the knees and calves and the edge of the seat. A small pillow behind the resident's lower back may provide support.
30. Arrange the resident's robe and clothing and cover the resident's legs with a bath blanket. Make sure the bath blanket does not touch the floor or the wheels of the chair.
31. Recheck that any tubing is secure and in place. If you have any concerns, ask a licensed nursing staff member to check that the IV or other tubing is working properly. If the resident has a urinary drainage bag, be sure it is positioned below the bladder.
32. Observe the resident for signs of discomfort or dizziness.
33. If transporting a resident using a wheelchair, push the wheelchair from behind and keep your body close to the chair. When entering an elevator, pull the wheelchair in backward. When leaving an elevator, wait until everyone leaves and then push the Open button, turn the wheelchair around, and pull the wheelchair out of the elevator backward.

Follow-Up

34. Make sure that the resident's body is in alignment and that the resident is safe and comfortable.
35. Place the call light and personal items within reach.
36. Conduct a safety check before leaving the room. The room should be clean and free from clutter or spills.
37. Wash your hands or use hand sanitizer before leaving the room.

Reporting and Documentation

38. Report any specific observations, complications, or unusual responses to the licensed nursing staff. Document this information, along with the care provided, in the chart or EMR.

Procedure

Transferring a Resident to a Chair or Wheelchair Using a Lift

Rationale

Moving a weak or immobile resident with a lift promotes safety and comfort during the transfer process.

Preparation

1. Ask the licensed nursing staff if there are doctor's orders for the procedure, if there are any specific instructions listed in the plan of care, and if the resident can be moved into the positions required for this procedure.
2. Practice safety by asking for assistance from a coworker.
3. Wash your hands or use hand sanitizer before entering the room.
4. Knock before entering the room.
5. Introduce yourself using your first or preferred name and title. Explain that you work with the licensed nursing staff and will be providing care.
6. Greet the resident and ask the resident to state his full name, if able. Then check the resident's identification bracelet.
7. Use Mr., Mrs., or Ms. and the resident's last name when conversing.
8. Explain the procedure in simple terms, even if the resident is not able to communicate or is disoriented. Ask permission to perform the procedure.
9. Bring the necessary equipment into the room. Place the following items in an easy-to-reach place:
   - lift
   - the appropriate size and type of sling for the resident's weight and size (consult a licensed nursing staff member if you are unsure what is appropriate)
   - a chair or wheelchair
   - a bath blanket

The Procedure

10. Provide privacy by closing the curtains, using a screen, or closing the door to the room.
11. Position the chair or wheelchair next to the bed and stabilize the chair for safety. If transferring the resident into a wheelchair, lock the wheels of the wheelchair and raise the footplates. Be sure the front swivel wheels of the wheelchair face forward.
12. Lock the bed wheels.
13. Maintain safety during the procedure. If there are side rails, raise and lock the rails on the opposite side of the bed from where you will be working. Lower the rail on the side where you are working.
14. Be sure any tubing, such as IVs or urinary drainage bags, are not moved or pulled out of place or kinked during or after positioning.
15. Roll the resident toward you and position the sling under him. You may need to roll the resident from side to side to get the sling into place beneath him. The lower part of the sling should rest behind the resident's knees, and the upper part should rest beneath the resident's shoulders.
16. Position the lift bar and frame over the bed in an open position. Lock the lift's wheels.
17. Attach the sling to the lift following the instructions in the manufacturer's handbook.
18. Make sure the open ends of the lift's hooks that will attach to the sling face away from the resident.
19. Ask the resident to fold his arms across his chest.

    > **Best Practice:** Talk to the resident as you lift him free of the bed. Talking to the resident will help lower anxiety.

20. When the lift holds the resident freely above the bed and is stable, move the resident away from the bed. Your coworker should support the resident's legs.
21. Position the resident above the chair or wheelchair.

(continued)

Transferring a Resident to a Chair or Wheelchair Using a Lift *(continued)*

22. Gently lower the resident as your coworker guides him into the chair or wheelchair. If the resident is being lowered into a chair, be sure the chair will not move.
23. Make sure the resident's feet and hands are positioned comfortably.
24. Lower the lift's bar so you can easily unhook the sling.
25. Follow your facility's policy to determine if the sling can be left beneath the resident.
26. Recheck that any tubing is secure and in place. If you have any concerns, ask a licensed nursing staff member to check that the IV or other tubing is working properly. If the resident has a urinary drainage bag, be sure it is positioned below the bladder.
27. Cover the resident with a blanket. Make sure the blanket does not touch the floor.
28. Remove, clean, and store equipment in the proper location. Remove soiled linens and discard disposable equipment.

Follow-Up

29. Wash your hands to ensure infection control.
30. Make sure the resident is comfortable and place the call light and personal items within reach.
31. Conduct a safety check before leaving the room. The room should be clean and free from clutter or spills.
32. Wash your hands or use hand sanitizer before leaving the room.

Reporting and Documentation

33. Report any specific observations, complications, or unusual responses to the licensed nursing staff. Document this information, along with the care provided, in the chart or EMR.

Procedure

Transferring a Resident from a Bed to a Stretcher

Rationale

Transferring a resident in one smooth or pivoting motion promotes safety.

Preparation

1. Ask the licensed nursing staff if there are doctor's orders for the procedure, if there are any specific instructions listed in the plan of care, and if the resident can be moved into the positions required for this procedure.
2. Practice safety by asking for assistance from a coworker.
3. Wash your hands or use hand sanitizer before entering the room.
4. Knock before entering the room.
5. Introduce yourself using your first or preferred name and title. Explain that you work with the licensed nursing staff and will be providing care.
6. Greet the resident and ask the resident to state his full name, if able. Then check the resident's identification bracelet.
7. Use Mr., Mrs., or Ms. and the resident's last name when conversing.
8. Explain the procedure in simple terms, even if the resident is not able to communicate or is disoriented. Ask permission to perform the procedure.
9. Bring the necessary equipment into the room. Place the following items in an easy-to-reach place:
   - stretcher
   - bath blanket
   - a pillow, if needed
   - a draw sheet, slide board, or other assistive device, if needed

The Procedure

10. Provide privacy by closing the curtains, using a screen, or closing the door to the room.
11. Lock the bed wheels and then raise the bed to hip level.
12. Maintain safety during the procedure. If there are side rails, raise and lock the rails on the opposite side of the bed from where you will be working. Lower the rail on the side where you are working.
13. Be sure any tubing, such as IVs or urinary drainage bags, are not moved or pulled out of place or kinked during or after positioning.
14. Position the stretcher alongside the resident's bed as close to the bed as possible. Lock the stretcher wheels or set the brake.
15. Lower the head of the bed to be as flat as possible. Raise the bed so it is even with the stretcher.

16. Stand at the side of the bed. The stretcher should be between your body and the resident's bed. Your coworker should stand at the other side of the resident's bed.

17. If there is a draw sheet on the bed, untuck it. If there is no draw sheet, place one on the bed, under the resident.

18. Ask the resident to move closer to the edge of the bed and closer to the stretcher, if able.

> **Best Practice:** Ask the resident to do as much of the transfer as possible while assisting with the draw sheet.

19. If the resident is too weak to assist with the transfer, instruct him to place his arms across his chest and tuck his chin to his chest to avoid hyperextending his neck.

> **Best Practice:** You can use a plastic or wooden slide board to assist in moving the resident. This device is placed between the bed and stretcher from the resident's back extending from the resident's shoulder to his hips.

20. On the count of three, move or slide the resident gently and smoothly from the bed to the stretcher with the draw sheet or slide board. You will usually transfer the lower body of the resident first and then move the upper body. Some residents will need to be transferred in one motion to prevent injury.

21. Recheck that any tubing is secure and in place. If you have any concerns, ask a licensed nursing staff member to check that the IV or other tubing is working properly. If the resident has a urinary drainage bag, be sure it is positioned below the bladder.

22. Cover the resident with a sheet or bath blanket to ready him for transport. Fasten safety straps, if available.

23. Raise the side rails of the stretcher and release the brake.

24. Position yourself at the head of the stretcher and push the stretcher so that the resident's feet face forward. Keep your body close to the stretcher as you transport the resident to the appropriate location in the healthcare facility.

Follow-Up

25. Make sure that the resident's body is in alignment and that the resident is safe and comfortable. Place the call light and personal items within reach.

26. Conduct a safety check before leaving the room. The room should be clean and free from clutter or spills.

27. Wash your hands or use hand sanitizer before leaving the room.

Reporting and Documentation

28. Report any specific observations, complications, or unusual responses to the licensed nursing staff. Document this information, along with the care provided, in the chart or EMR.

BECOMING A HOLISTIC NURSING ASSISTANT

Caring for Immobile Residents

Immobility can affect residents physically, emotionally, psychologically, and socially. Effects may include feelings of powerlessness, decreased ability to hear sounds and sense touch, and depression, which may result in limited social interaction. These effects are difficult to overcome alone, so holistic nursing assistants should pay special attention and use the following guidelines when caring for immobile residents:

- Always try to think ahead about the needs of immobile residents.
- Provide social stimulation by greeting, smiling, and talking with residents.
- During your shift, regularly check in to see how assigned residents are doing.
- Be sure the tone of your voice is friendly and at a moderate level.

- When appropriate, gently touch residents when speaking with them.
- Brighten the room with soft lighting and make sure the room is clean and organized. Remove any unneeded linen and supplies.
- Provide reading materials, music, and enjoyable television programs.
- When appropriate, transport residents to areas for socializing.
- Encourage family members and friends to visit often.

Apply It

1. Which of these guidelines would you be most comfortable following?
2. Which guidelines might be more difficult to follow? Explain your reasons and describe what you can do to overcome this difficulty.

How Can Comfort Be Promoted?

Positioning can promote resident relaxation, sleep, and overall comfort. As a holistic nursing assistant, you should use the resident's preferred position for rest, if possible. Follow doctors' orders for turning, if specified. Use comfortable bedding, and straighten and change soiled linens as necessary (**Figure 14.14**). Bedding should not be too tight, rub, or irritate the skin. Remove any items in the bed that may cause discomfort. Change the resident's positions for maximum comfort and support. Encourage residents who are mobile to change their positions often. Support residents with pillows, blankets, or rolls, as appropriate. Let the licensed nursing staff know if a resident complains of pain or discomfort from tubes and drains.

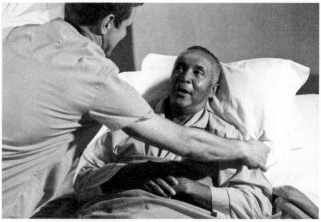

kali9/E+ via Getty Images

Figure 14.14 Straightening and changing linens can help promote comfort and maintain a resident's skin integrity.

SECTION 14.1 **Review and Assessment**

Key Terms Mini Glossary

ankylosis the stiffening or immobility of a joint.

body alignment the optimal (best) placement of all body parts such that bones are in their proper places and muscles are used efficiently.

contracture the tightening or shortening of a body part (such as a muscle, a tendon, or the skin) due to lack of movement.

foot drop a condition of paralysis or weakness in the front muscles of the foot and ankle; results in the dragging of the foot and toes.

orthostatic hypotension a condition in which a person feels dizzy when standing due to a fall in blood pressure.

syncope temporary unconsciousness; fainting.

trochanter rolls soft rolls that are placed along the body and that span from above the hip to above the knee; prevent external (outer) rotation of the hips; are usually premade or made from a towel or bath blanket and are usually 12–14 inches long.

Apply the Key Terms

Identify the key terms used in each sentence.

1. The nursing assistant uses correct body alignment to be sure the resident's body parts are in their proper places and his muscles are being used efficiently.
2. Mr. K's feet and toes are dragging due to foot drop.
3. When Mrs. L was positioned, the nursing assistant placed trochanter rolls along her body to prevent external rotation of her hips.
4. It is important to dangle a resident before asking them to stand to prevent orthostatic hypotension.
5. A new resident is being cared for by a nursing assistant. The resident has trouble ambulating because of ankylosis and a contracture.

Know and Understand the Facts

1. What are the benefits of good body alignment?
2. List three body positions that can be used to position residents.
3. Identify three resident-handling guidelines to follow when preparing to position a resident.

Analyze and Apply Concepts

1. Why is it important for residents to change positions? How often should positioning be done?
2. Explain how to turn a resident safely.
3. Describe what may happen if a resident stands too quickly. What can be done to prevent this reaction?
4. Describe the steps for using a lift.

Think Critically

Read the following care situation. Then answer the questions that follow.

Today, Lisa will be taking care of Mrs. G, who is 85 years old and does not speak English well. Lisa has been asked to transfer Mrs. G from her bed to a wheelchair. Mrs. G's two daughters are visiting and appear very protective of their mother. They are speaking Spanish to her when Lisa enters the room.

1. What can Lisa do to include Mrs. G's daughters in the transfer process?
2. What two actions should Lisa take to be sure the transfer is performed safely?

Ambulation and Assistive Ambulatory Devices

Objectives

To achieve the objectives for this section, you must successfully:

- **describe** the importance and stages of ambulation.
- **recognize** the limitations residents may have when ambulating.
- **explain** how to assist residents when they ambulate.
- **identify** the steps needed to assist residents with canes, walkers, and crutches.

Key Terms

Learn these key terms to better understand the information presented in the section.

assistive devices
axilla

Questions to Consider

- Have you ever had an injury that prevented you from walking for a period of time?
- When you were injured, was it difficult to do the things you like to do?
- Did you use crutches or a cane? Did it take time for you to become comfortable using your crutches or cane? How did people react to you? Were they respectful of your problem or were they unwilling to help? How did their treatment make you feel?

What Are the Stages of Ambulation?

Ambulation, or the ability to walk around, is important for achieving well-being. Ambulation improves circulation and muscle tone, preserves lung tissue and airway function, and helps promote muscle and joint mobility. As a nursing assistant, you will often assist a resident safely through three stages that lead to ambulation:

1. dangling
2. standing
3. ambulating

If you are helping someone ambulate, there are safety precautions you should take during ambulation. These include the following:

- Remove any small rugs or electrical cords on the floor, clean up any spills, and move anything that may cause a fall.
- Be sure there are nonslip bath mats in the bathroom. Grab bars, a raised toilet seat, and a shower tub seat are also helpful, if needed.

THINK ABOUT THIS

On average, children first walk independently when they are 11 months old. By adulthood, the average walking speed is about 3.1 miles per hour (mph), though the walking speed for older adults is slower. Walking speed varies depending on a person's height, weight, age, fitness level, effort, and culture. The ground surface and load a person is carrying also influence walking speed.

- Make sure personal items are easy to reach.
- Encourage the resident to use a fanny pack, apron, or other carrying case to help carry objects during ambulation.

How Should a Nursing Assistant Assist with Ambulation?

To prepare for any procedure in which you will assist a resident with ambulation, you should be familiar with the abbreviations and acronyms related to resident mobility (**Figure 14.15**). You should also be able to perform the following actions:

- Ask the resident if he or she is feeling any pain. If the resident is feeling pain, alert the licensed nursing staff about the resident's pain before beginning ambulation.
- Gather the appropriate supplies, equipment, and coworkers, if needed. Make sure you know how equipment works and understand the procedure for using it. If other healthcare staff are needed to conduct a procedure, make sure they know what to do.

Abbreviations and Acronyms Related to Resident Mobility

Abbreviation or Acronym	Meaning
amb	ambulation
BR	bed rest
BRP	bathroom privileges
HOB	head of bed
OOB	out of bed
up ad lib	up as desired
W/C	wheelchair

Goodheart-Willcox Publisher

Figure 14.15 Nursing assistants should be familiar with terminology related to mobility.

- Organize the physical environment and equipment for safe completion of the procedure. Lock the wheels of the bed or chair, put the bed or stretcher at the correct height, and make sure any electronic mobile equipment is charged. Identify and remove any tripping hazards such as electrical cords, throw rugs, and clutter.
- Tell the resident what actions you expect from him or her. Then show the resident what to do and help the resident during the procedure.
- When assisting residents, use good posture and proper body mechanics.
- If a resident begins to collapse during ambulation, do not try to carry, hold up, or catch her. Rather, assume a broad stance and place your preferred foot slightly ahead of the other and between the resident's legs. Move her close to you using the gait belt. You can guide her body by holding her at the waist or gently under the axilla (armpit), allowing her to slide down against your leg (**Figure 14.16**). Ease the resident slowly to the floor, using your body as an incline. If necessary, lower your body along with the resident's. Remember to always use proper body mechanics.
- If family members or friends would like to assist with ambulation, they may do so as long as a member of the licensed nursing staff has given permission and they understand and are comfortable with the procedure.

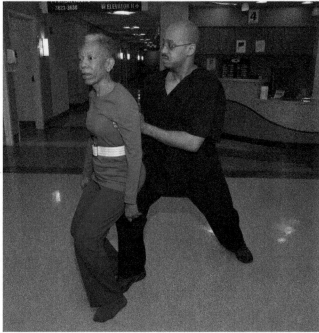

Wards Forest Media, LLC

Figure 14.16 If a resident begins to collapse, let the resident slide down against your leg and ease the resident to the floor. Call for help and report it to the licensed nursing staff.

When people do not feel well, they often want to stay in bed. Therefore, assisting with mobility is one of the most important responsibilities of holistic nursing assistants. The following procedure provides information about how to help residents move out of their beds and ambulate.

Procedure

Helping a Resident Ambulate

Rationale
Assisting a resident with ambulation can improve the resident's mental and physical health.

Preparation
1. Ask the licensed nursing staff if there are doctor's orders for the procedure, if there are any specific instructions listed in the plan of care, and if the resident can be moved into the positions required for this procedure.
2. Wash your hands or use hand sanitizer before entering the room.
3. Knock before entering the room.
4. Introduce yourself using your first or preferred name and title. Explain that you work with the licensed nursing staff and will be providing care.
5. Greet the resident and ask the resident to state her full name, if able. Then check the resident's identification bracelet.
6. Use Mr., Mrs., or Ms. and the resident's last name when conversing.
7. Explain the procedure in simple terms, even if the resident is not able to communicate or is disoriented. Ask permission to perform the procedure.

8. Bring the necessary equipment into the room. Place the following items in an easy-to-reach place:
   - a robe, if needed to ensure that the resident is not exposed, or properly fitting clothing
   - nonslip, properly fitting, low-heeled footwear
   - a gait belt (in good condition and functional)

The Procedure

9. Provide privacy by closing the curtains, using a screen, or closing the door to the room.
10. If the resident is in bed, lock the bed wheels and then lower the bed to its lowest position.
11. Maintain safety during the procedure. If the resident is in a bed with side rails, raise and lock the rails on the opposite side of the bed from where you will be working. Lower the rail on the side where you are working.
12. If the resident is in bed, assist her to a dangling position on the side of the bed. The resident may also be seated in a chair.
13. Help the resident put on nonslip, properly fitting shoes and a robe, if needed.
14. Apply the gait belt around the resident's waist over her clothing, if needed. The buckle of the gait belt should be in the front. Thread the belt through the teeth of the buckle and through the belt's two loops to lock it.
15. Check that the belt is snug, but that there is still enough room for you to place your fingers under the belt.
16. Face the resident and take hold of the gait belt using an underhand grasp above each hipbone for greater safety.
17. Signal the resident that it is time to stand. Using the gait belt, assist the resident to a standing position. Lift the resident using your arm and leg muscles. Bend your knees and keep your back straight. Do not twist your body.
18. Continue holding on to the gait belt while the resident gains her balance. Stand knee to knee or toe to toe with the resident to maintain stability of the resident's legs. Have the resident stand erect with her head up and back straight.
19. Walk behind and to one side of the resident during ambulation.
20. Hold on to the gait belt directly from behind. Watch for signs of possible resident collapse. *Do not attempt to catch a resident who begins to collapse during ambulation. Instead, slowly ease the resident to the floor using your body as an incline.*
21. Determine if the resident has a weak side. If the resident does, position yourself accordingly:
    - If the resident has a weak right side, stand behind and slightly to the right of her (**Figure 14.17A**).
    - If the resident has a weak left side, stand behind and slightly to the left of her (**Figure 14.17B**).

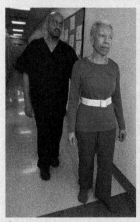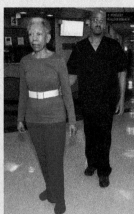

A   **B**   *Wards Forest Media, LLC*

Figure 14.17

22. Let the resident set the pace and keep a firm grasp on the gait belt, if used.
23. Encourage the resident to ambulate the ordered distance, but be observant. Watch for signs of resident fatigue. If collapse occurs, follow the steps discussed earlier.
24. When ambulation is complete, help the resident return to her room or bed. Remove the gait belt and the resident's robe and shoes.
25. If the resident returns to her bed, check to be sure the bed wheels are locked. Then reposition the resident and ensure the bed is in a low position.
26. Follow the plan of care to determine if the side rails should be raised or lowered.
27. Remove, clean, and store equipment in the proper location. Remove soiled linens and discard disposable equipment.

Follow-Up

28. Wash your hands to ensure infection control.
29. Make sure the resident is comfortable and place the call light and personal items within reach.
30. Conduct a safety check before leaving the room. The room should be clean and free from clutter or spills.
31. Wash your hands or use hand sanitizer before leaving the room.

Reporting and Documentation

32. Report any specific observations, complications, or unusual responses to the licensed nursing staff. Document this information, along with the care provided, in the chart or EMR.

How Are Assistive Devices Used During Ambulation?

Some residents require *assistive devices* for ambulation because they can bear only a limited amount of weight on their legs and feet. These assistive devices include canes, crutches, and walkers. The type of device used depends on how much support is needed.

Ambulating with a Cane

Canes are very useful for residents who have had surgery and are not yet able to maintain balance or who need extra stability. Older adults may use a cane if they have recovered from a stroke and are not yet able to fully ambulate. They may also use a cane if they have arthritis that results in restricted movement.

Several types of canes help residents ambulate (**Figure 14.18**). The type of cane chosen depends on the resident's preferred grip, balancing ability,

and need. To ambulate successfully with a cane, a resident must have a well-fitting cane and use it properly (**Figure 14.19**). When a resident stands up straight with the arms at the sides, the top of the cane should be in line with the resident's wrist. The resident should be able to slightly bend his or her elbow while using the cane. The resident should always hold the cane with his or her stronger hand (the hand *opposite* the side that needs more support).

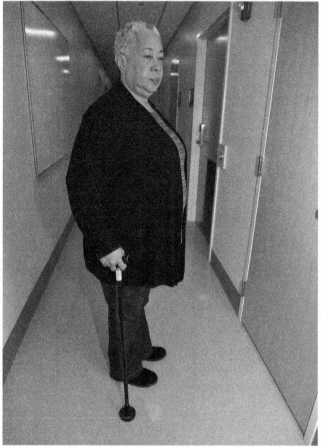

Wards Forest Media, LLC

Figure 14.19 Correct cane fit is important for resident safety. The resident should be able to bend his or her elbow slightly while using the cane.

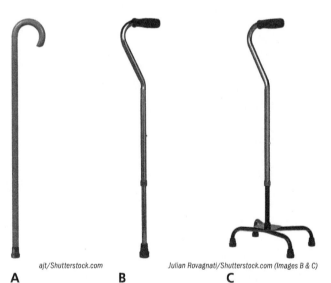

ajt/Shutterstock.com   *Julian Rovagnati/Shutterstock.com (Images B & C)*

A   B   C

Figure 14.18 The types of canes include C canes (A), functional grip canes (B), and quad canes (C).

Procedure

Providing Assistance with a Cane

Rationale

Assisting a resident who is ambulating with a cane reduces the chance of injury and promotes safe ambulation by helping the resident achieve balance and giving support.

Preparation

1. Ask the licensed nursing staff if there are doctor's orders for the procedure, if there are any specific instructions listed in the plan of care, and if the resident can be moved into the positions required for this procedure.

Procedure

2. Wash your hands or use hand sanitizer before entering the room.
3. Knock before entering the room.
4. Introduce yourself using your first or preferred name and title. Explain that you work with the licensed nursing staff and will be providing care.
5. Greet the resident and ask the resident to state her full name, if able. Then check the resident's identification bracelet.
6. Use Mr., Mrs., or Ms. and the resident's last name when conversing.
7. Explain the procedure in simple terms, even if the resident is not able to communicate or is disoriented. Ask permission to perform the procedure.
8. Bring the necessary equipment into the room. Place the following items in an easy-to-reach place:
   - a robe, if needed to ensure the resident is not exposed, or properly fitting clothing
   - nonslip, properly fitting, low-heeled footwear
   - a cane with one or four tips for added support (free from flaws, cracks, bends, or missing parts)
   - a gait belt (in good condition and functional)

The Procedure

9. Provide privacy by closing the curtains, using a screen, or closing the door to the room.
10. If the resident is in bed, lock the bed wheels and then lower the bed to its lowest position.
11. Maintain safety during the procedure. If the resident is in a bed with side rails, raise and lock the rails on the opposite side of the bed from where you will be working. Lower the rail on the side where you are working.
12. If the resident is in bed, assist her to a dangling position on the side of the bed. The resident may also be seated in a chair.
13. Help the resident put on nonslip, properly fitting shoes and a robe, if needed.
14. Apply the gait belt, if needed. Put the belt around the resident's waist over her clothing with the buckle in the front. Thread the belt through the teeth of the buckle and through the belt's two loops to lock it. Make the belt snug, but leave enough room to place your fingers under the belt.
15. The resident should hold the cane on her stronger side.
16. Face the resident and take hold of the gait belt using an underhand grasp for greater safety.

17. Using the gait belt, assist the resident to a standing position. Lift the resident using your arm and leg muscles. Bend your knees and keep your back straight. Do not twist your body.
18. Continue holding onto the gait belt while the resident gains her balance. Stand knee to knee or toe to toe with the resident to maintain stability of the resident's legs. Have the resident stand erect with her head up and back straight.
19. Position the cane and stabilize the resident with the cane before ambulation begins.
20. During ambulation, the resident should move the cane forward about 6–10 inches (**Figure 14.20**).

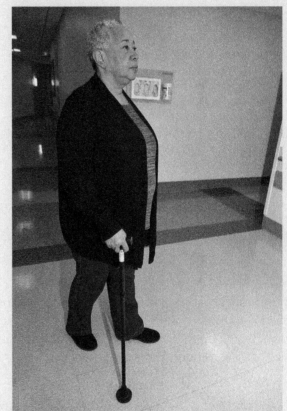

Figure 14.20   *Wards Forest Media, LLC*

21. After moving the cane forward, the resident should follow, first with the weak leg and then with the strong leg.
22. If using a gait belt, stand slightly behind and on the weaker side of the resident to provide additional support as needed.
23. Grasp the gait belt directly from behind using an underhand grip, if needed.
24. Encourage the resident to use handrails, if available.

(continued)

Providing Assistance with a Cane *(continued)*

25. Let the resident set the pace and keep a firm grasp on the gait belt, if used. Encourage her to ambulate the ordered distance, but be observant. Watch for signs of resident fatigue or possible collapse. *Do not attempt to catch a resident who begins to collapse during ambulation. Instead, slowly ease the resident to the floor, using your body as an incline.*
26. If it is allowed, and the resident is strong enough, assist her with climbing stairs with a cane. Before beginning, check to be sure that she can walk safely on flat surfaces.
27. Have the resident grasp the handrail (if possible) with the hand on her weak side. Ask her to hold the cane in her opposite, strong hand.
28. The resident should climb each stair using her strong leg first. Once the resident is balanced, she can move the cane up the stair, followed by her weak leg. She can repeat these steps to move up the stairs.
29. To come down stairs, the resident should place the cane on each stair first, followed by her weaker leg and then her stronger leg. Remind her to face forward and "go up with the good, down with the bad."
30. When the ambulation is complete, help the resident return to her room or bed. Remove the gait belt, if used, and her robe, cane, and shoes.
31. If the resident returns to her bed, check to be sure the bed wheels are locked. Then reposition the resident and ensure the bed is in the low position.
32. Follow the plan of care to determine if the side rails should be raised or lowered.
33. Remove, clean, and store equipment in the proper location. Remove soiled linens and discard disposable equipment.

Follow-Up

34. Wash your hands to ensure infection control.
35. Make sure the resident is comfortable and place the call light and personal items within reach.
36. Conduct a safety check before leaving the room. The room should be clean and free from clutter or spills.
37. Wash your hands or use hand sanitizer before leaving the room.

Reporting and Documentation

38. Report any specific observations, complications, or unusual responses to the licensed nursing staff. Document this information, along with the care provided, in the chart or EMR.

Ambulating with a Walker

Some residents need more support with ambulation than a cane can provide. Older adults may use walkers when they begin to lose their balance or stability and need extra assistance. For these residents, a *walker* is often a better option than a cane. A walker lets residents use their arms to take all or some of their weight off their lower body, but the resident must be able to pick up the walker. Different types of walkers can be used, depending on the resident's need (**Figure 14.21**).

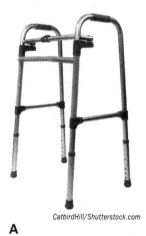
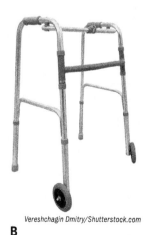
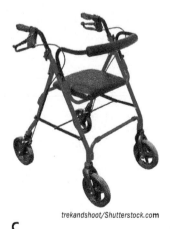

CatbirdHill/Shutterstock.com   Vereshchagin Dmitry/Shutterstock.com   trekandshoot/Shutterstock.com

A   **B**   **C**

Figure 14.21 The standard, pickup walker (A) must be picked up during ambulation. Rolling walkers may have two wheels (B) or four wheels (C).

A walker must fit the resident properly (**Figure 14.22**). The handles or top of the walker should be even with the resident's wrist when the resident is standing in an upright position with arms relaxed at the sides. When the resident holds onto the walker, his or her elbows should be bent in a comfortable and natural position. The resident should never stoop over while using the walker.

A resident should never try to climb stairs or use an escalator with a walker. Nursing assistants must closely monitor a resident ambulating with a walker. If the resident appears tired and weak, ambulation must stop to allow the resident time to rest.

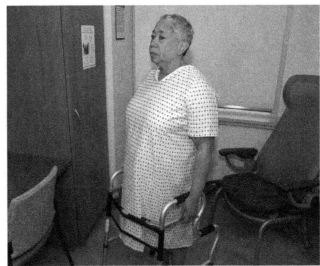

Wards Forest Media, LLC

Figure 14.22 The top of a correctly fitted walker should be even with the wrists.

Procedure

Providing Assistance with a Walker

Rationale
Assisting a resident to correctly use a walker reduces the chance of injury and promotes safe ambulation.

Preparation
1. Ask the licensed nursing staff if there are doctor's orders for the procedure, if there are any specific instructions listed in the plan of care, and if the resident can be moved into the positions required for this procedure.
2. Wash your hands or use hand sanitizer before entering the room.
3. Knock before entering the room.
4. Introduce yourself using your first or preferred name and title. Explain that you work with the licensed nursing staff and will be providing care.
5. Greet the resident and ask the resident to state her full name, if able. Then check the resident's identification bracelet.
6. Use Mr., Mrs., or Ms. and the resident's last name when conversing.
7. Explain the procedure in simple terms, even if the resident is not able to communicate or is disoriented. Ask permission to perform the procedure.

8. Bring the necessary equipment into the room. Place the following items in an easy-to-reach place:
   - a robe or properly fitting clothing
   - nonslip, properly fitting, low-heeled footwear
   - a standard or rolling walker
   - gait belt (in good condition and functional)

The Procedure
9. Provide privacy by closing the curtains, using a screen, or closing the door to the room.
10. If the resident is in bed, lock the bed wheels and then lower the bed to its lowest position.
11. Maintain safety during the procedure. If the resident is in a bed with side rails, raise and lock the rails on the opposite side of the bed from where you will be working. Lower the rail on the side where you are working.
12. If the resident is in bed, assist her to a dangling position on the side of the bed. The resident may also be seated in a chair.
13. Help the resident put on nonslip, properly fitting shoes and a robe, if needed.
14. Apply the gait belt, if needed. Put the belt around the resident's waist, over her clothing, with the buckle in the front. Thread the belt through the teeth of the buckle and through the belt's two loops to lock it. Make the belt snug, but leave enough room to place your fingers under the belt. Review the *Helping a Resident Ambulate* procedure for instruction on gait belt use.
15. Position the seated resident so she is centered in front of and inside the frame of the walker.

(continued)

Providing Assistance with a Walker *(continued)*

16. Place the walker about one step ahead of the seated resident and make sure the legs of the walker are level on the ground and stable.

17. Have the resident use both hands to grip the top of the walker for support. Then have the resident stand and walk into the walker. The resident should take the first step with her weaker leg. The heel of the foot should touch the ground first, and the foot should flatten.

18. The resident should take her next step with her strong leg. As the resident ambulates, position yourself behind and slightly to the side of her.

19. The resident should step with her weak leg and then with her strong leg again. This sequence should be repeated. Do not hurry the resident.

20. Make sure the resident does not step all the way to the front bar of the walker. Have her take small steps when she turns.

21. Let the resident set the pace and keep a firm grasp on the gait belt, if used.

22. Encourage the resident to ambulate the ordered distance, but be observant. Watch for signs of resident fatigue or possible collapse. *Do not attempt to catch a resident who begins to collapse during ambulation. Instead, slowly ease the resident to the floor, using your body as an incline.*

23. To assist the resident into a sitting position, first make sure the chair is stable (will not move). Have the resident stand with her back to the chair (**Figure 14.23A**). The resident should be close enough to sit down on the chair. Have the resident slide her weaker leg forward and shift her weight to the stronger leg. Have her switch hands from the walker to the arms of the chair and sit down slowly (**Figure 14.23B**).

24. To assist the resident in getting up from a chair, put the walker in front of the chair. Have the resident move forward in the chair, place her hands on the arms of the chair, and push up. She should then move her hands to the grips of the walker. The resident should stand for enough time to gain stability and balance before beginning to ambulate.

25. When ambulation is complete, help the resident return to her room or bed. Remove the gait belt, if used, and the resident's robe, walker, and shoes.

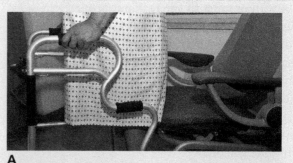

A

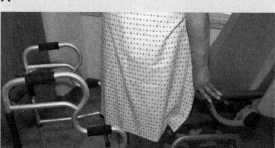

B

Figure 14.23

Wards Forest Media, LLC

26. If the resident returns to her bed, check to be sure the bed wheels are locked. Then reposition the resident and ensure the bed is in the low position.

27. Follow the plan of care to determine if the side rails should be raised or lowered.

28. Remove, clean, and store equipment in the proper location. Remove soiled linens and discard disposable equipment.

Follow-Up

29. Wash your hands to ensure infection control.

30. Make sure the resident is comfortable and place the call light and personal items within reach.

31. Conduct a safety check before leaving the room. The room should be clean and free from clutter or spills.

32. Wash your hands or use hand sanitizer before leaving the room.

Reporting and Documentation

33. Report any specific observations, complications, or unusual responses to the licensed nursing staff. Document this information, along with the care provided, in the chart or EMR.

Ambulating with Crutches

Crutches are often used by residents who have short-term conditions such as a sprained ankle or broken leg. Crutches can also assist residents with amputations or disabilities because they provide better support over time. Residents need upper body strength to use crutches. When using crutches, residents should support their weight on the handholds of the crutches, rather than placing their weight on the axillas.

Several different types of crutches may be used depending on the need (**Figure 14.24**). Before a resident can ambulate with crutches, the fit and size of the crutches must be checked. Also check for flaws (cracks in wooden crutches and bends in metal crutches) and tighten all the bolts on the crutches,

if appropriate. Some healthcare facilities do not allow nursing assistants to help a resident ambulate with crutches. Nursing assistants should always check facility policies and procedures and be trained before assisting residents ambulating with crutches.

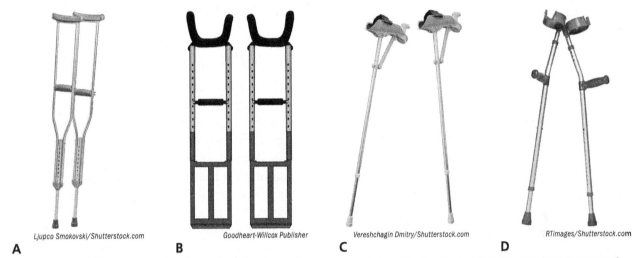

Ljupco Smokovski/Shutterstock.com   *Goodheart-Willcox Publisher*   *Vereshchagin Dmitry/Shutterstock.com*   *RTimages/Shutterstock.com*

A   **B**   **C**   **D**

Figure 14.24 The different types of crutches include standard underarm crutches (A), strutter crutches (B), platform crutches (C), and forearm crutches (D).

SECTION 14.2 **Review and Assessment**

Key Terms Mini Glossary

assistive devices used for support during ambulation because residents can bear only a limited amount of weight on their legs and feet; includes canes, crutches, and walkers.

axilla the armpit.

Apply the Key Terms
Write a sentence using each key term properly.
1. axilla
2. assistive devices

Know and Understand the Facts
1. Explain why it is important for residents to ambulate regularly.
2. What are the three stages of ambulation?
3. Identify three safety precautions to follow when helping residents ambulate with assistive devices.

Analyze and Apply Concepts
1. What should a nursing assistant do if a resident collapses during ambulation?
2. Describe the steps to follow when assisting a resident ambulating with a cane.

3. Explain the steps to follow when assisting a resident ambulating with a walker.

Think Critically
Read the following care situation. Then answer the questions that follow.

Mrs. B must now use a cane. Up until now she has been able to ambulate well but recently she has been having problems with her balance. Because of this, it is important that Mrs. B walk well with her cane. She dislikes using the cane fitted for her, but is willing to use the cane that belonged to her husband.

1. If Mrs. B uses her husband's cane, what guidelines could be used to make sure the cane fits Mrs. B properly?
2. How will you know if Mrs. B is able to ambulate safely with her cane?
3. What instructions can you provide about ambulating with a cane that will be important for Mrs. B to know?

Objectives

To achieve the objectives for this section, you must successfully:

- **define** rehabilitation and restorative care.
- **put** antiembolism stockings on a resident.
- **explain** range-of-motion exercises residents may need.
- **list** the types of assistive devices used for rehabilitation and restorative care.

Key Terms

Learn these key terms to better understand the information presented in the section.

atony	prosthetic
embolus	restorative care
orthotic	thrombus

Questions to Consider

- Have you ever had a goal that took a long time to achieve? What challenges or barriers made the goal difficult to achieve? Did any barriers keep you from accomplishing your goal? How did those barriers make you feel?
- What course of action did you take to achieve your long-term goal? If you did not achieve your goal, did you have to settle for something less? Was that good enough?

What Are Rehabilitation and Restorative Care?

Rehabilitation and restorative care work together to help residents regain lost abilities, maintain abilities, and prevent further loss of abilities. Rehabilitation services help residents maintain, regain, or improve skills that have been lost or impaired because of illness, trauma, or disability. These skills are usually functions of daily life, such as mobility, speech, or cardiac rehabilitation (in which an exercise program helps strengthen the cardiovascular system). Rehabilitation may be necessary after a serious accident, brain or spine injury, bone fracture, surgery, or the diagnosis of a degenerative disorder.

Restorative care goes beyond rehabilitation and has two goals. The first is to preserve and support improvements accomplished by rehabilitation. The second is to offer adjustments and improvements that help residents to live as independently as possible. The purpose of restorative care is to increase residents' self-esteem and to help them achieve and maintain the highest possible physical, mental, and psychosocial function.

Older adults most often require both rehabilitation and restorative care. This care is usually given after an older adult has suffered a stroke. Older adults who have hip fractures or coronary artery disease or who have been immobile or bedridden will receive this care.

Rehabilitation and Restorative Care Providers

There are OBRA requirements for specific rehabilitation and restorative services in nursing facilities. A doctor must order rehabilitation and restorative care that may last only a few weeks or can occur over a long period of time due to the type or chronic nature of the disease or condition. These services may be provided by the facility, by external providers, or by both. Services may include a variety of therapies and activities such as physical therapy, occupational therapy, speech therapy, or activity or recreational therapy. These services are included in a resident's plan of care.

Residents and their families are important factors in the success of this care. A resident's positive attitude, coping skills, willingness to participate, and family support can make a difference. A resident's age and overall health status can also influence progression.

The healthcare providers involved in rehabilitation and restorative care are important to the care's success. The physical therapist can provide range-of-motion exercises, muscle strengthening, and general conditioning exercises. Some treatments that physical therapists use include heat and water therapy, electric nerve therapy, traction, and massage therapy. Occupational therapists provide support with ADLs, which include bathing, dressing, cooking, and eating. Occupational therapists also teach residents and their family members how to use assistive devices, such as special eating utensils, for maximum independence. Speech therapists help residents with communication. For example, after a stroke, residents may have difficulty speaking or swallowing. The activity director or recreational therapist provides programs and activities that promote socialization, encourage mobility, and help to improve self-esteem.

The Nursing Assistant's Role

Holistic nursing assistants play an important role in rehabilitation and restorative care. Whenever a resident is not with a physical therapist, occupational therapist, or speech therapist, the resident will usually require follow-up and practice with ADLs (for example, eating, hygiene, communicating, and ambulating) according to the plan of care.

Nursing assistants must remember to promote independence. Residents who feel more in control of their lives will have a sense of achievement and self-worth. View each situation from the residents' perspective. Focus on their abilities and encourage them to make their own decisions, when appropriate. Listen, and have them talk about their feelings. Offer encouragement, be respectful, celebrate successes, observe resident progress, and provide ongoing documentation.

What Are Some Ways to Increase Circulation and Exercise?

Regular exercise helps maintain joint mobility and helps prevent contractures, *atony* (lack of strength),

and atrophy of muscles. It also stimulates circulation to prevent the formation of a *thrombus* (immobile blood clot) or *embolus* (mobile blood clot). One way to improve circulation is using antiembolism stockings. Exercise also improves coordination, and builds and maintains muscle strength. Exercise can be accomplished through range-of-motion (ROM) exercises.

Antiembolism Stockings

Risks for deep vein thrombosis (DVT), or blood clots that may break loose and travel through the bloodstream to cause a pulmonary embolus (PE) or a stroke, are high when a resident is immobile. The use of compression devices, including sequential compression devices (SCD) and antiembolism stockings, helps reduce these risks. If an SCD is used, follow the facility procedure. After the device is put in place, remain in the room for one full cycle (60–90 seconds) to be sure the device is working properly. The plan of care will determine the wearing schedule for antiembolism stockings.

Procedure

Applying Antiembolism Stockings

Rationale
When a resident is not active, elastic stockings are applied to promote circulation in the legs and feet.

Preparation
1. Ask the licensed nursing staff if there are doctor's orders for the procedure, if there are any specific instructions listed in the plan of care, and if the resident can be moved into the positions required for this procedure.
2. Wash your hands or use hand sanitizer before entering the room.
3. Knock before entering the room.
4. Introduce yourself using your first or preferred name and title. Explain that you work with the licensed nursing staff and will be providing care.
5. Greet the resident and ask the resident to state his full name, if able. Then check the resident's identification bracelet.
6. Use Mr., Mrs., or Ms. and the resident's last name when conversing.

7. Explain the procedure in simple terms, even if the resident is not able to communicate or is disoriented. Ask permission to perform the procedure.
8. Bring the necessary equipment into the room. Place the following items in an easy-to-reach place:
   - antiembolism stockings of the proper size and length (**Figure 14.25**)
   - disposable gloves, if needed

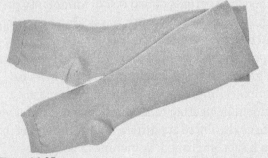

Figure 14.25   *Geo-grafika/Shutterstock.com*

The Procedure
9. Provide privacy by closing the curtains, using a screen, or closing the door to the room.
10. Lock the bed wheels and then raise the bed to hip level.

(continued)

Applying Antiembolism Stockings (continued)

11. Maintain safety during the procedure. If there are side rails, raise and lock the rails on the opposite side of the bed from where you will be working. Lower the rail on the side where you are working.
12. Wash your hands or use hand sanitizer to ensure infection control.

    Best Practice: Wear disposable gloves only if required for infection prevention and control.

13. Assist the resident into a supine position.
14. Expose one leg by fanfolding the linens toward the opposite leg. Make sure the leg is dry and free from lotion, ointments, or oils.
15. Take one stocking. Gather or turn the stocking inside out to the heel.
16. Slip the foot of the stocking over the resident's toes, foot, and heel (**Figure 14.26**).

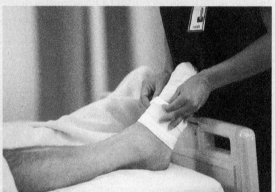

Figure 14.26   © Tori Soper Photography

17. Roll the stocking up the leg to the knee or thigh, depending on the length ordered. Be sure the stocking is properly placed. The toes may be covered or uncovered, depending on the stocking.
18. Repeat steps 14–17 to apply a stocking to the other leg.

    Best Practice: Check a resident's stockings often. Stockings should be smooth and wrinkle free and should not apply pressure to the toes. Also check circulation in the toes. Note sensation, if any swelling, and the temperature of the skin. Adjust the stockings as needed.

19. Check to be sure the bed wheels are locked, then reposition the resident and lower the bed.
20. Follow the plan of care to determine if the side rails should be raised or lowered.

Follow-Up

21. Wash your hands to ensure infection control.
22. Make sure the resident is comfortable and place the call light and personal items within reach.
23. Conduct a safety check before leaving the room. The room should be clean and free from clutter or spills.
24. Wash your hands or use hand sanitizer before leaving the room.

Reporting and Documentation

25. Report any specific observations, complications, or unusual responses to the licensed nursing staff. Document this information, along with the care provided, in the chart or EMR.

Range-of-Motion Exercises

When long periods of bed rest or immobility prevent regular exercise or activity, physical and emotional outcomes can include the loss of muscle mass or depression. *Range-of-motion (ROM) exercises* can help improve heart and lung function, increase flexibility, improve a resident's mood, and aid a resident in meeting rehabilitation and restorative care goals. There are different ways these exercises can be accomplished. Sometimes a continuous passive motion (CPM) machine is used to move a knee or a leg through a range of motion for a period of time while the resident relaxes. For the most part, however, the resident's doctor will determine which of the following three types of ROM exercises are appropriate. Nursing assistants will usually help residents perform these exercises:

- **Active range of motion (AROM):** uses the full range of motion of one or more body parts. The resident does not require physical help to perform exercises. Nursing assistants may need to remind or observe the resident to make sure exercises are done correctly.
- **Active-assistive range of motion (AAROM):** is used when a resident needs help achieving the full range of motion for one or more body parts. This may be because the muscles are too weak or stiff. Nursing assistants help with range of motion by encouraging normal muscle function.
- **Passive range of motion (PROM):** is used when a resident cannot move one or more body parts. Nursing assistants perform the full range of motion without any help from the resident. Passive exercises will not preserve muscle mass, but they will keep joints flexible.

Active-assistive and passive ROM exercises are performed slowly and gently to avoid hurting the resident or harming joints and bones. If a resident is in pain, the exercises must stop, and the licensed nursing staff should be notified. Sometimes weights are used with active and active-assistive range of motion. Some residents may need to wear a splint or brace to support their limbs during ROM exercises. Parallel bars and gait belts also help provide stability and balance and assist movement.

ROM exercises require residents to perform a variety of body movements. Some of these body movements are described in **Figure 14.27**.

Contraindications for ROM Exercises

It is important to remember that there may be *contraindications* for ROM exercises, or situations in which ROM exercises should not be used. ROM exercises may be contraindicated for residents with heart and respiratory diseases and conditions. This is because heart and respiratory problems may make the heart beat too fast and cause shortness of breath, chest pain, and fatigue. ROM exercises can also put stress on the soft tissues of joints and on bony structures. Therefore, ROM exercises should not be performed if joints are swollen or inflamed or if a muscle or bone near the joint has been injured.

General Guidelines for ROM Exercises

Before you conduct ROM exercises with a resident, you should familiarize yourself with the following general guidelines and with your facility's policies:

- **Follow a schedule:** ROM exercises should be performed at least twice a day. Immobile residents must have their joints exercised once every eight hours to prevent contractures. Performing ROM exercises as a resident bathes is beneficial because warm water relaxes the muscles and can reduce muscle spasms. Exercising before bedtime is another option.
- **Use the best approach:** Discussing the importance with residents may make them more willing to participate and have them help as much as possible. Remove pillows and supportive devices so there are no barriers to movement. Begin with exercises in the neck and work your way down the body. Exercise each joint through its range of motion a minimum of three to five times. Be respectful during ROM. If possible, the resident should be dressed in comfortable clothing, which allows free movement. If the resident is in a gown, be sure to keep body parts covered, when needed. For example, when exercising a leg, expose only one leg at a time, keeping the other leg covered

Body Movements

Movement	Description	Example
flexion	the act of bending a joint	bending the arm at the elbow
extension	the act of straightening a joint	lowering the arm back down at the elbow
hyperextension	an exaggerated, or extreme, extension	moving the arm from the side so that it extends behind the body
abduction	lateral (sideways) movement away from the midline (an invisible line running vertically through the body)	moving the leg away from the body
adduction	lateral movement toward the midline of the body	moving the leg toward the body
rotation	turning of a body part around an axis, or fixed point	rotating the ankle outward so that the foot moves away from the body
circumduction	rotating a body part in a complete circle	moving the pointer finger in a circular motion
supination	rotating a body part away from the body	rotating the forearm so that the palm faces upward
pronation	rotating a body part toward the body	rotating the forearm so that the palm faces downward

Goodheart-Willcox Publisher

Figure 14.27 Some body movements involved in ROM activities include flexion, extension, hyperextension, abduction, adduction, rotation, circumduction, supination, and pronation.

with a bath blanket. Do not exercise the resident to the point of fatigue. During PROM, make sure you support the extremity involved. Move each joint until you feel slight resistance, returning it to a neutral position when you are done.

- **Pay attention:** If performed incorrectly, ROM exercises can cause injury. Check with the licensed

nursing staff for specific instructions or limitations. For example, some facilities do *not* allow nursing assistants to exercise the neck. Remember to only exercise the joints that require exercise. Always stop and let the licensed nursing staff know if the resident complains of pain.

Procedure

Performing Range-of-Motion Exercises

Rationale

Range-of-motion (ROM) exercises are important for maintaining resident flexibility, preserving movement, and preventing skin inflammation or injury, such as a decubitus ulcer.

Preparation

1. Ask the licensed nursing staff if there are doctor's orders for the procedure, if there are any specific instructions listed in the plan of care, and if the resident can be moved into the positions required for this procedure.
2. Wash your hands or use hand sanitizer before entering the room.
3. Knock before entering the room.
4. Introduce yourself using your first or preferred name and title. Explain that you work with the licensed nursing staff and will be providing care.
5. Greet the resident and ask the resident to state her full name, if able. Then check the resident's identification bracelet.
6. Use Mr., Mrs., or Ms. and the resident's last name when conversing.
7. Explain the procedure in simple terms, even if the resident is not able to communicate or is disoriented. Ask permission to perform the procedure.
8. Bring the necessary equipment into the room. Place the following items in an easy-to-reach place:
   - towels or bath blankets

The Procedure

9. Provide privacy by closing the curtains, using a screen, or closing the door to the room.
10. Lock the bed wheels and then raise the bed to hip level.

11. Maintain resident safety during the procedure. If there are side rails, raise and lock the rails on the opposite side of the bed from where you will be working. Lower the rail on the side where you are working.

   | **Best Practice:** Wear disposable gloves only if required for infection prevention and control.

12. Exercising the neck
   - **Exercise the neck *only* if your facility allows it and if you have been instructed to do so.**
   - Support the resident's head and jaw with both hands (**Figure 14.28**). The head should be in a neutral position to start.

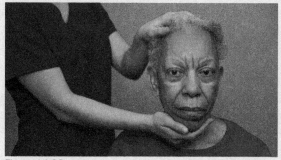

Figure 14.28   *Wards Forest Media, LLC*

   - Flexion—bring the head forward (**Figure 14.29**). Unless contraindicated, the chin should touch the chest.
   - Extension—bring the head back (**Figure 14.30**). Avoid hyperextending the neck, or extending the neck beyond its normal limits.

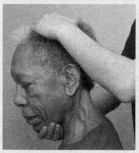
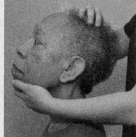

Wards Forest Media, LLC   *Wards Forest Media, LLC*
Figure 14.29   Figure 14.30

- Rotation—turn the head from side to side (**Figure 14.31**).

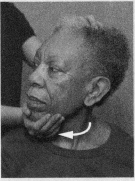 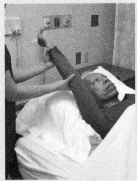

Figure 14.31 *Wards Forest Media, LLC*

- Lateral flexion—move the head to the right and to the left (**Figure 14.32**).

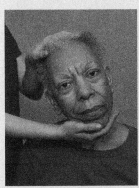 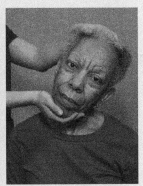

Figure 14.32 *Wards Forest Media, LLC*

13. Help the resident into the supine position (flat on the back) and provide a pillow for comfort, if appropriate.
14. Fanfold the top linens to the foot of the bed. Expose only the body part being exercised. Use a bath blanket or towel to cover an exposed body part for modesty or warmth.

> **Best Practice:** When exercising limbs, perform all of the steps listed here on one side of the body. Then move to the other side.

15. Exercising the shoulder
    - Grasp and support the resident's wrist with one hand. Grasp and support the resident's elbow with your other hand.
    - Flexion—raise the arm straight out in front of the resident and over the head (**Figure 14.33**).

- Extension—bring the arm down to the side (**Figure 14.34**).

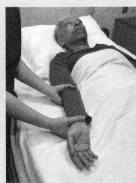 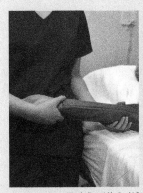

Wards Forest Media, LLC   *Wards Forest Media, LLC*
Figure 14.33   Figure 14.34

- Abduction—move the straight arm away from the side of the body (**Figure 14.35**).
- Adduction—move the straight arm to the side of the body (**Figure 14.36**).

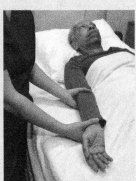

Wards Forest Media, LLC   *Wards Forest Media, LLC*
Figure 14.35   Figure 14.36

- Internal rotation—bend the elbow (**Figure 14.37**). Unless contraindicated, place the elbow at the same level as the shoulder. Move the forearm down toward the body.
- External rotation—move the forearm toward the head (**Figure 14.38**).

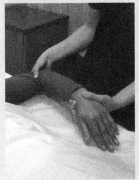 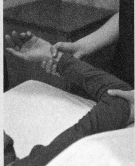

Wards Forest Media, LLC   *Wards Forest Media, LLC*
Figure 14.37   Figure 14.38

(continued)

Performing Range-of-Motion Exercises *(continued)*

16. Exercising the elbow
    - Grasp and support the resident's wrist with one hand. Grasp and support the resident's elbow with your other hand.
    - Flexion—bend the arm to touch the same-side shoulder, if possible (**Figure 14.39**).
    - Extension—straighten the arm (**Figure 14.40**).

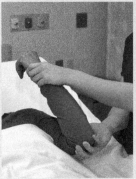

Wards Forest Media, LLC   *Wards Forest Media, LLC*

Figure 14.39   Figure 14.40

17. Exercising the forearm
    - Grasp and support the resident's wrist with one hand. Grasp and support the resident's elbow with your other hand.
    - Pronation—turn the hand so the palm is facing down.
    - Supination—turn the hand so the palm is facing up (**Figure 14.41**).

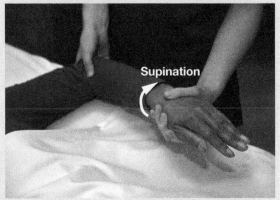

Supination

Figure 14.41   *Wards Forest Media, LLC*

18. Exercising the wrist (**Figure 14.42**)
    - Hold the resident's wrist with both of your hands.
    - Flexion—bend the hand down.
    - Extension—straighten the hand.
    - Radial flexion—with the hand straight up, turn the hand toward the thumb approximately 20°, as if the resident is waving.
    - Ulnar flexion—with the hand straight up, turn the hand toward the little finger approximately 30°.

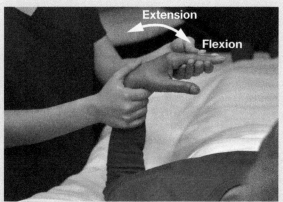

Extension

Flexion

Figure 14.42   *Wards Forest Media, LLC*

19. Exercising the thumb
    - Hold the resident's hand with one hand. Grasp the resident's thumb with your other hand.
    - Abduction—move the thumb out, away from the index finger (**Figure 14.43**).
    - Adduction—move the thumb in, toward the index finger (**Figure 14.44**).

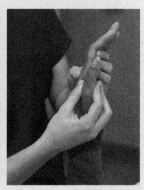

Wards Forest Media, LLC   *Wards Forest Media, LLC*

Figure 14.43   Figure 14.44

    - Opposition—touch each fingertip with the thumb (**Figure 14.45**).

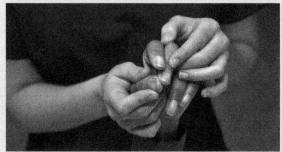

Figure 14.45   *Wards Forest Media, LLC*

    - Flexion—bend the thumb into the hand (**Figure 14.46**).
    - Extension—move the thumb out to the side of the fingers (**Figure 14.47**).

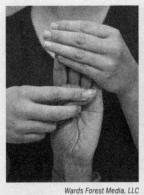
Wards Forest Media, LLC

Figure 14.46

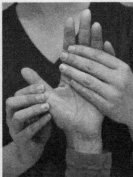
Wards Forest Media, LLC

Figure 14.47

20. Exercising the fingers
   - Abduction—spread the fingers and the thumb apart.
   - Adduction—bring the fingers and thumb together (**Figure 14.48**).

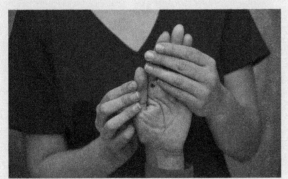

Figure 14.48   Wards Forest Media, LLC

   - Flexion—curl the fingers up to make a fist (**Figure 14.49**).
   - Extension—open the hand so the fingers, hand, and arm are straight (**Figure 14.50**).

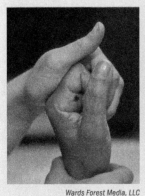
Wards Forest Media, LLC

Figure 14.49

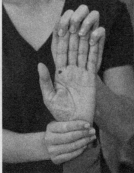
Wards Forest Media, LLC

Figure 14.50

21. Exercising the hip
   - Support the leg by placing one hand on top of the resident's thigh and your other hand under the resident's calf. If needed, cover the other leg with a bath blanket.

- Flexion—raise the leg and bend the knee (**Figure 14.51**).

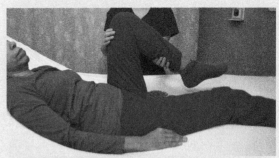

Figure 14.51   Wards Forest Media, LLC

- Extension—straighten the leg (**Figure 14.52**).

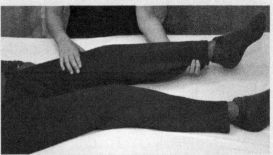

Figure 14.52   Wards Forest Media, LLC

- Abduction—move the leg away from the body (**Figure 14.53**).

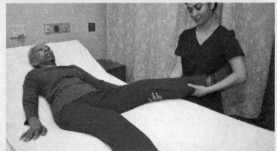

Figure 14.53   Wards Forest Media, LLC

- Adduction—move the leg toward the other leg (**Figure 14.54**).

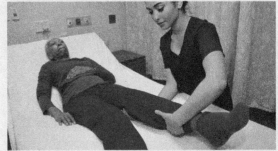

Figure 14.54   Wards Forest Media, LLC

(continued)

Performing Range-of-Motion Exercises *(continued)*

- Internal rotation—turn the leg inward (**Figure 14.55**).

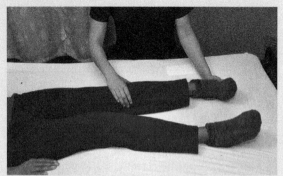

Figure 14.55
Wards Forest Media, LLC

- External rotation—turn the leg outward (**Figure 14.56**).

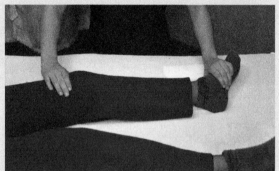

Figure 14.56
Wards Forest Media, LLC

22. Exercising the knee
    - Support the knee by placing one hand under the resident's knee and your other hand under the resident's ankle.
    - Flexion—bend the knee (**Figure 14.57**).

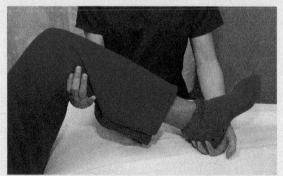

Figure 14.57
Wards Forest Media, LLC

- Extension—straighten the knee (**Figure 14.58**).

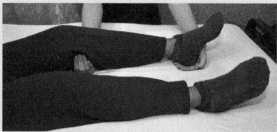

Figure 14.58
Wards Forest Media, LLC

23. Exercising the ankle
    - Support the foot and ankle by placing one hand under the resident's foot and your other hand under the resident's ankle.
    - Dorsal flexion—pull the foot forward and push down on the heel at the same time (**Figure 14.59**).
    - Plantar flexion—turn the foot down or point the toes (**Figure 14.60**).

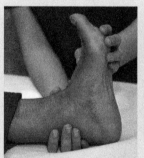
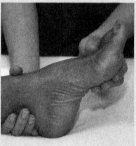

Wards Forest Media, LLC   *Wards Forest Media, LLC*

Figure 14.59   Figure 14.60

24. Exercising the foot
    - Support the foot and ankle by placing one hand under the resident's foot and your other hand under the resident's ankle.
    - Pronation—turn the outside of the foot up and the inside down (**Figure 14.61**).
    - Supination—turn the inside of the foot up and the outside down (**Figure 14.62**).

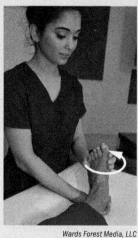
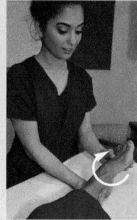

Wards Forest Media, LLC   *Wards Forest Media, LLC*

Figure 14.61   Figure 14.62

25. Exercising the toes
    - Flexion—curl the toes (**Figure 14.63**).
    - Extension—straighten the toes (**Figure 14.64**).

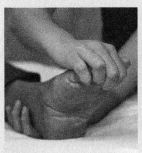 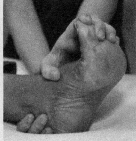

Wards Forest Media, LLC   *Wards Forest Media, LLC*
Figure 14.63   Figure 14.64

- Abduction—spread the toes apart (**Figure 14.65**).

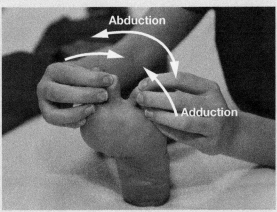

Figure 14.65   *Wards Forest Media, LLC*

- Adduction—pull the toes together.

26. Cover the exposed part of the resident's body and raise the side rail, if used.
27. Go to the other side of the bed and lower the side rail, if it is up.
28. Repeat exercises for the shoulder, elbow, forearm, wrist, fingers, hip, knee, ankle, foot, and toes on the other side of the body. Start with the shoulder and work your way down the body.
29. Check to be sure the bed wheels are locked, then reposition the resident and lower the bed.
30. Follow the plan of care to determine if the side rails should be raised or lowered.
31. Remove, clean, and store equipment in the proper location. Remove soiled linens and discard disposable equipment.

Follow-Up

32. Wash your hands to ensure infection control.
33. Make sure the resident is comfortable and place the call light and personal items within reach.
34. Conduct a safety check before leaving the room. The room should be clean and free from clutter or spills.
35. Wash your hands or use hand sanitizer before leaving the room.

Reporting and Documentation

36. Report any specific observations, complications, or unusual responses to the licensed nursing staff. Document this information, along with the care provided, in the chart or EMR.

What Assistive Devices Help Achieve Independent Living?

Many assistive devices can help residents function safely and independently in healthcare facilities. Some devices assist with ambulation, others help with ADLs, and still others make life easier and more enjoyable. Some examples of assistive devices include:

- walkers and canes
- shower chairs
- grab bars on the side and back of the bathtub or toilet
- graspers or reachers to lift items up from the floor
- special eating utensils with built-up handles to help people feed themselves
- cups with lids and specialized plates with deep centers
- special combs and brushes
- shoehorns to help people put on their shoes
- raised sitting chairs, raised toilet seats (**Figure 14.66**), and chair leg extenders
- large-print books and audio books
- large clocks, large telephone dials, and flashing lights to signal a telephone ring

Two other specialized types of assistive devices are prosthetic devices and orthotic devices.

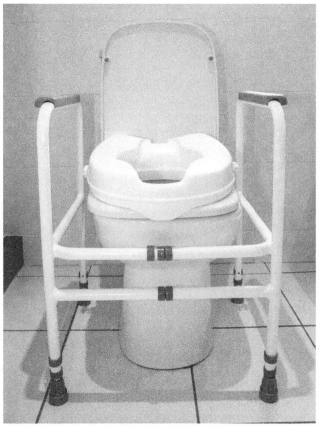

Figure 14.66 Raised toilet seats can help prevent falls in the bathroom.

Prosthetic Devices

A *prosthetic* is an artificial device designed to replace a missing body part. Arm and leg prosthetics are attached to the remaining limb and come in a wide variety, permitting different levels of activity. Arm prosthetics include hand and elbow prosthetics. An artificial hand helps a person grip objects or may lengthen a missing finger. Elbow prosthetics can provide a movable elbow joint. Lower-limb prosthetics include above-the-knee and below-the-knee devices (**Figure 14.67**). Prosthetics may use fluid hydraulics or microprocessors to create natural movement or may be made from rubber and wood.

Other prosthetics include *dentures*, which may replace all or some of a person's teeth and gums. Artificial eyes typically consist of glass or plastic prostheses made to look like eyes and are placed in the eye sockets. A person with a prosthetic of any kind often undergoes physical therapy to learn how to use the new device.

Orthotic Devices

An *orthotic* is a device that supports, aligns, or corrects a weak, immobile, injured, or deformed body part. Orthotics can improve joint movement or support the spine and other extremities. These devices come into direct contact with the body. Commonly used orthotics include casts, shoe inserts, and splints. Most orthotics can be purchased from a pharmacy and then fitted to the resident, but some are custom made. Uncomfortable orthotics can cause additional problems, so proper fit is very important.

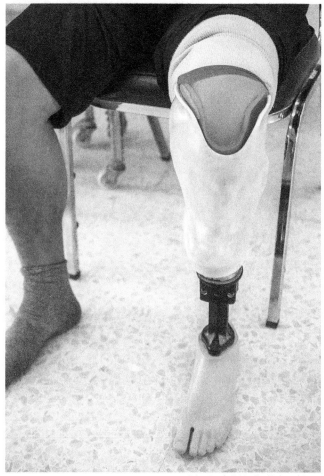

Figure 14.67 Prosthetic devices can promote function even after a limb or other body part is removed.

Digital ROM Exercise

For the past few months, healthcare staff at a local nursing home have encouraged immobile residents to play games and puzzles on tablets. This exercise has improved resident involvement, mobility, and dexterity (flexibility). Tablets' touch screens, puzzles, and games have helped reeducate residents who have suffered a stroke or have dementia. This way, older adults who are not mobile enough to play active video games can still be involved and learn using tablets. The swipe, tap, and slide functionality of the tablet allows these residents to play a game of checkers, even if they cannot pick up a checker piece.

Apply It

1. If you were a nursing assistant at this facility, how might you help residents use a tablet, even if they are not familiar with this technology?
2. What strategies could you use to include the use of tablets with physical exercises?

SECTION 14.3 Review and Assessment

Key Terms Mini Glossary

atony a lack of sufficient muscular strength.

embolus a mass (most commonly a blood clot) that travels through the blood and can become trapped in a blood vessel and obstruct blood flow.

orthotic a device that supports, aligns, or corrects a weakened, immobile, injured, or deformed part of the body.

prosthetic an artificial device designed to replace a missing body part.

restorative care care that assists with any adjustments and improvements that help residents live as independently as possible.

thrombus a blood clot that forms within a blood vessel and does not travel through the blood.

Apply the Key Terms

An incorrect key term is used in each of the following statements. Identify the incorrect key term and then replace it with the correct term.

1. Rehabilitation is care that assists with any adjustments and improvements that help residents live as independently as possible.
2. Mr. H has a prosthetic that helps support and align his weakened knee.
3. A thrombus is a blood clot that travels through a blood vessel and can obstruct the flow of blood.
4. Because of diabetes, Mrs. N requires an orthotic to replace the leg that was amputated.
5. The type of blood clot that does not travel through the blood is called an embolus.

Know and Understand the Facts

1. Describe the difference between rehabilitation and restorative care.
2. Identify two members of the healthcare team who provide rehabilitation or restorative care.
3. What are the three types of range-of-motion exercises?
4. Name six assistive, prosthetic, or orthotic devices.

Analyze and Apply Concepts

1. Why are range-of-motion exercises important for rehabilitation and restorative care?
2. Explain the steps needed to perform range-of-motion exercises on a resident's shoulder.

Think Critically

Read the following care situation. Then answer the questions that follow.

Han, a nursing assistant, has been asked to do ROM exercises with Mrs. F, a resident recovering from a broken hip. She complains of pain and is afraid to do ROM exercises on her own. Her doctor believes that exercising her hip will help her become more independent.

1. What should Han do when he meets Mrs. F for the first time?
2. Describe the ROM for exercising the hip.
3. How should Han respond to Mrs. F's complaints of pain when doing range-of-motion exercises?

Key Points

Reviewing the key points for this chapter will help you practice more safely and competently as a holistic nursing assistant and will help you prepare for the certification competency examination.

- Changing residents' positions on a regular basis helps restore body function, prevents deformities, relieves pressure, maintains skin integrity, and helps achieve comfort.
- Ambulation improves circulation and muscle tone, preserves lung tissue and airway function, and safeguards muscle and joint mobility.
- Moving and exercising the joints using range-of-motion (ROM) exercises can increase heart and lung function and improve muscle strength.
- Rehabilitation and restorative care work together to help residents regain lost abilities, maintain abilities, and prevent further loss of abilities.

Action Steps to Holistic Care

Review the information in this chapter. Complete the following activities.

1. Prepare a short paper or digital presentation that describes why body alignment is important and how it is maintained when residents are positioned, turned, dangled, and transferred. Discuss what actions ensure a safe environment for the resident.

2. With a partner, prepare a poster about assisting residents with canes, walkers, and crutches. Include the key steps and the actions that need to be taken to ensure safety.

3. Find two pictures in a magazine, in a newspaper, or online that best represent ways residents can become as independent as possible. Explain why you selected these images.

4. Research current scientific information about different types of prosthetic and orthotic devices. Write a brief report describing three current facts about prosthetics and orthotics that were not discussed in this chapter.

Building Math Skill

Lonnie is caring for Ms. E. The doctor ordered that she be repositioned every two hours. She was last repositioned at 5 a.m. Lonnie is working on the 7 a.m.-to-7 p.m. shift. How many times will Lonnie need to reposition Ms. E during his shift?

Preparing for the Certification Competency Examination

To prepare for the nursing assistant certification competency examination, you will need to know content found in this chapter. This content may be tested in the knowledge (written or oral) and skills (hands-on demonstration) portions of the exam. The following areas will be emphasized:

- body positions
- procedures for positioning, turning, lifting, and transferring
- supportive equipment and assistive devices
- effects of limited mobility
- safe ambulation
- ambulation with canes, walkers, and crutches
- rehabilitation and restorative care
- passive and active range of motion

These sample test questions are similar to ones you will find on the certification competency exam. See how well you can answer them. Be sure to select the *best* answer.

1. A nursing assistant can help a resident perform active ROM exercises by
   A. helping the resident learn how to perform the exercises
   B. watching the resident perform the exercises
   C. taking the resident outdoors for stimulation and fresh air
   D. moving the resident to the dining room in a wheelchair

2. Which device is used to maintain proper foot alignment and prevent foot drop?
   A. headboard
   B. backboard
   C. bed board
   D. footboard

3. Nursing assistants should lift and move residents on the count of
   A. five
   B. two
   C. three
   D. four

4. The compression device that helps circulation and reduces the risk of DVT is
   A. a gait belt
   B. an orthotic
   C. antiembolism stockings
   D. graspers and reachers

5. Which of the following statements is true about range-of-motion (ROM) exercises?
   A. They are performed just once a day.
   B. They are best performed starting from the bottom of the body.
   C. They are often performed during ADLs, such as bathing or dressing.
   D. They require at least 10 repetitions of each exercise.

6. During ambulation, a gait or transfer belt is often
   A. worn around the nursing assistant's waist for back support
   B. used to keep the resident positioned properly
   C. removed before walking
   D. worn around the resident's waist and used to hold onto the resident

7. Mrs. S is a resident who can move on her own with some assistance. What should a nursing assistant do to help her reposition in bed?
   A. assist Mrs. S in bending her knees and pushing up with her feet
   B. keep your knees straight while lifting her up under her arms
   C. use a gait or transfer belt to assist with repositioning
   D. pull the resident up holding one side of the draw sheet at a time

8. Which type of services helps residents maintain, restore, or improve skills and functioning for daily living?
   A. restorative care
   B. rehabilitation
   C. range of motion
   D. prosthetic devices

9. Mrs. A is a new cane user. A nursing assistant is helping her ambulate for the first time. What is an important guideline to maintain safety?
   A. When Mrs. A stands straight, her arms should be rigid at her sides.
   B. Mrs. A's elbow should be fully bent when she is using the cane.
   C. The cane should always be held in Mrs. A's stronger hand.
   D. The cane should always be held in Mrs. A's weaker hand.

10. Mr. D uses a walker. To use the walker correctly he should
    A. take his first step with his weaker leg
    B. take his first step with his stronger leg
    C. take his first step with his toe touching the ground first
    D. take his first step with the heel of his foot touching the ground last

11. Mr. O is experiencing shortening and tightening of his wrist due to lack of movement. What is this condition?
    A. atrophy
    B. atony
    C. ankylosis
    D. contracture

12. If a resident is seated in his bed with the head of the bed raised 45°, this position is called
    A. supine position
    B. Fowler's position
    C. Sims' position
    D. lateral position

13. When a limb or joint is moved beyond its normal range of motion, this is called
    A. flexion
    B. distal
    C. proximal
    D. hyperextension

14. A nursing assistant is caring for Ms. T, who is bedridden. How often should Ms. T be repositioned?
    A. every hour
    B. every 15 minutes
    C. every two hours
    D. every three hours

15. Which of the following is an artificial device designed to replace a missing body part?
    A. prosthetic
    B. orthotic
    C. atonic
    D. dystonic

Did you have difficulty with any of the questions? If you did, review the chapter to find the correct answer(s).

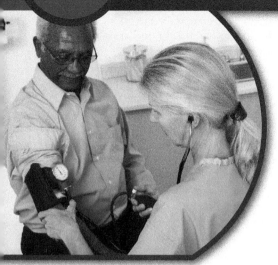

gchutka/Signature collection via Getty Images

Chapter Outline

Section 15.1
Measuring and Recording
Vital Signs

Section 15.2
Measuring and Recording
Height and Weight

Welcome to the Chapter

This chapter provides the knowledge and skills needed to measure the vital signs of temperature, pulse, respirations, and blood pressure. It also contains information about using a pulse oximeter to measure how well oxygen is being carried to body tissues, and about measuring height and weight. You will learn to effectively use these skills when providing care and will understand why accuracy in taking, measuring, and documenting this information is so important.

The information and procedures presented in this chapter will help you build the knowledge and skills needed to become a holistic nursing assistant. Check with your instructor to ensure these procedures are within your state's regulations for nursing assistant practice. The topics discussed in the chapter are highlighted on the Providing Holistic Care Framework.

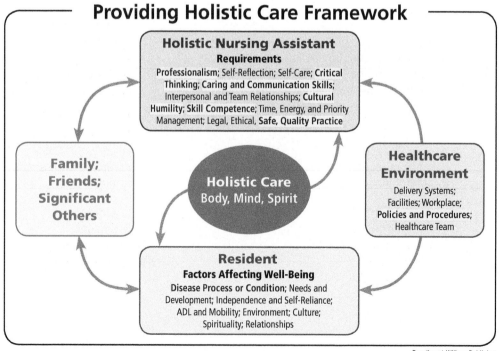

Goodheart-Willcox Publisher

Measuring and Recording Vital Signs

Objectives

To achieve the objectives for this section, you must successfully:

- **discuss** the purpose and importance of taking vital signs.
- **identify** the normal and abnormal ranges of vital signs.
- **describe** the locations and methods used to take vital signs.
- **list** the equipment needed to take vital signs.
- **describe** the importance of using a pulse oximeter.
- **explain** how to measure and document vital signs accurately and effectively.

Key Terms

Learn these key terms to better understand the information presented in the section.

apical pulse	hypotension
apnea	hypoventilation
aural	hypoxia
axillary temperature	probe
bradycardia	radial pulse
bradypnea	stertorous breathing
carotid pulse	stethoscope
Celsius (C)	systolic blood pressure
diastolic blood pressure	tachycardia
dyspnea	tachypnea
Fahrenheit (F)	temporal arteries
hyperventilation	tympanic temperature

Questions to Consider

- When was the last time someone measured your body's vital signs of temperature, pulse, respirations, and blood pressure?
- Did you know why your vital signs were being taken and why they were important? For example, were you sick? Were your vital signs measured for a physical exam?
- What was it like to have your vital signs measured?

Why Are Vital Signs Important?

Taking the vital signs of body temperature, pulse, respirations, and blood pressure are important skills for a holistic nursing assistant to learn. Vital signs can help doctors diagnose specific diseases, determine treatments and medications, and evaluate the effectiveness of treatments and medications. For example, a high body temperature can be a signal that a resident has an infection. If temperature starts to lower once treatment begins, this typically means the body is fighting the infection and the resident is getting better.

Vital signs are usually taken in a doctor's office during an exam, during admission to a healthcare facility, or once a day in long-term care facilities (more frequently when necessary). For each vital sign, well-established guidelines help nursing assistants determine whether the measurements are in a normal range.

Facility guidelines impact how vital signs are documented. Some facilities use paper forms for all residents on a shift and then transfer the measurements to each resident's chart or EMR. Other facilities use a specific form for each resident or enter vital signs into a resident's electronic record immediately.

How Is Temperature Measured and Recorded?

When you take a resident's temperature, you are measuring body heat, including how much body heat is produced and lost. Temperature is recorded in degrees (°) and is measured using either the Fahrenheit or the Celsius scale. The *Fahrenheit (F)* scale is used mostly in the United States, while the *Celsius (C)*, or *centigrade*, scale is used in other parts of the world (**Figure 15.1**).

Locations for Taking Temperature

Temperature can be taken using several different body locations using a thermometer:

- **Oral temperature:** taken under the tongue, or *sublingually.* This is the most common method of taking a temperature. Ask the resident to close his or her mouth completely while breathing through the nose. Wait at least 15 minutes after a resident has eaten, had something to drink, or smoked before using an oral thermometer. Oral temperature is not appropriate for residents who are receiving oxygen, who are coughing or sneezing, who are agitated or comatose, who have had mouth surgery, who may bite the thermometer, or who cannot follow instructions due to cognitive impairment.

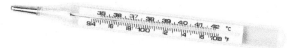

catshila/Shutterstock.com

Figure 15.1 In the Fahrenheit (°F) scale, water freezes at 32° and boils at 212°. In the Celsius (°C) scale, water freezes at 0° and boils at 100°.

- **Rectal temperature:** taken by inserting a lubricated thermometer one inch or less into the anus for 3 to 5 minutes. Rectal temperatures should not be taken if a resident has diarrhea, hemorrhoids, rectal bleeding, or has had rectal surgery. Rectal temperatures are also not advised for residents with certain heart conditions, because taking a rectal temperature can stimulate the vagus nerve and cause a temporary decrease in heart rate and blood pressure.
- *Axillary temperature:* taken by placing a thermometer into the axilla. Wait 15 minutes after the resident has washed or applied deodorant to the underarm to take an axillary temperature. Do not use this location if the resident has had breast or chest surgery.
- *Tympanic temperature:* taken in the ear, the thermometer must be placed properly in the ear for an accurate reading. If the resident has been sleeping or resting on one ear, use the opposite ear to get an accurate reading. Do not use a tympanic thermometer if there is drainage from the ear.
- **Temporal temperature:** taken on the forehead, where the temperature of the *temporal arteries* on each side of the head can be measured. Use only the area of the forehead that is bare—if a hat, wig, or bandage covers the forehead, it can affect the temperature.

Rectal and temporal artery temperatures provide more accurate measurements than temperatures at other sites.

A resident's body temperature can change slightly (by 1°F) during a day due to the dilation (expansion) of blood vessels. How much a resident eats or drinks, the external temperature, and age can also affect temperature. An older person may not adjust as quickly to changes in temperature and may often express feelings of being cold.

Pyrexia (fever) is caused by the body heating up to protect itself. Pyrexia can be a sign of an infection, some other disease process, an injury, or a possible reaction to a medication. *Hypothermia*, although uncommon, is a body temperature below 95°F (35°C). Average temperature ranges also vary based on the type of thermometer used (**Figure 15.2**).

Nondigital Thermometers

Nondigital thermometers can be used to take oral, rectal, or axillary temperatures. **Figure 15.1** earlier in this section shows a nondigital thermometer. These thermometers are tubes filled with a liquid (colored alcohol) that expands and moves up or down in response to heat. The bulb at the end of the thermometer is inserted into the body. The bulb of a rectal thermometer is thicker and wider than the bulb of an oral thermometer. Some thermometers are marked with a colored dot—blue for oral or axillary, and red for rectal.

Average Ranges of Body Temperature

Thermometer	Twelve Years and Older
Oral	97.6°F–99.6°F (36.4°C–37.5°C)
Rectal	98.6°F–100.6°F (37.0°C–38.1°C)
Tympanic	98.6°F–100.4°F (37.0°C–38.0°C)
Axillary	96.6°F–98.6°F (35.9°C–37.0°C)
Temporal Artery	97.2°F–100.1°F (36.2°C–37.8°C)

Goodheart-Willcox Publisher

Figure 15.2 Average temperatures for people twelve years and older vary based on the type of thermometer used.

It is important to correctly place each nondigital thermometer for the appropriate amount of time. Oral thermometers should be held in place for 3 minutes. Rectal thermometers should be placed in the anus for 3 to 5 minutes. Axillary thermometers take 5 minutes or longer to measure temperature.

Do not shake a thermometer when removing it. To read a nondigital thermometer, look at the thermometer's scale. Be sure the scale is visible so you can determine the level of liquid on the scale. The liquid level shows the resident's temperature.

Digital Thermometers

Digital thermometers are used to take oral, rectal, axillary, or tympanic temperatures and can take temperature in a few seconds. They are handheld, have a digital display, and are connected to an electronic unit (**Figure 15.3**).

Instead of a bulb, digital thermometers have a *probe*, which measures temperature. The probe of a thermometer is the tip. Probes are often marked by color—blue for oral or axillary, and red for rectal. The tip of a tympanic thermometer is short and is shaped to fit comfortably inside the external ear canal. A new cover should be placed on the probes or tip of a digital thermometer and should be discarded after each use (**Figure 15.4**). Once the probe or tip of the digital thermometer is inserted, the digital display should show the temperature reading within 20–60 seconds.

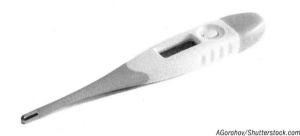

AGorohov/Shutterstock.com

Figure 15.3 A digital thermometer shows temperature on a digital display.

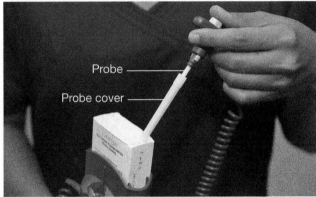

Probe

Probe cover

Wards Forest Media, LLC

Figure 15.4 A probe cover protects the probe of the thermometer. A new probe cover should be used for each reading.

Whether you use a nondigital or digital thermometer will depend on what is available in the healthcare facility where you work. As a nursing assistant, you will follow a specific procedure for taking, measuring, and documenting a temperature. Always identify the type of thermometer used when documenting, and report any irregularities to the licensed nursing staff.

Procedure

Using a Digital Oral Thermometer

Rationale

Body temperature that is outside the normal range can be a sign of a disease or condition or the result of an injury. The decision to use an oral thermometer is based on the need for accuracy and the age and condition of the resident. An oral thermometer is accurate for adults, as long as the adult keeps his or her mouth closed during the reading. Always follow the thermometer manufacturer's instructions and facility policy.

Preparation

1. Ask the licensed nursing staff if there are doctor's orders for the procedure, if there are any specific instructions listed in the plan of care, and if the resident can be moved into the positions required for this procedure.
2. Wash your hands or use hand sanitizer before entering the room.
3. Knock before entering the room.
4. Introduce yourself using your first or preferred name and title. Explain that you work with the licensed nursing staff and will be providing care.
5. Greet the resident and ask the resident to state his full name, if able. Then check the resident's identification bracelet.

(continued)

Using a Digital Oral Thermometer *(continued)*

6. Use Mr., Mrs., or Ms. and the resident's last name when conversing.
7. Explain the procedure in simple terms, even if the resident is not able to communicate or is disoriented. Ask permission to perform the procedure.
8. Bring the necessary equipment into the room. Place the following items in an easy-to-reach place:
   - a digital thermometer
   - the appropriate probe attachment (the *blue* probe for an oral temperature)
   - disposable probe covers
   - disposable gloves, if appropriate
   - pen and pad, form, or digital device for documenting the temperature
9. Be sure the resident has not eaten, had something to drink, smoked, or chewed gum for at least 15 minutes prior to taking the oral temperature.

The Procedure

10. Provide privacy by closing the curtains, using a screen, or closing the door to the room.
11. If the resident is in bed, lock the bed wheels and then raise the bed to hip level.
12. Maintain safety during the procedure. If the resident is in a bed with side rails, raise and lock the rails on the opposite side of the bed from where you will be working. Lower the rail on the side where you are working.
13. Position the resident comfortably.

> **Best Practice:** Let the resident know how long the thermometer will be in place. Ask the resident not to talk while the reading is being taken.

14. Place a disposable probe cover over the *blue* probe. Start the thermometer and wait until it shows it is ready.

> **Best Practice:** Wear disposable gloves only if required for infection prevention and control.

15. Have the resident open his mouth and lift his tongue. Slowly insert the covered probe into the mouth until the tip of the probe touches the base of the mouth under the tongue and to one side (**Figure 15.5**). Have the resident lower his tongue and close his mouth.

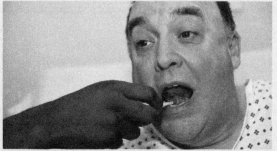

Figure 15.5   *Wards Forest Media, LLC*

16. Hold the probe in place in the mouth until you hear or see the signal that the reading is complete (**Figure 15.6**).

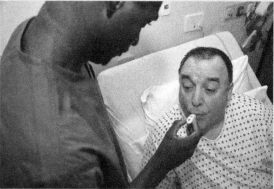

Figure 15.6   *Wards Forest Media, LLC*

17. Remove the thermometer from the resident's mouth and read the temperature on the display screen.
18. Do not touch the used probe cover with your bare hands. Dispose of the probe cover safely in a waste container or per facility policy.
19. If the resident is in bed, check to be sure the bed wheels are locked. Then reposition the resident and lower the bed.
20. Follow the plan of care to determine if the side rails should be raised or lowered.
21. Clean the probe according to facility policy and return the probe to its storage compartment on the thermometer.
22. Wash your hands or use hand sanitizer to ensure infection control.
23. Document the temperature on a pad, on a form, or in the electronic record according to facility policy.
24. Return the thermometer to a charging location per facility policy, if appropriate.

Follow-Up

25. Make sure the resident is comfortable and place the call light and personal items within reach.
26. Conduct a safety check before leaving the room. The room should be clean and free from clutter or spills.
27. Wash your hands or use hand sanitizer before leaving the room.

Reporting and Documentation

28. Report any specific observations, complications, or unusual responses to the licensed nursing staff. Document this information in the chart or EMR.

Procedure

Using a Digital Rectal Thermometer

Rationale

Body temperature that is outside the normal range can be a sign of a disease or condition or the result of an injury. The decision to use a rectal thermometer is based on the need for accuracy and the age and condition of the resident. Always follow the thermometer manufacturer's instructions and facility policy.

Preparation

1. Ask the licensed nursing staff if there are doctor's orders for the procedure, if there are any specific instructions listed in the plan of care, and if the resident can be moved into the positions required for this procedure.
2. Wash your hands or use hand sanitizer before entering the room.
3. Knock before entering the room.
4. Introduce yourself using your first or preferred name and title. Explain that you work with the licensed nursing staff and will be providing care.
5. Greet the resident and ask the resident to state her full name, if able. Then check the resident's identification bracelet.
6. Use Mr., Mrs., or Ms. and the resident's last name when conversing.
7. Explain the procedure in simple terms, even if the resident is not able to communicate or is disoriented. Ask permission to perform the procedure.
8. Bring the necessary equipment into the room. Place the following items in an easy-to-reach place:
   - a digital thermometer
   - the appropriate probe attachment (the *red* probe for a rectal temperature)
   - disposable probe covers
   - disposable gloves
   - water-soluble (dissolves in water) lubricating gel
   - tissues or toilet paper
   - pen and pad, form, or digital device for documenting temperature
   - sheet or drape

The Procedure

9. Provide privacy by closing the curtains, using a screen, or closing the door to the room.
10. If the resident is in bed, lock the bed wheels and then raise the bed to hip level.

11. Maintain safety during the procedure. If the resident is in a bed with side rails, raise and lock the rails on the opposite side of the bed from where you will be working. Lower the rail on the side where you are working.
12. Wash your hands or use hand sanitizer to ensure infection control.
13. Put on disposable gloves.
14. Place a disposable probe cover over the *red* probe. Start the thermometer and wait until it shows it is ready.
15. Assist the resident into a side-lying or lateral position. Have the resident bend her upper leg up to her stomach as far as possible. Help, if needed.
16. If the resident is covered by a drape or top sheet, fold it back to expose the buttocks. Expose only the area necessary for the procedure. Keep the rest of the resident covered to protect her privacy.
17. Apply enough water-soluble lubricating gel (about the size of a quarter) for comfortable entry.

   > **Best Practice:** To lubricate the end of the covered probe, you may put the gel directly on the probe or you may use tissue or toilet paper to apply the lubricant.

18. With one hand, gently raise the upper buttock to expose the anal area.
19. With the other hand, gently insert the rectal probe one inch or less into the anus.
20. Hold the probe in place until you hear or see the signal that the reading is complete.
21. Remove the thermometer and read the temperature on the display screen.
22. Dispose of the probe cover safely in a waste container or per facility policy.
23. Wipe the lubricant off the resident and discard the tissue or toilet paper.
24. Clean the probe with alcohol according to facility policy. Return the probe to its storage compartment on the thermometer.
25. Remove and discard your gloves and wash your hands or use hand sanitizer to ensure infection control.
26. Document the temperature on a pad, on a form, or in the electronic record according to facility policy.
27. If the resident is in bed, check to be sure the bed wheels are locked. Then reposition the resident and lower the bed.
28. Follow the plan of care to determine if the side rails should be raised or lowered.

(continued)

Using a Digital Rectal Thermometer *(continued)*

29. Return the thermometer to a charging location per facility policy.

Follow-Up

30. Make sure the resident is comfortable and place the call light and personal items within reach.

31. Conduct a safety check before leaving the room. The room should be clean and free from clutter or spills.

32. Wash your hands or use hand sanitizer before leaving the room.

Reporting and Documentation

33. Report any specific observations, complications, or unusual responses to the licensed nursing staff. Document this information in the chart or EMR.

Procedure

Using a Digital Axillary Thermometer

Rationale

While axillary temperature is not as accurate as other temperatures, the axilla (*armpit*) can often be more easily reached than other locations. Always follow the thermometer manufacturer's instructions and facility policy.

Preparation

1. Ask the licensed nursing staff if there are doctor's orders for the procedure, if there are any specific instructions listed in the plan of care, and if the resident can be moved into the positions required for this procedure.
2. Wash your hands or use hand sanitizer before entering the room.
3. Knock before entering the room.
4. Introduce yourself using your first or preferred name and title. Explain that you work with the licensed nursing staff and will be providing care.
5. Greet the resident and ask the resident to state his full name, if able. Then check the resident's identification bracelet.
6. Use Mr., Mrs., or Ms. and the resident's last name when conversing.
7. Explain the procedure in simple terms, even if the resident is not able to communicate or is disoriented. Ask permission to perform the procedure.
8. Bring the necessary equipment into the room. Place the following items in an easy-to-reach place:
   - a digital thermometer
   - the appropriate probe attachment (the *blue* probe for an axillary temperature)
   - disposable probe covers
   - disposable gloves, if appropriate
   - a towel
   - pen and pad, form, or digital device for documenting temperature

The Procedure

9. Provide privacy by closing the curtains, using a screen, or closing the door to the room.
10. If the resident is in bed, lock the bed wheels and then raise the bed to hip level.
11. Maintain safety during the procedure. If the resident is in a bed with side rails, raise and lock the rails on the opposite side of the bed from where you will be working. Lower the rail on the side where you are working.

   > **Best Practice:** Wear disposable gloves only if required for infection prevention and control.

12. Help the resident remove any clothing to expose his upper arm area.
13. Dry the axilla with the towel.
14. Place a disposable probe cover over the *blue* probe. Start the thermometer and wait until it shows it is ready.
15. Place the covered probe in the center of the axilla.
16. Place the resident's arm across his chest while holding the probe in place (**Figure 15.7**).

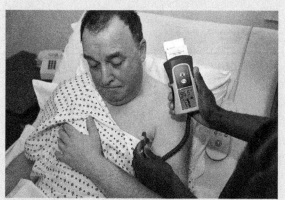

Figure 15.7

Wards Forest Media, LLC

17. Hold the probe in place in the axilla until you hear or see the signal that the reading is complete.
18. Remove the thermometer from the axilla and read the temperature on the display screen.

| **Best Practice:** Do not touch the probe cover.

19. Dispose of the probe cover safely in a waste container or per facility policy.
20. Clean the probe with alcohol according to facility policy. Return the probe to its storage compartment on the thermometer.
21. Wash your hands or use hand sanitizer to ensure infection control.
22. Document the temperature on a pad, on a form, or in the electronic record.
23. Assist the resident in replacing and securing his clothing.
24. If the resident is in bed, check to be sure the bed wheels are locked. Then reposition the resident and lower the bed.

25. Follow the plan of care to determine if the side rails should be raised or lowered.
26. Return the thermometer to a charging location per facility policy.

Follow-Up
27. Make sure the resident is comfortable and place the call light and personal items within reach.
28. Conduct a safety check before leaving the room. The room should be clean and free from clutter or spills.
29. Wash your hands or use hand sanitizer before leaving the room.

Reporting and Documentation
30. Report any specific observations, complications, or unusual responses to the licensed nursing staff. Document this information in the chart or EMR.

Disposable Oral Thermometers

Disposable oral thermometers are used to reduce the risk of cross- or re-infection and to measure the temperature of residents in isolation (**Figure 15.8**). They are plastic or paper and are discarded once used. The dots on the thermometer change color to show body temperature.

Tympanic Thermometers

A *tympanic thermometer* measures the temperature of **aural** blood vessels, or blood vessels in the ear. Tympanic temperature is taken on the tympanic membrane, or *eardrum*. Tympanic thermometers are usually battery-operated, are handheld, and have a digital display on the handle (**Figure 15.9**). Placement of the tympanic thermometer is very important for getting an accurate reading. Too much wax in the ears can interfere with the reading. Do not use this type of thermometer if the resident has a sore ear, has an ear infection, or has had ear surgery.

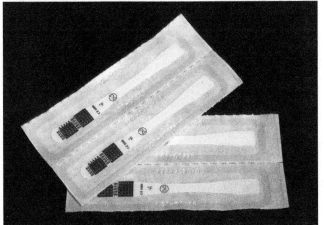

Wards Forest Media, LLC

Figure 15.8 Disposable oral thermometers are used once and then discarded. This helps prevent infections from spreading in healthcare facilities.

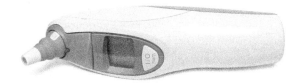

luk/Shutterstock.com

Figure 15.9 Tympanic thermometers are handheld and are inserted into the ear to measure tympanic temperature.

Procedure

Using a Digital Tympanic Thermometer

Rationale

Tympanic (*ear*) thermometers are another choice for taking temperatures. Placement is most important for an accurate reading. Always follow the thermometer manufacturer's instructions and facility policy.

Preparation

1. Ask the licensed nursing staff if there are doctor's orders for the procedure, if there are any specific instructions listed in the plan of care, and if the resident can be moved into the positions required for this procedure.
2. Wash your hands or use hand sanitizer before entering the room.
3. Knock before entering the room.
4. Introduce yourself using your first or preferred name and title. Explain that you work with the licensed nursing staff and will be providing care.
5. Greet the resident and ask the resident to state his full name, if able. Then check the resident's identification bracelet.
6. Use Mr., Mrs., or Ms. and the resident's last name when conversing.
7. Explain the procedure in simple terms, even if the resident is not able to communicate or is disoriented. Ask permission to perform the procedure.
8. Bring the necessary equipment into the room. Place the following items in an easy-to-reach place:
   - a digital tympanic thermometer
   - disposable plastic tympanic covers
   - disposable gloves, if necessary
   - pen and pad, form, or digital device for documenting the temperature

The Procedure

9. Provide privacy by closing the curtains, using a screen, or closing the door to the room.
10. If the resident is in bed, lock the bed wheels and then raise the bed to hip level.
11. Maintain safety during the procedure. If the resident is in a bed with side rails, raise and lock the rails on the opposite side of the bed from where you will be working. Lower the rail on the side where you are working.

    Best Practice: Wear disposable gloves only if required for infection prevention and control.

12. Check the lens of the tympanic thermometer to make sure it is clean and intact.
13. Position the resident's head so that the ear being used for the procedure is directly in front of you.
14. Place the disposable plastic cover on the tympanic thermometer.
15. Pull the outer ear up and back to open the ear canal (**Figure 15.10**).

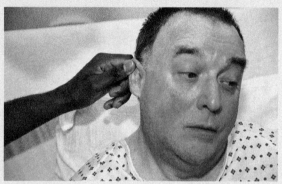

Figure 15.10   *Wards Forest Media, LLC*

16. Gently insert the covered tympanic thermometer into the ear until it seals the ear canal (**Figure 15.11**).

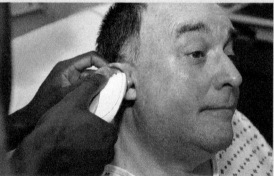

Figure 15.11   *Wards Forest Media, LLC*

17. Start the thermometer.
18. Hold the probe in place in the ear until you hear or see the signal that the reading is complete.
19. Remove the thermometer and read the temperature on the display screen.

    Best Practice: Do not touch the plastic tympanic cover.

20. Dispose of the plastic tympanic cover safely in a waste container or per facility policy.
21. Clean the tympanic thermometer according to facility policy.
22. Wash your hands or use hand sanitizer to ensure infection control.

23. Document the temperature on a pad, form, or in the electronic record.
24. If the resident is in bed, check to be sure the bed wheels are locked. Then reposition the resident and lower the bed.
25. Follow the plan of care to determine if the side rails should be raised or lowered.
26. Return the thermometer to a charging location per facility policy.

Follow-Up

27. Make sure the resident is comfortable and place the call light and personal items within reach.
28. Conduct a safety check before leaving the room. The room should be clean and free from clutter or spills.
29. Wash your hands or use hand sanitizer before leaving the room.

Reporting and Documentation

30. Report any specific observations, complications, or unusual responses to the licensed nursing staff. Document this information in the chart or EMR.

Temporal Artery Thermometers

Temporal artery thermometers use the surface temperature of the temporal arteries on either side of the head to measure body temperature (**Figure 15.12**). The device is swept across the forehead to read the resident's temperature. This type of temperature is often more accurate than an oral temperature because it is not affected by what a resident eats or drinks.

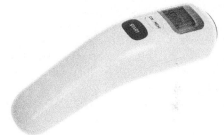

Michael Dechev/Shutterstock.com

Figure 15.12 Temporal artery thermometers measure the temperature of the temporal arteries on either side of the forehead.

Procedure

Using a Digital Temporal Artery Thermometer

Rationale

The temporal artery thermometer, used on the forehead, is less invasive than other methods because it does not need to enter a body cavity. Always follow the thermometer manufacturer's instructions and facility policy.

Preparation

1. Ask the licensed nursing staff if there are doctor's orders for the procedure, if there are any specific instructions listed in the plan of care, and if the resident can be moved into the positions required for this procedure.
2. Wash your hands or use hand sanitizer before entering the room.
3. Knock before entering the room.
4. Introduce yourself using your first or preferred name and title. Explain that you work with the licensed nursing staff and will be providing care.

5. Greet the resident and ask the resident to state his full name, if able. Then check the resident's identification bracelet.
6. Use Mr., Mrs., or Ms. and the resident's last name when conversing.
7. Explain the procedure in simple terms, even if the resident is not able to communicate or is disoriented. Ask permission to perform the procedure.
8. Bring the necessary equipment into the room. Place the following items in an easy-to-reach place:
   • a temporal artery thermometer
   • a pen and pad, form, or digital device for documenting the temperature

The Procedure

9. Provide privacy by closing the curtains, using a screen, or closing the door to the room.
10. If the resident is in bed, lock the bed wheels and then raise the bed to hip level.
11. Ensure safety during the procedure. If the resident is in a bed with side rails, raise and secure the rails on the opposite side of the bed from where you will be working. Lower the rail on the side where you are working.

(continued)

Using a Digital Temporal Artery Thermometer *(continued)*

> **Best Practice:** Wear disposable gloves only if required for infection prevention and control.

12. Position the resident comfortably.
13. Help or have the resident turn so that his forehead faces you.
14. Start the thermometer and wait until it shows it is ready.
15. Place the probe in the middle of the resident's forehead (**Figure 15.13A**). Then slowly move the thermometer across the forehead toward the ear, stopping in front of the ear (**Figure 15.13B**).

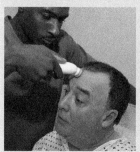 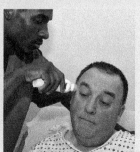

A **B** *Wards Forest Media, LLC*
Figure 15.13

16. Wait until you see or hear the signal that the temperature is complete.
17. Wash your hands or use hand sanitizer to ensure infection control.
18. Document the temperature on a pad, on a form, or in the electronic record.
19. If the resident is in bed, check to be sure the bed wheels are locked. Then reposition the resident and lower the bed.
20. Follow the plan of care to determine if the side rails should be raised or lowered.
21. Clean and store the temporal artery thermometer according to the facility policy.

Follow-Up

22. Make sure the resident is comfortable and place the call light and personal items within reach.
23. Conduct a safety check before leaving the room. The room should be clean and free from clutter or spills.
24. Wash your hands or use hand sanitizer before leaving the room.

Reporting and Documentation

25. Report any specific observations, complications, or unusual responses to the licensed nursing staff. Document this information in the chart or EMR.

What Is a Pulse?

When you take (measure) a *pulse,* you are feeling or hearing the pressure of blood against the wall of an artery as the heart *beats.* Pulse is an important vital sign because it shows how well the cardiovascular system is working. It is very important if a resident has a heart or respiratory condition.

Pulse Locations

There are several locations in which an artery comes close enough to the surface of the skin that you can feel a pulse (**Figure 15.14**). These are the three pulses most commonly used:

- *Radial pulse*: taken by feeling the radial artery located at the wrist (thumb side of the hand) on bare skin. Two fingers are gently placed on the radial artery to take the pulse. If a resident has an IV in one arm, do not use that arm when taking the pulse.
- *Apical pulse*: taken by listening to the apical artery located at the *apex* of the heart. It is usually taken if radial pulse is difficult to count or if a resident is unconscious. This pulse is taken using a **stethoscope**, or a medical device for listening to sounds in the body through bare skin.

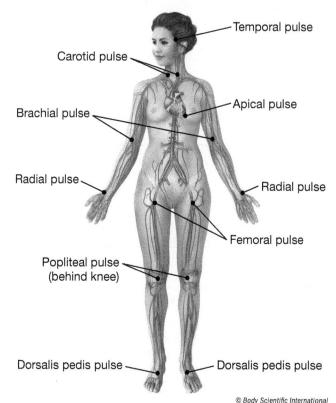

© Body Scientific International

Figure 15.14 Pulse can be measured at all of the locations shown here.

• *Carotid pulse*: taken by feeling the carotid artery. It is usually taken when a resident is unconscious (for example, during CPR).

Of these three, the radial and apical arteries are used most often. A nursing assistant may also measure pulse at the brachial arteries.

The Stethoscope

A stethoscope is used to help measure an apical pulse. It is also used when taking blood pressure, which is discussed later in this section. The stethoscope increases the sound of a pulse and transfers it to the user's ears. The diaphragm, or larger, flat surface of the stethoscope makes sound louder, while the bell on the other side helps you hear fainter sounds (**Figure 15.15**).

Before using a stethoscope, always disinfect the earpieces, diaphragm, and bell by rubbing them lightly with antiseptic or alcohol wipes. When cleaning the earpieces with alcohol, give the alcohol time to evaporate, as it can be painful in the ear canal. Wipe the tubing if it has come in contact with the resident or bed linen.

Pulse Rate Measurements

Pulse rate is measured by feeling or hearing the pulse and counting the number of beats in one minute using a watch with a second hand. Pulse rate is reported in *beats per minute*, or *bpm* (for example, *72 beats per minute* or *72 bpm*).

Resting pulse is taken when a resident is breathing normally and resting (sitting in a chair or in bed). The average range for the resting pulse rate in adults is 60–100 bpm.

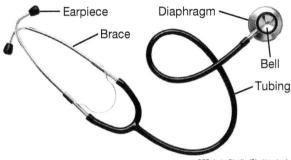

279photo Studio/Shutterstock.com

Figure 15.15 Place the earpieces of the stethoscope firmly in your ear canals, making sure they fit snugly. Rub the diaphragm gently to make sure you can hear sounds clearly through the stethoscope.

Pulse rate can be affected by activity, anxiety, excitement, pain, fever, medications, sleep patterns, and diseases or health conditions. For instance, during exercise, the average person's pulse rate may range from 90 to 120 beats per minute. A pulse that is slow (fewer than 60 beats per minute) is called **bradycardia**. A pulse that is fast (100 beats or more per minute) is called **tachycardia**.

When taking a pulse, remember that you are not only counting the number of beats, but also listening for the rhythm (pauses between beats). The rhythm may be described as normal (*regular*) or intermittent (*irregular*). The quality of the pulse can be full (*bounding*) or weak (*thready*). A thready pulse is hard to feel. When you think about all of these factors, you might report a pulse as *82 bpm and regular*.

Pulse is documented in a resident's electronic record or a form provided by the healthcare facility. Any irregularities of the pulse must be reported to the licensed nursing staff.

Procedure

Measuring a Radial Pulse

Rationale

Counting a radial pulse is the most common method of measuring heart rate and its quality. A pulse that falls outside the normal range may be a sign of a health issue, disease, or condition.

Preparation

1. Ask the licensed nursing staff if there are doctor's orders for the procedure, if there are any specific instructions listed in the plan of care, and if the resident can be moved into the positions required for this procedure.

2. Wash your hands or use hand sanitizer before entering the room.
3. Knock before entering the room.
4. Introduce yourself using your first or preferred name and title. Explain that you work with the licensed nursing staff and will be providing care.
5. Greet the resident and ask the resident to state her full name, if able. Then check the resident's identification bracelet.
6. Use Mr., Mrs., or Ms. and the resident's last name when conversing.

(continued)

Measuring a Radial Pulse *(continued)*

7. Explain the procedure in simple terms, even if the resident is not able to communicate or is disoriented. Ask permission to perform the procedure.
8. Bring the necessary equipment into the room. Place the following items in an easy-to-reach place:
   - a watch or clock with a second hand (not a digital watch)
   - pen and pad, form, or digital device for documenting the pulse

The Procedure

9. Provide privacy by closing the curtains, using a screen, or closing the door to the room.
10. If the resident is in bed, lock the bed wheels and then raise the bed to hip level.
11. Maintain safety during the procedure. If the resident is in a bed with side rails, raise and lock the rails on the opposite side of the bed from where you will be working. Lower the rail on the side where you are working.
12. Have the resident sit or lie down. Select the hand and arm you will use to take the pulse.

> **Best Practice:** If the resident has an IV in one arm, do not use that arm to take the pulse. Also, do not take the pulse on a weak arm. Some residents may have an arm that has been weakened by a stroke.

13. Position the hand and arm so they are well supported and rest comfortably.
14. Locate the radial artery by placing your middle finger and index finger toward the inside of the resident's wrist on the thumb side (**Figure 15.16**).

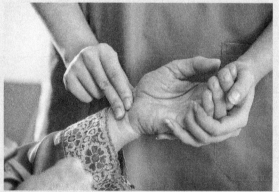

Figure 15.16   *Tyler Olson/Shutterstock.com*

> **Best Practice:** Do not use your thumb to feel for pulse. The thumb has its own pulse, which can be confused with the pulse you are taking.

15. Press your fingers gently on bare skin until you feel the pulse. Also, note the rhythm and quality of the pulse.
16. Start taking the pulse when you note the position of the second hand on your watch (**Figure 15.17**). Count pulse beats for one full minute or for 30 seconds and multiply the result by 2. Follow the facility policy. Counting for one full minute is more accurate and should be done if the pulse rhythm seems weak or irregular.

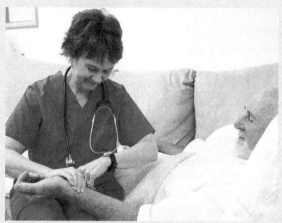

Figure 15.17   *Lisa F. Young/Shutterstock.com*

17. Document the pulse on a pad, on a form, or in the electronic record.
18. If the resident is in bed, check to be sure the bed wheels are locked. Then reposition the resident and lower the bed.
19. Follow the plan of care to determine if the side rails should be raised or lowered.

Follow-Up

20. Wash your hands to ensure infection control.
21. Make sure the resident is comfortable and place the call light and personal items within reach.
22. Conduct a safety check before leaving the room. The room should be clean and free from clutter or spills.
23. Wash your hands or use hand sanitizer before leaving the room.

Reporting and Documentation

24. Report any specific observations, complications, or unusual responses to the licensed nursing staff. Document this information in the chart or EMR.

Procedure

Measuring an Apical Pulse

Rationale
Apical pulse is usually taken if you want more information than a radial pulse can provide or if it is not possible to take a radial pulse. A pulse outside the normal range may be a sign of a health issue, medical disease, or condition.

Preparation
1. Ask the licensed nursing staff if there are doctor's orders for the procedure, if there are any specific instructions listed in the plan of care, and if the resident can be moved into the positions required for this procedure.
2. Wash your hands or use hand sanitizer before entering the room.
3. Knock before entering the room.
4. Introduce yourself using your first or preferred name and title. Explain that you work with the licensed nursing staff and will be providing care.
5. Greet the resident and ask the resident to state his full name, if able. Then check the resident's identification bracelet.
6. Use Mr., Mrs., or Ms. and the resident's last name when conversing.
7. Explain the procedure in simple terms, even if the resident is not able to communicate or is disoriented. Ask permission to perform the procedure.
8. Bring the necessary equipment into the room. Place the following items in an easy-to-reach place:
   - a stethoscope
   - antiseptic wipes
   - a watch or clock with a second hand (not a digital watch)
   - pen and pad, form, or digital device for documenting the pulse rate

The Procedure
9. Provide privacy by closing the curtains, using a screen, or closing the door to the room.
10. If the resident is in bed, lock the bed wheels and then raise the bed to hip level.
11. Maintain safety during the procedure. If the resident is in a bed with side rails, raise and lock the rails on the opposite side of the bed from where you will be working. Lower the rail on the side where you are working.
12. Have the resident sit or lie down.
13. Clean the earpieces and diaphragm of the stethoscope with an antiseptic wipe.

14. Warm the diaphragm of the stethoscope by rubbing it in the palms of your hands.
15. Place the earpieces of the stethoscope in your ears.
16. Uncover the left side of the resident's chest. Avoid any overexposure.
17. Place the diaphragm of the stethoscope on the left side of the chest, under the breast, or just below the left nipple (**Figure 15.18**).

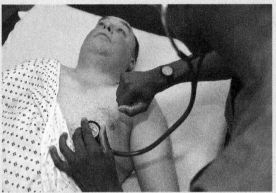

Figure 15.18   *Wards Forest Media, LLC*

> **Best Practice:** If the heartbeat is difficult to hear, have the resident turn slightly to the left or sit upright.

18. Note the position of the second hand on your watch. Count the heartbeats for 1 full minute. Note the rhythm and quality.
19. Cover the resident's chest.
20. Document the pulse on a pad, on a form, or in the electronic record.
21. If the resident is in bed, check to be sure the bed wheels are locked. Then reposition the resident and lower the bed.
22. Follow the plan of care to determine if the side rails should be raised or lowered.

Follow-Up
23. Wash your hands to ensure infection control.
24. Make sure the resident is comfortable and place the call light and personal items within reach.
25. Conduct a safety check before leaving the room. The room should be clean and free from clutter or spills.
26. Wash your hands or use hand sanitizer before leaving the room.

Reporting and Documentation
27. Report any specific observations, complications, or unusual responses to the licensed nursing staff. Document this information in the chart or EMR.

What Is the Rate of Respiration?

The *rate of respiration* is the measurement of a resident's breathing cycle (inhalation followed by exhalation). Respiration rate helps determine a resident's level of *blood oxygenation*, or how well oxygen is supplied to body cells. Respiration rate also provides information about conditions such as asthma, heart disease, and even infections. A normal adult respiration rate is 12–20 breaths per minute.

Finding the Rate of Respiration

To determine the rate of respiration, document the number of full breaths (each rise and fall of the chest) taken in one minute. Typically, this involves counting respirations for 15 seconds and multiplying the result by 4. Some healthcare facilities require nursing assistants to count respirations for 30 seconds and then multiply the result by 2. If respirations are irregular, the nursing assistant should count the number of full breaths for 1 full minute using a watch with a second hand.

It is best to count respiration rate with no warning immediately after pulse is taken. This way, the resident is breathing as he or she normally would. After taking the pulse, switch to counting respirations without mentioning the change to the resident. A resident who knows his or her respirations are being counted may subconsciously change his or her breathing, giving an inaccurate result.

Observing how well a resident is breathing is just as important as determining the number of breaths. When counting respirations, also observe the following:

- Is the breathing regular or irregular?
- Is the resident experiencing *hyperventilation* (deep, rapid breathing) or *hypoventilation* (slow, shallow breathing)?
- Is the breathing rapid (called *tachypnea*), deep and labored (called *dyspnea*), or unusually slow (called *bradypnea*)?
- Is the breathing noisy like snoring (called *stertorous breathing*)?
- Are there periods of no breathing at all (called *apnea*)?

Procedure

Counting Respirations

Rationale

Counting respirations involves measuring the number of inhalations and exhalations in 1 minute. A respiration rate that is outside the normal range may be a sign of a health issue, medical disease, or condition.

Preparation

1. Ask the licensed nursing staff if there are doctor's orders for the procedure, if there are any specific instructions listed in the plan of care, and if the resident can be moved into the positions required for this procedure.
2. Wash your hands or use hand sanitizer before entering the room.
3. Knock before entering the room.
4. Introduce yourself using your first or preferred name and title. Explain that you work with the licensed nursing staff and will be providing care.
5. Greet the resident and ask the resident to state his or her full name, if able. Then check the resident's identification bracelet.

6. Use Mr., Mrs., or Ms. and the resident's last name when conversing.
7. Explain the procedure in simple terms, even if the resident is not able to communicate or is disoriented. Ask permission to perform the procedure.
8. Bring the necessary equipment into the room. Place the following items in an easy-to-reach place:
   - a watch or clock with a second hand (not a digital watch)
   - a pen and pad, form, or digital device for documenting the respiration rate

The Procedure

9. Provide privacy by closing the curtains, using a screen, or closing the door to the room.
10. If the resident is in bed, lock the bed wheels and then raise the bed to hip level.
11. Maintain safety during the procedure. If the resident is in a bed with side rails, raise and lock the rails on the opposite side of the bed from where you will be working. Lower the rail on the side where you are working.
12. Have the resident sit or lie down.

13. The best time to count respirations is immediately after counting pulse rate. It is best not to tell residents you are counting respirations. When residents know their breathing is being observed, they may change their breathing patterns.

   > **Best Practice:** Depending on which pulse was taken, keep your fingers on the wrist or keep the stethoscope on the chest while counting respirations.

14. Begin counting respirations when the chest rises. Each rise and fall of the chest counts as one respiration. Note the regularity and depth of respirations, the expansion of the chest, and any pain or difficulty breathing.

15. Note the position of the second hand on your watch and count respirations for 1 full minute. Some facilities allow nursing assistants to count respirations for 15 seconds and multiply the result by 4 or count respirations for 30 seconds and multiply the result by 2. Follow the facility policy. Counting respirations for 1 full minute should be done if the respiration is irregular.

16. Let the licensed nursing staff know immediately if the resident complains of pain or difficulty breathing.

17. Document the respiration rate on a pad, on a form, or in the electronic record.

18. If the resident is in bed, check to be sure the bed wheels are locked. Then reposition the resident and lower the bed.

19. Follow the plan of care to determine if the side rails should be raised or lowered.

Follow-Up

20. Wash your hands to ensure infection control.

21. Make sure the resident is comfortable and place the call light and personal items within reach.

22. Conduct a safety check before leaving the room. The room should be clean and free from clutter or spills.

23. Wash your hands or use hand sanitizer before leaving the room.

Reporting and Documentation

24. Report any specific observations, complications, or unusual responses to the licensed nursing staff. Document this information in the chart or EMR.

Using a Pulse Oximeter

Another way to measure how well oxygen is being used in the body is to determine oxygen saturation (levels) in the blood. A *pulse oximeter* is commonly used when vital signs are being measured and is also used to measure oxygen effectiveness for a resident receiving oxygen.

A pulse oximeter is applied to the finger (or sometimes the earlobe or toe). It uses infrared light that passes through the body tissue of the finger. A pulse oximeter's digital display will show the amount of oxygen in the blood as a percentage (**Figure 15.19**). A normal reading is 95 percent to 100 percent oxygen in the blood. A reading below 85 percent is too low a level and is called *hypoxia* (not enough oxygen in the body). Oxygen saturation in the blood is documented as SpO_2.

Using a pulse oximeter has very few risks. If improperly placed, the pulse oximeter may give an inaccurate reading. If a pulse oximeter is used continuously, pay attention to the skin around and under the device and check for possible irritation.

Respirations (rate, regularity, and depth) and pulse oximeter percentages are documented on a form provided by the healthcare facility or in the

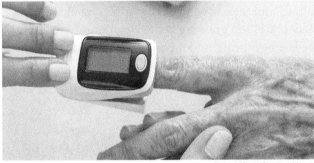

Click and Photo/Shutterstock.com

Figure 15.19 The pulse oximeter is placed on the finger and measures oxygen saturation in the blood.

electronic record. Any irregularities must be reported to the licensed nursing staff.

How Is Blood Pressure Measured?

Blood pressure is the force of blood pushing against the body's arterial walls. Measuring blood pressure is important. If a resident has **hypotension** (blood pressure that is too low), the body may not be getting enough oxygen and nutrients. The opposite of hypotension is *hypertension* (blood pressure that is too high), which may place too much pressure on the walls of the arteries (**Figure 15.20**). This pressure can

Blood Pressure Classification

Hypotension	Normal	Prehypertension	Hypertension
<90/60 mmHg	90–120/60–80 mmHg	120–129/<80 mmHg	Stage 1: 130–139/80–90 mmHG Stage 2: >140/90 mmHg

Goodheart-Willcox Publisher

Figure 15.20 The normal blood pressure range is below 120/80 mmHg.

cause a stroke or other cardiovascular problems. High or low blood pressure can also be a sign of, or cause, certain diseases and conditions, such as heart disease, kidney damage or failure, various injuries, or dizziness.

Measuring Blood Pressure

A blood pressure reading is made up of two pressure levels, which are measured as the heart beats. The first is *systolic blood pressure*, which is pressure when the heart muscle contracts and pushes blood through the artery. The second is *diastolic blood pressure*, which is pressure when the heart muscle relaxes. These pressure levels are measured using a stethoscope and a sphygmomanometer.

Both pressure levels are measured in *millimeters of mercury (mmHg)*. Systolic blood pressure is the higher number and the first beat heard (as a tapping sound) and measured (as 120 mmHg, for example). Diastolic blood pressure is the lower number and is the last beat heard and measured (as 80 mmHg, for example). For someone with these measurements, blood pressure would be documented as the fraction 120/80 mmHg. The normal blood pressure range for adults are systolic pressure 90–120 and diastolic 60–80.

Knowing Factors That Affect Blood Pressure

Many factors can affect blood pressure. These factors include the following:
- **Diet**: diets high in salt and fat may lead to higher blood pressure.
- **Weight**: being overweight can lead to higher blood pressure.
- **Exercise**: systolic blood pressure may be higher if a resident does not exercise or exercised right before blood pressure was taken.
- **Race**: African-Americans are more likely to have high blood pressure and at an earlier age compared to Caucasians or people of Hispanic descent.
- **Time of day**: blood pressure may be lower in the morning than later in the day and may be higher after a meal.

BECOMING A HOLISTIC NURSING ASSISTANT
Taking Vital Signs

To provide holistic care when measuring and recording vital signs, you can use the following guidelines:
- Know the function of and the normal ranges for different vital signs.
- Demonstrate skill and proficiency.
- Make sure measurements are accurate. Repeat the measurement if you are unsure of a reading. Explain to the resident that you want to take an accurate reading.
- Ask a member of the licensed nursing staff for help if you have trouble measuring a vital sign. *Never* make up a reading.
- Quickly report any abnormal results to the licensed nursing staff.

- When appropriate, give residents choices about the procedure. For example, you might let the resident choose the arm used to measure blood pressure or choose whether to sit up or lie down.
- Know that vital signs can change and are unique to each resident, the resident's environment, and factors of daily living such as diet and exercise.
- Maintain a professional and patient attitude when taking vital signs. Never show frustration or concern if you are having difficulty measuring a vital sign or if a vital sign is not in a normal range.

Apply It
1. Would any of these guidelines be challenging for you to follow? Explain your answer.
2. In your opinion, which guidelines would require more attention or practice on your part?

- **Position**: blood pressure may be higher if a resident is lying down and lower if a resident is standing up.
- **Cigarettes and alcohol**: using cigarettes and alcohol can increase blood pressure.
- **Drugs or medications**: some medications and drugs can make blood pressure higher or lower.
- **Stress, fear, or pain**: blood pressure may be higher if a resident is feeling stress, fear, or pain.

Taking a Resident's Blood Pressure

Blood pressure can be measured manually or electronically. Both ways are accurate; however, electronic devices reduce potential human error. Equipment may be movable, on a wall mount, or part of an electronic vital sign monitoring machine. Other types of blood pressure equipment include home blood pressure monitoring equipment with a cuff and digital monitoring device. Some have technology that links to smartphones. New wearable blood pressure technology is built into digital wristwatches, offering continuous or intermittent (not continuous) monitoring 24/7.

When taking a resident's blood pressure, be sure to check the equipment, make sure the resident is relaxed, and be prepared to perform the procedure. Avoid using an arm with an IV, cast, wound, or injury to take blood pressure. Residents who have had a mastectomy should not have blood pressure taken on the same side as the breast removal.

It is important to recheck a blood pressure reading if you are not sure the measurement is accurate or if you cannot hear the sounds clearly. You should recheck blood pressure if you suspect an error or faulty equipment, if this is the first time the blood pressure is high or low for this resident, or you notice a change in the resident's normal blood pressure.

When taking a manual blood pressure measurement, you will need a stethoscope and a *sphygmomanometer* (*sphygm/o* = pulse; *man/o* = pressure; *-meter* = measure). Two main types of sphygmomanometers are used to measure blood pressure (**Figure 15.21**):

- **Manual aneroid sphygmomanometer**: is movable and has a round dial and a needle that points to the numbers. You will need to use a stethoscope when using this device.
- **Electronic sphygmomanometer**: has a digital display and is found in many healthcare facilities. You will not need a stethoscope when using this device.

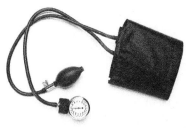

sirtravelalot/Shutterstock.com

A

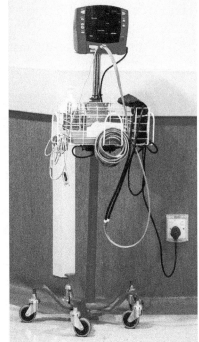

MALASIA/Shutterstock.com

B

Figure 15.21 Both manual (A) and electronic (B) sphygmomanometers can be used to measure blood pressure.

A sphygmomanometer has two parts: the measuring device and the cuff. When applying a blood pressure cuff, check that it is the right size. If the cuff is too small or too large, the blood pressure reading will not be accurate. The inflatable part of the cuff should cover two-thirds of the distance from the elbow to the shoulder. You should be able to fit your fingers between the closed cuff and the skin. No matter what type of device you use, be sure it is in working order before taking blood pressure.

THINK ABOUT THIS

The Centers for Disease Control and Prevention recently reported that 75 million American adults (29 percent) have high blood pressure. This means that about one in every three adults has hypertension. Approximately one-half (54 percent) of those with high blood pressure have their condition under control.

Before taking blood pressure, have residents relax or rest for a few minutes (5 minutes). This will help you get a reading that is most normal for the resident. The blood pressure reading may not be accurate if the resident has just been exercising, is in pain, is feeling anxious, or has recently had physical therapy. If possible, wait at least 30 minutes after these events before taking a routine blood pressure measurement. Also make sure the room or area in which blood pressure is taken is quiet. This will help you better hear through the stethoscope.

Other tips to be sure blood pressure measurement is as accurate as possible include:

- Have residents empty their bladder before you take their blood pressure. A full bladder can add 10–15 mmHg.
- Put the cuff on a bare arm; measuring over clothing can add 10–40 mmHg.
- Support the arm at heart level. Failing to support the arm can add 10 mmHg.
- Support the back. An unsupported back can add 5–10 mmHg.
- Never let residents' feet dangle or cross their legs. Crossing legs can add 2–8 mmHg.
- Do not converse with residents while taking a blood pressure. Doing this can add 10–15 mmHg.

Procedure

Taking a Blood Pressure

Rationale

Blood pressure measures the force of blood pushing against the body's arterial walls. A blood pressure reading outside the normal range may be a sign of a disease or health issue.

Preparation

1. Ask the licensed nursing staff if there are doctor's orders for the procedure, if there are any specific instructions listed in the plan of care, and if the resident can be moved into the positions required for this procedure.
2. Wash your hands or use hand sanitizer before entering the room.
3. Knock before entering the room.
4. Introduce yourself using your first or preferred name and title. Explain that you work with the licensed nursing staff and will be providing care.
5. Greet the resident and ask the resident to state his full name, if able. Then check the resident's identification bracelet.
6. Use Mr., Mrs., or Ms. and the resident's last name when conversing.
7. Explain the procedure in simple terms, even if the resident is not able to communicate or is disoriented. Ask permission to perform the procedure.
8. Bring the necessary equipment into the room. Place the following items in an easy-to-reach place:
   - a sphygmomanometer
   - an appropriately sized cuff
   - a stethoscope, if using a manual sphygmomanometer
   - antiseptic wipe(s)
   - disposable paper cover, if needed
   - a pen and pad, form, or digital device for documenting the blood pressure

The Procedure: Manual Device

9. Provide privacy by closing the curtains, using a screen, or closing the door to the room.
10. Clean the cuff with an antiseptic wipe or cover it with a disposable paper cover.
11. Have the resident rest quietly and lie comfortably on the bed or sit in a chair. Make sure the room is quiet.
12. When appropriate, let the resident choose which arm he wants you to use for taking blood pressure and whether he wants to sit up or lie down.
13. If the resident is in bed, lock the bed wheels and then raise the bed to hip level. If he is on an examining table, stand next to him or sit in a chair in front of him so you can get a clear view of the dial.
14. Clean the earpieces of the stethoscope with an antiseptic wipe and warm the diaphragm with your hands before cleaning it with antiseptic wipes.
15. Position the resident's arm so it rests level with the heart with the palm turned upward. Provide support, if needed (**Figure 15.22**).

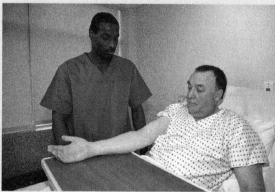

Figure 15.22   *Wards Forest Media, LLC*

Best Practice: Expose the upper arm so that you can place the cuff on bare skin.

16. Unroll the blood pressure cuff and loosen the valve on the bulb of the sphygmomanometer by turning it counterclockwise (**Figure 15.23**).

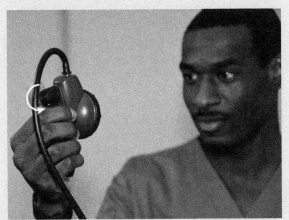

Figure 15.23 *Wards Forest Media, LLC*

17. Squeeze the cuff to expel any remaining air.
18. With your fingertips, locate the brachial artery at the inner aspect of the elbow (**Figure 15.24**).

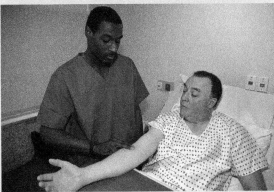

Figure 15.24 *Wards Forest Media, LLC*

19. Place the center of the cuff, usually marked with an arrow, above the brachial artery. (**Figure 15.25**).

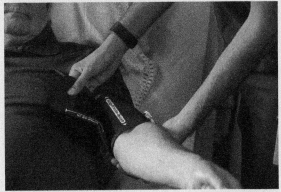

Figure 15.25 *© Tori Soper Photography*

20. Wrap the cuff smoothly and snugly around the exposed arm about 1 inch above the elbow. Do not wrap the cuff around clothing. Make sure the cuff is not too snug (**Figure 15.26**).

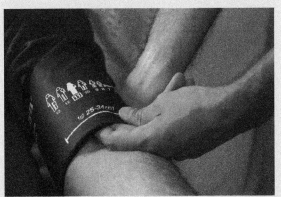

Figure 15.26 *© Tori Soper Photography*

21. Close the valve on the bulb of the sphygmomanometer by turning it clockwise. Be careful not to turn it too tightly.
22. Place the earpieces of the stethoscope in your ears.
23. Find the brachial pulse.
24. Place the warmed diaphragm of the stethoscope over the brachial artery.
25. Keep the measuring scale level with your eyes.
26. Inflate the cuff to 180 mmHg. You should not be able to hear the resident's pulse. If you do, inflate the cuff to 200 mmHg.

Best Practice: The stethoscope diaphragm should be held firmly against the skin close to the cuff, but should not be placed under the cuff (**Figure 15.27**).

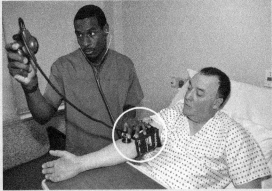

Figure 15.27 *Wards Forest Media, LLC*

27. Deflate the cuff by slowly turning the valve on the bulb of the sphygmomanometer counterclockwise at an even rate of 2–4 millimeters per second.

(continued)

Taking a Blood Pressure *(continued)*

28. Listen carefully while the cuff is deflating. Note the dial reading when you hear the first sound (beat). This is the systolic blood pressure.
29. Continue deflating the cuff slowly and evenly. Note the dial reading when the sound (beat) disappears. This is the diastolic blood pressure.
30. Remove the stethoscope earpieces from your ears. Completely deflate the cuff and remove it from the arm.
31. Document the blood pressure on a pad, on a form, or in the electronic record.
32. Report abnormal results to the appropriate licensed nursing staff member immediately.
33. Return the cuff to its case or wall mount.
34. Clean the earpieces and diaphragm of the stethoscope with antiseptic wipes. Discard the disposable cover, if used.
35. Return the stethoscope and cuff case (if appropriate) to their storage locations.
36. If the resident is in bed, check to be sure the bed wheels are locked. Then reposition the resident and lower the bed.
37. Follow the plan of care to determine if the side rails should be raised or lowered.

The Procedure: Electronic Device

38. Provide privacy by closing the curtains, using a screen, or closing the door to the room.
39. Bring the electronic blood pressure unit near the resident and plug it into a source of electricity.
40. Clean the cuff with an antiseptic wipe or cover it with a disposable paper cover.
41. Have the resident rest quietly and lie comfortably on the bed or sit in a chair.
42. If the resident is in bed, lock the bed wheels and then raise the bed to hip level. If he is on an examining table, stand next to him or sit in a chair in front of him so you can get a clear view of the digital display.
43. Remove any restrictive clothing from the resident's arm. Ask the resident which arm he would prefer, if appropriate.
44. Locate the *Power* switch and turn on the machine.
45. Squeeze any excess air out of the blood pressure cuff.
46. Connect the cuff to the connector hose.
47. Wrap the cuff smoothly and snugly around the resident's exposed arm. Do not wrap the cuff around clothing. Make sure the cuff is not too snug.

48. Make sure the arrow marked on the outside of the cuff is correctly placed over the brachial artery.
49. Make sure the connector hose between the cuff and the machine is not kinked.
50. Press the *Start* button. The cuff should begin to inflate and then deflate as the reading is being taken.
51. You will see or hear a signal when the reading is complete.
52. If you are taking periodic, automatic measurements, set the machine for the designated frequency of blood pressure measurements. The upper and lower alarm limits for systolic, diastolic, and mean blood pressure readings are set according to facility policy.
53. Document the blood pressure on a pad, on a form, or in the electronic record.
54. Report abnormal results to the licensed nursing staff immediately.
55. Clean the tubing and cuff with an antiseptic wipe. Discard the disposable cover, if used.
56. Remove the machine and place it in its appropriate storage location.
57. If the cuff is to remain on the arm between blood pressure readings, loosen it. Remove the cuff at least every two hours and rotate to the other arm, if possible. Evaluate the skin for redness or irritation. Report any abnormal observations to the licensed nursing staff.
58. If the resident is in bed, check to be sure the bed wheels are locked. Then reposition the resident and lower the bed.
59. Follow the plan of care to determine if the side rails should be raised or lowered.

Follow-Up

60. Wash your hands to ensure infection control.
61. Make sure the resident is comfortable and place the call light and personal items within reach.
62. Conduct a safety check before leaving the room. The room should be clean and free from clutter or spills.
63. Wash your hands or use hand sanitizer before leaving the room.

Reporting and Documentation

64. Report any specific observations, complications, or unusual responses to the licensed nursing staff. Document this information in the chart or EMR.

SECTION 15.1 **Review and Assessment**

Key Terms Mini Glossary

apical pulse a measurement of heartbeat taken by listening to the apex of the heart (to the left of the sternum slightly under the left breast) with a stethoscope.

apnea a lack of breathing.

aural relating to the ear or the sense of hearing.

axillary temperature a measurement of body temperature taken by placing a thermometer under the axilla.

bradycardia an abnormally slow pulse (fewer than 60 beats per minute).

bradypnea abnormally slow breathing.

carotid pulse a measurement of heartbeat taken by feeling the carotid artery, which is located on the neck by the trachea below the angle of the jaw.

Celsius (C) a temperature measurement scale in which the freezing point of water is 0° and the boiling point is 100° under normal atmospheric pressure; also called *centigrade*.

diastolic blood pressure the pressure of blood against the arteries when the heart muscle relaxes.

dyspnea difficult breathing or shortness of breath.

Fahrenheit (F) a temperature measurement scale in which the freezing point of water is 32° and the boiling point is 212° under normal atmospheric pressure.

hyperventilation deep, rapid breathing.

hypotension low blood pressure.

hypoventilation slow, shallow breathing.

hypoxia a lack of adequate oxygen supply in the body.

probe a long, thin, medical instrument used to measure temperature.

radial pulse a measurement of heartbeat taken by feeling the radial artery, which is located on the inside of the thumb side of the wrist.

stertorous breathing a type of breathing that sounds like snoring.

stethoscope a medical device used to listen to body sounds such as breathing, heartbeat, and lung and bowel sounds; has two earpieces connected by flexible tubing and a diaphragm and bell at the end.

systolic blood pressure the pressure of blood against the arteries when the heart muscle contracts and pushes blood out to the body.

tachycardia an abnormally fast pulse (more than 100 beats per minute).

tachypnea rapid, shallow breathing.

temporal arteries arteries located on each side of the head.

tympanic temperature a measurement of body temperature taken by placing a thermometer into the ear.

Apply the Key Terms

Write a sentence using each key term properly.

1. stethoscope
2. axillary temperature
3. bradycardia
4. diastolic blood pressure
5. hypoxia

Know and Understand the Facts

1. Identify two reasons why vital signs are measured.
2. Identify the locations where a pulse can be measured.
3. List the equipment needed to measure a blood pressure manually.
4. A resident has a blood pressure of 140/95 mmHg. Is this within the normal range?

Analyze and Apply Concepts

1. What should a nursing assistant do if a vital sign does not seem to be accurate?
2. What should a nursing assistant do if a vital sign is significantly higher or lower than it was when taken at an earlier time?

3. What equipment is needed to take a rectal temperature?
4. Which steps must always be performed to make sure blood pressure is measured accurately?
5. List two important descriptions that should be documented when measuring a pulse.

Think Critically

Read the following care situation. Then answer the questions that follow.

Seiji, a nursing assistant at the city rehabilitation facility, was taking Mr. L's vital signs. When Seiji finished, he realized that Mr. L's vital signs were very different from those taken the day before. Yesterday, Mr. L's blood pressure and pulse were much lower. Seiji used a different sphygmomanometer and stethoscope, so he thought that may be the problem.

1. What is the first action Seiji should take?
2. Should Seiji let the licensed nursing staff know about the change? If so, what should he say?
3. What should Seiji document in Mr. L's chart or electronic record?

Objectives

To achieve the objectives for this section, you must successfully:

- **describe** why height and weight measurements are important to know when providing care.
- **demonstrate** the skills needed to measure height and weight accurately and effectively for ambulatory, wheelchair-bound, and bedridden residents.

Key Terms

Learn these key terms to better understand the information presented in the section.

body mass index (BMI)
ideal body weight (IBW)
malnutrition

Questions to Consider

- How often do you weigh yourself? Do you keep track of your weight?
- Are you happy with your weight? If you are not, what changes would you like to make? How would you go about making these changes?

Why Is It Important to Measure Height and Weight?

Height and weight are usually measured on admission to a healthcare facility, during a resident's stay, and during a visit to a doctor's office. How often these measurements are taken (daily, weekly, or monthly) depends on doctors' orders for a health condition or disease. For example, a resident with kidney disease or congestive heart failure (CHF) may need to be weighed daily to help determine if he or she has *edema* (fluid build-up in the body tissues).

Height and weight measurements help healthcare staff to monitor a resident's health and determine nutritional status and medication dosages. The relationship between height and weight is also important because it can help determine a resident's overall health status. Height and weight are used to calculate ideal body weight (IBW) and body mass index (BMI). *Ideal body weight (IBW)* is the healthiest weight for an individual. *Body mass index (BMI)* is a number that determines whether a resident is a healthy weight, overweight, or underweight. This number is calculated by dividing weight in kilograms (kg)

by height in meters (m) squared. These calculations help a doctor plan calorie intake, protein, and fluid needs for a resident. Chapter 19 discusses BMI in more detail.

Measuring Height

Height can be measured in two ways. If a resident is able to walk, you can use an upright *balance scale* to measure height. If a resident is bedridden, you will need to use a tape measure. Height should be recorded in feet (') and inches (") or in centimeters (cm), depending on facility policy.

If a resident is able to walk, have the resident stand very straight on the center of the scale with arms and hands down at his or her sides. Lower the height bar until it rests on the top of the head. Read the height at the movable part of the ruler.

If a resident is bedridden, use a tape measure. If allowed, have the resident lie on his or her back, as straight as possible with arms straight at the sides and legs extended. Straighten and tighten the bedsheet. With the help of another healthcare staff member, extend the tape measure along the resident's side from the top of the head to the bottom of the heel (**Figure 15.28**). Measure the distance between the two points.

Measuring Weight

A resident's weight is often used to calculate medication dosage; accurate measurement is very important. Weight can also be a sign of certain conditions, such as *malnutrition* (poor nourishment) or edema. Weight

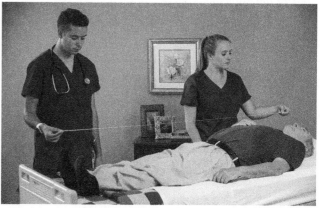

© Tori Soper Photography

Figure 15.28 To measure the height of a bedridden resident, use a tape measure.

can be measured using an upright balance or a digital scale for ambulatory residents (**Figure 15.29**). Chair and wheelchair scales may also be used. A hydraulic digital body lift or sling scale, a scale built into a bed, or a digital scale placed under the bed can be used if a resident is bedridden (**Figure 15.30**).

Weight should be measured at the same time each day. The resident should wear the same or similar clothing each time, and the same scale should be used, if possible. Be sure the resident has urinated before measurement. Always factor in additional items that may add weight, such as shoes, casts, catheters, colostomy bags, or other devices on the body. Weight should be measured in pounds (lbs) or in kilograms (kg), depending on facility policy.

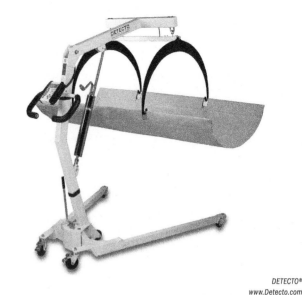

DETECTO®
www.Detecto.com

Figure 15.30 This is an example of a bed scale that can be used to weigh bedridden residents.

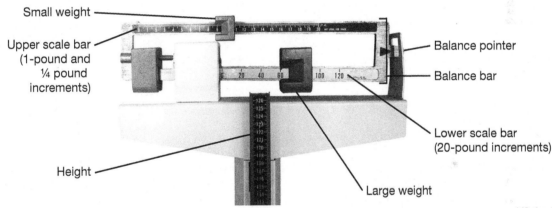

joklinghero/Shutterstock.com

Figure 15.29 A balance scale is used to measure weight. It can also measure height.

Procedure

Measuring the Height and Weight of Ambulatory Residents

Rationale

Height and weight measurements are used to calculate medication dosages and determine nutritional needs. Therefore, nursing assistants must measure and document height and weight accurately and according to facility policy.

Preparation

1. Ask the licensed nursing staff if there are doctor's orders for the procedure, if there are any specific instructions listed in the plan of care, and if the resident can be moved into the positions required for this procedure.

2. Wash your hands or use hand sanitizer before entering the room.
3. Knock before entering the room.
4. Introduce yourself using your first or preferred name and title. Explain that you work with the licensed nursing staff and will be providing care.
5. Greet the resident and ask the resident to state his or her full name, if able. Then check the resident's identification bracelet.
6. Use Mr., Mrs., or Ms. and the resident's last name when conversing.
7. Explain the procedure in simple terms, even if the resident is not able to communicate or is disoriented. Ask permission to perform the procedure.

(continued)

Measuring the Height and Weight of Ambulatory Residents *(continued)*

8. Ambulatory residents can walk to a scale placed in a central location within the facility. Bring the following items to the scale:
   • paper towel
   • a pen and pad, form, or digital device for documenting the height and weight

The Procedure

9. Provide privacy by closing the curtains, using a screen, or closing the door to the room.
10. Place a paper towel on the scale platform.
11. Raise the height bar above the level of the resident's head.
12. Help the resident remove her shoes or slippers and stand on the scale platform.
13. Ask the resident to stand up straight on the center of the scale with arms and hands down at the sides.
14. Lift the height bar, extend the arm, and then lower the arm until it rests on top of the resident's head (**Figure 15.31**).

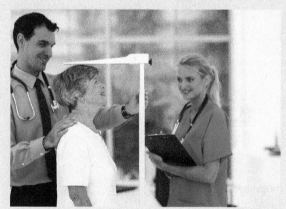

Figure 15.31   *michaeljung/Shutterstock.com*

15. Read the height at the movable part of the ruler (**Figure 15.32**).

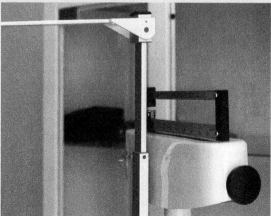

Figure 15.32   *Paolo_Toffanin/Signature collection via Getty Images*

16. Document the height on a pad, on a form, or in the electronic record.
17. Raise the height bar above the level of the resident's head. When it reaches a safe height, lower the arm and then return the height bar to its starting point.
18. Ask the resident to stand straight again with arms and hands at the sides.
19. Move the weights on the balanced scale bar to zero.
20. Move the lower and upper weights until the balance pointer is in the middle.

   > **Best Practice:** Move the large weight 50 pounds at a time until the weight bar falls. Then back the large weight up 50 pounds. Finally, move the small weight until the scale is balanced.

21. Add the amounts shown on the two bars together to determine the resident's weight (**Figure 15.33**).

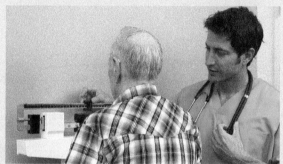

Figure 15.33   *inhauscreative/Signature collection via Getty Images*

22. Document the weight on a pad, on a form, or in the electronic record.
23. Help the resident step off the scale platform.
24. Assist the resident in putting on shoes or slippers.
25. Remove and discard the paper towel from the scale platform.
26. Assist the resident safely back to his room or bed.
27. If the resident is in bed, check to be sure the bed wheels are locked. Then reposition the resident and lower the bed.
28. Follow the plan of care to determine if the side rails should be raised or lowered.

Follow-Up

29. Wash your hands to ensure infection control.
30. Make sure the resident is comfortable and place the call light and personal items within reach.
31. Conduct a safety check before leaving the room. The room should be clean and free from clutter or spills.
32. Wash your hands or use hand sanitizer before leaving the room.

Reporting and Documentation

33. Report any specific observations, complications, or unusual responses to the licensed nursing staff. Document this information in the chart or EMR.

Procedure

Measuring the Height of Bedridden Residents

Rationale

Height measurements must be accurate for bedridden residents. The height measurement may be used when calculating medication dosages and residents' nutritional needs.

Preparation

1. Ask the licensed nursing staff if there are doctor's orders for the procedure, if there are any specific instructions listed in the plan of care, and if the resident can be moved into the positions required for this procedure.
2. Wash your hands or use hand sanitizer before entering the room.
3. Knock before entering the room.
4. Introduce yourself using your first or preferred name and title. Explain that you work with the licensed nursing staff and will be providing care.
5. Greet the resident and ask the resident to state his full name, if able. Then check the resident's identification bracelet.
6. Use Mr., Mrs., or Ms. and the resident's last name when conversing.
7. Explain the procedure in simple terms, even if the resident is not able to communicate or is disoriented. Ask permission to perform the procedure.
8. Bring the necessary equipment into the room. Place the following items in an easy-to-reach place:
   - a tape measure
   - a pen and pad, form, or digital device for documenting the height
9. You will need another person to assist in this measurement. Ask a coworker to help.

The Procedure

10. Provide privacy by closing the curtains, using a screen, or closing the door to the room.
11. Lock the bed wheels and then raise the bed to hip level.
12. Maintain safety during the procedure. If there are side rails, raise and lock the rails on the opposite side of the bed from where you will be working. Lower the rail on the side where you are working.
13. If allowed, have the resident lie on his back, as straight as possible, with his arms straight against his sides.

    | **Best Practice:** Straighten and tighten the bedsheet.

14. Extend the tape measure along the side of the resident from the top of his head to the bottom of his heel.
15. Measure the distance between the two points.
16. Document the height on a pad, on a form, or in the electronic record.
17. Check to be sure the bed wheels are locked, then reposition the resident and lower the bed.
18. Follow the plan of care to determine if the side rails should be raised or lowered.

Follow-Up

19. Wash your hands to ensure infection control.
20. Make sure the resident is comfortable and place the call light and personal items within reach.
21. Conduct a safety check before leaving the room. The room should be clean and free from clutter or spills.
22. Wash your hands or use hand sanitizer before leaving the room.

Reporting and Documentation

23. Report any specific observations, complications, or unusual responses to the licensed nursing staff. Document this information in the chart or EMR.

Procedure

Weighing Bedridden Residents Using a Hydraulic Digital Lift or Sling Bed Scale

Rationale

Weight measurements must be accurate for bedridden residents. The weight measurement may be used to calculate medication dosages and residents' nutritional needs.

Preparation

1. Ask the licensed nursing staff if there are doctor's orders for the procedure, if there are any specific instructions listed in the plan of care, and if the resident can be moved into the positions required for this procedure.
2. Wash your hands or use hand sanitizer before entering the room.

(continued)

Weighing Bedridden Residents Using a Hydraulic Digital Lift or Sling Bed Scale *(continued)*

3. Knock before entering the room.
4. Introduce yourself using your first or preferred name and title. Explain that you work with the licensed nursing staff and will be providing care.
5. Greet the resident and ask the resident to state her full name, if able. Then check the resident's identification bracelet.
6. Use Mr., Mrs., or Ms. and the resident's last name when conversing.
7. Explain the procedure in simple terms, even if the resident is not able to communicate or is disoriented. Ask permission to perform the procedure.
8. Bring the necessary equipment into the room. Place the following items in an easy-to-reach place:
   - a bed scale with the appropriate sling and attachments
   - a pen and pad, form, or digital device for recording the weight
9. You will need another person to assist in this measurement. Ask a coworker to help.

The Procedure

10. Provide privacy by closing the curtains, using a screen, or closing the door to the room.
11. Lock the bed wheels and then raise the bed to hip level.
12. Maintain safety during the procedure. If there are side rails, raise and lock the rails on the opposite side of the bed from where you will be working. Lower the rail on the side where you are working.
13. To be sure the measurement is accurate, balance the bed scale with the sling attached following the manufacturer's instructions.
14. Help the resident roll to one side. Position the sling beneath the resident's body lengthwise behind the shoulders, thighs, and buttocks. Be sure the sling is smooth.
15. Roll the resident back onto the sling and ensure that the sling is correctly positioned under the shoulders, thighs, and buttocks.
16. Center the bed scale over the bed. Carefully lower the arms of the scale and attach them securely to the sling bars.
17. Instruct the resident to keep her arms to her sides while she is being weighed.
18. Raise the sling so the resident's body and the sling hang freely over the bed.
19. Adjust the weights until the balance bar hangs freely on the end or read the digital display screen.
20. Document the weight on a pad, on a form, or in the electronic record.
21. Lower the resident back onto the bed and remove the sling.
22. Check to be sure the bed wheels are locked, then reposition the resident and lower the bed.
23. Follow the plan of care to determine if the side rails should be raised or lowered.

Follow-Up

24. Wash your hands to ensure infection control.
25. Make sure the resident is comfortable and place the call light and personal items within reach.
26. Conduct a safety check before leaving the room. The room should be clean and free from clutter or spills.
27. Wash your hands or use hand sanitizer before leaving the room.

Reporting and Documentation

28. Report any specific observations, complications, or unusual responses to the licensed nursing staff. Document this information in the chart or EMR.

Practicing Safety

Always be aware of safety issues when measuring a resident's height and weight, particularly if a resident is frail or has problems with fainting or dizziness.

Pay attention to infection control by washing your hands before and after these procedures. Document each procedure accurately and in a timely fashion. Notify the licensed nursing staff if there are any irregularities with your measurements.

HEALTHCARE SCENARIO

Bed Scales

A community hospital and health center recently purchased a new bed scale. Everyone is excited because the bed scale lets healthcare staff members easily weigh bedridden residents. The bed scale has a digital display, has a mat attached to the mattress, and is powered by a simple electrical cord. The bed scale can be left on the bed beneath the resident, if desired.

Apply It

1. What is the most important step a nursing assistant should take when using a new piece of equipment?
2. List the safety concerns the nursing assistant should be aware of when using this equipment.
3. What actions should be taken to be sure the resident is comfortable during the procedure?

SECTION 15.2 **Review and Assessment**

Key Terms Mini Glossary

body mass index (BMI) a number that uses height and weight to determine whether a person is a healthy weight, overweight, or underweight; determined by dividing weight in kilograms (kg) by height in meters (m) squared.

ideal body weight (IBW) the healthiest weight for an individual; determined primarily by height, but also takes gender, age, build, and muscular development into account using adjusted statistical tables.

malnutrition lack of proper nourishment due to inadequate or unbalanced intake of vitamins, minerals, and other nutrients or due to the body's inability to use nutrients.

Apply the Key Terms

Complete the following sentences using the key terms in this section.

1. A resident was not able to eat properly. He lacked proper nourishment and had an unbalanced intake of vitamins and minerals. The doctor was concerned that he had _____.
2. _____ uses height and weight to determine whether a person is a healthy weight, overweight, or underweight.
3. When a resident has the healthiest weight she can have for her age, gender, and muscular development, she has a(n) _____.

Know and Understand the Facts

1. Identify one purpose of measuring height.
2. Name one purpose of measuring weight.
3. What steps can be taken to make sure a resident is safe while using a bed scale?
4. What steps should be taken to be sure a resident's weight is accurate?

Analyze and Apply Concepts

1. What equipment should you assemble to measure the height of an ambulatory resident?

2. How do you measure weight using an upright, balance scale?
3. Explain how to measure the height of a bedridden resident.

Think Critically

Read the following care situation. Then answer the questions that follow.

Jessica and Juana, two nursing assistants, have been asked to weigh Mr. G using a bed scale. Mr. G was just admitted, is in pain, and has never been weighed with a bed scale. He is very overweight and tells Jessica he is embarrassed about his recent weight gain. As Jessica and Juana start to position Mr. G, Mr. G starts to cry and moan and says he does not want to be weighed.

1. How could Jessica and Juana respond to Mr. G using holistic communication skills?
2. Which is the best action for Jessica and Juana to take? Should they weigh Mr. G no matter what he does or says? Should they come back later and weigh Mr. G when he calms down? Should they tell the licensed nursing staff? Explain your choice.

Key Points

Reviewing the key points for this chapter will help you practice more safely and competently as a holistic nursing assistant and will help you prepare for the certification competency examination.

- Vital signs include temperature, pulse, respirations, and blood pressure. Vital signs provide information about health and the possible presence of a disease, infection, or injury.
- Body temperature is a person's body heat in degrees.
- Pulse measures the pressure of blood against the wall of an artery as the heart beats; it is an indicator of how well the cardiovascular system is working.
- Rate of respirations is a measurement of breathing. It indicates the quality of gas exchange and the cycle of inhalation followed by exhalation in the lungs.
- Blood pressure measures the force of blood against the body's arterial walls.
- Height and weight are used to determine medication dosage and nutritional status and can be a sign of overall health status.

Action Steps to Holistic Care

Review the information in this chapter. Complete the following activities.

1. With a partner, practice the procedure for measuring a radial pulse. Take turns practicing the procedure and evaluating each other's performance. Note any steps in the procedure that your partner performed incorrectly or forgot. Afterward, review any steps you may have performed inaccurately or forgotten.
2. Research the importance of the use of a pulse oximeter. Write a brief report describing three current facts not discussed in the chapter.

Building Math Skill

Mr. W was recently admitted to your skilled nursing facility. He is recovering from a stroke and was admitted to lose weight, improve his mobility, and stabilize his diabetes. His admission weight was 295 pounds. The doctor wants to carefully monitor his weight over the next week to see if the diet and activity plan ordered will be effective. These are the results according to Mr. W's weight log: Monday: 294; Tuesday: 293; Wednesday: 293; Thursday: 291; Friday: 292; Saturday: 292; Sunday: 291.

1. How many pounds did Mr. W lose during the first week on his diet and activity plan?
2. Which two days in a row did he have the greatest weight loss?
3. What is the percentage of weight loss since admission?

Preparing for the Certification Competency Examination

To prepare for the nursing assistant certification competency examination, you will need to know content found in this chapter. This content may be tested in the knowledge (written or oral) and skills (hands-on demonstration) portions of the exam. The following areas will be emphasized:

- normal ranges of vital signs
- purpose of taking vital signs and the factors affecting these measurements
- ways of measuring and recording body temperature, pulse (radial and apical), and respirations
- use of a pulse oximeter
- ways of measuring and recording blood pressure and any related precautions and contraindications
- ways of measuring and recording height and weight
- the importance of identifying and reporting abnormal findings

These sample test questions are similar to ones you will find on the certification competency exam. See how well you can answer them. Be sure to select the *best* answer.

1. When is the best time to count respirations?
   A. right before measuring temperature
   B. right after measuring blood pressure
   C. right after measuring pulse
   D. right before measuring pulse

2. Where is tympanic temperature taken?
   A. the axilla
   B. the anus
   C. the ear
   D. the forehead

3. A nursing assistant took Mrs. Z's blood pressure this morning and found that it was 165/110 mmHg, much higher than yesterday's measurement. What should the nursing assistant do next?
   A. take the blood pressure again and document only the second measurement
   B. take the blood pressure again and share both measurements with the licensed nursing staff
   C. document only the first blood pressure taken
   D. take blood pressure later in the day

4. Where should the stethoscope be placed when taking an apical pulse?
   A. above the diaphragm and sternum
   B. at the apex (bottom right) of the heart
   C. below the diaphragm and sternum
   D. at the apex (bottom left) of the heart

5. What is the medical term for high blood pressure?
   A. hypertension
   B. hypotachia
   C. hypotension
   D. hypertachia

6. Which of the following pulse rates is in the normal range for an adult?
   A. 52 bpm
   B. 70 bpm
   C. 125 bpm
   D. 105 bpm

7. According to Mr. Q's chart, he has a temperature of 100.8°F. What does this mean?
   A. His body temperature is low, indicating hypothermia. He should have his temperature taken again in the next few hours.
   B. His body temperature is in the normal range. No further action is required.
   C. His body temperature is high, which might mean he has a fever. He should have his temperature taken again in the next few hours.
   D. His body temperature is high, which might mean he has a fever. He should have his temperature taken again tomorrow.

8. Ms. V just ate breakfast. How long should a nursing assistant wait before measuring her oral temperature?
   A. 1–3 minutes
   B. 5–10 minutes
   C. 10–15 minutes
   D. 15–20 minutes

9. What is the level of blood pressure called when the heart muscle relaxes?
   A. embolic blood pressure
   B. diastolic blood pressure
   C. systolic blood pressure
   D. sclerotic blood pressure

10. Oxygen saturation in the blood is measured using a
    A. pulse oximeter
    B. sphygmomanometer
    C. stethoscope
    D. probe

11. How should a resident stand on a balance scale while his height is being measured?
    A. on the center of the scale with his arms at his sides
    B. facing the nursing assistant
    C. on the center of the scale with his arms raised
    D. at the back of the scale looking forward

12. Mr. A's blood pressure is 60/40 mmHg. Which of the following does he have?
    A. hypertension
    B. hypotachia
    C. hypotension
    D. hypertachia

13. Mrs. D's weight must be measured today. She is ambulatory, so the nursing assistant can use a balance scale. He should do all of the following except
    A. ask the resident to stand straight with her arms above her head
    B. move the weights on the balance scale bar to zero
    C. move the lower and upper weights until the balance pointer is in the middle
    D. add the amounts shown on the two bars to determine weight

14. A nursing assistant is taking rectal temperature. What must the nursing assistant remember about thermometer placement?
    A. The thermometer should be inserted 1½ inches into the anus and held in place for 3 to 5 minutes.
    B. The thermometer should be inserted 1 inch or less into the anus and held in place for 3 to 5 minutes.
    C. The thermometer should be inserted 1 inch or less into the anus and held in place for 2 minutes.
    D. The thermometer should be inserted 2 inches into the anus and held in place for 5 minutes or longer.

15. Ms. S has not been feeling well this morning. She states that she feels short of breath. The nursing assistant takes her pulse and it is 110 bpm. What is the medical term for a fast heart rate?
    A. bradycardia
    B. apnea
    C. dyspnea
    D. tachycardia

Did you have difficulty with any of the questions? If you did, review the chapter to find the correct answer(s).

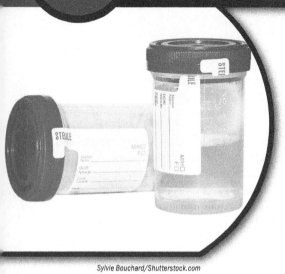

Sylvie Bouchard/Shutterstock.com

Chapter Outline

Section 16.1
Physical Examination

Section 16.2
Specimen Collection

Welcome to the Chapter

Physical examinations (PEs) are an important part of care, and nursing assistants are often responsible for preparing the equipment and supplies required for a physical examination. Physical examinations are conducted on an annual basis to check body system function and determine overall well-being. Examinations are also performed on an as-needed basis to evaluate specific complaints or injuries.

Collecting specimens is another important responsibility of nursing assistants. Specimens may be collected for diagnostic purposes or as part of a physical exam. The testing and analysis of specimens such as sputum, urine, and stool provide information for determining body system function, the presence of diseases and conditions, and monitoring well-being and the healing process.

The information and procedures presented in this chapter will help you build the knowledge and skills needed to become a holistic nursing assistant. Check with your instructor to ensure these procedures are within your state's regulations for nursing assistant practice. The topics discussed in the chapter are highlighted on the Providing Holistic Care Framework.

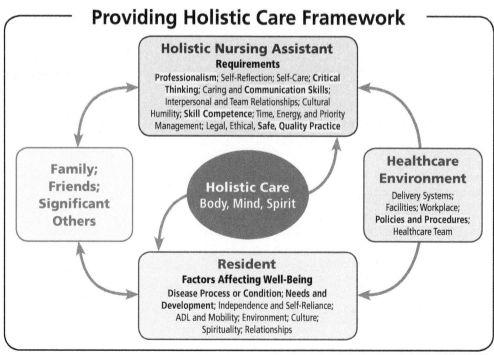

Providing Holistic Care Framework

Holistic Nursing Assistant
Requirements
Professionalism; Self-Reflection; Self-Care; **Critical Thinking**; Caring and **Communication Skills**; Interpersonal and Team Relationships; Cultural Humility; **Skill Competence**; Time, Energy, and Priority Management; Legal, Ethical, **Safe, Quality Practice**

Family; Friends; Significant Others

Holistic Care
Body, Mind, Spirit

Healthcare Environment
Delivery Systems; Facilities; Workplace; **Policies and Procedures**; Healthcare Team

Resident
Factors Affecting Well-Being
Disease Process or Condition; Needs and Development; Independence and Self-Reliance; ADL and Mobility; Environment; Culture; Spirituality; Relationships

Goodheart-Willcox Publisher

Physical Examination

Objectives

To achieve the objectives for this section, you must successfully:

- **discuss** the purpose of conducting physical examinations.
- **describe** the different types and importance of physical examinations.
- **identify** needed equipment and the draping procedures used to prepare residents for physical examinations.
- **explain** the procedure to prepare for physical examinations.

Key Terms

Learn these key terms to better understand the information presented in the section.

inspection	otoscope
laryngeal mirror	palpation
ophthalmoscope	speculum

Questions to Consider

- Think about the last time you had a physical examination. What was the reason for the examination?
- Do you wish you had known anything before, during, or after the examination?
- Were you nervous, worried, or uncomfortable about the examination? What would have made you feel more comfortable?

When and Where Are Physical Examinations Performed?

A *physical examination (PE)* is performed to determine the status or condition of body systems and functions. Some examinations may be performed annually, and others may be performed to evaluate a specific complaint or monitor a chronic disease.

Physical examinations usually take place in doctors' offices, but they may also be performed in a resident's room or exam room in a long-term care facility. In such cases, nursing assistants may prepare the room and resident for a physical examination. They may be asked to measure vital signs and drape (cover) the resident for the exam.

How Are Physical Examinations Performed?

A physical examination may be performed by a doctor, nurse practitioner, or physician assistant. These licensed healthcare providers review the resident's health history and information before beginning the examination.

Before the examination, vital signs are usually measured by a nursing assistant or medical assistant. Sometimes the healthcare provider will take vital signs. Other evaluations of body functions, called *health screening tests*, are also performed. These tests may include checking cholesterol levels, testing for osteoporosis, conducting Pap smears for female residents, and conducting prostate cancer screening for male patients. In a comprehensive exam, the healthcare provider examines each body system, starting at the resident's head and moving toward the feet. This is called a *head-to-toe examination*. The body is examined using visual *inspection* (for example, looking at the color of the skin or observing any bruising) and *palpation* (using the hands to feel an object such as a lump or mass in the body for size, shape or hardness). If a head-to-toe examination is not needed, the healthcare provider may examine only a specific body system.

What Types of Physical Examinations Are Performed?

There are several types of physical examinations:

- comprehensive, annual physical examinations, which usually include routine health screenings
- preemployment physical examinations
- travel physical examinations, which may include specific immunizations
- annual well-woman and well-man exams
- physical examinations needed to perform special diagnostic procedures or to examine specific body parts or functions

A physical examination may also be performed to screen for a disease, to evaluate a medical problem such as a respiratory issue or an injury for an early diagnosis and treatment, to update vaccinations, or to provide coaching for a healthier lifestyle.

How Do Nursing Assistants Prepare a Resident for an Examination?

Nursing assistants are responsible for preparing the exam room and gathering the needed equipment. A physical exam can also be performed in the resident's room. Depending on the type of examination, various equipment and screening tools may be needed:

- thermometer
- sphygmomanometer to measure blood pressure
- stethoscope to measure blood pressure, heart and lung sounds, and pulse
- tongue depressor to examine the throat
- *otoscope* to examine the ears (**Figure 16.1A**)
- *ophthalmoscope* to examine the eyes (**Figure 16.1B**)
- flashlight to examine pupils for dilation
- eye chart for vision screening
- *laryngeal mirror* to examine the mouth, tongue, and teeth (**Figure 16.1C**)
- tuning fork to test hearing (**Figure 16.1D**)
- percussion or *reflex hammer* to tap body parts to test reflexes (**Figure 16.1E**)
- vaginal *speculum* to examine the vagina and other parts of the female reproductive system (**Figure 16.1F**)
- nasal speculum
- sheets or drapes to cover the resident

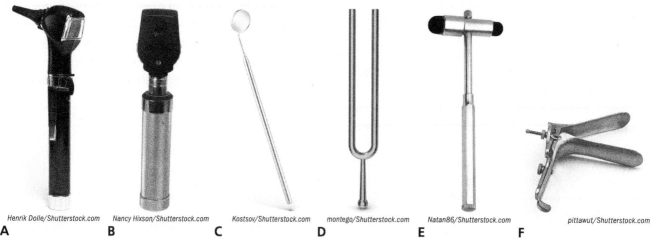

Henrik Dolle/Shutterstock.com   Nancy Hixson/Shutterstock.com   Kostsov/Shutterstock.com   montego/Shutterstock.com   Natan86/Shutterstock.com   pittawut/Shutterstock.com

A   **B**   **C**   **D**   **E**   **F**

Figure 16.1 For a physical examination, a healthcare provider may need an otoscope (A), ophthalmoscope (B), laryngeal mirror (C), tuning fork (D), reflex hammer (E), and vaginal speculum (F).

- disposable covering for the examination table
- containers for soiled instruments, gloves, tissues, and disposable covering and drapes
- disposable gloves
- lubricant
- alcohol wipes
- cotton-tipped applicators
- specimen containers and labels
- tissues
- paper towels

In some examinations, the resident stands on the floor or sits on the examining table. Draping is used to prepare for physical examinations when the resident is lying on an examining table. You learned about some of these positions in Chapter 14. The type of examination determines the positions and draping. Draping is important to prevent unnecessary exposure of the resident's body, to keep the resident comfortable, and to prevent chilling.

Draping a Resident in the Dorsal Recumbent Position

Dorsal recumbent position is used to examine the vagina or rectum. The resident lies flat on his or her back with the knees bent and feet flat on the table (**Figure 16.2**). A drape is placed in a diamond shape that covers the chest and perineal area (between the anus and scrotum on males and between the anus and vaginal opening on females).

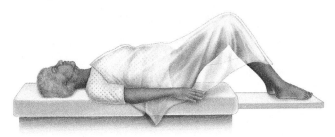
© Body Scientific International

Figure 16.2 In dorsal recumbent position, the drape should cover the chest and perineal area.

Draping a Resident in the Lithotomy Position

Lithotomy position is used to examine the vagina. The resident lies on her back, and her hips and buttocks are brought to the corners of the table (**Figure 16.3**). Her legs are bent, and her feet are placed in padded stirrups. A drape is placed in a diamond shape that covers the body, but not the head.

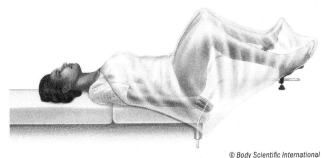
© Body Scientific International

Figure 16.3 In lithotomy position, the drape should cover the body, but not the head.

Draping a Resident in Fowler's Position

Fowler's position is often used to examine the legs and feet. The resident is seated on the table with the backrest at a 45° angle in Fowler's position (**Figure 16.4**). The legs are extended flat on the table. A drape should cover the lower abdomen and legs.

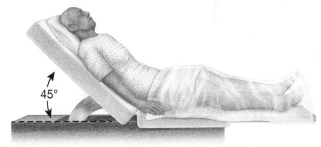
© Body Scientific International

Figure 16.4 In Fowler's position, the drape should cover the legs.

Draping a Resident in the Knee-Chest Position

Knee-chest position is used to examine the rectum. The resident kneels on the table with buttocks raised (**Figure 16.5**). The head remains on the table, the arms are extended above the head, and the elbows are bent. The head is turned to one side. A pillow under the head may provide comfort. A drape covers the back and legs.

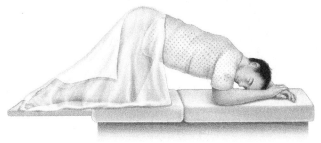
© Body Scientific International

Figure 16.5 In knee-chest position, the drape should cover the buttocks and legs.

BECOMING A HOLISTIC NURSING ASSISTANT

The Physical Examination

Several important approaches can help holistic nursing assistants prepare a resident for physical examination:

- Maintain a calm, friendly attitude. Use nonverbal communication, such as smiling or gently patting the arm, to demonstrate understanding.
- Bring the necessary paperwork or chart. If electronic health records are used, prepare the appropriate screen using a digital device.
- Cover the examining table with a disposable sheet. Prepare the equipment and instruments needed for the specific exam. Lay out the equipment and instruments so they are easy to reach during the examination.
- Prepare the drapes necessary for the exam. Have the resident remove only the clothes required by the examination. Be sure there is adequate lighting.
- Maintain excellent hand hygiene when preparing the room, when positioning and draping the resident, and after the examination is complete.
- Assist with dressing, undressing, or positioning the resident on the examination table, as needed. This is especially important for older adults.

- Be respectful when positioning and draping. Avoid unnecessary exposure of the resident. Also be aware of the room temperature. Ask if the resident needs extra drapes for comfort.
- Provide clear instructions. Be patient and be aware of the resident's level of health literacy. Use simple terms that are easily understood.
- Be sensitive to residents who are confused or who speak a different language. The resident may need an interpreter before and during the examination.
- Be aware that residents with disabilities may have difficulty moving during the examination. Maintain safety at all times and provide assistance, when needed.
- Pay attention during the examination. Some parts of the exam may be uncomfortable or painful for the resident, who may be too ill to tolerate the entire examination. Provide support if this happens.

Apply It

1. What concerns might a resident and his or her family have during an examination?
2. What approaches could you take to help lessen these concerns?

Draping a Resident in the Prone Position

Prone position is used to examine the spine and legs. The resident lies on his or her abdomen with arms and hands to each side (**Figure 16.6**). The head is turned to one side. A drape extends from the shoulders to the legs and may cover the feet.

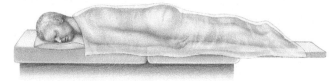

© Body Scientific International

Figure 16.6 In prone position, the drape should cover the shoulders and legs.

Draping a Resident in Sims' Position

Sims' position is usually used to examine the rectum and sometimes the vagina. It is a left side-lying position (**Figure 16.7**). The resident's left arm is bent and behind the back, while the right arm can be positioned comfortably resting on the table or pillow. The upper knee is bent, raised toward the chest, and supported by a pillow. A pillow under the bottom of the foot should make sure the toes do not touch the table. A drape extends from the shoulders to the toes.

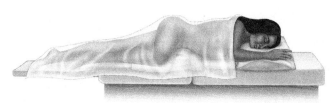

© Body Scientific International

Figure 16.7 In Sims' position, the drape should extend from the shoulders to the toes.

Draping a Resident in the Supine Position

Supine position is used to examine the front of the body and breasts. The resident lies flat on his or her back with the arms at each side (**Figure 16.8**). A drape extends from under the armpits to the toes.

When a physical examination is complete, a doctor, nurse practitioner, or physician assistant reviews the results. Recommendations are given for treatments and follow-up visits.

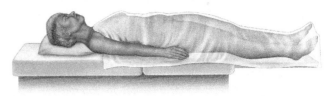

© Body Scientific International

Figure 16.8 In supine position, the drape should extend from under the armpits to the toes.

SECTION 16.1 **Review and Assessment**

Key Terms Mini Glossary

inspection the visual examination of a body part.

laryngeal mirror a medical instrument used to examine the mouth, tongue, and teeth.

ophthalmoscope a medical instrument used to examine the eyes.

otoscope a medical instrument used to examine the ears.

palpation the use of the hands to feel an object, such as a lump or mass in the body, to determine its size, location, shape, or hardness.

speculum a medical instrument used to examine the vagina or other body cavities.

Apply the Key Terms

Complete the following sentences using the key terms in this section.

1. A medical instrument used to examine the ears is called a(n) _____.
2. A(n) _____ is a medical instrument used to examine the mouth, tongue, and teeth.
3. A medical instrument used to examine the eyes is called a(n) _____.
4. The doctor used _____ to feel the swollen lump on Mr. G's leg.

Know and Understand the Facts

1. Name one purpose of conducting an annual physical examination.
2. Identify two types of examinations.
3. Identify two pieces of equipment typically used for physical examinations.

Analyze and Apply Concepts

1. Explain how to drape a resident in the supine and Sims' positions.
2. Explain how to drape a resident for the knee-chest and lithotomy positions.

3. Discuss four responsibilities a nursing assistant may have when preparing a resident for a physical examination.

Think Critically

Read the following care situation. Then answer the questions that follow.

Ms. I is a frail, 75-year-old resident at the long-term care facility where you work. This morning, she was crying and complaining about trouble breathing and itching on her abdomen and under her breasts. When you give Ms. I care, you notice a rash in those areas. When Ms. I urinates, her urine is cloudy and slightly brown. Ms. I's doctor is coming to see her this morning. When he arrives, he decides to conduct a physical examination in the exam room down the hall.

1. What is the first thing you should do to prepare for the physical examination?
2. What exam equipment do you think the doctor will need?
3. How should you position and drape Ms. I?
4. What safety measures will be most important for the physical examination?

Specimen Collection

Objectives

To achieve the objectives for this section, you must successfully:

- **explain** the purpose and importance of collecting specimens.
- **identify** the types of specimens and the tests used for analysis.
- **discuss** why accurate specimen collection is important.
- **demonstrate** the procedures for collecting sputum, urine, and stool specimens.

Key Terms

Learn these key terms to better understand the information presented in the section.

glucometer
guaiac test
occult blood
point-of-care
testing (POCT)
specimens
sputum

Questions to Consider

- Have you ever had to provide a specimen, or sample, as part of a physical examination, procedure, or to prepare for surgery? For example, have you been asked to give a doctor or nurse a small amount of urine for analysis?
- When providing a specimen, did you understand how to make sure the specimen was taken properly and did not become contaminated? Were the instructions clear? If they were not, what might the doctor or nurse have said or done differently?

Why Are Specimens Collected?

Specimens are samples of a body substance. They are collected so that specific tests can be done to provide information about a resident's health. Commonly collected specimens include *sputum* (a blend of saliva and mucus that is also called *phlegm*), urine, and stool (*feces*). There is a standard method and purpose for collecting each specimen (**Figure 16.9**). Specimens are tested and analyzed for several important reasons:

- Specimen collection is an important health screening tool that is used during a physical examination.
- Specimens can be tested to determine the presence of a specific pathogen. For example, if a urinary tract infection (UTI) is suspected, a urine specimen can help with diagnosis.
- Testing specimens can help identify the type of treatment needed (for example, the antibiotic to destroy a pathogen found).
- The results of specimen testing provide necessary information prior to a procedure or surgery, particularly if results are outside the normal range.

Specimen collection can occur in the place where a resident is receiving care. This is called *point-of-care testing (POCT)*. For example, a nursing assistant may use a medical instrument called a *glucometer* to measure blood sugar in a resident's room. Other specimens may need to go to a clinical laboratory

Specimen Collection

Specimen Type	Collection Method	Tests	Purpose
Sputum	Coughing	Routine sputum culture	To detect an infection and identify any pathogens (bacteria, viruses, or fungi)
Urine	Urination; removal from urinary catheter	Dipstick; urine straining; routine urinalysis; midstream clean catch for urine culture; 24-hour urine specimen collection	To diagnose diseases or cancer, monitor disease status or body system function, and detect the presence of medications and drugs
Stool	Feces; colostomy or ileostomy bag	Fecal occult blood test; stool culture; stool DNA test with immunochemical test	To detect blood in the stool, detect the presence of an infection, and screen for and diagnose diseases (such as colorectal cancer)

Goodheart-Willcox Publisher

Figure 16.9 The three types of specimens that are commonly collected and tested are sputum, urine, and stool.

for analysis. Specimens are sent to a laboratory in special, labeled containers with laboratory *requisition forms* (or *laboratory slips*) that are filled out by the laboratory or a licensed nursing staff member.

When results are returned from the laboratory, they will be reported within certain ranges. Results are usually communicated as *positive* (indicating the presence of an infection or disease) or *negative* (indicating that results are within normal range). The use of these terms can be confusing for residents. Some residents may think that negative results are "bad," when negative results are actually a good outcome. If a resident is confused, inform a licensed nursing staff member so he or she can follow up with the resident. It is *not* within a nursing assistant's scope of practice to explain test results to a resident.

Valid test results depend on accurate specimen collection. Because important decisions are made based on test results, the results must be accurate.

Valid results also depend on the proper and accurate labeling and handling of specimens. Information must be printed on specimen container labels. Hand hygiene must be used effectively to avoid introducing pathogens, procedures for specimen collection must be performed accurately and according to facility policy, and specimens must be properly labeled and handled effectively.

How Are Sputum Specimens Collected?

As a nursing assistant, you will likely care for residents with respiratory infections or diseases such as bronchitis, COPD, pneumonia, and tuberculosis. A *sputum specimen* is collected to identify an infection or determine if a known infection is improving or gone. A nursing assistant or respiratory therapist may collect a sputum specimen. Sputum is collected when a resident coughs.

Procedure

Collecting a Sputum Specimen

Rationale
Sputum specimens are typically collected when a resident has a respiratory disease or condition. Sputum is expelled (removed) from the lungs or bronchial tubes by coughing.

Preparation
1. Ask the licensed nursing staff if there are doctor's orders for the procedure, if there are any specific instructions listed in the plan of care, and if the resident can be moved into the positions required for this procedure.
2. Wash your hands or use hand sanitizer before entering the room.
3. Knock before entering the room.
4. Introduce yourself using your first or preferred name and title. Explain that you work with the licensed nursing staff and will be providing care.
5. Greet the resident and ask the resident to state her full name, if able. Then check the resident's identification bracelet.
6. Use Mr., Mrs., or Ms. and the resident's last name when conversing.

7. Explain the procedure in simple terms, even if the resident is not able to communicate or is disoriented. Ask permission to perform the procedure.
8. Bring the necessary equipment into the room. Place the following items in an easy-to-reach place:
   - sputum specimen container and lid (**Figure 16.10**)

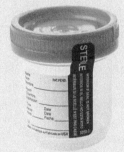

Figure 16.10   © Tori Soper Photography

   - label
   - disposable gloves
   - cup of water
   - emesis basin
   - paper towel
   - tissues
   - completed laboratory requisition form
   - specimen transport bag with a biohazard label, if needed (**Figure 16.11**)

(continued)

Collecting a Sputum Specimen *(continued)*

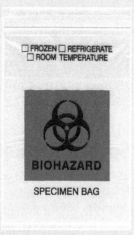

☐ FROZEN ☐ REFRIGERATE
☐ ROOM TEMPERATURE

BIOHAZARD

SPECIMEN BAG

ipkoe/Signature collection via Getty Images
Figure 16.11

9. Ask the licensed nursing staff if PPE should be worn during the procedure. If you need a face mask or other PPE, don these items according to the procedures in Chapter 8.
10. Complete the label by printing the resident's name and room number, the time and date of the specimen collection, and the doctor's name (**Figure 16.12**). Place the label on the specimen container. Some labels may request additional information, such as birth date or other identifiers. Be sure the name on the label matches the resident's identification.

> *Helen Johns*
> *Room 117*
> *0630, 8/15/2021*
> *Dr. Lynton*

Figure 16.12   *Goodheart-Willcox Publisher*

Best Practice: It is best to collect sputum specimens in the early morning, before the resident has had anything to eat.

The Procedure

11. Provide privacy by closing the curtains, using a screen, or closing the door to the room.
12. Lock the bed wheels and then raise the bed to hip level.
13. Maintain safety during the procedure. If there are side rails, raise and lock the rails on the opposite side of the bed from where you will be working. Lower the rail on the side where you are working.
14. Wash your hands or use hand sanitizer to ensure infection control.
15. Put on disposable gloves and any other PPE, as required by the licensed nursing staff.

16. Position the resident in Fowler's position or have the resident sit on the side of the bed. These positions make it easier for the resident to cough.
17. Ask the resident to rinse her mouth with water and spit into the emesis basin.

   > **Best Practice:** A steam-like mist may be used to loosen sputum prior to collection. A resident who is well hydrated prior to the collection may find it easier to cough because the fluids will help thin out the sputum.

18. Give the resident the sputum specimen container. Instruct her not to touch the inside of the container or lid. Place the lid on top of a paper towel on the overbed table.
19. Have the resident take three deep breaths with her mouth open and then cough deeply to bring up sputum. Ask the resident to cover her mouth with a tissue, using her other hand, while coughing. Then instruct her to spit the sputum into the container. Collect 1–2 tablespoons of sputum, unless otherwise instructed.
20. Put the lid on the sputum specimen container immediately.
21. Remove and discard your gloves.
22. Wash your hands or use hand sanitizer to ensure infection control.
23. Put on a new pair of disposable gloves.
24. Double-check that the specimen identified on the label matches the specimen collected.
25. Attach the requisition form to ensure that the specimen container is complete and ready for transport to the laboratory. Make sure the lid is placed tightly on the container.
26. Place the sputum specimen container in a specimen transport bag. Use a biohazard bag or label, if needed. Do not let the specimen container touch the outside of the bag.
27. Check to be sure the bed wheels are locked, then reposition the resident and lower the bed.
28. Follow the plan of care to determine if the side rails should be raised or lowered.
29. Offer the resident a glass of water and an emesis basin to cleanse the mouth. An ambulatory resident can do this in the bathroom.
30. Remove, clean, and store equipment in the proper location. Remove soiled linens and discard disposable equipment.

Follow-Up

31. Remove and discard your gloves.
32. Wash your hands to ensure infection control.
33. Make sure the resident is comfortable and place the call light and personal items within reach.
34. Conduct a safety check before leaving the room. The room should be clean and free from clutter or spills.

35. Wash your hands or use hand sanitizer before leaving the room.
36. Send or take the labeled sputum specimen container to the laboratory or another assigned location with the requisition form. Sputum must be tested before it begins to dry.

Reporting and Documentation

37. Report any specific observations, complications, or unusual responses to the licensed nursing staff. Document this information, along with the procedure, in the chart or EMR.

How Are Urine Specimens Collected?

After blood, urine is the second-most collected specimen. Urine specimens are tested in three ways:

- **Observation of clarity, color, and odor:** healthy urine is usually transparent, amber in color, and odorless. The more hydrated a resident is, the clearer urine will be. Most changes in urine color are temporary and caused by food colors or medications. However, if a resident is dehydrated, urine will be concentrated and orange in color. Any lasting abnormal urine color may be the sign of a disease or condition. For example, red urine usually indicates the presence of blood in the urine. Cloudy urine with pus or mucus might be caused by a UTI. A foul odor, such as a fishy smell, may be a sign of a bladder infection.
- **Dipstick examination:** nursing assistants may also be asked to test a urine specimen using a *dipstick reagent,* or *test strip* (**Figure 16.13**). This test typically shows if urine is concentrated or acidic or has abnormal amounts of protein, ketones, bilirubin, sugar, and white or red blood cells (evidence of blood).

- **Microscopic examination in a laboratory:** specimens or cultures are viewed through a microscope to identify substances in the urine.

Types of Urine Specimens

There are three types of urine specimens that nursing assistants may need to collect:

- **Routine specimens:** used to identify any abnormalities in different components of the urine. Once a specimen is collected, routine urinalysis identifies chemicals and medications in the urine, the presence of infection, and can help diagnose diseases (such as diabetes). Routine urinalysis is usually performed as part of a physical examination, on admission to a hospital, or before surgery.
- **Midstream specimens:** are free from pathogens (also called *clean-catch specimens*). Before collection, the perineal area is cleansed with disposable wipes or washcloths with soap and water (**Figure 16.14**). Then, the specimen is collected midway through urination after a short stream of urine has exited the urethra. This keeps microorganisms from the skin of the vagina or penis from contaminating the

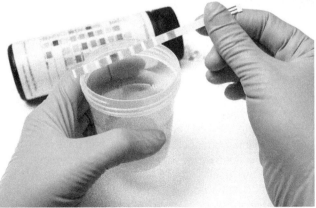

AlexRaths/Essentials collection via Getty Images

Figure 16.13 A dipstick reagent contains chemicals that change color depending on the presence of particular substances in the urine.

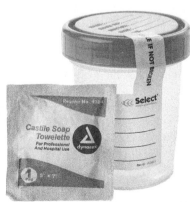

© *Tori Soper Photography*

Figure 16.14 A urine collection kit consists of a specimen container and wipe.

specimen. The last part of the stream of urine is not collected. The collection container is considered sterile. Midstream specimens are used to identify an infection as well as conditions such as kidney stones.

- **Twenty-four-hour specimens:** are usually used to check kidney function. All urine expelled over a full 24-hour period is collected. The urine is stored in a container kept in ice (**Figure 16.15**).

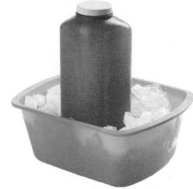

© Tori Soper Photography

Figure 16.15 A 24-hour collection container should be placed in ice.

Procedure

Collecting Urine Specimens

Rationale

Urine specimens help identify abnormalities, diseases, or infections in the urinary system. They can also identify the presence of chemicals and medications in the body. Proper collection of urine specimens is necessary to get accurate results. Various methods, including routine collection, midstream collection, and 24-hour collection, are used.

Preparation

1. Ask the licensed nursing staff if there are doctor's orders for the procedure, if there are any specific instructions listed in the plan of care, and if the resident can be moved into the positions required for this procedure.
2. Wash your hands or use hand sanitizer before entering the room.
3. Knock before entering the room.
4. Introduce yourself using your first or preferred name and title. Explain that you work with the licensed nursing staff and will be providing care.
5. Greet the resident and ask the resident to state his full name, if able. Then check the resident's identification bracelet.
6. Use Mr., Mrs., or Ms. and the resident's last name when conversing.
7. Explain the procedure in simple terms, even if the resident is not able to communicate or is disoriented. Ask permission to perform the procedure.

The Procedure: Routine Urine Specimen

8. Bring the necessary equipment into the room. Place the following items in an easy-to-reach place:
   - urinary hat (**Figure 16.16**)

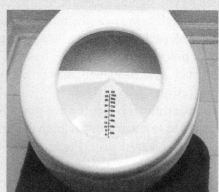

Figure 16.16 robeo/Essentials collection via Getty Images

   - bedpan or urinal and cover
   - disposable gloves
   - urine specimen container and lid
   - label
   - urine graduate
   - completed laboratory requisition form
   - specimen transport bag with a biohazard label, if needed
   - pen and form or digital device for recording the intake and output (I&O)
   - paper towel
9. Complete the label by printing the resident's name and room number, the time and date of the specimen collection, and the doctor's name. Place the label on the specimen container. Be sure the name on the label matches the resident's identification.
10. Provide privacy by closing the curtains, using a screen, or closing the door to the room.

11. Wash your hands or use hand sanitizer to ensure infection control.

12. Put on disposable gloves.

13. Have the resident urinate into a urinary hat placed in the front half of the toilet, into a bedpan, or into a urinal. Because the resident has not had much to drink yet, the first urination of the morning is best for this test. The urine will not be dilute (watered down) so any pathogens or abnormalities will be more visible.

14. Ask the resident not to have a bowel movement or to put toilet paper into the urine specimen. Provide a bag or waste container for the toilet paper.

15. If the resident used a bedpan or urinal, cover it and take it into the bathroom. If measuring the resident's input and output (I&O), pour the urine from the bedpan or urinal into a clean graduate (**Figure 16.17**). (You will learn how to measure I&O in Chapter 20.)

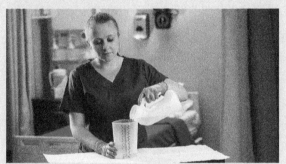

Figure 16.17   © Tori Soper Photography

16. Remove and discard your gloves.

17. Wash your hands or use hand sanitizer to ensure infection control.

18. Put on a new pair of gloves.

19. Note the total urine output amount and document it on the paper or electronic intake and output form.

20. Place a paper towel on a flat surface.

21. Remove the lid from the urine specimen container and place it, inside facing up, on the paper towel. Carefully pour about 120 mL of the urine directly from the graduate into the specimen container. If I&O is not measured, you may pour the urine directly from the urinal into the specimen container (**Figure 16.18**). To avoid contamination, do not touch the inside of the specimen container or lid.

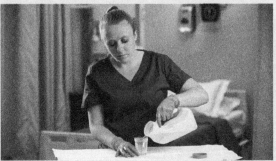

Figure 16.18   © Tori Soper Photography

22. Put the lid on the specimen container. Double-check that the specimen identified on the label matches the specimen collected. Make sure the lid is placed tightly on the container.

23. Attach the requisition form to ensure that the specimen container is complete and ready for transport to the laboratory.

24. Place the specimen container in a specimen transport bag. Use a biohazard bag or label, if needed. Do not let the specimen container touch the outside of the bag.

25. Empty the rest of the urine into the toilet.

26. Remove, clean, and store equipment in the proper location. Remove soiled linens and discard disposable equipment.

27. Remove and discard your gloves.

28. Wash your hands or use hand sanitizer to ensure infection control.

29. Put on a new pair of gloves.

30. Assist the resident with hand washing and hygiene, as needed.

31. If the resident is in bed, check to be sure the bed wheels are locked, then reposition the resident and lower the bed.

32. Follow the plan of care to determine if the side rails should be raised or lowered.

The Procedure: Midstream Urine Specimen

33. Bring the necessary equipment into the room. Place the following items in an easy-to-reach place:
    - midstream specimen kit, packaged in a sterile wrapper (including specimen container, label, disposable wipes, and disposable gloves)
    - several washcloths
    - soap
    - disposable gloves
    - completed laboratory requisition form
    - specimen transport bag with a biohazard label, if needed

34. Complete the label by printing the resident's name and room number, the time and date of the specimen collection, and the doctor's name. Place the label on the specimen container. Be sure the name on the label matches the resident's identification.

35. Provide privacy by closing the curtains, using a screen, or closing the door to the room.

36. Wash your hands or use hand sanitizer to ensure infection control.

37. Put on disposable gloves.

38. Assist the resident to the bathroom or provide a bedside commode, bedpan, or urinal.

(continued)

Collecting Urine Specimens *(continued)*

Best Practice: Explain the procedure, and if appropriate, allow the resident to collect the specimen. Otherwise, assist the resident with the procedure.

39. Have the resident clean the perineal area with disposable wipes or a washcloth, soap, and warm water. Provide assistance, if needed.
    A. **Female:** Use one hand to separate the labia with a wipe. This hand is now contaminated and should not touch anything sterile. Hold a wipe in the other hand and clean down the urethral area from front to back. Use a clean wipe for each wipe. Separate the labia to collect the urine specimen.
    B. **Male:** Hold the penis with one hand. If the penis is not circumcised, pull back the foreskin. The hand holding the penis is now contaminated and should not touch anything sterile. Clean the penis in a circular motion starting at the urethral opening. Start at the center and work outward. Use a clean wipe for each wipe.
40. Remove and discard your gloves.
41. Wash your hands or use hand sanitizer to ensure infection control.
42. Open the midstream specimen kit on the bathroom counter or on the overbed table. Open the packaging and keep the contents on top of the sterile wrapper.
43. Put on a new pair of gloves.
44. Open the specimen container and place the lid on the sterile wrapper, with the inside of the lid facing up. Open the wipes in the kit.
45. Make sure the toilet paper and specimen container are within reach.
46. Ask the resident to start a stream of urine and then stop urinating.
47. Have the resident hold the specimen container, if able, to catch the next stream of urine. Hold the specimen container yourself if the resident is unable.
48. After obtaining the specimen, remove the container before the flow of urine stops. The specimen should contain only urine that passes during the middle of urination.
49. Put the lid on the specimen container immediately. Do not allow anything to touch the inside of the container. Make sure the lid is placed tightly on the container.
50. Double-check that the specimen identified on the label matches the specimen collected.
51. Attach the requisition form to ensure that the specimen container is complete and ready for transport to the laboratory.

52. Place the specimen container in a specimen transport bag. Use a biohazard bag or label, if needed. Do not let the specimen container touch the outside of the bag.
53. Remove, clean, and store equipment in the proper location. Remove soiled linens and discard disposable equipment.
54. Remove and discard your gloves.
55. Wash your hands or use hand sanitizer to ensure infection control.
56. Put on a new pair of gloves.
57. Assist the resident with hand washing and hygiene, as needed.
58. If the resident is in bed, check to be sure the bed wheels are locked, then reposition the resident and lower the bed.
59. Follow the plan of care to determine if the side rails should be raised or lowered.

The Procedure: 24-Hour Urine Specimen

60. Bring the necessary equipment into the room. Place the following items in an easy-to-reach place:
    - a 24-hour urine collection container
    - pan and ice
    - label
    - disposable gloves
    - urinary hat
    - sign for the room to indicate a 24-hour urine collection
    - completed laboratory requisition form
    - pen and form or digital device for recording the collection and I&O
61. Complete the label by printing the resident's name and room number, the time and date of the specimen collection, and the doctor's name. Place the label on the specimen container. Be sure the name on the label matches the resident's identification.
62. Place the 24-hour urine collection container in the bathroom in a pan of ice.
63. Post a sign over the bed or in the bathroom about the specimen collection, as instructed by the licensed nursing staff.
64. Be sure the resident understands that, for the next 24 hours, all urine needs to be saved and poured into the designated container in the bathroom.
65. Provide privacy by closing the curtains, using a screen, or closing the door to the room.
66. Wash your hands or use hand sanitizer to ensure infection control.
67. Put on disposable gloves.
68. Before collection begins, the resident should urinate and discard the urine. This will make sure the bladder is completely empty and is the start of the 24-hour collection. Note the date and time on the appropriate form or in the electronic record.

69. Have the resident urinate into the urinary hat in the toilet. Ask the resident not to put toilet paper into the pan and to notify you when done. If the resident is not ambulatory, collect the urine from the bedside commode, bedpan, or urinal.
70. If the resident is on I&O, measure all the urine and document it before pouring it into the 24-hour collection container.
71. Maintain fresh ice in the pan under the specimen container.
72. At the end of the 24 hours, have the resident urinate one more time and pour the urine into the container.
73. Double-check that the specimen identified on the label matches the specimen collected. Make sure the lid is placed tightly on the container.
74. Attach the requisition form to ensure the specimen container is complete and ready for transport to the laboratory.
75. Remove the sign about the 24-hour urine collection from the room.
76. Remove and discard your gloves. Perform hand hygiene and put on a new pair of gloves.
77. Assist the resident with hand washing and hygiene, as needed.
78. Check to be sure the bed wheels are locked, then reposition the resident and lower the bed.
79. Follow the plan of care to determine if the side rails should be raised or lowered.
80. Remove, clean, and store equipment in the proper location. Remove soiled linens and discard disposable equipment.

Follow-Up
81. Remove and discard your gloves.
82. Wash your hands to ensure infection control.
83. Make sure the resident is comfortable and place the call light and personal items within reach.
84. Conduct a safety check before leaving the room. The room should be clean and free from clutter or spills.
85. Wash your hands or use hand sanitizer before leaving the room.
86. Send or take the labeled urine specimen containers to the laboratory with the requisition form or store the specimen according to instructions from the licensed nursing staff.

Reporting and Documentation
87. Report any specific observations, complications, or unusual responses to the licensed nursing staff. Document this information, along with the procedure, in the chart or EMR.

Urine Specimen Straining

Occasionally, urine specimens need to be strained. Urine straining is usually done when a resident has kidney or bladder stones that need to be retrieved for testing. Urine is collected and strained through a strainer. It continues to be strained until all stones have been collected or until a licensed nursing staff member ends the collection. The stones are put into a container and sent to the laboratory per facility policy.

How Are Stool Specimens Collected and Tested?

Three different tests may be performed to examine stool (*feces*) specimens. One is the fecal *occult blood* test, which detects blood in the stool. Stool specimens may also be used to screen for and diagnose possible infection. A third test examines stool specimens for signs of colon cancer or the presence of noncancerous *polyps*, or growths.

Procedure

Collecting a Stool Specimen

Rationale
Proper collection of a stool specimen is necessary for accurate screening and diagnosis.

Preparation
1. Ask the licensed nursing staff if there are doctor's orders for the procedure, if there are any specific instructions listed in the plan of care, and if the resident can be moved into the positions required for this procedure.
2. Wash your hands or use hand sanitizer before entering the room.

(continued)

Collecting a Stool Specimen (continued)

3. Knock before entering the room.

4. Introduce yourself using your first or preferred name and title. Explain that you work with the licensed nursing staff and will be providing care.

5. Greet the resident and ask the resident to state her full name, if able. Then check the resident's identification bracelet.

6. Use Mr., Mrs., or Ms. and the resident's last name when conversing.

7. Explain the procedure in simple terms, even if the resident is not able to communicate or is disoriented. Ask permission to perform the procedure.

8. Bring the necessary equipment into the room. Place the following items in an easy-to-reach place:
   • disposable specimen pan
   • bedpan and cover or commode
   • disposable gloves
   • stool specimen container and lid
   • label
   • toilet paper
   • wooden tongue blade
   • plastic bag or waste container for disposal
   • completed laboratory requisition form
   • specimen transport bag with a biohazard label, if needed

9. Complete the label by printing the resident's name and room number, the time and date of the specimen collection, and the doctor's name. Place the label on the specimen container. Be sure the name on the label matches the resident's identification.

The Procedure

10. Provide privacy by closing the curtains, using a screen, or closing the door to the room.

11. Wash your hands or use hand sanitizer to ensure infection control.

12. Put on disposable gloves.

13. If the resident is ambulatory, have her use the toilet in the bathroom. Ask the resident to urinate first and flush the toilet. Then ask the resident to stand. Place a disposable specimen pan in the back half of the toilet. Ask the resident to have a bowel movement into the specimen pan.

14. If the resident is not ambulatory, have her use a bedside commode or bedpan and urinate first. Discard the urine. If the resident uses a bedside commode, place a disposable specimen pan in the back half of the bucket. Then instruct the resident to have a bowel movement into the disposable specimen pan or into the bedpan.

15. Provide a plastic bag or waste container to dispose of toilet paper.

16. If a bedside commode or bedpan was used, cover the disposable specimen pan or bedpan and take it into the bathroom.

17. Use a wooden tongue blade to remove about two teaspoons of stool from the bedpan or disposable specimen pan (**Figure 16.19**). Observe the stool for color, amount, and quality. The sample should be about the size of a walnut. Try to remove stool from two different places. Include any pus, mucus, or blood present in the stool.

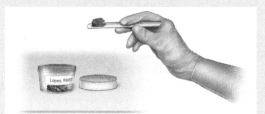

Figure 16.19 · © *Body Scientific International*

> **Best Practice:** Only formed or hardened stool can be used for the specimen. To avoid contamination, do not touch the inside of the specimen container or lid.

18. Put the lid on the specimen container. Make sure the lid is placed tightly on the container.

19. Double-check that the specimen identified on the label matches the specimen collected.

20. Attach the requisition form to ensure that the specimen container is complete and ready for transport to the laboratory.

21. Place the specimen container in a specimen transport bag. Use a biohazard bag or label, if needed. Do not let the specimen container touch the outside of the bag.

22. Wrap the wooden tongue blade in toilet paper. Discard it in a plastic bag or waste container. Empty the remaining stool into the toilet.

23. Remove and discard your gloves. Perform hand hygiene and put on a new pair of gloves.

24. Assist the resident with hand washing and hygiene, as needed.

25. Check to be sure the bed wheels are locked, then reposition the resident and lower the bed.

26. Follow the plan of care to determine if the side rails should be raised or lowered.

27. Remove, clean, and store equipment in the proper location. Remove soiled linens and discard disposable equipment.

Follow-Up

28. Remove and discard your gloves.
29. Wash your hands to ensure infection control.
30. Make sure the resident is comfortable and place the call light and personal items within reach.
31. Conduct a safety check before leaving the room. The room should be clean and free from clutter or spills.
32. Wash your hands or use hand sanitizer before leaving the room.

33. Send or take the labeled stool specimen container to the laboratory with the requisition form or store the specimen according to instructions from the licensed nursing staff.

Reporting and Documentation

34. Report any specific observations, complications, or unusual responses to the licensed nursing staff. Document this information, along with the procedure, in the chart or EMR.

Fecal Occult Blood Test (FOBT)

The *fecal occult blood test (FOBT)*, or **guaiac test**, is a POCT that can be performed at the bedside. The resident should avoid certain foods (such as red meat, horseradish, and broccoli) and medications (such as aspirin, ibuprofen, and vitamin C supplements) three days before the test. This will help prevent inaccurate results.

To perform a FOBT, you will need a *Hemoccult kit*. The Hemoccult kit contains a *Hemoccult slide*, which has front and back portions covered with a paper flap and a developer solution. During a FOBT, a stool sample is applied to special guaiac paper on the front of the Hemoccult slide. Then the back flap of the Hemoccult slide is opened, and the developer solution is applied to the back side of the paper. This solution creates a chemical reaction that shows the presence of occult blood.

Nursing assistants may not be allowed to perform this test in some states or facilities. If nursing assistants are allowed to perform this test, they should follow facility policy and package directions, along with these general steps:

1. Practice hand hygiene and standard precautions.
2. Maintain privacy and check the resident's identification.

3. Provide an explanation of the procedure you will be performing.
4. Get a Hemoccult kit, paper towel, and wooden tongue blade. Open the Hemoccult kit.
5. Label the outside of the Hemoccult slide with the resident's name, the date, and the time the specimen was collected.
6. Place a paper towel on a flat surface. Open the front flap of the Hemoccult slide, exposing the guaiac paper.
7. Using the wooden tongue blade, collect a small amount of stool from a fresh stool specimen.
8. Smear a small amount of stool in Box A on the Hemoccult slide (**Figure 16.20**).

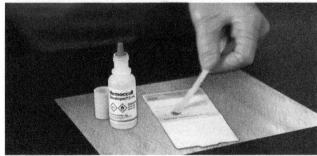

© Tori Soper Photography

Figure 16.20 A small amount of stool should be smeared on the Hemoccult slide using a wooden tongue blade.

HEALTHCARE SCENARIO
Colorectal Screening

A new colorectal screening test that uses stool samples can detect the presence of red blood cells and DNA mutations (changes) that may show certain types of abnormal growths. These abnormal growths may be a sign of cancer, such as colon cancer. Residents with positive test results are asked to undergo a diagnostic *colonoscopy* (visual examination of the colon using a scope).

Apply It

1. Why is this new test important?
2. How might this test affect the number of people who are screened for colorectal cancer?

9. Repeat the procedure using stool from a different part of the stool specimen. Smear the stool in Box B on the Hemoccult slide.

10. Close the front flap of the Hemoccult slide and turn the slide over to the back side.

11. Open the back flap of the Hemoccult slide. Apply two drops of the developer solution to each box on the guaiac paper and wait 30–60 seconds before reading the results (**Figure 16.21**). If the slide turns blue, occult blood is present in the stool (considered *guaiac positive*). If the slide does not change color, there is no occult blood in the stool (considered *guaiac negative*).

12. Dispose of the Hemoccult slide in the appropriate container, according to the facility's policy.

13. Report the results to the licensed nursing staff and document the results and care given in the chart or EMR.

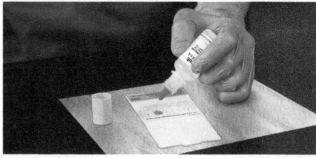

© Tori Soper Photography

Figure 16.21 The developer solution is applied to the Hemoccult slide to help detect occult blood.

SECTION 16.2 **Review and Assessment**

Key Terms Mini Glossary

glucometer a medical device that measures blood sugar levels.

guaiac test a diagnostic procedure used to identify fecal occult blood.

occult blood the presence of very small amounts of blood in the stool.

point-of-care testing (POCT) specimen collection at the place in which a resident is receiving care.

specimens samples of a body substance.

sputum a blend of saliva and mucus; also called *phlegm*.

Apply the Key Terms

An incorrect key term is used in each of the following statements. Identify the incorrect key term and then replace it with the correct term.

1. Collecting a sputum specimen is a diagnostic procedure used to help identify fecal occult blood.

2. When testing occult blood, the nursing assistant collects a blend of saliva and mucus.

3. Point-of-care testing is a specific measure to show that there is a small amount of blood in the stool.

4. A glucometer is a sample of body substances.

5. When a nursing assistant is performing a guaiac test, she is using a medical device that measures blood sugar levels.

Know and Understand the Facts

1. Explain why specimen collection is important.

2. Identify and describe three types of specimens that are collected.

3. Why is a sputum specimen collected?

4. Why is a midstream urine specimen collected?

5. Identify two reasons why accurate specimen collection is very important.

Analyze and Apply Concepts

1. Explain how to position and assist a resident when collecting a sputum specimen.

2. Describe how to clean a female resident for a midstream urine specimen collection.

3. Explain the steps to collect a stool specimen.

4. Describe the guidelines for performing an FOBT.

Think Critically

Read the following care situation. Then answer the questions that follow.

Mrs. Z was admitted to a long-term care facility last week. She is not happy about being in the facility and hopes to leave soon. She has mild dementia and a slight limp from a stroke last year. She is an anxious woman who does not often smile and complains a lot about her health. Today, Mrs. Z says she has itching and burning when she urinates. Mrs. Z's stomach has been upset for days, and she is sure she is bleeding when she has a bowel movement. Mrs. Z and her daughter want to know what you are going to do about her pain and concerns. The daughter has already called Mrs. Z's doctor.

1. What should you tell Mrs. Z you are going to do about her pain and concerns?

2. What should you be observing, given Mrs. Z's complaints?

3. If the doctor orders an FOBT and midstream urine specimen for Mrs. Z, how should you prepare Mrs. Z for specimen collection?

Key Points

Reviewing the key points for this chapter will help you practice more safely and competently as a holistic nursing assistant and will help you prepare for the certification competency examination.

- Physical examinations help determine the status of body systems and screen for and diagnose diseases.
- Specimens may be collected as part of a health screening, or to identify the presence of pathogens or necessary treatments. Valid test results depend on accurate specimen collection.
- The three most commonly collected types of specimens are sputum, urine, and stool. Sputum is collected when a resident coughs. Urine can be collected as a routine specimen, midstream specimen, or 24-hour specimen. Some urine specimens need to be strained. Stool is collected and tested in a fecal occult blood test (FOBT) or using a stool DNA test.

Action Steps to Holistic Care

Review the information in this chapter. Complete the following activities.

1. With a partner, select one type of physical examination. Prepare a poster that identifies four facts residents and the public should know.

2. With a partner, write a song or a poem about the process used to drape a resident for a physical examination. Include the reasons why this information is important.

3. Find two pictures in a magazine, in a newspaper, or online of a physical examination. Describe the type of exam, any nonverbal communication, and discuss what message is being shown about the exam.

4. Research and write a brief report describing three current facts about urine specimen collection not covered in the chapter.

5. Create a poster or digital presentation that describes each of the specimen collections discussed in the chapter. Include when, why, and how each specimen is collected, and any best practice guidelines the nursing assistant should follow for accurate collection.

Building Math Skill

Teresita is helping with a 24-hour urine specimen collection for Mrs. Y. The collection started 9 a.m. yesterday and it is now 8:45 a.m. the next day. Mrs. Y needs to urinate. Teresita makes sure Mrs. Y urinates into a hat and pours the urine into a graduate to be measured. After noting the amount, 250 mL, she pours it into the iced 24-hour urine container, which already contains 1675 mL of urine. When the 24-hour urine collection ends, how many milliliters will she record?

Preparing for the Certification Competency Examination

To prepare for the nursing assistant certification competency examination, you will need to know content found in this chapter. This content may be tested in the knowledge (written or oral) and skills (hands-on demonstration) portions of the exam. The following areas will be emphasized:

- preparation for physical examinations
- specimen collection
- standard precautions during specimen collection
- specimen sources
- tests used to examine specimens
- specimen collection procedures for sputum, urine, and stool
- accurate documentation

These sample test questions are similar to ones you will find on the certification competency exam. See how well you can answer them. Be sure to select the *best* answer.

1. Which medical instrument is used to examine the ears?
   A. ophthalmoscope
   B. glucometer
   C. otoscope
   D. speculum

2. If a doctor uses her hands to feel a body part, she is performing
   A. palpation
   B. percussion
   C. inspection
   D. observation

(Continued)

3. A nursing assistant helping Dr. James with a physical examination wants to be sure the resident, Mrs. E, is comfortable. What is the best approach the nursing assistant can take?
   A. make sure Mrs. E dresses and undresses herself
   B. double-drape Mrs. E to maintain her privacy
   C. stand behind Dr. James so Mrs. E can hear the instructions
   D. make sure the drape covers Mrs. E properly and keeps her warm

4. What makes a dipstick urine test different from other urine tests?
   A. The dipstick is checked every hour for 24 hours.
   B. The dipstick test uses a chemical strip that changes color.
   C. The dipstick test is done in a sterile environment.
   D. Urine is collected only from a urinary catheter.

5. Which position is usually used to examine a resident's legs and feet?
   A. Fowler's position
   B. prone position
   C. knee-chest position
   D. lithotomy position

6. Sputum is collected when a resident
   A. urinates
   B. coughs
   C. sneezes
   D. blinks

7. A resident was just told his test results were negative. What does this mean?
   A. The test results were within normal range.
   B. The test results were not within normal range.
   C. The test results were unclear.
   D. The test results need to be repeated.

8. How do nursing assistants use a biohazard specimen bag when collecting specimens?
   A. Nursing assistants use it to store equipment.
   B. Nursing assistants put the specimen container in it for storage.
   C. Nursing assistants put the specimen container in it for transport.
   D. Nursing assistants use it to dispose of unused items.

9. Mr. P has been having rectal bleeding, and the doctor wants to examine him. Which of the following positions may be used?
   A. prone position
   B. supine position
   C. Sims' position
   D. Fowler's position

10. How does the procedure for midstream urine collection differ from that of routine collection?
    A. The container is sterile.
    B. Only the last part of the stream is saved.
    C. The perineal area must be cleansed.
    D. Midstream collection is done only in the morning.

11. Which of the following is the one way to identify if there is blood in the stool?
    A. midstream collection
    B. stool DNA test
    C. fecal occult blood test
    D. stool culture

12. Which of the following is an example of point-of-care testing?
    A. performing a lung scan
    B. taking a blood pressure
    C. having a bowel culture
    D. using a glucometer

13. What might a nursing assistant be asked to do to retrieve a kidney or bladder stone from urine?
    A. culture the urine
    B. strain the urine
    C. store the urine
    D. heat the urine

14. The doctor wants to examine Ms. R's eyes. Which medical instrument will he need?
    A. ophthalmoscope
    B. glucometer
    C. otoscope
    D. speculum

15. Mr. L is having a 24-hour urine collection. What is the most important action to take to get an accurate test result?
    A. The container should be shaken.
    B. The container should have a lid.
    C. The container should be kept warm.
    D. The container should be kept iced.

Did you have difficulty with any of the questions? If you did, review the chapter to find the correct answer(s).

17 Restful Environment

Welcome to the Chapter

When people are admitted to a long-term care facility, they enter a different and unknown environment. Holistic nursing assistants who are familiar with the organization of residents' rooms will be best able to help residents feel more comfortable. In this chapter, you will learn about typical room arrangements, call light use, and ways to respond to requests. You will also learn about the types of beds used in healthcare facilities, and how to make an occupied, unoccupied (closed and open), and surgical bed. Holistic nursing assistants can promote comfort by establishing an environment that is relaxing, is restful, and encourages sleep. One way to create a relaxing and restful environment is to give residents back rubs.

The information and procedures presented in this chapter will help you build the knowledge and skills needed to become a holistic nursing assistant. Check with your instructor to ensure these procedures are within your state's regulations for nursing assistant practice. The topics discussed in the chapter are highlighted on the Providing Holistic Care Framework.

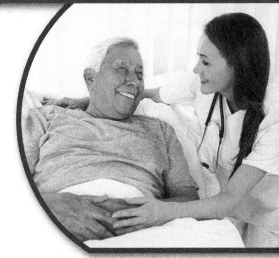

Andrey_Popov/Shutterstock.com

Chapter Outline

Section 17.1
The Resident's Room

Section 17.2
Promoting Comfort, Relaxation, Rest, and Sleep

Providing Holistic Care Framework

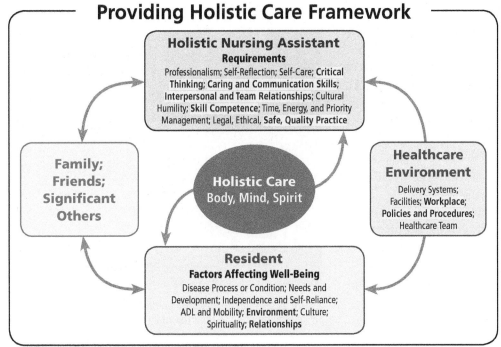

Holistic Nursing Assistant
Requirements
Professionalism; Self-Reflection; Self-Care; **Critical Thinking; Caring and Communication Skills; Interpersonal and Team Relationships;** Cultural Humility; **Skill Competence;** Time, Energy, and Priority Management; Legal, Ethical, **Safe, Quality Practice**

Family; Friends; Significant Others

Holistic Care
Body, Mind, Spirit

Healthcare Environment
Delivery Systems; Facilities; **Workplace; Policies and Procedures;** Healthcare Team

Resident
Factors Affecting Well-Being
Disease Process or Condition; Needs and Development; Independence and Self-Reliance; ADL and Mobility; **Environment;** Culture; Spirituality; **Relationships**

Goodheart-Willcox Publisher

The Resident's Room

Objectives

To achieve the objectives for this section, you must successfully:

- **identify** the equipment typically found in a resident's room.
- **explain** how to respond to communication call systems.
- **describe** the different types of beds commonly found in healthcare facilities.
- **demonstrate** how to make an occupied, unoccupied, and surgical bed.

Key Terms

Learn these key terms to better understand the information presented in the section.

bath blanket
disposable
  protective pad

draw sheet
traction

Questions to Consider

- Think about the last time you visited someplace new. Did you feel out of place or lost? Did you experience any feelings of fear, confusion, or insecurity?
- What helped you feel better? Did anyone help you? If so, what did he or she say or do?

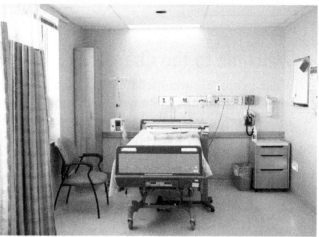

Tyler Olson/Shutterstock.com

Figure 17.1 Like most rooms in a healthcare facility, this room contains a chair, overbed table, bedside stand, and privacy curtain.

What Does a Resident's Room Look Like?

Rooms in healthcare facilities are often arranged in a similar manner. Most healthcare facilities do not have a lot of space, so rooms are designed as efficiently as possible. Rooms must be arranged to meet the needs of the healthcare providers and the residents (**Figure 17.1**).

Most facilities offer private or semiprivate rooms. A private room holds only one resident, and a semiprivate room holds two residents. Rooms often include separate bathrooms with safety features such as handrails, and a small closet or wardrobe to store personal items.

To provide residents with privacy, curtains enclose the area around the bed. A half curtain may provide privacy between two residents in a room, or a full curtain may surround each personal area. In some private rooms, a curtain near the doorway may maintain privacy from people in the hallway. When there are no curtains, screens may be used.

Room Equipment

Each room will have a bed, sometimes called a *hospital bed* due to its style and function (not to the type of facility). A movable *overbed table* is used for personal care and can hold a meal tray. A *bedside stand*, which may be movable or built into the wall, usually holds personal items and supplies. One or two chairs are normally located next to the bed. On the wall opposite the bed, there may be a communication board, which contains important information that is updated each shift (**Figure 17.2**). Most rooms also have a television.

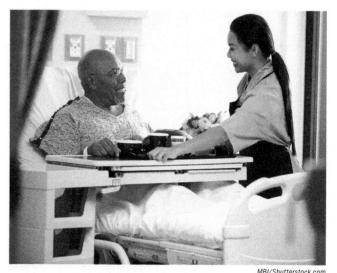

MBI/Shutterstock.com

Figure 17.2 If the resident will be eating in his room, the overbed table may be used to hold the meal tray.

Many times rooms in long-term care facilities look like a bedroom in a home (**Figure 17.3**). This is because residents often stay in a facility for a long time. Residents have the right to use personal items, including furniture, as space permits and as long as they do not interfere with the rights, health, and safety of other residents. A call light is usually placed near or on the bed so residents can communicate with healthcare providers.

Many rooms have equipment or lighting attached to the wall behind the bed. This may include oxygen and blood pressure equipment. Other equipment or supplies may be needed because of a resident's disease or condition. These supplies may include extra towels or blankets, *traction* equipment (weights, pulleys, and tape that help treat muscular and skeletal disorders), a blood pressure machine, or a bedside commode for residents who cannot easily walk to the bathroom.

Call Lights

As you learned in Chapter 4, answering a call light quickly and keeping it within the resident's reach helps keep residents safe. Use of a call light can prevent residents from wandering, becoming confused, or unsafely getting out of bed. There are many types of communication systems, and they can be wired or wireless (**Figure 17.4**). Call lights are found in resident rooms, and emergency call lights are also found in resident bathrooms, usually near the toilet.

Sometimes it may seem like a resident uses a call light too often or unnecessarily. Frequent call light use may be the result of fear or anxiety, past experiences with long wait times, or boredom. No

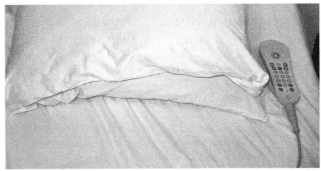

Wards Forest Media, LLC

A

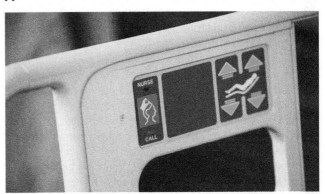

© Tori Soper Photography

B

Figure 17.4 There are many different types of call lights: A—handheld remote; B—call button integrated into the side rail on a bed.

matter how many times there is a call, remember that the resident is in need. It is your responsibility to respond and deliver safe, quality care. Regular rounding may also reduce unnecessary call light use, as residents know they will interact with the staff periodically throughout each shift.

What Types of Beds Are Used in Healthcare Facilities?

There are two different bed types that permit a resident's position to be changed in bed: electric and manual. An *electric bed* can be raised or lowered and allows the head and foot to be repositioned. Controls for an electric bed may be at the side of the bed, in a

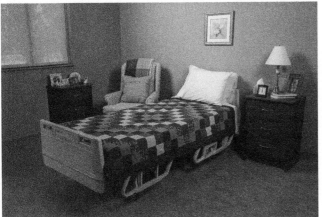

© Tori Soper Photography

Figure 17.3 In a long-term care facility, a resident's room may be arranged to look like a typical bedroom with storage and furnishings.

THINK ABOUT THIS

The average wait time for a response to a call light is five minutes. The next time you are in pain or need to go to the bathroom, watch a clock and wait five minutes before doing anything. What impact did waiting five minutes have? Did you want to do something before the time was up? How do you think a resident feels waiting so long for a response?

BECOMING A HOLISTIC NURSING ASSISTANT

Answering Call Lights

These guidelines will help improve the quality of care you provide, will promote resident safety and comfort, and will reduce the number of unnecessary calls. In facilities, a call light may cause a light to turn on above or on the side of the door to the resident's room and may be accompanied by a ringing sound outside the room. In other facilities, staff members carry mobile electronic devices, such as pagers or cell phones, which receive the alert.

When you answer a call light, do so quickly and according to facility policy and procedure. If the call comes from a resident's bathroom, consider it an emergency and respond immediately. Be courteous when responding to the call. Many call lights now have an intercom that allows nursing staff members to talk to the resident. If you use the intercom, make sure you can be heard. Do not rely only on the intercom to respond to a resident's needs. If the call comes from a bathroom, never use the intercom. Go directly to the room.

When you enter a resident's room, be polite and attentive to the resident's requests. If you feel the resident has inconvenienced you, your body language may tell the resident how you feel. Be sure your nonverbal communication is as considerate as your words.

The following guidelines can help you respond well to and reduce a resident's need to use the call light:

- Observe the resident's position and ask if the resident is comfortable each time you leave the room. Reposition the resident, if needed.
- Make sure the resident can reach the call light. For example, if a resident has a weak left arm and hand, place the call light on his or her right, or stronger, side.
- Put the telephone, TV remote control, and bed light switch within the resident's reach.
- Place the overbed table next to the bed, if needed.
- Position the tissue box and drinking water so they can be easily reached.
- Put the waste container next to the bed.
- Ask about the resident's pain level. If the resident is experiencing pain, notify the licensed nursing staff immediately.

Before leaving the room, ask the resident if there is anything else you can do before you go. Be sincere and show interest in the resident's response. If appropriate, remind the resident that you (or another member of the nursing staff) will be back again to check on him or her during your shift.

Apply It

1. A resident has used the call light five times in the last hour. When you answered the last call light, the resident requested ice for his water and help picking up a piece of paper he could not reach. When the call light goes on for the sixth time, what should you do?
2. What actions can you take to help reduce a resident's frequent use of the call light?

---

hand controller, or sometimes at the foot of the bed. This type of bed can allow residents to control their positions.

Manual beds are not used as often as electric beds. The position of a manual bed is changed by turning a crank located at the end of the bed. For safety reasons, the crank must be in the down position when not in use. Some types of specialty beds are made for residents over 500 pounds or to eliminate pressure points.

Beds have wheels at each corner that can be locked or unlocked using a foot lever by each wheel or a lever under the bed near the wheels (**Figure 17.5**). Beds also have a mattress that may be covered with plastic. Beds in some long-term care facilities may not have side rails or may have an ambulatory assist rail (to help the resident get in and out of bed). If the bed does have side rails, these may span the length of each side of the bed, may be found only at the top of the bed, or at the top and bottom of the bed

(**Figure 17.6**). Side rails can be raised or lowered with a release lever.

Because different brands of beds may be used in the same facility, take time to locate all lock and release levers each time you deliver care.

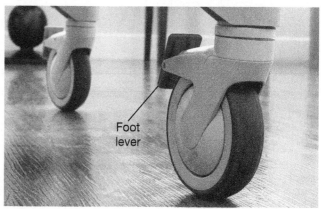

Foot lever

Figure 17.5 Each bed wheel has a foot lever that locks or unlocks it.

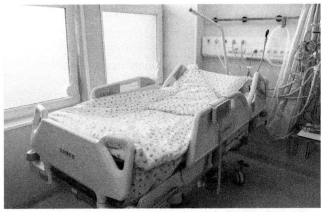

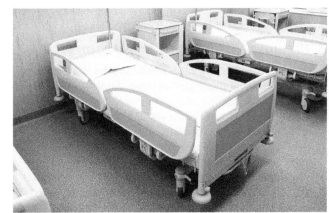

A

B

Figure 17.6 Many beds have side rails that may span only the top of the bed (A) or the full length of the bed (B).

What Is the Proper Way to Make a Bed?

As a nursing assistant, you will be making *occupied beds*, or beds with residents in them, because residents are *bedridden*, (they are not able to get in or out of bed). If a resident is bedridden, you will need to change the linens while the resident is still in bed. You also need to know how to make *unoccupied* and *surgical beds*. Unoccupied beds can be made closed or open. If a bed will not be occupied for an extended period of time, it should be made *closed* with the top linens pulled up. A closed bed may also be made in preparation for a new admission. *Open* beds have the top linens pulled down because they will soon be occupied. If a resident has left her bed for the day, the bed should be remade open. An open bed promotes comfort and allows the resident to get in and out of bed easily.

There are times when you will be asked to make a surgical bed. A surgical bed has linens opened lengthwise (**Figure 17.7**). This allows for a safe and comfortable transfer.

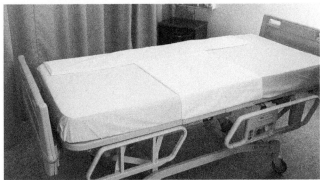

Figure 17.7 When a surgical bed is made, it allows for easy and safe transfer of the resident in and out of bed.

Linens

Before you begin making a bed, familiarize yourself with the linens you will be using. Some healthcare facilities use only bottom and top flat sheets to make beds; however, many facilities now use a fitted bottom sheet and flat top sheets. In addition to flat and fitted sheets, blankets, and pillowcases, you may use the following special types of linens and bed coverings:

- *Draw sheet*: also called a *pull sheet*, *turning sheet*, or *lift sheet*, this sheet is either smaller in size than a regular-size flat sheet or is a flat sheet folded in half. It is placed lengthwise over the middle of the bottom sheet. A draw sheet has several uses. It can keep the mattress and bottom sheets dry and can be used to turn or move a resident in bed.
- *Bath blanket*: this regular-size blanket is usually made from cotton or another absorbent material and is used to keep residents warm during a bed bath. It may also be used as a protective covering to maintain resident modesty and warmth during various procedures.
- *Disposable protective pad*: sometimes called an *incontinence pad*, this small, often multi-layered, leakproof, highly absorbent pad is made from washable cotton or a disposable, paperlike material. It is placed under a resident's buttocks and on top of the draw sheet. Disposable protective pads are used to promote the comfort of incontinent residents, absorb drainage, and prevent the bed from becoming soiled during procedures.

Personal Space and Possessions

Personal space is the area around a person in which he or she feels most comfortable. An unfamiliar person entering this space may feel threatening. When residents are in a new place or are frightened or sick, they tend to become withdrawn and narrow their personal space. Personal items become a very important part of their personal space. Residents may be concerned about the security of their personal items in different and unfamiliar environments. This is particularly true for older adults. They may also keep their personal items close to them. It is not unusual for a resident to keep a favorite blanket or family photo close. The narrowing of personal space is often a defense mechanism and is meant to protect the resident and his or her personal items. Residents from certain cultures may especially value particular religious objects and other special possessions. Do not move these items out of the way, go through them, or store them without permission. Move items carefully so they will not fall or break.

Apply It

1. Have you ever had to be very close to other people, such as in a crowded elevator? How did you feel? Were you uncomfortable? If so, what did you do?
2. Do you position special items in a certain way? If so, has someone ever moved these items? How did that feel?

Mitered Corners

When making a bed, a flat or fitted bottom sheet may be used, depending on facility preference. If a flat sheet is used, make the bed with mitered corners. This prevents skin irritation or rubbing by keeping the flat sheet tucked securely and neatly under the mattress. **Figure 17.8** shows the process of making a mitered corner.

Mitered Corners

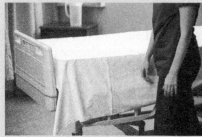

A. Tuck the top of the flat sheet underneath the head of the mattress and the bottom of the sheet underneath the foot of the mattress. The sides of the sheet should remain untucked.

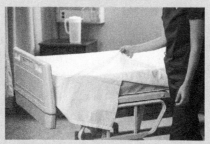

B. Start at one corner of the bed. Grasp the hem of the sheet with one hand, approximately a foot in from the end of the bed, and pull it up vertically, creating a triangle. Place the triangle on top of the mattress.

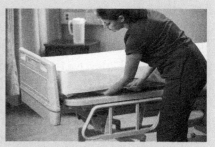

C. Tuck the hanging, or bottom, part of the sheet underneath the mattress with both hands.

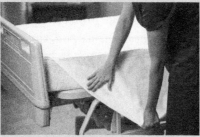

D. Lift the triangle corner of the sheet off the mattress with one hand and tightly pull it down toward the floor. Smooth out any wrinkles with your other hand.

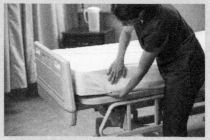

E. Tuck the sheet under the mattress tightly with one hand, while smoothing out the mitered corner with the other hand. Miter each corner of the bed.

Figure 17.8 Mitered corners should be used with a flat bottom sheet, top sheet, and bedspread.

Pillowcases

Changing a pillowcase is an important part of making a bed. A pillowcase is often covered with pathogens. Changing the pillowcase regularly and when it appears to be soiled is an important part of infection prevention and control.

To change a pillowcase when the resident is in bed, ask the resident to raise his or her head and assist, if needed. The resident may have more than one pillow on his or her bed. If possible, leave a pillow under the resident's head while you change another pillowcase. If there is only one pillow, keep the resident flat in bed after removing it to avoid neck injury. Discard the used pillowcase in the laundry hamper. To maintain infection prevention and control, do not shake the pillowcase or pillow and do not let them touch your scrubs.

A pillowcase can be changed in two ways (**Figure 17.9**). There is no best method. Often nursing assistants select the method that is easiest or most comfortable, or simply continue using the method they learned first.

Guidelines for Bed Making

Whether you are making an open, closed, or surgical bed, the following guidelines can help you provide holistic care and promote safety:

- Pay attention to the condition of the bed. Are the linens very wrinkled or messy? Are the linens soiled? If so, remake the bed with fresh, clean linens.
- Always ask for help if you need it. You may need help if making a bed containing an overweight resident.
- If residents have dressings, tubes, or an IV, be sure not to dislodge these devices when changing the linens.

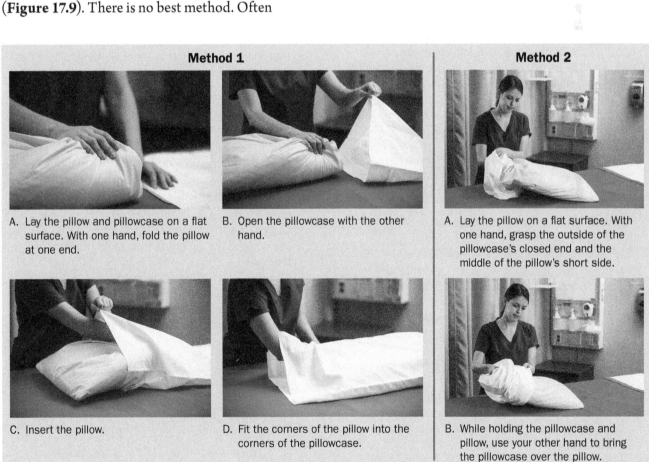

Method 1

A. Lay the pillow and pillowcase on a flat surface. With one hand, fold the pillow at one end.

B. Open the pillowcase with the other hand.

C. Insert the pillow.

D. Fit the corners of the pillow into the corners of the pillowcase.

Method 2

A. Lay the pillow on a flat surface. With one hand, grasp the outside of the pillowcase's closed end and the middle of the pillow's short side.

B. While holding the pillowcase and pillow, use your other hand to bring the pillowcase over the pillow.

© Tori Soper Photography

Figure 17.9 There are two methods for changing a pillowcase that may be used in healthcare facilities.

- Be mindful of fragile skin as you move a resident in bed and make sure the skin is not scraped or bruised.
- Make sure the bed linen is not too tight around and on top of the feet, particularly if the resident is an older adult. To prevent this from happening, create a *toe pleat*. Fold the linen at the top of the resident's feet. Then grasp the fold and lift it gently so the resident can move his or her feet freely (**Figure 17.10**).
- Always follow facility policy and consider safety and comfort during and after bed-making procedures.

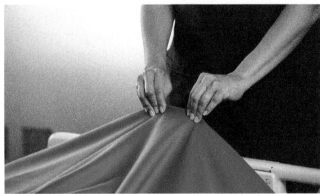

© Tori Soper Photography

Figure 17.10 A toe pleat can prevent bed linens from being too tight around and on top of the feet.

Procedure

Making an Occupied Bed

Rationale

An occupied bed is made when a resident is not able or permitted to be out of bed. Making an occupied bed provides an opportunity to observe the resident's skin. Alert the licensed nursing staff if you observe any redness, sores, or decubitus ulcers.

Preparation

1. Ask the licensed nursing staff if there are doctor's orders for the procedure, if there are any specific instructions listed in the plan of care, and if the resident can be moved into the positions required for this procedure.
2. Wash your hands or use hand sanitizer before entering the room.
3. Knock before entering the room.
4. Introduce yourself using your first or preferred name and title. Explain that you work with the licensed nursing staff and will be providing care.
5. Greet the resident and ask the resident to state his full name, if able. Then check the resident's identification bracelet.
6. Use Mr., Mrs., or Ms. and the resident's last name when conversing.
7. Explain the procedure in simple terms, even if the resident is not able to communicate or is disoriented. Ask permission to perform the procedure.
8. Bring the necessary equipment into the room. Place the following items in an easy-to-reach place:
   - laundry hamper
   - 1 bath blanket
   - 1 bottom sheet (flat or fitted)
   - 1 top, flat sheet
   - 1 cotton draw sheet, if needed
   - 1 disposable protective pad, if needed
   - 1 bedspread, if used
   - 2 blankets
   - pillowcases, depending on how many pillows are being used

   Best Practice: Once you bring linens into a room, the linens cannot be used for another resident, not even a roommate. Never bring in more linens than you need. Remove any unused linens, as they are considered contaminated.

The Procedure

9. Provide privacy by closing the curtains, using a screen, or closing the door to the room.
10. Lock the bed wheels and then raise the bed to hip level.
11. Maintain safety during the procedure. If there are side rails, raise and lock the rails on the opposite side of the bed from where you will be working. Lower the rail on the side where you are working.
12. Be sure any tubing, such as IVs or urinary drainage bags, is not moved, pulled out of place, or kinked during or after the procedure.

    Best Practice: Wear disposable gloves only if required for infection prevention and control.

13. Arrange the clean linens in the order they will be used.
14. Remove the call light from the bed.
15. Make sure the bed is flat, unless otherwise indicated by the plan of care.

16. Loosen the top linens from the foot of the bed.

Best Practice: Never shake any linens, whether they are clean or dirty. Shaking them can spread pathogens.

17. Place the bath blanket over the top linens (blanket and top sheet).
18. Ask the resident to hold the top edge of the bath blanket, or tuck it under the resident's shoulders.
19. Remove the top linens from under the bath blanket. Be careful not to expose the resident.
20. Place the top linens in the laundry hamper.
21. Make the bed one side at a time. If the mattress has slipped out of place, ask a coworker to help you move it to the head of the bed before continuing.
22. Ask the resident to turn toward the side of the bed farthest from you and grasp the side rail, if used.
23. Help the resident turn, if necessary. Keep the resident covered with the bath blanket.
24. Move the pillow with the resident and adjust it under the head for comfort.
25. Starting at the head of the bed, loosen the soiled bottom linens. Remove and dispose of the disposable protective pad, if used.
26. Roll the soiled bottom linens toward the resident and tuck them against his back (**Figure 17.11**). *Note:* The bath blanket has been removed in these images to show the procedure more clearly.

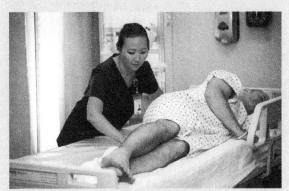

Figure 17.11 © Tori Soper Photography

27. Place a clean bottom sheet on top of the mattress. If using a fitted bottom sheet, pull the corners of the sheet tightly and smoothly over the corners of the mattress. Smooth the sheet and tuck it tightly under the top and side of the mattress. If using a flat sheet, place the center fold next to the resident. The narrow hem should come to the foot edge of the mattress. Tuck the top of the sheet under the head of the mattress. Make a mitered, or square, corner and tuck the sheet under the side of the mattress, working toward the foot of the bed.

28. If used, position the draw sheet with the center fold next to the resident. Tuck it under the mattress.
29. Ask the resident to roll toward you and over all of the soiled linens. Assist the resident, if needed. Move the pillow and bath blanket with the resident.
30. Raise and lock the side rail, if used. Then go to the opposite side rail and lower it.
31. Remove the soiled bottom linens by rolling the edges inward and toward you. Put the soiled linens in the laundry hamper.

Best Practice: Never allow soiled linens to touch your scrubs.

32. Pull the clean bottom sheet into place as quickly as possible (**Figure 17.12**). If using a fitted bottom sheet, pull the corners of the sheet tightly and smoothly over the corners of the mattress. Smooth the sheet and tuck it tightly under the top and side of the mattress. If using a flat sheet, tuck the sides under the mattress at the head and foot of the bed. Make a mitered corner at each end. Pull the sheet tight and tuck it under the mattress from top to bottom.

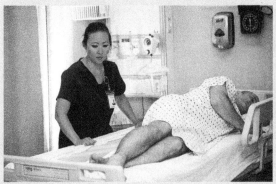

Figure 17.12 © Tori Soper Photography

33. If used, pull the draw sheet tight and tuck it in. Place a disposable protective pad on top of the draw sheet and under the resident's buttocks, if needed.
34. Ask the resident to lie on his back in the center of the bed. Assist him into this position if he cannot move himself.
35. Change the pillowcases and place the pillows under the resident's head. Discard the used pillowcases in the laundry hamper.

Best Practice: When changing pillowcases, help the resident move his head, if needed. Have the resident raise his head when you remove the pillow and help, if needed. When the pillow is removed, keep the resident flat in bed to avoid neck injury.

36. Place the clean top sheet over the resident.

(continued)

Making an Occupied Bed *(continued)*

37. Remove the bath blanket. Discard the bath blanket in the laundry hamper.
38. Place the blanket and bedspread (if used) on the resident. Tuck these in at the bottom of the bed and make mitered corners.
39. If needed, create room for the toes by making toe pleats in the top linens.
40. Recheck that any tubing is in place. If you have any concerns, ask a licensed nursing staff member to check that the IV or other tubing is working properly. If the resident has a urinary drainage bag, be sure it is positioned below the bladder.
41. Once the resident is positioned comfortably, lower the bed.
42. Follow the plan of care to determine if the side rails should be raised or lowered.

Follow-Up
43. Wash your hands to ensure infection control.
44. Make sure the resident is comfortable and place the call light and personal items within reach.
45. Conduct a safety check before leaving the room. The room should be clean and free from clutter or spills.
46. Wash your hands or use hand sanitizer before leaving the room.

Reporting and Documentation
47. Report any specific observations, complications, or unusual responses to the licensed nursing staff. Document this information, along with the care provided, in the chart or EMR.

Procedure

Making an Unoccupied Bed

Rationale
An unoccupied bed may be made open or closed. A closed bed is made with the top linens pulled to the head of the bed. An open bed is made with the top linens fanfolded at the foot of the bed.

Preparation
1. Wash your hands or use hand sanitizer before entering the room.
2. If the room is occupied, knock before entering. If you know the room is vacant, skip ahead to step 7.
3. Introduce yourself using your first or preferred name and title. Explain that you work with the licensed nursing staff and will be providing care.
4. Greet the resident and ask the resident to state his or her full name, if able. Then check the resident's identification bracelet.
5. Use Mr., Mrs., or Ms. and the resident's last name when conversing.
6. Explain the procedure in simple terms, even if the resident is not able to communicate or is disoriented. Ask permission to perform the procedure.
7. Bring the necessary equipment into the room. Place the following items in an easy-to-reach place:
   - laundry hamper
   - mattress pad, if used
   - 1 bottom sheet (flat or fitted)
   - 1 top sheet
   - 1 cotton draw sheet, if needed
   - 1 disposable protective pad, if needed
   - 1 bedspread, if used
   - 2 blankets
   - pillowcases, depending on how many pillows are being used

The Procedure
8. Lock the bed wheels and then raise the bed to hip level or a comfortable working level. Lower the side rails, if present.

   Best Practice: Wear disposable gloves only if required for infection prevention and control.

9. Arrange the clean linens in the order they will be used.
10. Remove the soiled linens by rolling the edges inward. Deposit them in the laundry hamper.

    Best Practice: Never allow soiled linens to touch your scrubs.

11. If the mattress has slid down, move it back to the head of the bed.
12. To save time and energy, work on one side of the bed until that side is complete. Then go to the other side of the bed.
13. If used, place the mattress pad even with the top of the mattress and unfold it. Pull the corners of the mattress pad tightly and smoothly over the corners of the mattress.
14. Place the bottom sheet on top of the mattress pad. Unfold the sheet lengthwise. The center fold should be in the middle of the bed, and the hem stitching should face the mattress pad. The small hem should be at the foot of the bed.

15. If using a fitted bottom sheet, pull the corners of the sheet tightly and smoothly over the corners of the mattress. Smooth the sheet and tuck it tightly under the top and side of the mattress. If using a flat sheet, make a mitered corner. Tuck the sheet in at the head of the bed and along the side of the bed to the foot. Repeat this step on the other side of the bed.

16. If used, place a draw sheet on the bed (**Figure 17.13**). Tuck it under the mattress. Place a disposable protective pad on top of and in the center of the draw sheet.

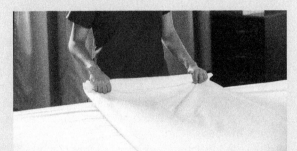

Figure 17.13   © Tori Soper Photography

17. Unfold and apply the top sheet with the wrong side up. Place the hem even with the upper edge of the mattress and the center fold in the center of the bed.

18. Keeping the blanket centered, spread it over the top sheet and foot of the mattress. Do the same with the bedspread, if used.

19. Tuck the top sheet, blanket, and bedspread (if used) under the mattress at the foot of the bed.

20. If making a closed bed, make a mitered corner at the foot of the bed and tuck in the sides of the top sheet, blanket, and bedspread, if used (**Figure 17.14**). Fold the top sheet back over the blanket to make an 8-inch cuff at the head of the bed.

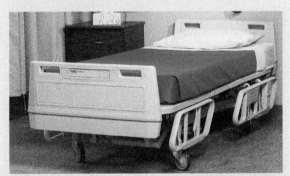

Figure 17.14   © Tori Soper Photography

21. If making an open bed, do not tuck in the sides of the bedspread (if used), blanket, and top sheet. Instead, face the head of the bed and grasp these linens with both hands. Fanfold the bed linens to the foot of the bed (**Figure 17.15**). Smooth the hanging sheet on both sides of the bed.

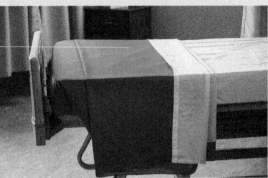

Figure 17.15   © Tori Soper Photography

22. Insert the pillows into the pillowcases.

23. Place the pillows at the head of the bed. The open ends of the pillowcases should face away from the door.

24. Check to be sure the bed wheels are locked, then lower the bed to its lowest position.

Follow-Up

25. Wash your hands to ensure infection control.

26. Place the call light on the bed.

27. Replace the bedside stand next to the bed if it was moved to make the bed.

28. Place the chair in its assigned location.

29. Place the overbed table over the foot of the bed, opposite the chair.

30. Take the laundry hamper to the proper location.

31. Conduct a safety check before leaving the room. The room should be clean and free from clutter or spills.

32. Wash your hands or use hand sanitizer before leaving the room.

Reporting and Documentation

This is an accepted, standard procedure. It does not need to be reported or documented.

Procedure

Making a Surgical Bed

Rationale

Properly arranging bed linens when a surgical bed is needed to promote a quick and smooth transfer.

Preparation

1. Wash your hands or use hand sanitizer before entering the room. You do not need to knock, because the room will be unoccupied.
2. Bring the necessary equipment into the room. Place the following items in an easy-to-reach place:
   - laundry hamper
   - mattress pad, if used
   - 1 bottom sheet (flat or fitted)
   - 1 top sheet
   - 1 draw sheet, if needed
   - disposable protective pad, if needed
   - 1 bedspread, if used
   - 2 blankets
   - pillowcases, depending on how many pillows are being used

The Procedure

3. Lock the bed wheels and then raise the bed to hip level or a comfortable working level.

   Best Practice: Wear disposable gloves only if required for infection prevention and control.

4. Arrange the clean linens in the order they will be used.
5. Strip the bed and deposit used linens in the laundry hamper.
6. Wash your hands or use hand sanitizer to ensure infection control.
7. Make the bottom layer of the bed like an unoccupied, closed bed. Start by placing the mattress pad, if used, even with the top of the mattress and unfolding it. Pull the corners of the mattress pad tightly and smoothly over the corners of the mattress.
8. Place the bottom sheet on top of the mattress pad. Unfold the sheet lengthwise. The center fold should be in the middle of the bed, and the hem stitching should face the mattress pad. The small hem should be at the foot of the bed.

9. If using a fitted bottom sheet, pull the corners of the sheet tightly and smoothly over the corners of the mattress. Smooth the sheet and tuck it tightly under the top and side of the mattress. If using a flat sheet, make a mitered corner. Tuck the sheet in at the head of the bed and along the side of the bed to the foot.
10. If used, place a draw sheet on the bed. Tuck it under the mattress. Place a disposable protective pad on top and in the center of the draw sheet, if needed.
11. Make the top layer of the bed like an unoccupied, closed bed, but do not tuck in the bottom sheet, blanket(s), and bedspread. Start by unfolding and applying the top sheet with the wrong side up. Place the hem even with the upper edge of the mattress so the center fold is in the center of the bed.
12. Keeping the blanket centered, spread it over the top sheet and foot of the mattress. Do the same with the bedspread, if used.
13. Fold the top linens back from the foot of the bed and onto the bed, even with the edge of the mattress.
14. Fanfold the top linens lengthwise away from the side of the bed where the stretcher will be placed. (The stretcher is usually positioned on the side of the bed nearest the door.) This leaves that side of the bed open to receive the patient.
15. Put the pillowcases on the pillows according to procedure and place the pillows upright against the headboard. This will help prevent the patient's head from hitting the headboard during transfer from the stretcher to the bed.
16. Leave the wheels of the bed locked and raise the bed to its highest position.
17. Leave both side rails down.
18. Move furniture away from the bed to make room for the stretcher.

Follow-Up

19. Place the call light on the bedside stand or under the pillow until the patient comes to the room.
20. Return the laundry hamper to the proper location.
21. Conduct a safety check before leaving the room. The room should be clean and free from clutter or spills.
22. Wash your hands or use hand sanitizer before leaving the room.

Reporting and Documentation

This is an accepted, standard procedure. It does not need to be reported or documented.

How Can Nursing Assistants Promote a Healing Environment?

One of your most important responsibilities as a holistic nursing assistant is to promote and maintain a healing environment. A *healing environment* is one that pays attention to the individual rights of residents and humanizes their experience. Part of promoting a healing environment is understanding how rooms are arranged, responding to call lights, and making sure the resident's bed is made properly with clean linen. As you learned in Chapters 3 and 4, federal and state laws, regulations, and standards also protect resident rights and outline care requirements. The following guidelines include these laws, regulations, and standards and will help you promote a safe, healing environment for residents:

- Always try to respond to resident preferences.
- Organize the room to be sure residents stay safe.
- Keep the resident's room clean. If you see something on the floor, pick it up using gloves or a paper towel. Always wash your hands after throwing something away.
- Maintain proper temperature and ventilation in resident rooms. OBRA regulations require that room temperature be kept between 71°F and 81°F. Older adults may want the room to be on the warm side of that range. Keeping the door open or opening a window can provide airflow, if appropriate.

- Reduce odors in resident rooms. Proper ventilation can help prevent odors from becoming an issue. Odor control may be needed after elimination, during dressing changes, and if there are soiled linens.
- Keep noise to a minimum. A quiet environment promotes healing. Residents can use headphones to watch television or listen to music.
- Check for enough safe electrical outlets to prevent the use of extension cords.
- Provide sufficient lighting so that residents can read easily and function even with impaired vision. Lighting should not be so glaring that it is uncomfortable.
- Make sure residents are able to use the telephones in their rooms comfortably and privately.
- Look at the seating in the room. It should be at the right height to support residents and allow for easy wheelchair transfer.
- Keep the room free from clutter and allow enough space for the resident to get up and ambulate or freely maneuver with ambulation equipment.
- Pay attention to any physical disabilities and provide the required equipment. For example, you may need to provide adaptive devices for reaching for or picking up items.
- Respect the resident's personal items. Do not move a personal item without a reason or the resident's permission.
- Above all, be respectful and treat residents with dignity.

HEALTHCARE SCENARIO

Facility Design

Last week, a local architecture firm received a best design award for its work on the community's long-term care facility. The firm is known for its work in healthcare and employs two nurses to provide information about resident needs. To win this award, the facility design needed to be beneficial to residents, promote a healing environment, and meet the needs of a long-term stay. Firms that competed for this award were asked to reconfigure the arrangement of resident rooms and redesign the nurses' station, dining room, and recreation rooms in the long-term care facility. Many of the residents in the long-term care facility are over the age of 80, have lived in the facility with their spouses for at least one year, and use a walker or wheelchair.

Apply It

1. What areas do you think the firm concentrated on to respond to residents' needs effectively?
2. How do you think resident rooms should be arranged to make sure they have a safe and comfortable environment?
3. How do you think the dining room and recreation rooms should be designed to respond to residents' needs?
4. What features do you think would promote a healing environment for these residents?

SECTION 17.1 Review and Assessment

Key Terms Mini Glossary

bath blanket a blanket, usually made from cotton or another absorbent material, that keeps a resident warm during a bed bath; may also be used as a protective covering to maintain resident modesty and warmth during various procedures.

disposable protective pad a pad that is small, often multilayered, leakproof, and highly absorbent; can be placed under the buttocks of incontinent residents, used to absorb drainage, or used during procedures to prevent the bed from becoming soiled; also called an *incontinence pad*.

draw sheet a small, flat sheet or a regular-size flat sheet folded in half and placed lengthwise over the middle of the bottom sheet of the bed; is used to help turn a resident in bed; also called a *pull sheet*, *turning sheet*, or *lift sheet*.

traction weights, pulleys, and tape used to exert a slow, gentle pull; used to treat a muscular or skeletal disorder, such as a fracture, and to bring displaced bones back into place.

Apply the Key Terms

Identify the key term used in each sentence.

1. The nursing assistant used a draw sheet—a small, flat sheet or regular-sized sheet folded in half—to help turn a resident in bed.
2. A multilayered, leakproof, and highly absorbent disposable protective pad is placed under the resident's buttocks to absorb drainage and to prevent the bed from becoming soiled.
3. When a nursing assistant wants to maintain resident modesty and keep the resident warm, she will use a bath blanket made from cotton or another absorbent material.
4. Traction exerts a slow, gentle pull using weights, pulleys, and tape to treat muscular or skeletal disorders.

Know and Understand the Facts

1. List three types of equipment typically found in a resident's room.
2. Explain the primary function of a call light.
3. Identify three different types of linens used when making a bed.
4. Identify three important guidelines for making beds.
5. Describe how to make a mitered corner.
6. Select one method for changing a pillowcase, and then describe the procedure.
7. Explain why it is important to create a toe pleat after making an occupied bed.

Analyze and Apply Concepts

1. Explain when and how to respond to a call light.
2. What can be done if a resident seems to be overusing the call light system?

3. Describe the differences between making an occupied and unoccupied bed.
4. List four guidelines for promoting a healing environment.

Think Critically

Read the following care situation. Then answer the questions that follow.

Farah has been asked to make Mrs. G's bed. Mrs. G has diabetes and is quite overweight. She is bedridden today after a procedure to clean a wound on her leg. The wound now has a dressing, and Mrs. G also has an IV. Farah knows she will need to make an occupied bed. Farah also knows that Mrs. G is not always comfortable being taken care of and is protective of her personal possessions.

1. Which steps of the bed-making procedure should Farah be especially aware of when making Mrs. G's bed?
2. How should Farah handle Mrs. G's IV and dressing as she makes the bed?
3. Given that Mrs. G has diabetes and is overweight, are there any special steps Farah should take during and after the bed-making procedure?
4. What should Farah do to keep Mrs. G comfortable during care and maintain respect for her personal possessions?

Promoting Comfort, Relaxation, Rest, and Sleep

Objectives

To achieve the objectives for this section, you must successfully:

- **discuss** how comfort, relaxation, rest, and sleep contribute to healing and better health.
- **describe** ways holistic nursing assistants can provide comfort, and promote relaxation, rest, and sleep.
- **demonstrate** how and when to give appropriate and effective back rubs.

Key Terms

Learn these key terms to better understand the information presented in the section.

dysrhythmia
fatigue

hallucinations
sleep deprivation

Questions to Consider

- Sleep is an important part of maintaining a healthy life balance. How many hours do you sleep each night? Do you get too little, too much, or just the right amount of sleep?
- If you do not get enough sleep, what keeps you from sleeping? Is lack of sleep something you developed recently or have you experienced it your whole life? Have your sleeping patterns affected your life while awake?
- If you want to change your sleeping patterns, what could you do differently?

How Can Nursing Assistants Provide a Comfortable, Relaxing Environment?

Providing a comfortable environment is an important part of giving holistic care. Residents find comfort in different ways. It is a personal experience. They may see an object, the presence of family and friends, a particular food, or the memory of good health as comforting. For those who have chronic pain, remembering a time when they were pain-free can bring comfort.

Comfort

To promote and give comfort, holistic nursing assistants must observe for levels of comfort. Holistic nursing assistants should ask residents what is comfortable for them. Be sensitive to any culturally relevant issues related to comfort, identify and perform actions that promote comfort, and ask if these actions are effective.

Holistic nursing assistants can create a healing environment by providing books or magazines to read, suggesting social activities of interest, encouraging residents to spend time with family members, turning on a favorite television program, playing music, repositioning residents, or suggesting a nap. Keeping noise levels down is also an important part of promoting a comfortable environment. Regular exposure to a noisy environment can lead to hearing impairment and loss and hypertension.

In Chapter 10, you learned about the importance of relieving pain to achieve comfort. Helping residents with pain relief is an important part of holistic care and will promote comfort.

Relaxation

Relaxation is another important part of healing. Relaxing reduces stress hormones and provides a healthy internal and external environment.

Relaxation is a personal experience. What some people find relaxing may not be relaxing for others. For example, some people find exercise relaxing, while others think it is tiring and stressful. When a resident is seriously ill or in pain, it may be challenging to relax.

Some pain-relief approaches, such as deep breathing and soothing music, can help a resident relax. One technique is *mindful presence,* the practice of checking your body for thoughts and feelings of stress and then consciously letting go of these stressful feelings and thoughts. Many people also find yoga or meditation relaxing. As a holistic nursing assistant, you can relax by showing residents you feel grateful for each day, laughing out loud, giving a reassuring smile, and simply providing a human touch. These actions may result in residents feeling relaxed as well. In response, residents may sigh, let out a deep breath, sit back, loosen their shoulders, and laugh and smile back at you (**Figure 17.16**).

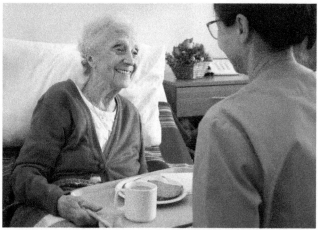

FredFroese/Signature Collection via Getty Images

Figure 17.16 If you are relaxed, residents will sense that and feel more comfortable in their environment.

Why Are Rest and Sleep Important?

There is a difference between rest and sleep, but both rest and sleep are very important to health and well-being. *Rest* can occur at any time and is usually the result of *fatigue* (extreme tiredness). *Sleep*, however, is necessary for survival and must occur daily. Sleep restores the body's energy, helps repair muscle tissue, and releases hormones that promote growth in children and young adults.

Circadian Rhythm

The body has a natural sleep-wake cycle called *circadian rhythm*. Circadian rhythm is controlled by structures in the brain that help regulate sleepiness and wakefulness over 24 hours. Circadian rhythm responds to light, causing people to sleep when it is dark and be awake when it is light. As people age, their circadian rhythm can change, causing residents to develop sleep problems or disorders. Residents who have vision problems and cannot detect light may also have trouble sleeping due to disrupted circadian rhythm.

Sleep Deprivation

When people get too little sleep, they may experience **sleep deprivation**. Recent research has found that one in three adults does not get the recommended seven hours of sleep each night. When people get too little sleep, they usually need even more sleep to make up for loss of sleep. Insufficient sleep causes a person to be drowsy and makes it difficult to concentrate.

Ongoing sleep deprivation can cause memory problems and unsafe physical performance. It can also cause mood swings and **hallucinations** (visual, verbal, or physical perceptions that are not real, but are mistaken for reality). Sleeping problems are common among people with heart disease, diabetes, Alzheimer's disease, stroke, cancer, and mental disorders such as depression and schizophrenia. Sleep deprivation can increase a person's risk for obesity, headaches, and epileptic seizures.

The quality of sleep is important to health. During sleep, a person goes through five stages of sleep and then keeps cycling through them. The number of sleep cycles (each lasting about 90–110 minutes) a person has and the lengths of the sleep stages can be affected by a person's age; the time of day or night; recent amounts of sleep, exercise, and stress; and environmental conditions (such as room temperature and lighting).

Sleep Disorders

Nearly 70 million people in the United States have sleep disorders. The most common sleep disorders are insomnia, sleep apnea, narcolepsy, and restless legs syndrome (RLS). Sleep disorders can have significant effects on residents and their mobility, ability to manage ADLs, and general health and well-being.

Insomnia

Insomnia is a sleep disorder that causes people to not be able to fall or stay asleep. One in 10 US adults has *chronic insomnia*, which is defined as one episode of sleeplessness each week. Between 20 and 30 percent of adults experience temporary insomnia at any given time. Sleep medications may be prescribed to treat insomnia, but insomnia is best helped by healthy sleep habits.

Sleep Apnea

Interrupted breathing during sleep is called *sleep apnea* or *obstructive sleep apnea*. Sleep apnea may cause periodic gasping, snorting, or snoring. For about 10–20 seconds, a person may struggle to breathe. Blood oxygen will decrease, and the person will wake up enough to resume breathing. This may occur many times during the sleep cycle, leaving people with feelings of irritability, depression, and a morning headache.

People with sleep apnea have increased risks for stroke or heart attack. Sleep apnea may be the result of obesity and can be treated through losing weight or sleeping on the side. A *continuous positive airway pressure (CPAP) machine* can help with breathing by increasing pressure on the throat, preventing it from collapsing (**Figure 17.17**). Surgery may be needed to treat sleep apnea in some cases. People with sleep apnea should not take sleep medications that prevent them from waking during the night. In the United States, approximately 12–18 million people have sleep apnea, and one-quarter of these people are middle-age men.

Narcolepsy

Severe daytime sleepiness with uncontrollable, sometimes sudden periods of sleep is called *narcolepsy*. Signs of narcolepsy include sudden loss of voluntary muscle control and feelings of weakness ranging from slurred speech to collapse, hallucinations, or sleep paralysis. Episodes of narcolepsy are sometimes called *sleep attacks*. These attacks may last several seconds or minutes during the day. After episodes end, recovery is usually rapid.

Narcolepsy is usually treated with prescription medications that help people avoid falling asleep at inappropriate times. Scheduled naps are also helpful.

Restless Legs Syndrome (RLS)

Restless legs syndrome (RLS) causes an unpleasant creeping, crawling, and prickling sensation in the legs and feet. This feeling makes people want to move their legs to find relief. One in 10 people in the United States have RLS, which is usually inherited.

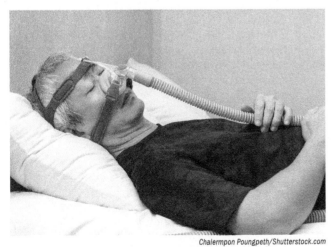

Chalermpon Poungpeth/Shutterstock.com

Figure 17.17 The CPAP machine helps treat sleep apnea by preventing the throat from collapsing.

Constant leg movements, aches, and pains can make it challenging to fall and stay asleep, leading to insomnia. Symptoms can occur at any age, but RLS is more common among older adults. RLS can often be relieved with prescription medications.

Healthy Sleep Habits

Good sleep habits can help people get the sleep they need. Some good sleep habits include the following:

- Set a regular schedule for going to sleep and waking up.
- Limit the number and length of naps during the day. A short nap may be restful, but too many naps can make it hard to sleep at night.
- Avoid large meals, caffeinated drinks (coffee or tea), chocolate, and soft drinks before going to bed. Some medications may also cause sleeplessness.
- Relax before bed and sleep in a comfortable, quiet, and dark environment with a temperature conducive to sleep.
- Use restful activities such as warm baths, deep breathing, and activities that lead to relaxation and sleep.
- Read or listen to music to encourage sleep.
- Exercise during the day, but not during the five to six hours before going to sleep.

Evening Care

Helping residents feel relaxed is particularly important in the evening, before residents go to bed. Holistic nursing assistants can help create a relaxing, restful environment by providing evening care, or *p.m. care*, and giving a back rub.

Evening care typically includes routine vital signs, if ordered; assisting with elimination and measuring output; helping with hygiene and oral care; and assisting in changing soiled pajamas and linen. Other duties may include straightening bed linens; arranging pillows and assistive devices; and providing fresh drinking water, unless the resident is NPO (*nothing by mouth*) for an ordered procedure the next day (**Figure 17.18**).

Back Rubs

Giving a *back rub*, if appropriate, is another common nursing assistant responsibility. A back rub should *not* be performed without permission from

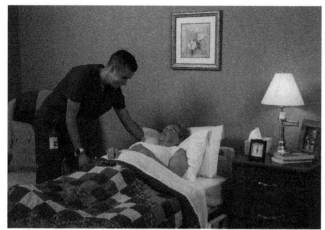

© Tori Soper Photography

Figure 17.18 Evening care helps get a resident ready to go to bed. Evening care should promote relaxation and comfort at the end of the day.

the doctor or licensed nursing staff; if the resident refuses; or if there are burns on the back, rib or spinal fractures, pulmonary embolism, or open wounds. If the resident has hypertension or *dysrhythmia* (abnormal heart rhythm), measure the resident's pulse and blood pressure to be sure it is safe to give a back rub. Back rubs can be given during morning or evening care, after a bath, or after changing a resident's position.

Maintaining privacy during care is very important. For example, close the curtains around the resident. While giving care, talk with residents about the day's activities and experiences. Ask residents about their health or treatments, any problems they may have, their feelings, and any pain. Report residents' answers (particularly related to pain levels and difficulty sleeping) to the licensed nursing staff and document important details. Some residents may want to listen to music, read, or watch television prior to sleeping. Leaving the lights or any electronics on can disturb the sleep cycle. Make sure radio or television volumes are at a reasonable level and that controls are in reach. Also ask if the resident would like any other personal items nearby.

Evening care helps promote physical and emotional well-being at the end of the day. Be gentle and talk in soft tones when giving care.

Procedure

Giving a Back Rub

Rationale

Back rubs stimulate circulation to the skin and muscles, relieve muscle tension and stiffness, promote comfort and relaxation, help relieve pain, and offer nursing assistants an opportunity to observe the resident's skin for any redness or decubitus ulcers.

Preparation

1. Ask the licensed nursing staff if there are doctor's orders for the procedure, if there are any specific instructions listed in the plan of care, and if the resident can be moved into the positions required for this procedure.
2. Wash your hands or use hand sanitizer before entering the room.
3. Knock before entering the room.
4. Introduce yourself using your first or preferred name and title. Explain that you work with the licensed nursing staff and will be providing care.
5. Greet the resident and ask the resident to state his full name, if able. Then check the resident's identification bracelet.
6. Use Mr., Mrs., or Ms. and the resident's last name when conversing.
7. Explain the procedure in simple terms, even if the resident is not able to communicate or is disoriented. Ask permission to perform the procedure.
8. Bring the necessary equipment into the room. Place the following items in an easy-to-reach place:
   - a basin of warm water (100–105°F)
   - 1 hand towel
   - 2 bath towels
   - 1 bath blanket
   - body lotion (one the resident has used before or one that will not irritate the skin)
   - disposable gloves
   - laundry hamper

   Cover the overbed table with the hand towel and then place the needed equipment and linens on top of the overbed table.

The Procedure

9. Provide privacy by closing the curtains, using a screen, or closing the door to the room.

Best Practice: You should explain the procedure to the resident before starting. During the back rub, however, you may not want to talk with the resident. Silence can help create a relaxing environment. Pay special attention to the resident's behavior, attitude, responses to the procedure, and interactions with you.

10. Lock the bed wheels and then raise the bed to hip level.
11. Maintain safety during the procedure. If there are side rails, raise and lock the rails on the opposite side of the bed from where you will be working. Lower the rail on the side where you are working.
12. Be sure any tubing, such as IVs or urinary drainage bags, are not moved or pulled out of place or kinked during or after positioning.

Best Practice: Wear disposable gloves only if required for infection prevention and control.

13. Place the lotion bottle in the basin of warm water.
14. Make sure the room is at a comfortable temperature. Dim the lights, if appropriate.
15. Cover the resident with the bath blanket. If possible, ask the resident to hold the bath blanket while you fanfold the bed linens to the foot of the bed. Be sure the resident is not exposed.
16. If permitted, help the resident turn to the prone position. Otherwise, move him to a side-lying position facing away from you. Use whichever position is most comfortable and appropriate for the resident.
17. Expose the resident's back. Keep the rest of the body covered with the bath blanket.
18. Check the skin for signs of redness. Pay special attention to the coccyx (*tailbone*) and bony areas.
19. Pour a small amount of lotion into the palm of your hand. Rub your hands together and use friction to continue warming the lotion.
20. Keep your knees slightly bent and your back straight to maintain good body mechanics. Apply the warm lotion to the resident's back.
21. Starting from the sacral area, make small, circular motions with the palms of your hands (**Figure 17.19**). Stroke upward on both sides of the spine and be sure to always apply pressure *away* from the spine. Move your hands up to the back of the neck.

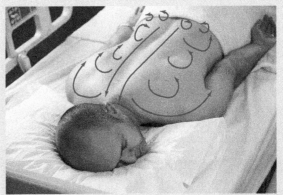

Figure 17.19   © Tori Soper Photography

22. Next, use firm, smooth strokes across and around the shoulders. Move down the upper arms, applying less pressure than on the shoulders.
23. Finally, using a circular motion, move your hands from the shoulders down the sides of the back to the buttocks.

Best Practice: Massage gently and move slowly to help the resident relax. Ask if you are applying too much or too little pressure during the back rub. Do not massage painful or red areas and stop if the resident complains of numbness or tingling in the arms and legs or if the lotion causes a rash or feeling of itchiness.

24. Repeat the procedure for 3 to 5 minutes, adding more warm lotion as needed. Complete the back rub by providing long, gentle strokes up from the lower back to the base of the neck and down again several times.
25. After completing the back rub, gently remove any excess lotion and pat the resident's skin dry with the bath towel.
26. Close or change the resident's gown or pajama top. Remove the bath blanket, straighten the linens, and tighten the bottom sheet.
27. Recheck that any tubing is in place. If you have any concerns, ask a licensed nursing staff member to check that the IV or other tubing is working properly. If the resident has a urinary drainage bag, be sure it is positioned below the bladder.
28. Check to be sure the bed wheels are locked, then reposition the resident and lower the bed.
29. Follow the plan of care to determine if the side rails should be raised or lowered.
30. Remove, clean, and store equipment in the proper location. Remove soiled linens and discard disposable equipment.

(continued)

Giving a Back Rub *(continued)*

Follow-Up

31. Wash your hands to ensure infection control.
32. Make sure the resident is comfortable and place the call light and personal items within reach.
33. Conduct a safety check before leaving the room. The room should be clean and free from clutter or spills.

34. Wash your hands or use hand sanitizer before leaving the room.

Reporting and Documentation

35. Report any specific observations, complications, or unusual responses to the licensed nursing staff. Document this information, along with the care provided, in the chart or EMR.

SECTION 17.2 **Review and Assessment**

Key Terms Mini Glossary

dysrhythmia an irregular or abnormal heart rhythm.

fatigue a feeling of extreme tiredness or exhaustion.

hallucinations visual, verbal, or physical perceptions of objects that are not real, but are mistaken for reality.

sleep deprivation a loss or deficiency of the recommended hours of sleep.

Apply the Key Terms

An incorrect key term is used in each of the following statements. Identify the incorrect key term and then replace it with the correct term.

1. Fatigue is an irregular or abnormal heart rhythm.
2. Mr. L has dysrhythmia. He tells the nursing assistant that he has visual, verbal, or physical perceptions of objects that are not real, but he thinks they are.
3. Hallucinations are a loss or deficiency of the recommended hours of sleep.
4. When a resident has dysrhythmia, he has a feeling of extreme tiredness or exhaustion.

Know and Understand the Facts

1. Describe two ways sleep contributes to health.
2. Discuss three actions holistic nursing assistants can take to promote and provide comfort and relaxation.
3. Describe one sleep disorder.
4. Name three good sleep habits.
5. Discuss two ways holistic nursing assistants can help promote relaxation.
6. How does circadian rhythm affect sleep?
7. When is performing a back rub inappropriate?

Analyze and Apply Concepts

1. Discuss why rest and sleep are important for older residents.
2. What are the responsibilities of providing evening or p.m. care?
3. Describe two best practices for performing a back rub.

Think Critically

Read the following care situation. Then answer the questions that follow.

Ms. M, an 82-year-old frail resident, had a stroke three months ago. The stroke caused her to fall, leaving her with a concussion and fractured right hip. She is making good progress but her mobility is limited. She seems to be depressed about her immobility and complains frequently that she cannot sleep at night, and is too uncomfortable to rest or relax during the day.

1. What do you know about rest and sleep that might help Ms. M?
2. What are three actions you could take to help her rest and sleep?
3. Describe the evening care you can provide Ms. M.

Key Points

Reviewing the key points for this chapter will help you practice more safely and competently as a holistic nursing assistant and will help you prepare for the certification competency examination.

- As a nursing assistant, you must promote and maintain a healing environment in the resident's room and create an atmosphere that responds to residents' rights and humanizes their experiences.
- Call lights should always be available and within easy reach for the resident. Answer the call light immediately, no matter how frequently it is used.
- Healthcare facilities have beds that can be repositioned electronically or manually. Bed wheels can be locked and unlocked with a foot lever.
- Occupied, unoccupied, and surgical beds must be made according to procedure. When making a bed, consider safety, ask for help, and take special care with residents who have dressings, tubes, IVs, or fragile skin.
- Promoting comfort, rest, relaxation, and sleep is necessary for healing and well-being.

Action Steps to Holistic Care

Review the information in this chapter. Complete the following activities.

1. Prepare a short paper or digital presentation that describes how call systems should be used to make sure there is a safe environment for residents.
2. Research recently developed call light technology and create a poster or digital presentation outlining two new types of technology. Explain how this technology is used and how it might improve response time and resident satisfaction.
3. With a partner, prepare a poster about making occupied, unoccupied, and surgical beds. Include the key steps and actions that ensure safety.
4. Practice the procedures for making a mitered corner and properly replacing a pillowcase. When you have finished, review your textbook to be sure the procedure was done properly. If you made a mistake, repeat the procedure until you can do it according to the procedure.
5. Find one picture in a magazine, in a newspaper, or online that you believe best represents a safe, comfortable resident's room. Explain why you selected the image.

Building Math Skill

Ms. N slept 6 hours last night. You know that each sleep cycle lasts 90 minutes. How many sleep cycles did Ms. N experience last evening?

Preparing for the Certification Competency Examination

To prepare for the nursing assistant certification competency examination, you will need to know content found in this chapter. This content may be tested in the knowledge (written or oral) and skills (hands-on demonstration) portions of the exam. The following areas will be emphasized:

- preparation of a room
- communication to meet resident needs
- safety and security of personal items
- occupied, unoccupied, and surgical bed making
- comfort, relaxation, rest, and adequate sleep
- evening, or p.m., care
- ways to perform a back rub

These sample test questions are similar to ones you will find on the certification competency exam. See how well you can answer them. Be sure to select the *best* answer.

1. Excessive tiredness and sudden muscle weakness during the day are symptoms of
   A. insomnia
   B. narcolepsy
   C. RLS
   D. sleep apnea

2. The type of bed that residents can control themselves is a(n)
   A. manual bed
   B. electronic bed
   C. occupied bed
   D. motorized bed

(Continued)

3. When should a nursing assistant consider a call light an emergency and respond immediately?
   A. when the resident is in bed
   B. when the resident is in a chair
   C. when the resident has visitors
   D. when the resident is in the bathroom

4. What can a nursing assistant do to avoid spreading pathogens when handling linens?
   A. keep linens close to his or her uniform
   B. avoid shaking linens out when placing them on the bed
   C. give dirty linens to another nursing assistant after removing them
   D. put clean linens on top of the laundry hamper

5. A nursing assistant fanfolds the top linens to the foot of the bed when making a(n)
   A. surgical bed
   B. occupied bed
   C. open, unoccupied bed
   D. closed, occupied bed

6. In his room, Mr. H has many personal items that sometimes get in the way of providing care. What should a nursing assistant do to safeguard these items and provide a comfortable environment for Mr. H?
   A. ask the family members to take many of these items home
   B. store the items in the resident's closet so they don't get in the way
   C. ask Mr. H if you can move his items and have him decide where
   D. while Mr. H is sleeping, move his items to other spots in the room

7. When a resident's call light goes off again for the fifth time in the morning, what should a nursing assistant do?
   A. go to the room to check on the resident
   B. wait before going to the room because it is likely not important
   C. ask another staff member to check the room
   D. check the resident's chart to see what might be wrong

8. Which of the following actions will help make residents' rooms more comfortable?
   A. offering residents drinking water often
   B. talking with residents about their families and friends
   C. keeping the room at a comfortable temperature
   D. conversing with residents during morning care

9. When a nursing assistant was making a bed, he brought in too many linens. What should he do with the unused, clean linens?
   A. use them for another bed in the room
   B. use them for the next room
   C. put them back in the linen closet
   D. discard them in the laundry hamper

10. What is the *most* important consideration when working with beds?
    A. bed cleanliness
    B. bed comfort
    C. bed safety
    D. bed location

11. Mrs. W was admitted to the long-term care facility two days ago. She is frightened about her stay and very concerned about her ill husband. She uses the call light often for what seem to be unimportant requests. What can a nursing assistant do to lessen her need to use the call light?
    A. ask if she needs anything else before leaving the room
    B. gently assure her that her husband will be fine
    C. ask her roommate to talk with her
    D. keep the television on to distract and entertain her

12. One primary purpose of an overbed table is to
    A. stack linens
    B. place meal trays
    C. place dressings
    D. place the resident's chart

13. A nursing assistant wants to be sure he gives a back rub that provides comfort. What should he do?
    A. place the lotion bottle in the basin of cool water
    B. have bright lights in the rooms so he can see the resident's back
    C. massage gently and move slowly to help the resident relax
    D. massage the resident's muscles firmly to provide comfort

14. What is the primary consideration when making a surgical bed?
    A. cleanliness
    B. comfort
    C. quality
    D. ease of transfer

15. To efficiently make a closed or open unoccupied bed, a nursing assistant should
    A. start from the top
    B. do one side at a time
    C. start from the bottom
    D. ask someone to help him or her

Did you have difficulty with any of the questions? If you did, review the chapter to find the correct answer(s).

Welcome to the Chapter

In this chapter, you will learn two important daily responsibilities of holistic nursing assistants: assisting with personal hygiene and grooming. Typically, these responsibilities start with a.m. care, or *morning care*. They may include shampooing, brushing, and combing hair; shaving; providing oral and denture care; giving fingernail and foot care; and performing perineal care. Assistance with dressing, undressing, and changing a gown or clothing (especially if there is an IV) may also be needed. In addition to a.m. care, some residents will also require a complete or partial bed bath or assistance with a tub bath or shower. At times, a therapeutic whirlpool or sitz bath may be ordered by a doctor.

A nursing assistant must also care for residents' skin. This chapter includes procedures that help maintain the skin's integrity, such as the use of warm moist compresses, warm soaks, an aquathermia pad, cold moist compresses, and ice packs.

The information and procedures presented in this chapter will help you build the knowledge and skills needed to become a holistic nursing assistant. Check with your instructor to ensure these procedures are within your state's regulations for nursing assistant practice. The topics discussed in the chapter are highlighted on the Providing Holistic Care Framework.

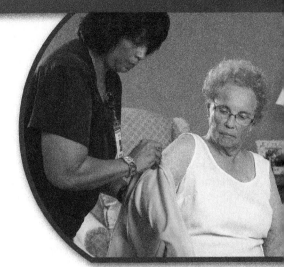

© Tori Soper Photography

Chapter Outline

Section 18.1
Bathing, Grooming, and Dressing

Section 18.2
Caring for the Skin

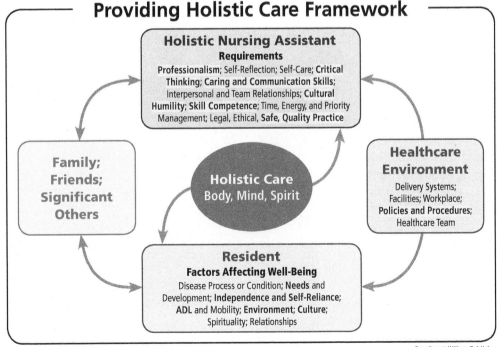

Providing Holistic Care Framework

Holistic Nursing Assistant
Requirements
Professionalism; Self-Reflection; Self-Care; Critical Thinking; Caring and Communication Skills; Interpersonal and Team Relationships; Cultural Humility; Skill Competence; Time, Energy, and Priority Management; Legal, Ethical, Safe, Quality Practice

Family; Friends; Significant Others

Holistic Care
Body, Mind, Spirit

Healthcare Environment
Delivery Systems; Facilities; Workplace; Policies and Procedures; Healthcare Team

Resident
Factors Affecting Well-Being
Disease Process or Condition; Needs and Development; Independence and Self-Reliance; ADL and Mobility; Environment; Culture; Spirituality; Relationships

Goodheart-Willcox Publisher

SECTION 18.1 Bathing, Grooming, and Dressing

Objectives

To achieve the objectives for this section, you must successfully:

- **describe** the principles of personal hygiene and grooming and their importance in daily care.
- **identify** ways to promote independence during personal hygiene and grooming.
- **demonstrate** personal hygiene and grooming responsibilities.
- **perform** the steps for providing oral and dental care, fingernail and foot care, and perineal care.

Key Terms

Learn these key terms to better understand the information presented in the section.

emesis basin	podiatrist
hemorrhoids	sitz bath
hygiene	skin integrity
perineal care	therapeutic
perineum	whirlpool

Questions to Consider

- Has someone ever had to help you with your daily hygiene or grooming, such as bathing, brushing your teeth, or dressing and undressing? If so, how did it feel to rely on someone else for an activity you usually do yourself?
- If you have never had help with daily hygiene or grooming, imagine what the experience might be like. How do you think it would make you feel?
- What actions could someone take to help another person accept and feel good about receiving assistance with daily hygiene?

Hygiene is routine actions such as bathing that promote and maintain cleanliness and health. Personal hygiene and grooming help create a healing, clean, relaxing environment. They also help maintain a resident's physical and emotional well-being and help improve quality of life by assisting residents so they look and feel their best.

What Are Personal Hygiene and Grooming Responsibilities?

When providing care to residents, nursing assistants have several personal hygiene and grooming responsibilities. These responsibilities include morning care, bathing, hair care and shaving, oral care, fingernail and foot care, dressing or undressing, and perineal care. *Perineal care* is care of the *perineum*, or the area between the thighs (including the coccyx, pubis, anus, urethra, and external genitals). In this section, you will learn about these responsibilities and the procedures for performing them properly.

Morning Care

Morning care, or *a.m. care*, promotes physical and emotional health at the start of the day. Morning care typically includes taking vital signs; assisting with elimination and measuring output; collecting specimens ordered by the doctor; helping residents wash their faces, comb their hair, and perform oral care; and if necessary, changing soiled pajamas. Other duties include straightening bed linens, changing soiled sheets or blankets, providing fresh drinking water, and arranging the bedside for breakfast, if the residents will be staying in their rooms (**Figure 18.1**).

Use these general guidelines when performing morning care. Wash your hands or use hand sanitizer prior to and after providing care, as well as when you enter and leave the room. This will help ensure infection control. Maintain a clean, safe environment while providing personal hygiene and grooming care. Once linens and gowns are taken out of the linen closet for a resident, they cannot be used for another resident unless they are washed first. Never

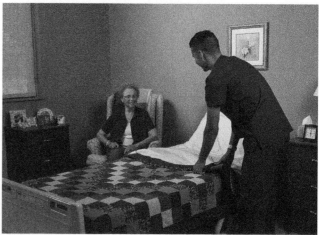

© Tori Soper Photography

Figure 18.1 One example of morning care is straightening a resident's bed linens.

use equipment that is intended for one resident on another resident without cleaning or disinfecting the equipment first. Never reuse soiled towels or linens. Always throw away disposable items after use.

Bathing

Bathing is very important. It helps maintain cleanliness and keeps residents free from sweat, irritation, and possible bacterial growth. Baths can also be pleasant, relaxing, and *therapeutic* (healing). During bathing, nursing assistants can observe a resident's *skin integrity* (condition of the skin), level of hydration, and muscle and joint movement. While daily bathing of the whole body may not be possible, it is important that the resident's hands, face, and genital areas be washed every day, and hand hygiene should be encouraged throughout the day.

Some residents are mobile enough to use a shower or take a tub bath. When showering, some residents may need a shower chair so they can sit in the shower. A chair may also be used as a fall-prevention strategy in case a resident gets tired during the shower. Place a nonslip bath mat on the floor outside the shower for safety. If the resident is taking a tub bath, place a towel in the tub so the resident can sit on it. All necessary towels, soap, and hygiene items should be within easy reach. Turn on the shower and adjust the water temperature or fill the tub half-full of water at a temperature of 100–105°F (the average water temperature for a tub bath or shower), or as directed by the licensed nursing staff. Make sure the grab bars in the shower and tub are within reach and that the resident knows where they are. Do not leave the resident unattended.

THINK ABOUT THIS

Hot tap water is a major cause of burn injury. Older adults are most at risk for scald burns. Hot water causes third-degree burns

- in one second at 156°F;
- in two seconds at 149°F;
- in five seconds at 140°F; and
- in 15 seconds at 133°F.

Bathing Residents with Limited Mobility

For residents who are not able to get out of bed, a doctor may order a *total bed bath*. During a total bed bath, the entire body is washed by a nursing assistant using washcloths and warm, soapy water in a washbasin or liquid, no-rinse soap. When a total bed bath is too exhausting for a resident, a *partial bed bath* may be given. A partial bed bath involves washing the face, hands, axilla, genitalia, back, and buttocks. The nursing assistant may provide only part of the bath for residents who can perform some bathing tasks themselves.

One alternative to a traditional bed bath is a *towel bath*. In a towel bath, a resident is bathed using a prepared, warm, moist bath towel containing a no-rinse soap solution. The resident is massaged through the towel and then dried with a bath blanket.

Another alternative to the bed bath is a *bag bath*, which is performed using a series of 10 washcloths. The washcloths are moistened with a no-rinse cleanser, placed in a bag, and warmed in a microwave, according to specific instructions. Each washcloth should be used for a different body area and then discarded into a bath basin. The next body part should be washed with a fresh cloth. Once the bath is complete, the resident should be dried with a bath blanket.

BECOMING A HOLISTIC NURSING ASSISTANT
The Personal Experience of Hygiene Care

Caring for another person's body is a very personal activity. To the resident, you may be a stranger, so you must ask the resident for permission to give care. Be aware of how and where you touch. Maintain professional boundaries and do not expose the resident or invade personal space. Respect that this is a private experience for the resident.

People can become frustrated and impatient when they are no longer able to care for themselves. Holistic caregiving requires that you safely promote independence and support personal and cultural desires and needs. It is important to talk with residents while giving care. Share information about the care being given and pay attention to your verbal and nonverbal communication and the responses you get during care.

Apply It

1. As a holistic nursing assistant, what can you do to maintain professional and personal boundaries during personal hygiene or grooming care?
2. What actions can a holistic nursing assistant take to provide comfort and relaxation during care?

Using Sitz Baths and Whirlpools

Some baths, such as sitz baths and whirlpools, are considered therapeutic. A *sitz bath* is a treatment in which a resident soaks in warm water that covers his or her perineal area. This helps reduce soreness, irritation, and burning from diseases and conditions such as diarrhea, *hemorrhoids* (inflamed veins around the anus or inside the rectum), and vaginal infections. When giving a sitz bath, use the plan of care to determine the appropriate water temperature. A sitz bath generally lasts 10–20 minutes. Always note the time the sitz bath begins and check on the resident every five minutes for safety. Make sure the resident is comfortable and provide warmth by placing a blanket around the resident's shoulders and over the legs, if needed. Stay with the resident if he or she is feeling weak or not steady.

A *whirlpool* is a bathtub that uses small jets to move warm water. The resident places his or her entire body or a body part into the tub for treatment as directed by the plan of care. A whirlpool helps decrease swelling and inflammation, eases muscle spasms and pain, and promotes healing.

No matter what type of bath is ordered, encourage residents to do as much of it themselves as they can. Keep residents warm and safe and maintain privacy. Use excellent body mechanics as you turn and position the resident. If the resident is extremely overweight or unconscious, be sure to ask for assistance, if needed.

Procedure

Giving a Total or Partial Bed Bath

Rationale

Bed baths clean the skin, control odor, and promote healing. They also give nursing assistants an opportunity to observe skin integrity. A total bed bath is given when an entire bath must be performed for an immobile resident. Partial bed baths are given to residents who cannot perform parts of the bath independently or who cannot tolerate a total bed bath.

Preparation

1. Ask the licensed nursing staff if there are doctor's orders for the procedure, if there are any specific instructions listed in the plan of care, and if the resident can be moved into the positions required for this procedure.
2. Wash your hands or use hand sanitizer before entering the room.
3. Knock before entering the room.
4. Introduce yourself using your first or preferred name and title. Explain that you work with the licensed nursing staff and will be providing care.
5. Greet the resident and ask the resident to state her full name, if able. Then check the resident's identification bracelet.
6. Use Mr., Mrs., or Ms. and the resident's last name when conversing.
7. Explain the procedure in simple terms, even if the resident is not able to communicate or is disoriented. Ask permission to perform the procedure.

Best Practice: To promote relaxation, be sure the room is at a comfortable temperature for the resident and that there are no drafts. Turn on the resident's favorite music at a low volume, if desired.

8. Bring the necessary equipment into the room. Place the following items in an easy-to-reach place:
   - bath blankets
   - disposable protective pad
   - disposable gloves
   - laundry hamper
   - clean bed linens

   Place the following items on a chair next to the bed:
   - several washcloths and hand towels
   - 2–3 bath towels
   - 2 clean gowns

   Arrange the towels, linens, and gowns in the order they will be used. Then place a hand towel on the overbed table. Place the following equipment and linens on the hand towel:
   - washbasin
   - liquid soap (no-rinse, if appropriate)
   - personal hygiene products, such as deodorant and lotion
   - cotton-tipped applicators

The Procedure

9. Provide privacy by closing the curtains, using a screen, or closing the door to the room.
10. Lock the bed wheels and then raise the bed to hip level.

11. Maintain safety during the procedure. If there are side rails, raise and lock the rails on the opposite side of the bed from where you will be working. Lower the rail on the side where you are working.

12. Wash your hands or use hand sanitizer to ensure infection control.

   Best Practice: Before beginning the bath, ask if the resident needs to use a bedpan or urinal. Also remove any jewelry except a wedding ring. Place jewelry in a safe and secure place.

13. Be sure any tubing, such as IVs or urinary drainage bags, are not moved or pulled out of place or kinked during or after positioning.

14. Put on disposable gloves.

15. Loosen and pull the bed linens out from under the mattress. Let them hang on all four sides of the bed.

16. Fanfold the bedspread and blanket to the foot of the bed, but leave the top sheet covering the resident.

17. Place the bath blanket over the top sheet. If possible, have the resident hold the bath blanket while you pull the top sheet out from under the bath blanket. If you will not be changing the bed linens, fanfold the top sheet to the foot of the bed. If you will be changing the bed linens, place the soiled top sheet in the laundry hamper.

18. Keep the resident covered with the bath blanket as you remove her gown and put it in the laundry hamper.

19. Fill the washbasin about two-thirds full of warm water. Check the water temperature. It should be 100–105°F. The water should feel comfortably warm to your elbow. You may also ask the resident to feel the water temperature, but always check it yourself first.

20. Place the washbasin on the overbed table, which should be covered with a hand towel. Be sure the washcloths and towels are easy to reach.

   Best Practice: Bathing starts at the top of the body. Begin with the face and proceed to the bottom of the body, section by section.

21. Check the position of the bed and resident. Position the resident so she is on the side of the bed closest to you. If necessary and permitted, adjust the bed so the resident is in a Fowler's position. Place a dry towel across her chest under the chin and another under her head.

22. Make a bath mitt with a washcloth (**Figure 18.2**).

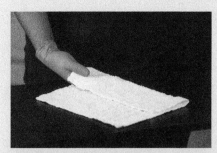
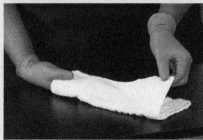
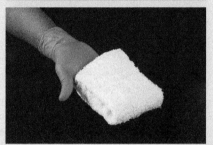

Figure 18.2   © Tori Soper Photography

23. Wet the bath mitt using only water, not soap. If the resident requests soap, keep the soap away from her eyes. Gently wash each eye from the inner corner to the outer corner (**Figure 18.3**). To prevent infection, use a different, clean part of the mitt for each wipe.

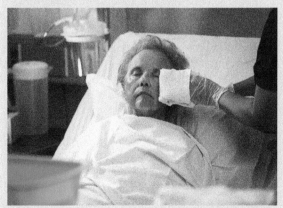

Figure 18.3   © Tori Soper Photography

(continued)

Giving a Total or Partial Bed Bath *(continued)*

24. Wash the entire face, ears, and neck with a new bath mitt. Rinse well to remove any soap used. Gently pat-dry the face, ears, and neck with a dry towel.

    Best Practice: Before washing each arm, place a dry towel under it.

25. Support the arm farthest from you. Wash the shoulder, axilla, arm, hand, and fingers with soap and water using a clean bath mitt. Wash the axilla thoroughly. Rinse and dry well.

26. Apply deodorant, unless directed otherwise.

27. Apply lotion to the resident's arm and hand, unless directed otherwise. Gently massage the lotion in a circular motion with the palm of your hand.

    Best Practice: Always warm lotion in your gloved hands before placing it on the resident.

28. Keep the resident warm by placing the dry arm under the bath blanket.

29. Support the arm nearest to you. Wash, rinse, dry, and apply lotion to the shoulder, axilla, arm, hand, and fingers using the same procedure.

30. Place a dry bath towel across the resident's chest and fold the bath blanket down to the pubic area.

    Best Practice: Never expose the resident. During the bath, observe the resident for redness, sores, or irritation on the skin, especially under breast tissue and skin folds or on bony projections. Take extra care around any dressings or catheters. Always check with the resident to be sure you are not rubbing too hard.

31. Lift the dry bath towel slightly and wash, rinse, and dry the chest and abdominal areas. Wash the navel and any creases in the skin with cotton-tipped applicators.

32. Apply lotion to the skin, unless directed otherwise. Gently massage the lotion in a circular motion with the palm of your hand.

33. Pull the bath blanket up and over the bath towel. Then remove the bath towel from beneath the bath blanket.

34. Lower the bed and raise the side rails for safety. Give the resident the call light.

35. Empty, rinse, and refill the washbasin about two-thirds full of warm water. Check the water temperature. It should be 100–105°F. The water should feel comfortably warm to your elbow. You may also ask the resident to feel the water temperature, but always check it yourself first.

36. Place the washbasin on the overbed table.

    Best Practice: If needed, remove your gloves and wash your hands before emptying the washbasin. Practice hand hygiene and put on a new pair of gloves after replacing the washbasin on the overbed table.

37. Place a dry towel under the resident's leg farthest from you. Be sure the genitalia are not exposed. Support the thigh and leg. Wash, rinse, and dry the thigh and leg well.

38. Apply lotion according to the plan of care. If lotion is used, gently massage it in a circular motion with the palm of your hand.

39. Wash, rinse, dry, and apply lotion to the thigh and leg nearest you using the same procedure. Then cover both legs with the bath blanket.

40. Expose the foot and thigh nearest you and bend the knee. Place the washbasin on top of a towel near the foot to be washed. Support the knee and place the resident's foot in the water (**Figure 18.4**). Using a bath mitt, wash and clean between the toes and under the toenails. Remove the foot from the water, then rinse and dry it well.

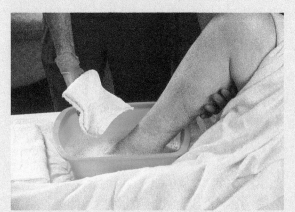

Figure 18.4   © Tori Soper Photography

41. Apply lotion according to the plan of care. If lotion is used, gently massage it in a circular motion with the palm of your hand. To prevent fungal infection, do not put lotion between the toes.

42. Wash, rinse, dry, and apply lotion to the other foot using the same procedure.

    Best Practice: Observe the toenails and the skin between the toes for redness and cracks.

43. Remove the washbasin and the towel.

44. Cover the resident's legs and feet with the bath blanket.

45. Lower the bed and raise the side rails for safety. Give the resident the call light.

46. Place any soiled linens in the laundry hamper.
47. Remove the soiled gloves and put on clean gloves.
48. Empty, rinse, and refill the washbasin about two-thirds full of warm water. Check the water temperature. It should be 100–105°F. The water should feel comfortably warm to your elbow. You may also ask the resident to feel the water temperature, but always check it yourself first.
49. Help the resident turn onto her side to expose her back and buttocks. Place a towel lengthwise next to her back. Wash, rinse, and dry the back of the neck, back, and buttocks (**Figure 18.5**).

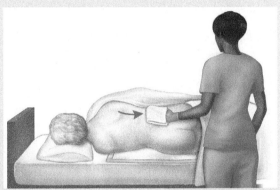

Figure 18.5   © Body Scientific International

50. Give the resident a back rub with warmed lotion.
51. Help the resident turn onto her back with a towel under her buttocks and upper legs.
52. Lower the bed and raise the side rails for safety. Give the resident the call light.
53. Empty, rinse, and refill the washbasin about two-thirds full of warm water. Check the water temperature. It should be 100–105°F. The water should feel comfortably warm to your elbow. You may also ask the resident to feel the water temperature, but always check it yourself first.

54. If there is no urinary catheter, offer the resident a clean, soapy washcloth to wash the genital area. If the resident cannot do this, perform perineal care, as outlined in the perineal care procedure later in this section.
55. Help the resident put on a clean gown or other clothing, as appropriate.
56. Recheck that any tubing is in place. If you have any concerns, ask a licensed nursing staff member to check that the IV or other tubing is working properly. If the resident has a urinary drainage bag, be sure it is positioned below the bladder.
57. Check to be sure the bed wheels are locked, then reposition the resident and lower the bed.
58. Follow the plan of care to determine if the side rails should be raised or lowered.
59. Remove, clean, and store equipment in the proper location. Remove soiled linens and discard disposable equipment.

Follow-Up

60. Remove and discard your gloves.
61. Wash your hands to ensure infection control.
62. Make sure the resident is comfortable and place the call light and personal items within reach.
63. Conduct a safety check before leaving the room. The room should be clean and free from clutter or spills.
64. Wash your hands or use hand sanitizer before leaving the room.

Reporting and Documentation

65. Report any specific observations, complications, or unusual responses to the licensed nursing staff. Document this information, along with the care provided, in the chart or EMR.

Hair Care

Another personal hygiene and bathing responsibility that nursing assistants have is shampooing, brushing, and combing residents' hair. People have different types of hair, and hair may be affected by age, genetics, medications, and skin conditions.

Baldness (*alopecia*) is progressive hair thinning. About 40 percent of women experience female pattern hair loss by menopause, and about 50 percent of men by the age of 50.

Hair also turns gray or white due to changes in melanin (pigment) production in the hair follicles.

Gray hair usually develops due to age and stress, though the cause is different for each individual. Most people 75 years of age or older have varying amounts of gray hair, and men tend to become grayer at a younger age than women.

Hair Conditions

Various hair conditions may affect hair care. The scalp may have lesions such as cuts, ulcerations or sores, scabs, or blisters, or may itch. Be careful and gentle when providing hair care if the resident has scalp lesions.

While some shedding of dead skin cells is normal, *dandruff* can occur due to excessive flaking of dead skin cells from the scalp, and there is usually redness and irritation. Dandruff is often a result of frequent exposure to extreme temperature variations (heat or cold) or certain triggers, such as stress.

Lice are parasites that crawl and can be spread by close human contact. Head lice attach their eggs to the base of the hair shaft on the scalp, usually around and behind the ears and near the neckline. Symptoms of head lice include a sense of something moving in the hair, itching, and sores on the head due to excessive scratching (which can lead to infection). Treatment includes over-the-counter or prescription medications. When using these products, carefully follow the instructions as directed. If a resident has lice, the hair should also be combed to check for lice every two to three days for two to three weeks after treatment.

Shampooing Hair

Some residents are able to shampoo their own hair while showering. Others may require assistance during their shower or bath, but are able to wash their hair independently. For bedridden residents, dry shampoo (in the form of a spray or powder) or liquid, no-rinse shampoo may be used. These residents may also have their hair shampooed in bed. The following procedure describes the steps for providing assistance with hair care for bedridden residents. This includes shampooing, combing, and brushing the hair.

Procedure

Providing Assistance with Hair Care

Rationale

Shampooing hair promotes cleanliness and comfort. The scalp is stimulated during shampooing, and this improves circulation.

Preparation

1. Ask the licensed nursing staff if there are doctor's orders for the procedure, if there are any specific instructions listed in the plan of care, and if the resident can be moved into the positions required for this procedure.
2. Wash your hands or use hand sanitizer before entering the room.

3. Knock before entering the room.

4. Introduce yourself using your first or preferred name and title. Explain that you work with the licensed nursing staff and will be providing care.

5. Greet the resident and ask the resident to state his full name, if able. Then check the resident's identification bracelet.

6. Use Mr., Mrs., or Ms. and the resident's last name when conversing.

7. Explain the procedure in simple terms, even if the resident is not able to communicate or is disoriented. Ask permission to perform the procedure.

8. Bring the necessary equipment into the room. Place the following items in an easy-to-reach place:
   - shampoo basin or tray; if inflatable, have the basin or tray ready (**Figure 18.6**).

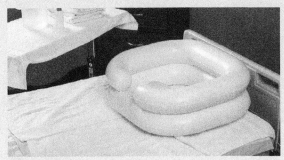

Figure 18.6   © Tori Soper Photography

- catch basin to collect used water
- 2 bath blankets
- waterproof pillow cover
- disposable protective pads or clean plastic trash bag
- a small washbasin, liquid soap, and antiseptic
- disposable gloves

Place the following items on the overbed table:
- 2 bath towels
- several washcloths
- shampoo and conditioner
- pitcher of warm water (100–105°F)
- washbasin with warm water (100–105°F) to refill the pitcher
- brush (without metal prongs that can damage the hair and scalp)
- comb (large-tooth comb for wet hair; avoid metal combs or combs with broken teeth that can tear individual hair strands and damage the scalp)
- several cotton balls or 2 × 2 gauze bandages
- hair dryer, if available and permitted
- personal hair products, if needed or desired
- handheld mirror

The Procedure

9. Provide privacy by closing the curtains, using a screen, or closing the door to the room.

10. Lock the bed wheels and then raise the bed to hip level.

11. Maintain safety during the procedure. If there are side rails, raise and lock the rails on the opposite side of the bed from where you will be working. Lower the rail on the side where you are working.

12. Wash your hands or use hand sanitizer to ensure infection control.

13. Put on disposable gloves.

14. Carefully comb, brush, or gently use your fingers to remove any tangles from the resident's hair prior to shampooing.

> **Best Practice:** Observe and report signs of skin breakdown, such as lesions or any other skin conditions, as you prepare to shampoo the hair.

15. Gently place a cotton ball or a 2 × 2 gauze bandage in each ear canal to prevent the entry of water.

16. Loosen the resident's gown at the neck.

17. Help the resident into a supine position and then lower the head of the bed.

18. Cover the resident with the bath blanket. Fanfold the top bed linens to the foot of the bed. Make sure the resident is not exposed.

19. Remove the pillow from under the resident's head and gently place the resident's head on the bed.

20. Place the disposable protective pad or plastic trash bag and then a towel on the bed beneath the resident's head and upper body.

21. Remove the pillowcase and replace it with the waterproof cover.

22. Place the pillow with the waterproof cover beneath the resident's shoulders so the resident's head is tilted slightly backward.

23. Place a bath towel around the resident's head and shoulders. There should be enough padding to provide comfort and prevent water leakage.

24. Raise the resident's head and slide the shampoo tray or basin under it. Be sure the basin tubing is connected to the catch basin.

25. Place a protective pad on the floor near the head of the bed. Put the catch basin on top of the pad.

26. Place a washcloth over the resident's eyes.

27. Check the water to be sure it is at a warm, but safe, temperature.

28. Using the pitcher, pour enough water to wet the hair (**Figure 18.7**). When needed, refill the pitcher using the washbasin filled with warm water.

(continued)

Providing Assistance with Hair Care *(continued)*

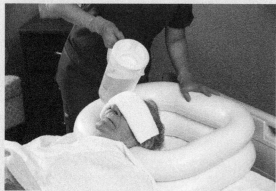

Figure 18.7   © Tori Soper Photography

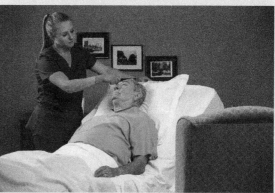

Figure 18.8   © Tori Soper Photography

29. Apply a small amount of shampoo to your hands and begin forming a lather. With both hands, apply the shampoo to the scalp using a massaging motion. Apply the shampoo from the scalp outward to the ends of the hair strands, and from the front to the back of the head. Lift the resident's head gently to shampoo the back of the head.

   Best Practice: Use your fingertips, not your fingernails. Be very careful if there are lesions on the scalp.

30. Rinse the resident's hair thoroughly, pouring warm water from the pitcher. Rinse from the hairline and work down to the ends of the hair strands. When needed, refill the pitcher using the washbasin filled with warm water. Check the water temperature.

31. If appropriate, apply conditioner and rinse thoroughly.

32. Remove and discard your gloves. Put on another pair of disposable gloves.

33. Dry the resident's forehead, ears, and neck with a clean bath towel. Remove the cotton balls or 2 × 2 gauze bandages from each ear canal.

34. Carefully remove the shampoo basin or tray and set it on the chair next to the bed. Be sure there is a dry bath towel under the resident's head.

35. Raise the head of the bed 60–90°, if appropriate.

36. Dry the resident's hair with a clean bath towel by blotting, not by rubbing.

37. If the hair is wet, comb it to remove tangles and then style the hair. Part the hair in sections. Comb each section separately using a downward motion and comb from underneath to remove any tangles (**Figure 18.8**). If the resident is able, have him move his head so you can get all angles. If the resident is unable, support his head while moving it.

Best Practice: Hair is fragile when it is wet. Do not brush wet hair because brushing can damage the hair. Instead, use a comb.

38. Brush the hair if it is dry and not tangled. Be slow and gentle. Have the resident move his head so you can get all angles. If the resident is unable, support his head while moving it.

   Best Practice: To prevent hair loss, do not brush or pull the hair too much during drying or styling. If caring for a resident undergoing chemotherapy, use a child or baby hair brush with softer bristles.

39. Style the resident's hair neatly. If a resident has long hair, suggest a loose braid to prevent snarls, knots, or tangles. Use a hair dryer only if available and permitted.

40. Remove the towel and let the resident use the handheld mirror, if desired, to view the hair. If a hair salon or barber shop is available in the facility, ask the resident if he might want to visit in the future.

41. Remove all equipment and used towels from the bed.

42. Assist with changing the resident's gown if it got wet during the procedure.

43. Remove the bath blanket and replace the linens.

44. Remove the waterproof cover, replace it with a clean pillowcase, and put the pillow under the resident's head.

45. Check to be sure the bed wheels are locked, then reposition the resident and lower the bed.

46. Follow the plan of care to determine if the side rails should be raised or lowered.

47. Remove, clean, and store equipment in the proper location. Clean the brush and comb in the bathroom. Use the washbasin of warm water and a small amount of liquid soap. You may also use a small amount of antiseptic. Quickly tap the brush or comb in the filled washbasin and then rinse with cool, running water. Let the brush and comb air-dry and then put them away. Remove soiled linens and discard disposable equipment.

Follow-Up

48. Remove and discard your gloves.
49. Wash your hands to ensure infection control.
50. Make sure the resident is comfortable and place the call light and personal items within reach.
51. Conduct a safety check before leaving the room. The room should be clean and free from clutter or spills.

52. Wash your hands or use hand sanitizer before leaving the room.

Reporting and Documentation

53. Report any specific observations, complications, or unusual responses to the licensed nursing staff. Document this information, along with the care provided, in the chart or EMR.

Shaving

Many men choose to shave daily, while others shave less regularly. Skin products and razors are chosen based on the resident's preference. Preshaving oil or shaving cream with aloe can soften skin and hair, and help prevent irritation, nicks, cuts, and razor bumps and burns. *Electric razors* are less irritating than blades and should be used if the resident is taking blood thinning medication to prevent blood clots from forming. If a blade is used, a *safety razor* with a single or double blade is better than multiblade razors (**Figure 18.9**).

If you are asked to help a resident shave, practice infection control and follow these guidelines:

- Make sure any dentures are in place before you begin.
- Before using a safety razor, soften the beard by placing wet, warm washcloths on the resident's face. Then generously apply shaving cream or gel to the areas that will be shaved. Rinse the razor often in warm water while shaving. When you are finished, rinse the skin thoroughly to remove any excess shaving cream.
- Before using an electric razor, ask the resident if he prefers a dry shave or one with preshave lotion. If lotion is desired, apply a generous amount on the areas that will be shaved.

- Hold the skin tight with the fingers of one hand and shave in the direction of hair growth (**Figure 18.10**). When shaving the chin or under the nose, ask the resident to hold that part of the skin tight. If there is facial hair, maintain the mustache or beard line.
- Shave lightly to prevent nicks or cuts. If a nick or cut occurs, apply pressure with a small piece of facial tissue. Report any nicks or cuts to the licensed nursing staff after you finish shaving.
- Apply aftershave lotion or powder, if the resident desires.
- Do not shave over any skin sores, moles, growths, acne, or bruises on the face.

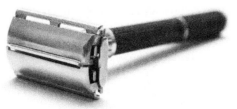

Digital Signal/Shutterstock.com

Figure 18.9 If a blade is used, safety razors are the safest option. Old razor blades should be disposed of in the sharps container.

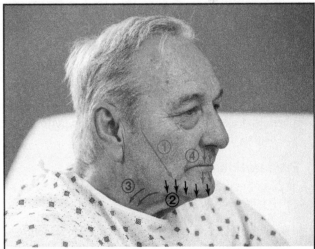

© Tori Soper Photography

1. Start at the sideburns and shave in downward strokes to the jawline.
2. Use short, downward strokes along the jawline.
3. Carefully shave the neck using gentle, downward strokes.
4. Use short strokes to shave above and below the lips.

Figure 18.10 Always shave in the direction of hair growth.

- Use a fine-tooth comb to straighten mustache hairs. Use a wide-tooth comb for a wet beard. Once dry, beards can be brushed. Wax or balm can be applied to the mustache or beard.
- Make sure any used razor blades are discarded in the sharps container.

Oral and Denture Care

At birth, humans have 20 deciduous teeth (commonly called *baby teeth*), which are eventually replaced by 32 permanent (*adult*) teeth. Some residents do not have all of their natural teeth. They may have bridges, partial dentures, or full dentures, which contain false teeth to replace missing teeth (**Figure 18.11**).

Dentures that have been properly cared for typically last about five years. As people age, so do their bones and gums, which may cause dentures to become loose. This can make it hard to chew and cause food to get caught between the gums and dentures. Because of these difficulties, residents may not receive adequate nutrients, which may cause lack of healing and weight loss. Poorly fitting dentures can cause mouth and gum irritation, sores, and infections; any cracks in dentures should be repaired.

Oral care and teeth cleaning are an important part of daily hygiene. They keep the mouth fresh, teeth and gums healthy, and remove any bad tastes from

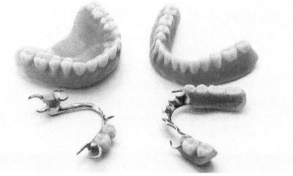

Bunwit Unseree/Shutterstock.com

Figure 18.11 Partial dentures replace some missing teeth and often have a metal or plastic base. Full dentures replace all natural teeth on the upper, lower, or both gums.

illnesses or medications. Good oral care can also help prevent dental cavities, tooth decay, bad breath, gum disease, and gum and bone infection. Oral care may be needed as often as every two hours if the resident is unable to take fluids by mouth.

Routine teeth cleaning consists of daily brushing and flossing in the morning and evening and after eating. Flossing is important, as it removes up to 80 percent of the film that hardens into plaque, which can stick to the teeth and become difficult to remove. Rinsing the mouth is also important. If dentures are worn, they must be cleaned properly and stored correctly when not being worn.

Procedure

Providing Oral Care

Rationale

Performing oral care helps reduce bacteria, provides moisture, freshens the mouth, makes food taste better, and cleans the teeth.

Preparation

1. Ask the licensed nursing staff if there are doctor's orders for the procedure, if there are any specific instructions listed in the plan of care, and if the resident can be moved into the positions required for this procedure.
2. Wash your hands or use hand sanitizer before entering the room.
3. Knock before entering the room.
4. Introduce yourself using your first or preferred name and title. Explain that you work with the licensed nursing staff and will be providing care.

5. Greet the resident and ask the resident to state her full name, if able. Then check the resident's identification bracelet.
6. Use Mr., Mrs., or Ms. and the resident's last name when conversing.
7. Explain the procedure in simple terms, even if the resident is not able to communicate or is disoriented. Ask permission to perform the procedure.
8. Bring the necessary equipment into the room. Some of these items may already be in the bedside stand or bathroom. Place a paper towel, towel, or disposable protective pad on the overbed table as an infection-control barrier before placing the following items:
   - soft-bristled toothbrush (always use soft-bristled for older adults)
   - toothpaste (with an American Dental Association seal)
   - mouthwash

- pitcher of fresh, cool water
- several disposable cups
- spoon or tongue blade
- disposable gloves
- *emesis basin*, which should be small and kidney shaped (**Figure 18.12**)

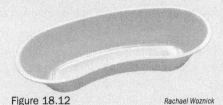

Figure 18.12   *Rachael Woznick*

- 2 washcloths
- 2–3 towels
- 2 face masks, if needed
- dental floss

> **Best Practice:** Replace a toothbrush every three to four months. Replace it sooner if the bristles become frayed.

The Procedure

9. Provide privacy by closing the curtains, using a screen, or closing the door to the room.
10. If the resident is able to sit in a chair, assist her to a chair and then place the overbed table with the equipment and linens in a comfortable position so she may brush her teeth.
11. If the resident is in bed and needs assistance, lock the bed wheels and then raise the bed to hip level.
12. Maintain safety during the procedure. If there are side rails, raise and lock the rails on the opposite side of the bed from where you will be working. Lower the rail on the side where you are working.
13. Raise the head of the bed to at least 60–90° and ensure that there is sufficient lighting to perform the procedure.
14. Wash your hands or use hand sanitizer to ensure infection control.
15. Put on disposable gloves.
16. Spread a towel across the resident's chest to protect her clothing and the top linen.
17. Fill a disposable cup half-full with water and half-full with mouthwash and mix with a spoon or tongue blade.
18. Have the resident take a mouthful from the cup and swish the mixture in her mouth.
19. Hold the emesis basin underneath the resident's chin so she can spit the mixture into the basin. Wipe the resident's mouth and chin dry.
20. Fill a disposable cup half-full with water. Wet the toothbrush in the water.

21. Put toothpaste on the wet toothbrush. If the resident is able, let her brush her own teeth. If she cannot, brush her teeth for her.
    A. Hold the brush at a 45° angle to the gum (**Figure 18.13**).

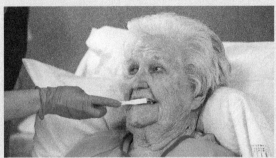

Figure 18.13   © *Tori Soper Photography*

    B. Starting at the back of the mouth, use gentle, circular motions to brush the outer surfaces, inner surfaces, and chewing surfaces of the teeth (**Figure 18.14**).

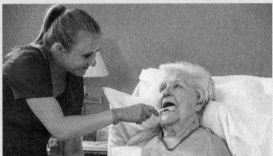

Figure 18.14   © *Tori Soper Photography*

    C. To clean the inside surfaces of the front teeth, tilt the brush vertically and make several up-and-down strokes.
    D. Brush the tongue to remove bacteria and keep the breath fresh, but do not brush so far back that gagging occurs.
22. During brushing, have the resident spit toothpaste and excess saliva into the emesis basin, as needed (**Figure 18.15**).

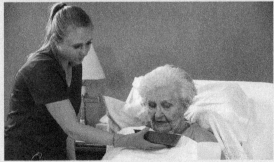

Figure 18.15   © *Tori Soper Photography*

(continued)

Providing Oral Care *(continued)*

23. When finished, help the resident rinse the toothpaste out of her mouth using the mouthwash solution or fresh water and the emesis basin. Then wipe her mouth.

24. If the resident is able, let her floss her teeth. If she is not able, floss her teeth for her. Put on a face mask before beginning, if needed.

> **Best Practice:** If the resident will floss independently, you may need to show her the proper way to floss.

A. Cut a piece of floss 18 inches long.
B. Wrap the ends of the floss around the middle finger of each hand. Place the other fingers out of the way and hold the dental floss stretched tight between the middle fingers (**Figure 18.16**).

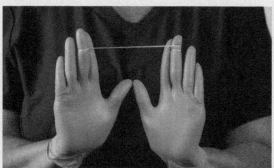

Figure 18.16   © Tori Soper Photography

C. Ask the resident to open her mouth.
D. Gently insert the floss between each pair of teeth. Do not press the floss into the gum. Slide the floss around both sides of each tooth. Discard the floss when completed.

E. When finished, offer the resident the mouthwash solution or fresh water to rinse the mouth.

> **Best Practice:** Let the licensed nursing staff know if the resident complains of pain or sensitivity, sores on the lips or mouth, cracked or bleeding lips or gums, bad breath that does not improve after oral care, or chipped or cracked teeth.

25. If the resident is in bed, check to be sure the bed wheels are locked. Then reposition the resident and lower the bed. If the resident is in a chair, help her back to bed, if desired.

26. Follow the plan of care to determine if the side rails should be raised or lowered.

27. Remove, clean, and store equipment in the proper location. Remove soiled linens and discard disposable equipment.

Follow-Up

28. Remove and discard your gloves.
29. Wash your hands to ensure infection control.
30. Make sure the resident is comfortable and place the call light and personal items within reach.
31. Conduct a safety check before leaving the room. The room should be clean and free from clutter or spills.
32. Wash your hands or use hand sanitizer before leaving the room.

Reporting and Documentation

33. Report any specific observations, complications, or unusual responses to the licensed nursing staff. Document this information, along with the care provided, in the chart or EMR.

Procedure

Cleaning and Storing Dentures

Rationale

Cleaning dentures keeps them intact, freshens the mouth, removes food particles that can cause irritation, and reduces bacteria on the dentures.

Preparation

1. Ask the licensed nursing staff if there are doctor's orders for the procedure, if there are any specific instructions listed in the plan of care, and if the resident can be moved into the positions required for this procedure.

2. Wash your hands or use hand sanitizer before entering the room.
3. Knock before entering the room.
4. Introduce yourself using your first or preferred name and title. Explain that you work with the licensed nursing staff and will be providing care.
5. Greet the resident and ask the resident to state his full name, if able. Then check the resident's identification bracelet.
6. Use Mr., Mrs., or Ms. and the resident's last name when conversing.
7. Explain the procedure in simple terms, even if the resident is not able to communicate or is disoriented. Ask permission to perform the procedure.

8. Bring the necessary equipment into the room. Put a paper towel, towel, or disposable protective pad on the overbed table as an infection-control barrier before placing the following items:
   - toothbrush or denture brush
   - denture cup and lid, labeled with the resident's name and room number (**Figure 18.17**)

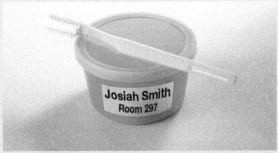

Figure 18.17   © Tori Soper Photography

   - toothpaste or denture cleaner
   - disposable cups
   - emesis basin
   - washcloths
   - mouthwash
   - denture solution
   - several towels
   - several packets of 2 × 2 gauze bandages
   - oral swabs
   - disposable gloves

The Procedure

9. Provide privacy by closing the curtains, using a screen, or closing the door to the room.
10. If the resident is able to sit in a chair, assist him to a chair and then place the overbed table with the equipment and linens in a comfortable position so he may clean his dentures.
11. If the resident is in bed and needs assistance, lock the bed wheels and then raise the bed to hip level.
12. Maintain safety during the procedure. If there are side rails, raise and lock the rails on the opposite side of the bed from where you will be working. Lower the rail on the side where you are working.
13. Raise the head of the bed, if permitted.
14. Wash your hands or use hand sanitizer to ensure infection control.
15. Put on disposable gloves.
16. Spread a towel across the resident's chest to protect his clothing and the top linen.
17. Place a washcloth in the bottom of the emesis basin.
18. Ask the resident to remove his dentures and place them in the emesis basin.

19. If the resident cannot remove his dentures, ask him to open his mouth. Remove his dentures for him.
    - A. Upper dentures: grasp the upper denture firmly using a 2 × 2 gauze bandage. Ease the denture downward and forward and then remove it from the mouth.
    - B. Lower dentures: grasp the lower denture firmly using a new 2 × 2 gauze bandage. Ease the denture upward and forward and then remove it from the mouth.
20. Place the dentures in the emesis basin on top of the washcloth. Never carry the dentures in your hands. Take the emesis basin, toothbrush or denture brush, and toothpaste or denture cleaner to the sink. Place the basin next to the sink.
21. If the resident wears full dentures, clean the resident's oral cavity after the dentures are removed. Clean the resident's oral cavity with oral swabs and half-strength mouthwash.
22. Place a washcloth in the bottom of the clean sink to protect the dentures from breaking or scratching in case they fall. Do not place the dentures in the sink.
23. Take one denture out of the emesis basin. Apply toothpaste or denture cleaner to the denture. Wet the toothbrush by immersing it in clean, running water. Make sure to brush away from you (**Figure 18.18**). Hold the denture low in the sink. With the denture in the palm of your hand, brush all surfaces until they are clean. Then rinse the denture thoroughly using cool, running water. Repeat the same procedure for a second denture.

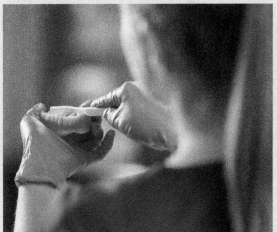

Figure 18.18   © Tori Soper Photography

Best Practice: Use cool or lukewarm water only. Hot water can damage dentures and cause them to lose their shape.

(continued)

Cleaning and Storing Dentures *(continued)*

Best Practice: Be sure to check the dentures for any cracks. Report cracks to the licensed nursing staff.

24. If the dentures will be stored, fill the labeled denture cup with cool water, mouthwash, or denture solution. Place the dentures in the cup and close the lid.

Best Practice: Always store dentures in liquid when they are out of the resident's mouth.

25. Leave the labeled denture cup with clean solution on the bedside stand, where it can be easily reached.
26. Check that the dentures are moist if reinserting them. If the resident is able, ask him to put the dentures back into his mouth. Assist, if needed. Check that the dentures fit correctly.
27. Remove and discard your gloves after either storing the dentures or inserting them into the resident's mouth.
28. Wash your hands or use hand sanitizer to ensure infection control.
29. Put on a new pair of gloves.
30. If the resident is in bed, check to be sure the bed wheels are locked. Then reposition the resident and lower the bed. If the resident is in a chair, help him back to bed, if desired.
31. Follow the plan of care to determine if the side rails should be raised or lowered.
32. Remove, clean, and store equipment in the proper location. Use disinfectant to clean the emesis basin. Remove soiled linens and discard disposable equipment.

Follow-Up

33. Remove and discard your gloves.
34. Wash your hands to ensure infection control.
35. Make sure the resident is comfortable and place the call light and personal items within reach.
36. Conduct a safety check before leaving the room. The room should be clean and free from clutter or spills.
37. Wash your hands or use hand sanitizer before leaving the room.

Reporting and Documentation

38. Report any specific observations, complications, or unusual responses to the licensed nursing staff. Document this information, along with the care provided, in the chart or EMR.

Fingernail Care

Fingernail care promotes cleanliness and helps prevent irritation or infection from torn or bleeding cuticles, cracked fingernails, or dirt under the fingernails. Smooth fingernails also prevent the skin from breaking if residents scratch themselves.

Fingernail care may be provided while the resident sits in a chair or with the resident in bed, with the head of the bed raised. Place a towel on top of the overbed table and then put the following items on the towel:

- washbasin with warm water (100–105°F)
- 1–2 emery boards
- nail clipper
- orangewood stick, if permitted
- 2–3 hand towels
- disposable protective pad
- several washcloths
- lotion
- disposable gloves
- soap

Practice hand hygiene before performing fingernail care and put on a pair of disposable gloves. Use the following guidelines to provide fingernail care:

1. Check the water temperature. It should be 100–105°F. The water should feel comfortably warm to your elbow. You may also ask the resident to feel the water temperature, but always check it yourself first. Add a small amount of soap to the washbasin.
2. Help the resident comfortably position his fingers in the washbasin to soak. If appropriate, use a rolled-up towel to support his wrists. Cover the resident's hands and the washbasin with a dry hand towel to retain the heat. Soak the resident's fingernails for approximately 5–10 minutes. If needed, remove the resident's hands and add more warm water.
3. Wash the resident's hands, cleaning under the fingernails.

4. If permitted, push the cuticles back gently with a washcloth or the dull end of an orangewood stick. Clean under each nail with an orangewood stick. Wipe the orangewood stick after cleaning each nail.

5. Remove the washbasin and dry the resident's hands thoroughly.

6. Use a nail clipper to cut the fingernails straight across, if permitted. Do not clip below the tips of the fingers (**Figure 18.19**).

7. Shape and smooth the fingernails with an emery board.

8. Apply lotion and gently massage the resident's fingers and hands. Remove extra lotion with a towel.

9. Let the licensed nursing staff know if you observe loose nails or dry, reddened, or irritated areas.

10. Remove, clean, and store equipment in the proper location. Disinfect the nail clippers. Remove soiled linens and discard disposable equipment.

11. Remove and discard your gloves. Then, wash your hands.

12. Making sure the resident is comfortable and place the call light and personal items within reach.

13. Conduct a safety check before leaving the room. The room should be clean and free from clutter or spills.

14. Wash your hands or use hand sanitizer before leaving the room.

15. Report any specific observations, complications, or unusual responses to the licensed nursing staff. Document this information, along with the care provided, in the chart or EMR.

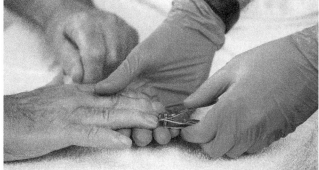

© Tori Soper Photography

Figure 18.19 When clipping a resident's fingernails, be very careful not to accidentally clip or damage the skin surrounding the fingernail.

Foot Care

As residents age, they may have more difficulty with their feet and toenails. For example, toenails may become thick and yellow, unattractive, and harder to keep clean and trimmed. *Calluses* (hard, rough areas on the skin on the heel or ball of the foot) and *corns* (small patches of thickened, dead skin with a hard center on the tops and sides of the foot) may form. The formation of a *bunion* (swelling on the joint of the big toe) is another concern. Some over-the-counter treatments are available for these foot problems.

Special foot care should be given to residents who have diabetes or peripheral vascular disease (PVD). These residents may have serious nerve damage, or *peripheral neuropathy*, which causes a loss of pain, heat, and cold sensitivity in the feet. The feet may also become numb, which can result in unnoticed sores and swelling of the feet. A **podiatrist** (a doctor who specializes in foot health) may regularly check resident's feet, particularly residents who require special foot care.

There are several ways to maintain good blood circulation and protect feet:

- Have the resident elevate his or her feet when sitting. The resident should wiggle his or her toes and move the feet up and down for 5 minutes two to three times daily. The legs should never be crossed for long periods.

- Encourage residents to wear comfortable shoes. Check the insides of shoes before residents put them on. Make sure the lining is smooth and there are no objects inside. Socks should also be worn, and residents should never walk barefoot.

- Protect the feet from hot and cold. Do not put feet into very hot water. Always test the temperature of water first. Never use hot water bottles, heating pads, or electric blankets on the feet.

Nursing assistants also provide daily foot care. This includes bathing the feet and keeping toenails trimmed, if permitted.

Procedure

Providing Foot Care

Rationale

Daily foot care promotes cleanliness and helps prevent infections and foot odor.

Preparation

1. Ask the licensed nursing staff if there are doctor's orders for the procedure, if there are any specific instructions listed in the plan of care, and if the resident can be moved into the positions required for this procedure.
2. Wash your hands or use hand sanitizer before entering the room.
3. Knock before entering the room.
4. Introduce yourself using your first or preferred name and title. Explain that you work with the licensed nursing staff and will be providing care.
5. Greet the resident and ask the resident to state his full name, if able. Then check the resident's identification bracelet.
6. Use Mr., Mrs., or Ms. and the resident's last name when conversing.
7. Explain the procedure in simple terms, even if the resident is not able to communicate or is disoriented. Ask permission to perform the procedure.
8. Bring the necessary equipment into the room. Place a paper towel, towel, or disposable protective pad on the overbed table as an infection-control barrier before placing the following items:
   - washbasin or foot bath with warm water (100–105°F)
   - 1–2 emery boards, nail clipper, and orangewood stick, if permitted
   - 2–3 hand towels
   - several washcloths
   - disposable protective pad
   - lotion
   - disposable gloves
   - soap

The Procedure

9. Provide privacy by closing the curtains, using a screen, or closing the door to the room.
10. If the resident is able to sit in a chair, assist her to a chair. Place a disposable protective pad on the floor in front of the chair.
11. If the resident is in bed, lock the bed wheels and then raise the bed to hip level.
12. Ensure safety during the procedure. If there are side rails, raise and secure the rails on the opposite side of the bed from where you will be working. Lower the rail on the side where you are working.
13. Raise the head of the bed.
14. Wash your hands or use hand sanitizer to ensure infection control.
15. Put on disposable gloves.
16. Place the washbasin or foot bath with warm water on top of the protective pad. Check the water temperature. It should be 100–105°F. The water should feel comfortably warm to your elbow. You may also ask the resident to feel the water temperature, but always check it yourself first. Add a small amount of soap to the washbasin or foot bath.
17. Help the resident comfortably position each foot in the washbasin or foot bath to soak. Each foot may need to be soaked separately if the resident is lying in bed. If the resident is sitting in a chair, both feet can be soaked at the same time.
18. Make sure the feet are completely covered by the water. Cover the feet and washbasin with a dry hand towel to retain heat.
19. Soak the feet for approximately 10–15 minutes. If needed, remove the feet and add more warm water.
20. Lift one foot out of the washbasin at a time and wash the entire foot. Clean between the toes and under the toenails with a soapy washcloth.
21. Rinse off all soap, especially between the toes.

> **Best Practice:** The feet should be inspected for irritation, redness, cracks, swelling, blisters, or breaks in the skin, especially around the toenails. If observed, immediately report these to the licensed nursing staff.

22. Push the cuticles back gently with a washcloth or the dull end of an orangewood stick, if permitted.
23. Remove the washbasin or foot bath and dry the feet thoroughly, especially between the toes.
24. Use a nail clipper to cut the toenails, if permitted. Trim the toenails straight across. Do not cut below the tips of the toes. Trimming the toenails is always easier after they have been soaked or bathed.
25. Shape and smooth any rough toenail edges with an emery board.
26. Apply lotion to the tops and soles of the feet and gently massage it into the skin (**Figure 18.20**). Never put lotion between the toes, as this can cause fungal growth. Gently remove any excess lotion with a dry, clean towel.

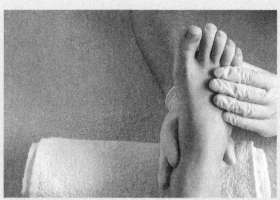

Figure 18.20   *FotoDuets/Shutterstock.com*

27. Remove and discard your gloves.
28. Wash your hands or use hand sanitizer to ensure infection control.
29. Put on a new pair of gloves.
30. If the resident is in bed, check to be sure the bed wheels are locked. Then reposition the resident and lower the bed. If the resident is in a chair, help her back to bed, if desired.

31. Follow the plan of care to determine if the side rails should be raised or lowered.
32. Remove, clean, and store equipment in the proper location. Disinfect the nail clippers. Remove soiled linens and discard disposable equipment.

Follow-Up
33. Remove and discard your gloves.
34. Wash your hands to ensure infection control.
35. Make sure the resident is comfortable and place the call light and personal items within reach.
36. Conduct a safety check before leaving the room. The room should be clean and free from clutter or spills.
37. Wash your hands or use hand sanitizer before leaving the room.

Reporting and Documentation
38. Report any specific observations, complications, or unusual responses to the licensed nursing staff. Document this information, along with the care provided, in the chart or EMR.

Perineal Care

Perineal care (sometimes called *peri care*) is the process of cleaning the genitals, or *external organs*, of the female and male reproductive systems, the urethral opening, and the anus. Perineal care should be performed daily to prevent infections, skin breakdown, and possible odor. It is also performed after elimination for residents who are immobile or who cannot provide this care for themselves, and each time a resident is incontinent. Residents who have a catheter require catheter care in addition to perineal care (see Chapter 20).

Procedure

Providing Female and Male Perineal Care

Rationale
Proper perineal care promotes cleanliness, provides comfort, and reduces the potential for infections.

Preparation
1. Ask the licensed nursing staff if there are doctor's orders for the procedure, if there are any specific instructions listed in the plan of care, and if the resident can be moved into the positions required for this procedure.

2. Wash your hands or use hand sanitizer before entering the room.
3. Knock before entering the room.
4. Introduce yourself using your first or preferred name and title. Explain that you work with the licensed nursing staff and will be providing care.
5. Greet the resident and ask the resident to state his or her full name, if able. Then check the resident's identification bracelet.
6. Use Mr., Mrs., or Ms. and the resident's last name when conversing.
7. Explain the procedure in simple terms, even if the resident is not able to communicate or is disoriented. Ask permission to perform the procedure.

(continued)

Providing Female and Male Perineal Care *(continued)*

8. Bring the necessary equipment into the room. Place a paper towel, towel, or disposable protective pad on the overbed table as an infection-control barrier before placing the following items:
   - washbasin
   - bath blanket
   - disposable gloves
   - soap
   - disposable protective pad
   - several washcloths
   - several hand towels
   - bedpan or urinal
   - laundry hamper

The Procedure: Female Perineal Care

9. Provide privacy by closing the curtains, using a screen, or closing the door to the room.
10. Lock the bed wheels and then raise the bed to hip level.
11. Maintain safety during the procedure. If there are side rails, raise and lock the rails on the opposite side of the bed from where you will be working. Lower the rail on the side where you are working.
12. Wash your hands or use hand sanitizer to ensure infection control.
13. Put on disposable gloves.
14. Position the resident on her back, if possible. Place the disposable protective pad under the resident's buttocks.
15. Cover the resident with a bath blanket. If possible, have the resident hold the bath blanket while you fanfold the bed linens to the foot of the bed. Be sure the resident is not exposed.
16. Offer the resident a bedpan. If the resident uses the bedpan or urinal, empty the contents and wash the bedpan or urinal. Remove and discard your gloves after assisting with toileting.
17. Wash your hands or use hand sanitizer to ensure infection control.
18. Put on a new pair of gloves.
19. Fill the washbasin with warm water. Check the water temperature. It should be 100–105°F. The water should feel comfortably warm to your elbow. You may also ask the resident to feel the water temperature, but always check it yourself first.
20. Ask the resident to bend her knees and separate her legs.

    Best Practice: If the resident cannot bend her knees and separate her legs, access the perineal area from a lateral, or side-lying, position with knees bent.

21. Move the linens down to the foot of the bed to expose only the perineal area. Keep the legs covered.
22. Wet a washcloth in the washbasin and apply a small amount of soap.

    Best Practice: Soap can be difficult to rinse from a female's perineal area. Use a small amount to avoid leaving residue, which can be irritating.

23. Gently separate the labia with one hand. Keep the labia separated as much as possible during the procedure.
24. Wash the outer folds of the labia (*labia majora*) and the inner folds (*labia minora*) using single, downward strokes from top to bottom or front to back (**Figure 18.21**).

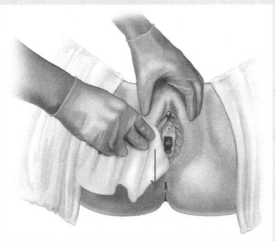

Figure 18.21   © Body Scientific International

25. With each downward stroke, turn the washcloth to a clean side or get a new washcloth. You will use several washcloths during this procedure. Avoid placing your fingers on an area after washing it.
26. Use a new washcloth with a small amount of soap to clean from the clitoris to the anus (down the center).
27. Fill the washbasin with fresh, warm water. Change your gloves, if needed.
28. Using fresh water and a clean washcloth, rinse the area thoroughly.
29. Gently pat the area dry with a towel.
30. Turn the resident onto her side away from you.
31. Apply soap to a wet washcloth.
32. With one hand, lift the upper buttock to expose the anus. Wash the anal area using gentle, front-to-back strokes from the vagina to the anus (**Figure 18.22**).

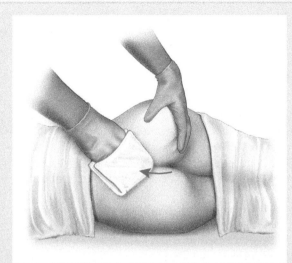

Figure 18.22   © Body Scientific International

33. Rinse and gently pat the area dry.
34. Reposition the resident so she is lying on her back.
35. Remove and dispose of the protective pad.
36. Remove and discard your gloves.
37. Wash your hands or use hand sanitizer to ensure infection control.
38. Put on a new pair of gloves.
39. Replace the top covers and remove the bath blanket.
40. Check to be sure the bed wheels are locked and then lower the bed.
41. Follow the plan of care to determine if the side rails should be raised or lowered.
42. Remove, clean, and store equipment in the proper location. Remove soiled linens and discard disposable equipment.

The Procedure: Male Perineal Care

43. Provide privacy by closing the curtains, using a screen, or closing the door to the room.
44. Lock the bed wheels and then raise the bed to hip level.
45. Ensure safety during the procedure. If there are side rails, raise and secure the rails on the opposite side of the bed from where you will be working. Lower the rail on the side where you are working.
46. Wash your hands or use hand sanitizer to ensure infection control.
47. Put on disposable gloves.
48. Position the resident on his back, if possible. Place the disposable protective pad under the resident's buttocks.
49. Cover the resident with a bath blanket. If possible, have the resident hold the bath blanket while you fanfold the bed linens to the foot of the bed. Be sure the resident is not exposed.

50. Offer the resident a bedpan or urinal. If the resident uses the bedpan or urinal, empty the contents and wash the bedpan or urinal. Remove and discard your gloves after assisting with toileting.
51. Wash your hands or use hand sanitizer to ensure infection control.
52. Put on a new pair of gloves.
53. Fill the washbasin with warm water. Check the water temperature. It should be 100–105°F. The water should feel comfortably warm to your elbow. You may also ask the resident to feel the water temperature, but always check it yourself first.
54. Ask the resident to bend his knees and separate his legs.

> **Best Practice:** If the resident cannot bend his knees and separate his legs, access the perineal area from a lateral, or side-lying, position with the knees bent.

55. Move the linens down to the foot of the bed to expose only the perineal area. Keep the legs covered.
56. Wet a washcloth in the washbasin and apply a small amount of soap.
57. Gently lift and hold the penis in one hand. Start at the tip of the penis (meatus) and wash on each side in a circular motion down the shaft of the penis to the base (**Figure 18.23**).

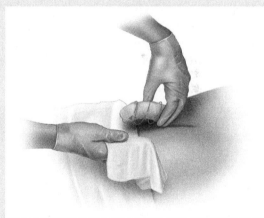

Figure 18.23   © Body Scientific International

58. If the penis is not circumcised, carefully pull back the foreskin while washing, rinsing, and drying the penis. If the foreskin will not retract, report this to the licensed nursing staff.
59. Lift and wash the scrotum. Also wash the inner thighs.
60. Fill the washbasin with fresh, warm water. Change your gloves, if needed.
61. Using fresh water and a clean washcloth, rinse the area thoroughly.
62. Gently pat the area dry with a towel.

(continued)

Providing Female and Male Perineal Care *(continued)*

63. Turn the resident onto his side away from you.
64. Apply soap to a wet washcloth.
65. Wash the anal area using gentle, front-to-back strokes.
66. Rinse and gently pat the area dry.
67. Reposition the resident so he is lying on his back.
68. Remove and dispose of the protective pad.
69. Remove and discard your gloves.
70. Wash your hands or use hand sanitizer to ensure infection control.
71. Put on a new pair of gloves.
72. Replace the top covers and remove the bath blanket.
73. Check to be sure the bed wheels are locked and then lower the bed.
74. Follow the plan of care to determine if the side rails should be raised or lowered.
75. Remove, clean, and store equipment in the proper location. Remove soiled linens and discard disposable equipment.

Follow-Up
76. Remove and discard your gloves.
77. Wash your hands to ensure infection control.
78. Make sure the resident is comfortable and place the call light and personal items within reach.
79. Conduct a safety check before leaving the room. The room should be clean and free from clutter or spills.
80. Wash your hands or use hand sanitizer before leaving the room.

Reporting and Documentation
81. Report any specific observations, complications, or unusual responses to the licensed nursing staff. Document this information, along with the care provided, in the chart or EMR.

Dressing and Undressing

As a nursing assistant, you will often assist in dressing and undressing residents. A person's clothing expresses his or her personal preferences and image. Residents often prefer to choose their clothing. Encourage residents to be as independent as possible during dressing and undressing by helping with buttons, snaps, or shoes, if needed. Special care is needed with residents who have an IV. See the Procedure: *Changing a Gown or Clothing with an IV.* Clothing with zippers, Velcro™ fasteners, elastic waistbands, and slip-on shoes can make it easier for residents to maintain some independence when dressing. Shoes or slippers should fit well and have nonskid soles or strips. This helps maintain safety so that residents do not slip or trip.

Procedure

Dressing and Undressing

Rationale
Residents in your care may require assistance during dressing and undressing. It is your responsibility to make sure these activities are performed safely.

Preparation
1. Ask the licensed nursing staff if there are doctor's orders for the procedure, if there are any specific instructions listed in the plan of care, and if the resident can be moved into the positions required for this procedure.
2. Wash your hands or use hand sanitizer before entering the room.
3. Knock before entering the room.
4. Introduce yourself using your first or preferred name and title. Explain that you work with the licensed nursing staff and will be providing care.
5. Greet the resident and ask the resident to state her full name, if able. Then check the resident's identification bracelet.
6. Use Mr., Mrs., or Ms. and the resident's last name when conversing.
7. Explain the procedure in simple terms, even if the resident is not able to communicate or is disoriented. Ask permission to perform the procedure.
8. Bring the necessary equipment into the room. Place the following items in an easy-to-reach place:
   • bath blanket, as needed
   • disposable gloves, if needed for infection control
   • laundry hamper
   • clothes, arranged in the order they will be put on

The Procedure: Dressing

9. Provide privacy by closing the curtains, using a screen, or closing the door to the room.

10. Lock the bed wheels and then raise the bed to hip level.

11. Maintain safety during the procedure. If there are side rails, raise and lock the rails on the opposite side of the bed from where you will be working. Lower the rail on the side where you are working.

   Best Practice: Wear disposable gloves only if required for infection prevention and control.

12. Assist the resident to a Fowler's position. Determine how high to raise the head of the bed based on resident comfort. If the resident is mobile, she may be dressed in a chair or while sitting on the edge of the bed.

13. If the resident is in bed, fanfold the top linens to the foot of the bed. Cover the resident with a bath blanket, as needed, for warmth, dignity, and privacy. Remove pajamas or clothing using the undressing procedure.

   Best Practice: To minimize stress, put clothing on the weak or painful side of the resident's body first and remove clothes from the unaffected or strong side first.

14. If the resident wears a bra, ask her to put her arms through the straps and then place her breasts in the breast cups. Ask the resident to lean forward, assisting as needed. Bring the sides of the bra together in the back and close the fasteners. Adjust, if needed.

15. To put on upper garments that open in the back, slip the clothing over the resident's hands (weak side first). Move the clothing up the arms and position it on the shoulders. Close the garment and any fasteners in the back.

16. To put on upper garments that open in the front, slide the clothing onto the weak or painful arm and shoulder first (**Figure 18.24A**). Bring the garment around the resident's back. Ask the resident to lower her head and shoulders so she can slide her stronger arm through the garment more easily (**Figure 18.24B**). Close the garment and any fasteners in the front.

17. To put on upper garments that slip over the head, put the neck of the garment over the resident's head. Slide the resident's weaker arm and shoulder into the garment. Raise the resident's head and shoulders and pull the garment toward the waist. Slide the arm and shoulder of the stronger arm through the garment. Close any fasteners.

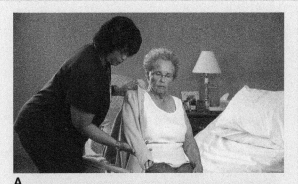

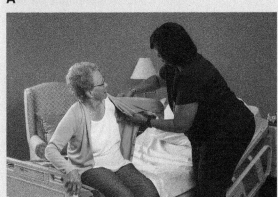

A

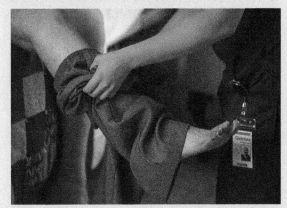

B

Figure 18.24

© Tori Soper Photography

18. Slide the resident's underwear and then pants over the feet and up the legs (**Figure 18.25**). Start with the weak or painful side first. Ask the resident to bend at the knees and lift her buttocks off the bed. Assist, if needed. Grasp the top of the garment with both hands and slide the garment over the resident's hips and buttocks toward the waist. Close any fasteners. If the resident is unable to assist, roll her from side to side to dress the lower body.

Figure 18.25

© Tori Soper Photography

19. Pull the resident's socks or stockings up over each foot. Adjust until the length of the sock or stocking is smooth.

(continued)

Dressing and Undressing *(continued)*

20. If the resident will be leaving her bed, put nonskid footwear on her feet and secure any fasteners. If she will be staying in bed, do not put on shoes.
21. If the resident is staying in bed, replace the top bed linens. Discard the bath blanket, if used, in the laundry hamper.
22. Check to be sure the bed wheels are locked, then reposition the resident and lower the bed.
23. Follow the plan of care to determine if the side rails should be raised or lowered.

The Procedure: Undressing

24. Provide privacy by closing the curtains, using a screen, or closing the door to the room.
25. Lock the bed wheels and then raise the bed to hip level.
26. Maintain safety during the procedure. If there are side rails, raise and lock the rails on the opposite side of the bed from where you will be working. Lower the rail on the side where you are working.

> **Best Practice:** Wear disposable gloves only if required for infection prevention and control.

27. Assist the resident to a Fowler's position. Determine how high to raise the head of the bed based on resident comfort. If the resident is mobile, she may be undressed in a chair or while sitting on the edge of the bed.
28. If the resident is in bed, fanfold the top linens to the foot of the bed. Cover the resident with a bath blanket, as needed, for warmth, dignity, and privacy.
29. If the resident's clothing opens in the back, raise the resident's head and shoulders or turn her slightly to the side away from you. This will make it easier to undo fasteners.
30. Pull the clothing to the resident's sides.
31. Remove the clothing from the resident's arms.
32. If the clothing does not open in the back, bring the clothing up to the resident's neck and remove over her head.

> **Best Practice:** Remember to remove clothing from the stronger arm first and then from the weaker arm. Do not force or overextend the arms.

33. Remove the resident's shoes and socks or stockings.
34. Undo clothing fasteners and remove the resident's belt. Ask the resident to lift her buttocks, assisting, if needed.
35. Grasp the top of the garment with both hands and slide the pants over the resident's buttocks and down toward the knees. If the resident is unable to assist, have her roll from side to side as you lower the pants. Slide the pants down the legs. Remove the clothing from the stronger leg first and then from the weaker leg. Never force or overextend the legs. Put on pajamas using the dressing procedure.

> **Best Practice:** Never pull, push, or roughly handle the resident when putting on or removing clothes.

36. Replace the top linens. Discard the bath blanket, if used, in the laundry hamper.
37. Check to be sure the bed wheels are locked, then reposition the resident and lower the bed.
38. Follow the plan of care to determine if the side rails should be raised or lowered.

Follow-Up

39. Wash your hands to ensure infection control.
40. Make sure the resident is comfortable and place the call light and personal items within reach.
41. Conduct a safety check before leaving the room. The room should be clean and free from clutter or spills.
42. Wash your hands or use hand sanitizer before leaving the room.

Reporting and Documentation

43. Report any specific observations, complications, or unusual responses to the licensed nursing staff. Document this information, along with the care provided, in the chart or EMR.

When delivering care, you may be asked to change a hospital gown or clothing when there is an IV. This needs to be done carefully so the IV insertion and tubing are not dislodged and so the IV pole remains in place. The procedure that follows should be used when the IV is hanging on an IV pole and gowns with snaps or Velcro™ at the sleeves and shoulders are not available. When an IV is running through an electric pump, a gown with snaps or Velcro™ at the sleeves and shoulders are required.

Procedure

Changing a Gown or Clothing with an IV

Rationale

A gown or clothing should be changed daily and whenever it becomes wet or soiled. Special care should be taken when the resident has an IV.

Preparation

1. Ask the licensed nursing staff if there are doctor's orders for the procedure, if there are any specific instructions listed in the plan of care, and if the patient can be moved into the positions required for this procedure.
2. Wash your hands or use hand sanitizer before entering the room.
3. Knock before entering the room.
4. Introduce yourself using your first or preferred name and title. Explain that you work with the licensed nursing staff and will be providing care.
5. Greet the resident and ask the resident to state his full name, if able. Then check the resident's identification bracelet.
6. Use Mr., Mrs., or Ms. and the resident's last name when conversing.
7. Explain the procedure in simple terms, even if the resident is not able to communicate or is disoriented. Ask permission to perform the procedure.
8. Bring the necessary equipment into the room. Place the following items in an easy-to-reach place:
   - bath blanket
   - 2 clean gowns or appropriate clothing
   - disposable gloves
   - laundry hamper

The Procedure

9. Provide privacy by closing the curtains, using a screen, or closing the door to the room.
10. Lock the bed wheels and then raise the bed to hip level.
11. Maintain safety during the procedure. If there are side rails, raise and lock the rails on the opposite side of the bed from where you will be working. Lower the rail on the side where you are working.
12. Wash your hands or use hand sanitizer to ensure infection control.
13. Put on disposable gloves.
14. Assist the resident to a Fowler's position. Determine how high to raise the head of the bed based on resident comfort.
15. Cover the resident with a bath blanket and fanfold the top bed linens to the foot of the bed.
16. If the resident is wearing a gown without snaps or fasteners at the neck, undo the gown ties at the neck and free the gown from underneath the body.
17. Slip the gown down the resident's arms. Make sure the bath blanket stays in place.
18. Remove the gown from the resident's arm without the IV and tubing. Move the gown across the resident's chest and lay it next to the other arm.
19. Gather the sleeve of the arm with the IV so there is no pull or pressure on the IV tubing. Slide the gown over the IV site and tubing (**Figure 18.26A**).
20. Carefully remove the resident's arm and hand from the sleeve.
21. Keep the sleeve gathered and slide your hand along the tubing to the IV bag. Remove the IV bag from the IV pole (**Figure 18.26B**). Never disconnect the IV tubing from its insertion site or the IV bag.

   Best Practice: Never lower the bag of IV fluid below the arm while changing the gown.

22. Slide the IV bag and tubing through the sleeve (**Figure 18.26C**). Hang the IV bag back on the pole.
23. To put a clean gown on the resident, gather the sleeve of the gown that will go on the arm with the IV.
24. Remove the IV bag from the pole (**Figure 18.26D**). Slide the sleeve over the IV bag and tubing at the shoulder part of the gown. Hang the IV bag back on the pole.
25. Slide the gathered sleeve over the IV tubing, the resident's hand and arm, and the IV site. Slide the sleeve onto the resident's shoulder.
26. Put the resident's other arm through the opposite sleeve and fasten the gown.
27. Replace the top linens and remove the bath blanket.
28. Check to be sure the bed wheels are locked, then reposition the resident and lower the bed.

(continued)

Changing a Gown or Clothing with an IV *(continued)*

29. Follow the plan of care to determine if the side rails should be raised or lowered.
30. Remove, clean, and store equipment in the proper location. Remove soiled linens and discard disposable equipment.

Follow-Up

31. Remove and discard your gloves.
32. Wash your hands to ensure infection control.
33. Make sure the resident is comfortable and place the call light and personal items within reach.

34. Conduct a safety check before leaving the room. The room should be clean and free from clutter or spills.
35. Wash your hands or use hand sanitizer before leaving the room.

Reporting and Documentation

36. Report any specific observations, complications, or unusual responses to the licensed nursing staff. Document this information, along with the care provided, in the chart or EMR.

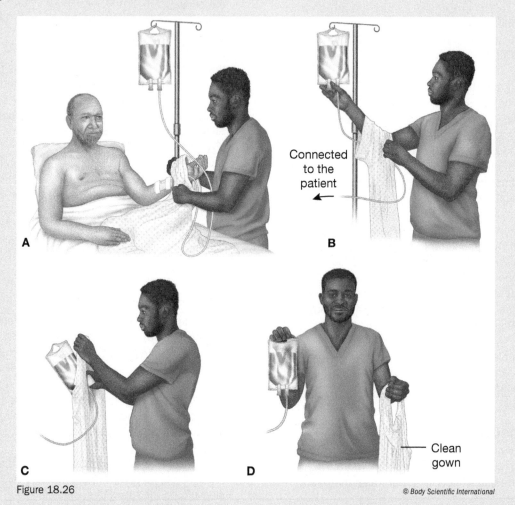

Connected to the patient

A

B

C

D

Clean gown

Figure 18.26

© Body Scientific International

SECTION 18.1 **Review and Assessment**

Key Terms Mini Glossary

emesis basin a small, usually kidney-shaped bowl often used for oral care or if the resident needs to vomit.

hemorrhoids swollen, inflamed veins found under the skin around the anus (external) or inside the rectum (internal); are caused by pressure from straining during bowel movements; may be itchy or painful at times and can cause rectal bleeding.

hygiene routine actions such as bathing that promote and maintain cleanliness and health.

perineal care hygiene care that involves cleansing the area between the thighs (the coccyx, pubis, anus, urethra, and external genitals).

perineum the area between the thighs; includes the coccyx, pubis, anus, urethra, and external genitals.

podiatrist a doctor who specializes in diagnosing and treating diseases and conditions that affect the feet.

sitz bath a type of therapeutic bath that soaks a person's perineum, buttocks, and sometimes hips in warm water.

skin integrity the condition of the skin; healthy skin is whole or intact without irritation, inflammation, or damage.

therapeutic having a healing effect on the body and mind.

whirlpool a type of bathtub used for therapeutic purposes; has small spray jets that swirl water.

Apply the Key Terms

Write a sentence using each key term properly.

1. therapeutic
2. skin integrity
3. perineal care
4. emesis basin
5. sitz bath

Know and Understand the Facts

1. List three reasons why personal hygiene and grooming are important.
2. What are two guidelines a holistic nursing assistant should follow to perform safe fingernail care?
3. Identify two important actions a holistic nursing assistant should take when giving oral care.
4. What special care is important when performing foot care?

Analyze and Apply Concepts

1. Identify two ways a holistic nursing assistant can encourage independence during personal hygiene and grooming.
2. Describe how to bathe the arm of a resident with limited mobility.
3. A resident is not able to wash her own hair. Describe the steps needed to assist her with hair care.
4. Identify two ways a holistic nursing assistant can show respect and maintain resident dignity during bathing.
5. Explain how to make a bathmit with a washcloth.

6. Identify three guidelines to follow when shaving a resident.
7. Explain how to perform male perineal care.
8. Explain how to perform female perineal care.
9. What is one best practice for changing a gown or clothing of a resident with an IV?

Think Critically

Read the following care situation. Then answer the questions that follow.

Mrs. B is 80 years old and was admitted to the hospital last night with pneumonia. She has diabetes, PVD, and arthritis. You have been assigned to help her with personal hygiene and grooming this morning. Mrs. B is having difficulty breathing and has an IV. She is also stiff from her arthritic joints. When you enter Mrs. B's room, you find that she is sleeping. She has a strong body odor, her hair is tangled, and she has very long, dirty fingernails.

1. If you could perform only one personal hygiene procedure, which would be the most important?
2. What steps would you need to take to perform the procedure?
3. What actions can you take to help Mrs. B be more comfortable when providing care?
4. Given Mrs. B's current condition, describe five safety and quality care issues you would need to be aware of when performing her personal hygiene and grooming.

Caring for the Skin

Objectives

To achieve the objectives for this section, you must successfully:

- **explain** the importance of maintaining skin integrity.
- **describe** how heat and cold applications can help and harm the skin.
- **demonstrate** safe skin care when using hot and cold therapies.

Key Terms

Learn these key terms to better understand the information presented in the section.

compresses	hydration
cryotherapy	pallor
cyanotic	tepid
gangrene	thermotherapy

Questions to Consider

- The next time you are with friends or family members, observe their skin. Look at their faces, arms, or legs. How would you describe their skin texture (smooth or rough), tone, and integrity? Is their skin dry or oily? Does their skin have marks such as freckles, moles, bumps, pimples, or a rash?
- Compare your skin with the skin of a person you are observing. What are the similarities and differences?
- How healthy do you think the person's skin is? How healthy is your skin? What makes the skin look healthy or unhealthy?

How Can Nursing Assistants Help Maintain Skin Integrity?

The skin is the largest organ in the human body. Skin that remains healthy and maintains its integrity is able to perform its important functions. This is especially important for older adults, whose skin is more likely to tear or bruise.

Nursing assistants can help maintain the skin integrity of residents by giving excellent skin care and carefully observing the skin, particularly when caring for residents with diabetes. You should also be especially careful with residents taking blood thinning and steroid medications, which cause bruising to occur more easily. Any changes in the skin must be reported immediately to the licensed

nursing staff. Following are several actions you should take as part of your care:

- Change a resident's position every two hours. When possible, and with a doctor's order, help residents ambulate and perform range-of-motion exercises.
- Avoid giving residents long baths, as these can remove oils from the skin. Use warm, rather than very hot, water.
- Use mild cleansers rather than strong soaps. Strong soaps have ingredients that can remove oil from the skin.
- Gently pat the skin dry after a bath or shower. This leaves some moisture on the skin.
- Regularly moisturize the skin, especially if it is dry. Do not put lotion between the toes, where fungus can grow. Give a very light massage, if appropriate, while applying lotion.
- If the resident is incontinent, use disposable protective pads. These can be removed and replaced more easily than linens.
- Keep linens neat and wrinkle free. Make sure linens are free from food crumbs and any other items that can place pressure on the skin.
- Keep the skin clean and dry. If the skin is covered with urine or feces due to incontinence, clean the skin immediately with mild soap and water and gently pat the area dry. Wear disposable gloves for infection control.
- Avoid dragging or pulling the resident during positioning. Friction can cause the skin to become red or irritated and experience shearing or tearing.

Pressure Points and Decubitus Ulcers

Residents who are immobile due to illness, who are in wheelchairs, or who need to use assistive devices are more vulnerable to changes in their skin integrity. As you learned in Chapter 10, *pressure points* are more likely to be at risk for changes in their skin integrity than other areas of the skin. If the skin is damaged in any way, *decubitus ulcers* can develop. The severity of decubitus ulcers ranges from stage 1 to stage 4 (as shown in **Figure 10.5**). Pressure points should be kept dry and clean. Any ulcers should be cleaned and dressed with bandages, and wet or creased dressings and bandages should be changed according to the plan of care.

Observing the skin carefully while performing personal hygiene, grooming, and any other procedures is the best way to identify any problems with the skin's integrity, including decubitus ulcers.

Observation of the Skin

Skin types can be normal, dry, oily, or combination. Skin type can change over time due to personal care, cosmetics used, environment, medications taken, hormones, and aging.

A person's skin type depends on

- the water content of the skin, which affects flexibility;
- oiliness, which affects texture; and
- sensitivity.

When observing the skin, always be sure there is bright light. Notice whether the skin is cool, warm, hot, moist, or dry. Look at the color of the skin, lips, and nail beds. Regularly check the skin for red areas, irritation, or skin breakdown at pressure points (see **Figure 10.5**).

If you notice red skin, immediately remove whatever is causing the pressure. Do not massage the area. Recheck the skin in 15 minutes. If the redness is gone, you do not need to take any other action. If the redness does not disappear after 15 minutes, talk with the licensed nursing staff about ways to provide relief.

Also check areas where body parts rub together, especially if the resident is obese. This includes under the breasts, between the folds of the abdomen, and between the buttocks and thighs.

Report to the licensed nursing staff if you observe any of the following:

- The skin has a ***pallor*** (unusually pale color), is flushed (red), or is ***cyanotic*** (blue due to insufficient oxygen).
- There are new abrasions, tears, bruises, rashes, and blisters.
- A blister has opened.
- There are new lumps and swollen or tender areas.
- There is new or increased drainage or bleeding.
- You smell unusual odors.
- The resident complains of itching or burning or is scratching or rubbing an area excessively.
- The scalp is flaky, itchy, or sore.
- Head lice are present.

When Are Heat Applications Helpful?

The use of heat on the skin to increase circulation and ease pain is called ***thermotherapy***. Heat has many healing qualities. It can reduce pain, relax muscles, improve flexibility, ease headaches, and help treat arthritis.

Care should be taken if the resident is sensitive to heat or cannot feel it, or has infections, tumors, open wounds, or stitches. Physical therapists often apply heat applications, but heat applications are applied by nursing assistants only based on a doctor's order and the plan of care. Heat applications may include warm, moist ***compresses*** (pads), warm soaks, and an aquathermia pad.

Types of Heat Applications

Heat applications can be moist or dry. Moist heat is usually preferred because it goes into the skin more effectively and is less drying. Heat applications include heating pads, heat wraps, and compresses or soaks. Sitz baths and the whirlpool tub are also considered heat applications. Heat applications that can raise body temperature include hot baths, saunas, steam baths, and hot showers. Some commercial, premoistened heat compresses are available and are packaged in foil. The *aquathermia pad*, or *K-pad*, provides dry heat to promote skin circulation by applying a constant temperature to a body part for a specified period of time (**Figure 18.27**).

Care for Heat Applications

The following guidelines will help make sure heat applications are helpful and not harmful:

- Practice safety when working with water. Prevent or clean up spills on or near the resident and your work area.

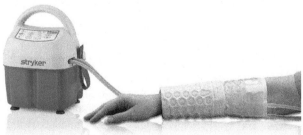

Copyright © 2017 Stryker

Figure 18.27 Use distilled water and provide a barrier such as a flannel cover to prevent the aquathermia pad from directly touching the resident's skin. Do not use pins. Check the pad for leaks and make sure the tubing and pad are level with the heating unit. The tubing should never hang below the bed.

- Make sure the heat application is warm, not hot. Maintain a consistent temperature, if possible.
- Apply heat for 15–20 minutes, unless the doctor orders a shorter or longer time, and check every five minutes to see how the resident's skin reacts to the heat application. Heat applications may be applied more than once a day, depending on the doctor's order.
- Never apply a heat application directly to the resident's skin. Always provide a barrier between the heat application and the skin.
- If using an aquathermia pad, set the temperature as directed by the licensed nursing staff. Check the skin underneath the pad for redness, swelling, or blisters. Stop the treatment and remove the pad if redness, swelling, or blisters appear or if the resident complains of pain, discomfort, or decreased sensation. Immediately notify the licensed nursing staff. Refill the heating unit if distilled water drops below the full line.
- Maintain resident *hydration* (a sufficient amount of fluid in body tissues), proper resident body position, and comfort during treatment with heat applications.

Further treatment may be required after a heat application. For example, dressings may need to be reapplied to the affected area. Review the procedures for changing dressings in Chapter 8.

Procedure

Using Warm, Moist Compresses

Rationale
The safe and proper application of warm, moist compresses promotes healing and eases pain.

Preparation
1. Ask the licensed nursing staff if there are doctor's orders for the procedure, if there are any specific instructions listed in the plan of care, and if the resident can be moved into the positions required for this procedure.
2. Wash your hands or use hand sanitizer before entering the room.
3. Knock before entering the room.
4. Introduce yourself using your first or preferred name and title. Explain that you work with the licensed nursing staff and will be providing care.
5. Greet the resident and ask the resident to state his full name, if able. Then check the resident's identification bracelet.
6. Use Mr., Mrs., or Ms. and the resident's last name when conversing.
7. Explain the procedure in simple terms, even if the resident is not able to communicate or is disoriented. Ask permission to perform the procedure.
8. Bring the necessary equipment into the room. Place a paper towel, towel, or disposable protective pad on the overbed table as an infection-control barrier before placing the following items:
   - washbasin
   - several gauze pads
   - 2–3 washcloths and hand towels
   - bath towel
   - plastic wrap, ties, tape, and rolled gauze, if needed
   - bath blanket
   - disposable protective pad
   - disposable gloves
   - laundry hamper

The Procedure
9. Provide privacy by closing the curtains, using a screen, or closing the door to the room.
10. Lock the bed wheels and then raise the bed to hip level.
11. Maintain safety during the procedure. If there are side rails, raise and lock the rails on the opposite side of the bed from where you will be working. Lower the rail on the side where you are working.
12. Position the resident properly for the procedure. The proper position will depend on the body part receiving the warm, moist compress.
13. Place a disposable protective pad under the body part that will receive the warm, moist compress and use the bath blanket to cover any other exposed areas.
14. Fill the washbasin one-half to two-thirds full of warm water. Check the water temperature. It should be 100–105°F. The water should feel comfortably warm to your elbow. You may also ask the resident to feel the water temperature, but always check it yourself first.
15. Wash your hands or use hand sanitizer to ensure infection control.

16. Put on disposable gloves.

17. Use a washcloth or gauze pad as a compress for the skin. Place the compress in the warm water and squeeze out any excess moisture.

18. Observe the application site for inflammation and skin color. Alert the licensed nursing staff if the skin is red or inflamed. Proceed only by direction.

19. If the skin is not red or inflamed, apply the compress to the body part. Note the time of application.

20. Cover the compress with plastic wrap and then a bath towel. You may also secure the bath towel in place with ties, tape, or rolled gauze. Follow instructions from the licensed nursing staff. Never put tape on the resident's skin.

21. Place the call light and personal items within reach. Place a glass of fresh water on the overbed table, if permitted.

22. Check to be sure the bed wheels are locked, then lower the bed.

23. Follow the plan of care to determine if the side rails should be raised or lowered. Unscreen the resident or open the door to the room, if appropriate.

24. Remove and discard your gloves.

25. Wash your hands or use hand sanitizer to ensure infection control.

26. Check on the resident every 5 minutes (**Figure 18.28**). Treatments usually last no longer than 20 minutes, unless otherwise ordered by the doctor.

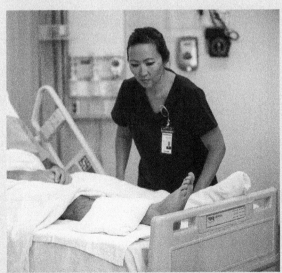

Figure 18.28   © Tori Soper Photography

Best Practice: Observe and check the following: Is the compress warm enough or too hot? Is there pain or burning at the site? Does the resident feel weak, faint, or drowsy? If there are any problems or complications, remove the application and report to the licensed nursing staff.

27. When it is time to remove the warm, moist compress, lock the bed wheels and then raise the bed to hip level.

28. Ensure safety during the procedure. If there are side rails, raise and lock the rails on the opposite side of the bed from where you will be working. Lower the rail on the side where you are working.

29. Wash your hands or use hand sanitizer to ensure infection control.

30. Put on disposable gloves.

31. Carefully remove the compress. Note the time the compress is removed. Observe the resident's response to the application.

32. Appropriately discard the compress. Remove the protective pad and change any wet linens. Assist with any further treatment as instructed by the licensed nursing staff.

33. Check to be sure the bed wheels are locked, then reposition the resident and lower the bed.

34. Follow the plan of care to determine if the side rails should be raised or lowered.

35. Remove, clean, and store equipment in the proper location. Remove soiled linens and discard disposable equipment.

Follow-Up

36. Remove and discard your gloves.

37. Wash your hands to ensure infection control.

38. Make sure the resident is comfortable and place the call light and personal items within reach.

39. Conduct a safety check before leaving the room. The room should be clean and free from clutter or spills.

40. Wash your hands or use hand sanitizer before leaving the room.

Reporting and Documentation

41. Report any specific observations, complications, or unusual responses to the licensed nursing staff. Document this information, along with the care provided, in the chart or EMR.

Procedure

Using Warm Soaks

Rationale

The safe and proper application of warm soaks promotes healing and eases pain. Warm soaks increase blood flow to the affected area.

Preparation

1. Ask the licensed nursing staff if there are doctor's orders for the procedure, if there are any specific instructions listed in the plan of care, and if the resident can be moved into the positions required for this procedure.
2. Wash your hands or use hand sanitizer before entering the room.
3. Knock before entering the room.
4. Introduce yourself using your first or preferred name and title. Explain that you work with the licensed nursing staff and will be providing care.
5. Greet the resident and ask the resident to state his full name, if able. Then check the resident's identification bracelet.
6. Use Mr., Mrs., or Ms. and the resident's last name when conversing.
7. Explain the procedure in simple terms, even if the resident is not able to communicate or is disoriented. Ask permission to perform the procedure.
8. Bring the necessary equipment into the room. Place a paper towel, towel, or disposable protective pad on the overbed table as an infection-control barrier before placing the following items:
   - washbasin or an arm or foot bath
   - disposable protective pad
   - bath blanket
   - several hand towels
   - disposable gloves

The Procedure

9. Provide privacy by closing the curtains, using a screen, or closing the door to the room.
10. If the resident is in bed, lock the bed wheels and then raise the bed to hip level.
11. Maintain safety during the procedure. If there are side rails, raise and lock the rails on the opposite side of the bed from where you will be working. Lower the rail on the side where you are working.
12. Wash your hands or use hand sanitizer to ensure infection control.
13. Put on disposable gloves.

14. Position the resident and body part for the procedure. If the resident cannot get out of bed, the soak may take place in bed. The soak may also take place out of bed, with the resident seated at the edge of the bed or in a chair.
15. Use a bath blanket to cover any exposed areas and provide warmth.
16. Fill the washbasin half-full with warm water. Check the water temperature. The water should feel comfortably warm to your elbow. You may also ask the resident to feel the water temperature, but always check it yourself first.
17. Put a disposable protective pad under the washbasin to catch any spills.
18. Place the affected body part into the warm water. Pad the edge of the washbasin with a towel. Note the time of the application.
19. Place the call light and personal items within reach. Place a glass of fresh water on the overbed table, if permitted.
20. If the resident is in bed, check to be sure the bed wheels are locked, then lower the bed. Follow the plan of care to determine if the side rails should be raised or lowered. If the resident is sitting in a chair or on the edge of the bed, be certain all safety precautions are in place. Unscreen the resident or open the door to the room, if appropriate.
21. Remove and discard your gloves.
22. Wash your hands or use hand sanitizer to ensure infection control.
23. Check on the resident every 5 minutes. Treatments usually last no longer than 15–20 minutes, unless otherwise ordered by the doctor. The water may have to be changed to maintain the desired warmth.

   > **Best Practice:** Observe and check the following: Is the water warm enough or too hot? Is there pain or burning? Does the resident feel weak, faint, or drowsy? If there are any problems or complications, remove the application and report to the licensed nursing staff.

24. When the warm soak is complete, lock the bed wheels and then raise the bed to hip level if the resident is in bed.
25. Ensure safety during the procedure. If there are side rails, raise and lock the rails on the opposite side of the bed from where you will be working. Lower the rail on the side where you are working.
26. Wash your hands or use hand sanitizer to ensure infection control.
27. Put on disposable gloves.

28. Remove the body part from the warm water and pat it dry with a clean hand towel (**Figure 18.29**). Note the time the soak was stopped. Assist with any further treatment as instructed by the licensed nursing staff.

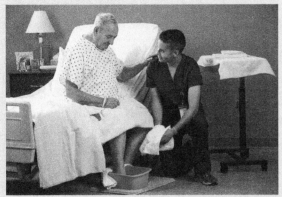

Figure 18.29   © Tori Soper Photography

29. Discard the water. Remove the protective pad and change any wet linens.
30. If the resident is in bed, check to be sure the bed wheels are locked. Then reposition the resident and lower the bed.

31. Follow the plan of care to determine if the side rails should be raised or lowered.
32. Remove, clean, and store equipment in the proper location. Remove soiled linens and discard disposable equipment.

Follow-Up
33. Remove and discard your gloves.
34. Wash your hands to ensure infection control.
35. Make sure the resident is comfortable and place the call light and personal items within reach.
36. Conduct a safety check before leaving the room. The room should be clean and free from clutter or spills.
37. Wash your hands or use hand sanitizer before leaving the room.

Reporting and Documentation
38. Report any specific observations, complications, or unusual responses to the licensed nursing staff. Document this information, along with the care provided, in the chart or EMR.

When Are Cold Applications Useful?

Cryotherapy is the use of cold applications to reduce swelling and ease pain. It is typically recommended for acute injuries during the first 24–48 hours after an injury. Cryotherapy is most effective for sprains, bumps, bruises, and soft-tissue injuries.

Physical therapists often apply cold applications, but nursing assistants may apply cold applications only based on a doctor's order and the plan of care. Cold applications can include cold, moist compresses and different types of ice packs. An *ice cap* is an ice pack used specifically for the head. It has a wide opening so it can be filled easily with ice chips. Another specialized ice pack is the *ice collar*, a narrow bag filled with ice that curves to fit the neck. A *tepid* (slightly warm) sponge bath may also be used to lower body temperature.

HEALTHCARE SCENARIO
Warm Soak Safety

A recent online news article told the story of Mr. W, who is 79 years old and a resident at a local healthcare facility. The nursing assistant caring for Mr. W was in a rush when she provided a warm soak for his feet, as ordered in his plan of care. Mr. W is diabetic, and warm soaks are an important part of his foot care. The nursing assistant prepared the warm soak, but did not feel the temperature of the water. She only asked Mr. W if the water was okay. Mr. W has PVD from diabetes and is not able to feel hot and cold. He put his feet in the water and said it was fine. Mr. W did not remove his feet until the nursing assistant returned 10 minutes later. When the nursing assistant came into the room, she found that Mr. W's skin was red and blistered.

Apply It
1. What did the nursing assistant do wrong?
2. What proper procedure should the nursing assistant have followed?
3. What should the nursing assistant do when she sees Mr. W's skin after the warm soak?

The following guidelines will help make sure cold applications are helpful and not harmful:

- Practice safety when working with water. Prevent or clean up spills on or near the resident and your work area.
- Apply cold compresses to injured areas for no more than 20 minutes at a time or as long as ordered by the doctor. The cold application can be removed for 10 minutes and then reapplied for 10 minutes. Check every 5 minutes to see how the resident's skin tolerates the cold application.
- Always cover the rest of the resident if he or she feels cold during the application.
- Always wrap ice packs in a thin covering such as a towel before applying them to the resident's body.
- Immediately stop a cold application if the resident complains of numbness or if the skin appears white or spotty.
- Stop the cold application if the resident complains of burning pain. Burning pain can be a sign of a lack of blood supply to the skin, which can lead to necrosis.
- Check for signs of *frostbite*, a condition in which the skin becomes too cold or frozen, red, and numb. *Frostnip* is the first stage of frostbite and can be treated by warming the skin. Severe frostbite can cause infection and **gangrene** (decay of body tissue) and can possibly require amputation.
- Maintain proper resident body position and comfort during treatment with cold applications.

Further treatment may be required after a cold application. For example, dressings may need to be reapplied to the affected area. Review the procedures for changing dressings in Chapter 8.

Procedure

Using Cold Applications

Rationale
Cold applications, such as moist compresses or an ice pack, help reduce swelling and bruising and ease pain when an acute injury occurs.

Preparation
1. Ask the licensed nursing staff if there are doctor's orders for the procedure, if there are any specific instructions listed in the plan of care, and if the resident can be moved into the positions required for this procedure.
2. Wash your hands or use hand sanitizer before entering the room.
3. Knock before entering the room.
4. Introduce yourself using your first or preferred name and title. Explain that you work with the licensed nursing staff and will be providing care.
5. Greet the resident and ask the resident to state her full name, if able. Then check the resident's identification bracelet.
6. Use Mr., Mrs., or Ms. and the resident's last name when conversing.
7. Explain the procedure in simple terms, even if the resident is not able to communicate or is disoriented. Ask permission to perform the procedure.
8. Bring the necessary equipment into the room. Place a paper towel, towel, or disposable protective pad on the overbed table as an infection-control barrier before placing the following items:
   - bath blanket
   - disposable protective pad
   - disposable gloves, if needed for infection control

When Using a Cold, Moist Compress
   - large basin with ice
   - small basin with cold water
   - several small towels and washcloths
   - gauze pads (appropriate size for the area receiving application)
   - bath towel

When Using an Ice Pack
   - 1 ice pack (ice bag, ice collar, ice glove, or ready-to-use disposable cold pack depending on the affected body part)
   - flannel cover
   - ties, tape, or rolled gauze
   - ice chips or crushed ice, if needed
   - large spoon, cup, or ice scooper, if needed
   - paper towels

Best Practice: During either cold application, ask the resident about the temperature of the compress or ice pack. Is it too cold? Does the resident feel numb or have any burning pain? Check often for red or pale skin. If there are any problems or complications, remove the application and report to the licensed nursing staff.

The Procedure

9. Provide privacy by closing the curtains, using a screen, or closing the door to the room.
10. If the resident is in bed, lock the bed wheels and then raise the bed to hip level.
11. Maintain safety during the procedure. If there are side rails, raise and lock the rails on the opposite side of the bed from where you will be working. Lower the rail on the side where you are working.
12. Position the resident and body part for the procedure. Depending on the body part receiving the application, the resident may be in bed, seated at the edge of the bed, or in a chair. The proper position will depend on the body part receiving the application.
13. If the resident is in bed, check to be sure the bed wheels are locked, then lower the bed. Follow the plan of care to determine if the side rails should be raised or lowered. If the resident is sitting in a chair or on the edge of the bed, be certain all safety precautions are in place.
14. Place a disposable protective pad under the body part that will receive the application and use the bath blanket to cover any other exposed area and provide warmth.

Using Cold, Moist Compresses

15. Pour the cold water from the small basin into the large basin with ice.
16. Use a washcloth or gauze pad as a compress for the skin. Place the compress in the cold water and thoroughly wring out the compress to remove excess moisture.
17. Gently apply the compress to the body part and wrap it with a towel (**Figure 18.30**). Work as quickly as possible to prevent temperature change. Note the time of the application.

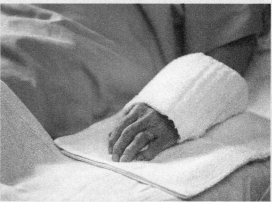

Figure 18.30   © Tori Soper Photography

18. Change the compress frequently. Continue the treatment as ordered, usually for 20 minutes.
19. Appropriately discard each compress. Remove the protective pad and change any wet linens. Assist with any further treatment as instructed by the licensed nursing staff.

Using an Ice Pack

20. If you are not using a disposable cold pack, fill an ice pack one-half full of crushed ice or ice chips using a spoon, cup, or ice scooper.
21. Remove excess air from the ice pack by twisting or squeezing it.
22. Place the cap or stopper on the ice pack tightly. Check for any leaks.
23. Dry the ice pack with towels. Place the ice pack in its cover.
24. Apply the ice pack to the body part. Note the time of application.
25. Secure the ice pack with ties, tape, or rolled gauze, if needed. Never apply tape to the resident's skin.
26. Place the call light and personal items within reach. Place a glass of fresh water on the overbed table, if permitted.
27. Check on the resident every 5 minutes. Treatments usually last no longer than 20 minutes, unless ordered by the doctor. Change the ice pack if the ice starts melting.
28. When the ice pack application is complete, lock the bed wheels and then raise the bed to hip level if the resident is in bed. Ensure safety during the procedure. If there are side rails, raise and secure the rails on the opposite side of the bed from where you will be working. Lower the rail on the side where you are working.

(continued)

Using Cold Applications (continued)

29. Remove the ice pack and pat the body part dry with a clean hand towel. Note the time the ice pack was removed. Assist with any further treatment as instructed by the licensed nursing staff.
30. Discard the water from the ice pack. Remove the protective pad and change any wet linens.
31. If the resident is in bed, check to be sure the bed wheels are locked. Then reposition the resident and lower the bed.
32. Follow the plan of care to determine if the side rails should be raised or lowered.
33. Remove, clean, and store equipment in the proper location. Remove soiled linens and discard disposable equipment.

Follow-Up

34. Wash your hands to ensure infection control.
35. Make sure the resident is comfortable and place the call light and personal items within reach.
36. Conduct a safety check before leaving the room. The room should be clean and free from clutter or spills.
37. Wash your hands or use hand sanitizer before leaving the room.

Reporting and Documentation

38. Report any specific observations, complications, or unusual responses to the licensed nursing staff. Document this information, along with the care provided, in the chart or EMR.

SECTION 18.2 Review and Assessment

Key Terms Mini Glossary

compresses pads of material; can be warm, cold, dry, or moist.
cryotherapy the use of cold applications to reduce swelling and ease pain.

cyanotic discolored and bluish due to insufficient oxygen.
gangrene a condition characterized by the death and decay of body tissue due to lack of blood supply.
hydration a sufficient amount of fluid in the body tissues.

pallor an unusually pale color of the skin.
tepid slightly warm.
thermotherapy the use of heat applications to increase circulation and ease pain.

Apply the Key Terms

Think about the definitions of the following key terms. Describe one difference between each pair of key terms.

1. pallor and tepid
2. thermotherapy and cryotherapy
3. compress and hydration
4. cyanotic and gangrene
5. tepid and cyanotic

Know and Understand the Facts

1. Identify four strategies for maintaining skin integrity.
2. When is it appropriate to use a heat application?
3. List three different heat applications.
4. Identify two different cold applications.

Analyze and Apply Concepts

1. Explain how heat and cold applications can be either helpful or harmful.

2. Discuss the steps for applying a warm, moist compress to a resident's ankle.
3. Discuss the steps for applying an ice pack to a resident's arm.

Think Critically

Read the following care situation. Then answer the questions that follow.

During Mrs. J's bath yesterday, her nursing assistant Iman noticed that Mrs. J's skin bruised more easily even though she was very gentle. Mrs. J's lips have a bluish color, and her skin is pale. Yesterday, Mrs. J hit her arm getting out of bed. The arm is swollen, and Mrs. J states it is painful. The doctor ordered cold, moist compresses for 15 minutes, three times a day. Mrs. J is assigned to Iman today.

1. When Iman noticed the changes in Mrs. J's skin, what should she have done?
2. Why might cold applications help Mrs. J?

Key Points

Reviewing the key points for this chapter will help you practice more safely and competently as a holistic nursing assistant and will help you prepare for the certification competency examination.

- Personal hygiene and grooming promote healing and physical and emotional well-being; create an environment of cleanliness, relaxation, and comfort; and help improve quality of life.
- Personal hygiene includes morning care; bathing; hand hygiene; shampooing, brushing, and combing hair; shaving; oral and denture care; fingernail and foot care; and perineal care. Nursing assistants may also assist with dressing and undressing residents and changing the gown or clothes of a resident with an IV.
- Maintaining skin integrity keeps the skin healthy. Nursing assistants must observe the skin regularly and immediately report any changes to the licensed nursing staff.
- Heat applications increase circulation, raise skin temperature, relax muscles, and ease pain. Cold applications are typically recommended for acute injuries because they reduce inflammation.

Action Steps to Holistic Care

Review the information in this chapter. Complete the following activities.

1. Select one personal hygiene procedure from this chapter. Prepare a short paper or digital presentation that identifies and describes the four most important practices in the procedure. Include one that promotes comfort and one that ensures safety.
2. Select one heat or cold application from this chapter. Prepare a poster that shows three facts that demonstrate proper procedure and safe application.
3. Find four pictures in a magazine, in a newspaper, or online: two that demonstrate good skin integrity and two that show poor skin integrity. Describe each image and explain why it was selected.
4. Select one cultural, ethnic, or religious group and describe its beliefs about personal hygiene and grooming. List two ways holistic nursing assistants can respect those beliefs when providing care.

Building Math Skill

Seth, the nursing assistant caring for Mr. Y, knows he has to place a warm, moist compress on Mr. Y's right lower leg during his shift. The doctor's order states that the compress needs to be on the leg for 20 minutes. Seth knows that he must check Mr. Y's skin under the compress every 5 minutes. How many times will he need to check during this procedure?

Preparing for the Certification Competency Examination

To prepare for the nursing assistant certification competency examination, you will need to know content found in this chapter. This content may be tested in the knowledge (written or oral) and skills (hands-on demonstration) portions of the exam. The following areas will be emphasized:

- principles of daily hygiene and grooming, including independence and self-reliance during these activities
- personal hygiene and grooming within a plan of care
- bathing, including a sitz bath and whirlpool
- hair care and shampooing, brushing, and combing hair
- shaving of male residents
- oral and denture care
- nail and foot care and important actions for residents with particular diseases and conditions
- dressing and undressing and changing gowns for residents with IVs
- skin integrity and the complications and effects of inadequate skin care
- applications of heat and cold

These sample test questions are similar to ones you will find on the certification competency exam. See how well you can answer them. Be sure to select the *best* answer.

1. To what angle should the head of the bed be raised for oral care?
   A. at least 20°
   B. at least 45°
   C. at least 15°
   D. at least 60°

2. A warm, moist compress is usually applied for
   A. 25 minutes
   B. 15 minutes
   C. 10 minutes
   D. 5 minutes

(Continued)

3. Mrs. R recently had a stroke, and her left side is paralyzed. When helping Mrs. R dress, which arm should the nursing assistant put into the sleeve of her pajama top first?
   A. right arm
   B. stronger arm
   C. stable arm
   D. weaker arm

4. A nursing assistant is providing a foot bath for Mr. U, a diabetic. Which of the following should the nursing assistant do?
   A. soak Mr. U's feet for at least 40 minutes
   B. use enough water to cover Mr. U's ankles
   C. make sure the water is not too hot
   D. strongly rub Mr. U's feet with a towel after the bath

5. One of the most important responsibilities holistic nursing assistants have when providing personal hygiene and grooming is
   A. discarding all dirty linens immediately
   B. encouraging resident independence and self-reliance
   C. giving clear instructions
   D. have residents' families help as much as possible

6. A new nursing assistant has been asked to wash Mrs. F's hair. She reviews the procedure for rinsing out shampoo and finds that she should
   A. start at the hairline and move down the strands of hair
   B. start from the bottom of the hair and work up to the top strands
   C. rinse from side to side and then rinse the hairline
   D. start in the middle of the scalp and move toward the hairline

7. When giving a total bed bath, the nursing assistant should
   A. start with the arms and then wash the legs and the rest of the body
   B. start with the abdomen, wash the arms and legs, and then wash the rest of the body
   C. start with the feet and work up the body to the face
   D. start at the top of the body, beginning with the face

8. Which of the following is an important guideline for giving foot care?
   A. apply lotion to the toes and feet and massage briskly
   B. apply lotion to the feet, toes, and between the toes
   C. apply lotion to the tops and soles of the feet, but not between the toes
   D. apply lotion to the tops and soles of the feet and between the toes

9. When performing female perineal care, a nursing assistant should
   A. place her fingers on the areas being washed
   B. wash the labia using downward strokes from top to bottom
   C. wash from the thighs in toward the labia
   D. wash the labia using upward strokes from bottom to top

10. When observing the skin of an older, frail, female resident, where should the nursing assistant look first?
    A. under the breasts
    B. between the legs
    C. around the neck and ears
    D. at the elbows and tailbone

11. One possible harmful effect of cold applications is
    A. frostbite
    B. cyanosis
    C. edema
    D. pallor

12. Which of the following is an important guideline for shaving?
    A. put a cool compress on the face and then shave in the direction of hair growth
    B. put a warm compress on the face and then shave opposite the direction of hair growth
    C. put a warm compress on the face and then shave in the direction of hair growth
    D. put a cool compress on the face and then shave opposite the direction of hair growth

13. What is the difference between a whirlpool and a sitz bath?
    A. A sitz bath is usually part of a total bed bath.
    B. A whirlpool has jets that swirl the water.
    C. A whirlpool is usually part of a total bed bath.
    D. A sitz bath has jets that swirl the water.

14. Yesterday, the doctor diagnosed Mrs. I with a sprained ankle. His order is to apply
    A. warm, moist compresses
    B. warm soaks
    C. a heating pad
    D. cold, moist compresses

15. Which of the following is included in a.m. care?
    A. oral care
    B. warm, moist compresses
    C. whirlpool
    D. cold, moist compresses

Did you have difficulty with any of the questions? If you did, review the chapter to find the correct answer(s).

Welcome to the Chapter

In Chapter 9, you learned about the structure and function of the *gastrointestinal system*, which provides the foundation for understanding nutrition and the importance of healthy eating. In this chapter, the focus is on the nutrients and foods that make up a well-balanced, healthy diet at different stages of life (called *life cycle nutrition*). You will also learn about the factors that can determine food preferences and about the influence of tradition and culture on food selection. You will become familiar with different eating and weight disorders, and therapeutic diets doctors may order for residents.

As a nursing assistant, you will be responsible for helping residents during mealtime. You may need to feed residents or help them with their meals, sometimes with adaptive and assistive eating devices. You will also need to understand and be comfortable with alternative feeding therapies and eating problems, which may include dysphagia, choking, and aspiration.

The information and procedures presented in this chapter will help you build the knowledge and skills needed to become a holistic nursing assistant. Check with your instructor to make sure these procedures are within your state's regulations for nursing assistant practice. The topics discussed in the chapter are highlighted on the Providing Holistic Care Framework.

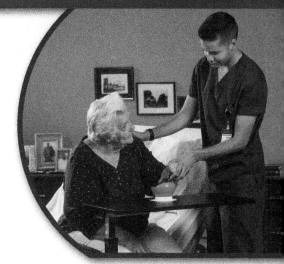
© Tori Soper Photography

Chapter Outline

Section 19.1
Food Preferences, Nutrition, and Eating Challenges

Section 19.2
Therapeutic Diets and Nutritional Support

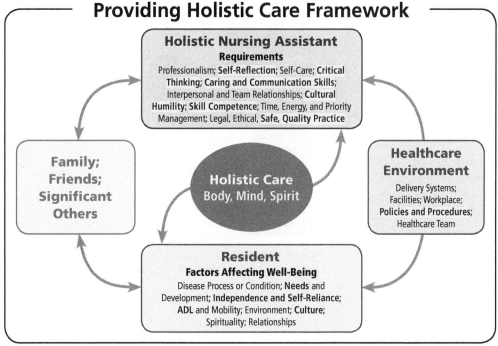

Providing Holistic Care Framework

Holistic Nursing Assistant
Requirements
Professionalism; **Self-Reflection**; Self-Care; **Critical Thinking**; **Caring and Communication Skills**; Interpersonal and Team Relationships; **Cultural Humility**; **Skill Competence**; Time, Energy, and Priority Management; Legal, Ethical, **Safe, Quality Practice**

Holistic Care
Body, Mind, Spirit

Family; Friends; Significant Others

Healthcare Environment
Delivery Systems; Facilities; Workplace; **Policies and Procedures**; Healthcare Team

Resident
Factors Affecting Well-Being
Disease Process or Condition; **Needs** and Development; **Independence and Self-Reliance**; **ADL** and Mobility; Environment; **Culture**; Spirituality; Relationships

Goodheart-Willcox Publisher

Food Preferences, Nutrition, and Eating Challenges

Objectives

To achieve the objectives for this section, you must successfully:

- **discuss** the factors that influence and the reasons behind individual food preferences and food selection.
- **identify** the components of a healthy diet.
- **explain** what nutrients are.
- **describe** different food or nutrient-related conditions, including obesity and weight loss in older adults.

Key Terms

Learn these key terms to better understand the information presented in the section.

calories	metabolism
carbohydrates	minerals
dehydration	nutrition
dietary fats	obesity
eating disorder	proteins
electrolytes	Recommended
hydrated	Dietary Allowances
legumes	(RDAs)
malabsorption	vitamins

Questions to Consider

- Think about the foods that you eat regularly. Do you eat healthfully? If you do not, what foods do you eat that are not good for you? Why do you eat these foods? Is it because they are easy to find? Do they taste so good that you do not want to give them up? Is eating these foods a family tradition?
- Do you snack? What snacks do you eat, and when do you eat them? Would you consider your snacks healthy? Why?

As a holistic nursing assistant, you need to understand the importance of nutrition and its impact on health and well-being. Good nutrition can influence the quality of people's lives as they age. Eating healthfully improves the healing process and is important for residents with chronic illnesses such as diabetes. Good nutrition should also be part of *your* daily life. When you eat healthfully, you will have the energy you need to provide safe, quality care.

Why Do People Have Different Food Preferences?

People often choose food they like, rather than foods that are healthy. They may like a particular food because they have an emotional connection to the food and they can relate it to a positive experience in their life. Some people may also find certain foods comforting. Food selection and food preferences are usually based on life habits and begin during childhood (**Figure 19.1**). These preferences are shaped by the food purchased by the family, dietary traditions, finances, and ethnic or religious customs. Preferences are also shaped by age, diseases or conditions, medications taken, and even the way food smells. Understanding *nutrition*, or how eating certain foods keeps the body healthy, may also influence food preferences. Food allergies, physical disabilities, time, food costs, advertisements for food, and dietary needs or restrictions also influence what people choose to eat.

Eating patterns, which describe how often and how fast people eat, are similarly affected by experience. Eating patterns become habits, guide food choice, influence how you eat foods, can affect your digestion, and can cause weight disorders.

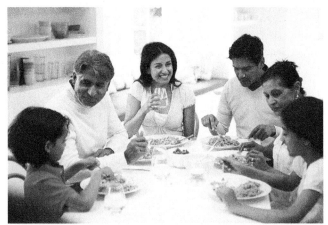
Monkey Business Images/Shutterstock.com

Figure 19.1 Family and culture have a significant impact on a person's eating patterns and food selections.

CULTURE CUES
Food Traditions

Cultural and religious groups typically have unique food traditions. Some traditional foods are served on holidays, celebrations, special occasions, or feast days. Many cultures also have customs that affect how and when food should be eaten and that identify acceptable or unacceptable foods. Some foods are eaten to communicate a person's social status, and some foods are symbolic, and represent maintaining health and having a long life. Food practices are not followed by all families and individuals in a culture. However, many people do follow all or some parts of their cultural or religious eating traditions.

As a holistic nursing assistant, you must be aware of, and sensitive to, residents' food traditions. Some food traditions promote residents' treatments, and other food traditions have a harmful effect. If you are not sure about a resident's food traditions,

you can check the plan of care. You can also ask the resident what eating traditions or customs he or she practices.

Apply It

1. What traditional foods and food aromas (smells) do you remember from your childhood?
2. List the foods that are special to your family traditions, culture, or religion.
3. Describe any cultural or religious food traditions your family has. Do you follow your family's cultural or religious food traditions? If you do, describe any challenges you have experienced in keeping these traditions.
4. Describe any cultural or religious food traditions that your friends follow. In what ways do these traditions differ from yours? How do you feel about the differences?

What Nutrients Are Most Important?

Eating a healthy diet means including the proper amounts of *nutrients* (substances needed for normal body function) in your diet. Nutrients are required for **metabolism**, which is the chemical process that converts nutrients into energy. During the process of metabolism, **calories** (units of energy) in food and fluids combine with oxygen to release energy that the body needs to function properly. Metabolism is also important for building, maintaining, and repairing body tissues.

The main nutrients your body needs are carbohydrates, dietary fats (*lipids*), proteins, vitamins, minerals, and water:

- **Carbohydrates:** the body's main source of energy, carbohydrates are found in *starches* (for example, potatoes, dried beans, oats, rice, pasta, or bread); *sugar* (found in milk and fruit, molasses, honey, and corn syrup), and *fiber* (found in fruits, vegetables, whole grains, nuts, and **legumes**, which are plants with pods that contain edible seeds). Carbohydrates need to be chosen wisely to achieve the best nutrition. Foods with added sugars and refined grains, such as white flour, white bread, and white rice, should be avoided. It is better to eat fruits, vegetables, and whole grains.

- **Dietary fats:** (also called *lipids*) provide energy for the body; assist in the absorption of vitamins A, D, E, and K; and make food taste better. There are three different types of fats: saturated fats (found in animal and dairy products, such as meats, butter, cream, and cheese), *trans* fats (found in cakes or cookies containing shortening or margarine), and unsaturated fats (found in olive, canola, safflower, peanut, and corn oils; most nuts; mayonnaise; avocados; and some fish). Eating too much saturated fat may raise cholesterol and increase the risk of developing type 2 diabetes. *Trans* fat may also increase the risk of cardiovascular disease. Unsaturated fats, however, have a positive impact on cholesterol levels and decrease the risk of cardiovascular disease and type 2 diabetes (**Figure 19.2**).

- **Proteins:** found in every cell, proteins also help produce energy. They are necessary for body structure and function as they carry oxygen and enzymes, promote growth and repair, and help maintain the body's fluid balance. Proteins are found in eggs, milk, soybeans, meat, poultry, seafood, vegetables, grains, processed soy products, nuts, and seeds.

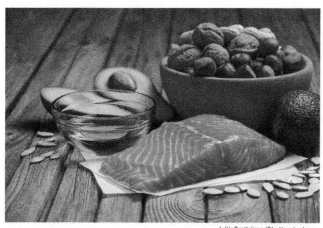

JulijaDmitrijeva/Shutterstock.com

Figure 19.2 Some examples of foods containing dietary fats are oil, fish, avocados, and nuts.

- *Vitamins*: play a role in the development and growth of cells and are needed for the body to function properly. Most vitamins cannot be made in the body. Instead, they must be part of the food you eat or taken as a vitamin supplement (typically in the form of a pill). *Fat-soluble vitamins* (vitamins A, D, E, and K) can be dissolved in fat and stored in the body. *Water-soluble vitamins* (B complex vitamins and vitamin C) dissolve in water, cannot be stored in the body, and are easily eliminated in the urine. There are **Recommended Dietary Allowances (RDAs)**, or recommended levels of intake for each vitamin. For example, if too much vitamin C is taken, it can cause an upset stomach and kidney stones. Some vitamins can also interfere with clinical tests and have harmful interactions with medications (for example, vitamins E and K for residents taking blood thinners). RDAs are different for each age group.
- *Minerals*: these are inorganic substances found in the body, meaning they do not come from a plant or an animal. Minerals help regulate energy and assist in metabolism. Calcium, sodium, iron, potassium, magnesium, fluorine, and zinc are all important minerals that contribute to body function. For example, *electrolytes* are minerals (such as sodium, calcium, and potassium), found in the blood, urine, tissues, and other body fluids, which have an electrical charge. Electrolytes help balance the amount of water in the body and also the body's acid/base balance (pH).

- **Water:** staying *hydrated*, or having enough fluid in the body, is very important for all age groups (**Figure 19.3**). Water is found in all the beverages you drink, as well as in fruits and vegetables. Breathing, sweating, and eliminating all remove water from the body. Proper hydration improves energy, mood, and how clearly people think. Even the smallest amount of *dehydration*, or lack of fluids, can slow down the body's metabolism and have a negative effect on the cardiovascular and central nervous systems. One simple way to determine dehydration is to check the color of a resident's urine. If the urine is pale yellow, there is sufficient hydration. If the color is closer to dark yellow or orange, more fluids are needed. See Chapter 20 for more information.

Many people also take one or more dietary supplements each day. Most supplements include vitamins and minerals, but can also include plant-based substances, herbs, and enzymes. Supplements are usually available as tablets, capsules, powders, drinks, or energy bars, and can be purchased over the counter at retail stores. Examples of supplements include echinacea, St. John's wort, turmeric, and probiotics. Supplements are meant to add to a person's diet, not take the place of healthy food selections. Supplements are *not* medicine. It is important to know what supplements residents are taking, because they may react negatively with the resident's ordered medications or diet.

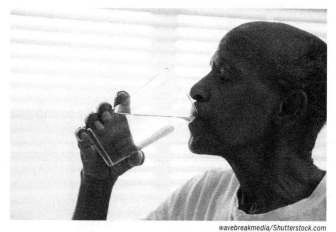

wavebreakmedia/Shutterstock.com

Figure 19.3 Hydration improves energy, mood, and thinking. It is essential to the body's functions.

Sometimes the body does not take in the nutrients it needs. *Malabsorption* can occur if the intestine fails to take in essential nutrients and fluids and transfer them to the bloodstream. Malabsorption can result from intestinal diseases, infections, inflammation, trauma, surgery, or nutritional deficiencies and can lead to weight loss and dehydration. This condition must be corrected, because it can lead to serious outcomes if essential nutrients are not consumed daily.

How Can People Choose Safe and Healthy Foods?

Both MyPlate and the *Dietary Guidelines for Americans* help people choose healthy foods in appropriate amounts. Your choices determine whether or not your body gets all of the nutrients it needs daily. When selecting foods, people can use food labels to determine the nutrients in a food. Food labels are important to review; they offer information about the food product. The labels are helpful to review when caring for residents who are on special diets or have dietary restrictions. Look at the serving size, number of calories in a serving, how these nutrients meet the recommended daily intake, and if they are appropriate for the resident's diet, according to the plan of care.

MyPlate

There are five main food groups—fruits, vegetables, grains, protein, and dairy, as shown in the MyPlate logo in **Figure 19.4**. *MyPlate* is a government resource that helps people learn about food groups, food selections, and the proper amounts of food to eat from each group to achieve a healthy diet.

MyPlate offers the following guidelines for selecting foods from the five food groups:

- **Fruits**: Vary food choices and pick potassium-rich fruits, such as bananas, orange juice, prunes and prune juice, dried peaches, and apricots. If choosing canned fruits, select fruits that are canned with 100 percent fruit juice or water, instead of syrup.

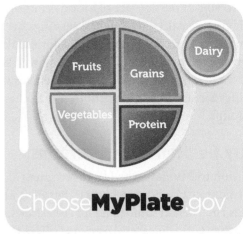

US Department of Agriculture

Figure 19.4 MyPlate is a food guidance system designed to help people make healthy nutritional choices.

- **Vegetables**: Vegetables are categorized into five groups: dark green vegetables, starchy vegetables, red and orange vegetables, beans and peas, and other vegetables. For the best nutrition, pick any vegetable or 100 percent vegetable juice.
- **Grains**: Grains are divided into two groups: whole grains and refined grains. Whole grains provide more dietary fiber. Instead of selecting refined grains like white rice and bread, choose whole grains, such as whole-wheat flour, bulgur (cracked wheat), oatmeal, whole cornmeal, and brown rice. Some people are *gluten sensitive* or *gluten intolerant*. These people have an abnormal immune response to gluten (protein found in wheat, barley, or rye) during digestion and suffer with pain, bloating, nausea, constipation or diarrhea. However, these people can eat grains such as rice, corn, or millet.
- **Protein**: Eat meat, poultry, seafood, beans and peas, eggs, processed soy products, nuts, and seeds. Select lean or low-fat meat and poultry. While people who are vegetarians do not eat meat, they can get the protein they need by eating beans and peas, processed soy products, and nuts and seeds.
- **Dairy**: This food group includes all liquid milk products and foods made from milk. Select fat-free or low-fat milk, yogurt, and cheese, as well as calcium-fortified soy milk. Some people are *lactose intolerant*, which means they have trouble digesting milk products. These people will need to drink or eat low-lactose or lactose-free milk products or soy beverages.

The *serving* or *portion size* of a food is important to achieving a healthy diet. Small servings or portions help reduce the number of calories taken in. Servings or portion sizes must be followed strictly when people are on special diets. **Figure 19.5** shows guidelines for servings and portion sizes in the five food groups.

Dietary Guidelines for Americans

In addition to MyPlate, the US government's Department of Health and Human Services also provides the *Dietary Guidelines for Americans*. The *Dietary Guidelines for Americans* offers the following guidance:

- Establish and follow healthy eating habits throughout your life to make sure you are getting the nutrition you need, maintaining a healthy weight, and to lower your risk of a chronic disease.
- Eat a variety of foods from all food groups, making sure to eat the proper amounts of foods that are rich in nutrients.
- Limit saturated fats, sodium, and foods with added sugar (such as soft drinks and desserts).
- Replace unhealthy food and beverage choices with nutrient-rich alternatives that fit within your cultural and personal preferences to make these changes more successful.

Food Safety

In addition to selecting proper foods to eat, *food safety* is an important part of healthy eating and dietary awareness. During the preparation and consumption of food, there is a risk for *foodborne illnesses*, which are diseases caused by pathogens or chemicals (such as pesticides) that contaminate food. There are more than 250 different foodborne illnesses.

Symptoms of foodborne illness include cramping, nausea, vomiting, and diarrhea. Sometimes the symptoms are mild, and other times they can be severe. Older people with weak immune systems are at greater risk.

Some government agencies are responsible for setting food safety standards, conducting needed inspections, guaranteeing that standards are met, maintaining a strong enforcement program to handle those who do not comply with standards, and providing food education. The government agencies involved in food safety include:

- the US Department of Agriculture (USDA)
- the Food and Drug Administration (FDA)
- the Centers for Disease Control and Prevention (CDC)
- the Environmental Protection Agency (EPA)
- the US Department of Health and Human Services (HHS)

What Can Happen When People Are Not Eating Healthfully?

It is not always easy to eat healthfully. Not only do people deal with their own food preferences, selections, and patterns, they are also exposed to a variety of food products through advertisements and at the grocery store. People of all ages can

Serving and Portion Size Guidelines

Food Group	Guidelines
Fruits	In general, 1 cup is equal to 1 cup of fruit, 1 cup of 100-percent fruit juice, or ½ cup of dried fruit.
Vegetables	In general, 1 cup is equal to 1 cup of raw or cooked vegetables, 1 cup of 100-percent vegetable juice, or 2 cups of raw leafy greens.
Grains	In general, 1 ounce-equivalent is equal to 1 slice of bread, 1 cup of ready-to-eat cereal, or ½ cup of cooked rice, cooked pasta, or cooked cereal.
Protein	In general, 1 ounce-equivalent is equal to 1 ounce of meat, poultry, or fish; ¼ cup cooked beans; 1 egg; 1 tablespoon of peanut butter; or ½ ounce of nuts or seeds.
Dairy	In general, 1 cup is equal to 1 cup of milk, yogurt, or soymilk (soy beverage); 1½ ounces of natural cheese; or 2 ounces of processed cheese.

Goodheart-Willcox Publisher

Figure 19.5 Understanding portion sizes is vital to getting adequate nutrition.

make unhealthy food choices, or have a troubled relationship with food. This can cause serious problems, particularly with older adults.

Overweight, Obesity, and Underweight

Today, the United States is facing an obesity epidemic, which is a significant health problem. *Obesity* is a health condition that occurs when a person's body weight is much greater than what is considered healthy for a certain height. Adults are not the only ones affected; childhood obesity is also a problem. Being obese results in serious diseases, such as diabetes and cardiovascular conditions.

A common way to measure if a person is underweight, at a healthy weight, overweight, or obese is to use *body mass index* or *BMI*. BMI is a calculation of a person's body fat based on an adult man's or woman's height (in meters) and current weight (in kilograms). To calculate BMI, divide a person's weight in kilograms by his or her height in meters squared [weight/(height)^2]. You can also calculate BMI using pounds and inches (**Figure 19.6**).

- A BMI less than 18.5 falls within the *underweight* range.
- A BMI between 18.5 and 24.9 indicates a healthy weight.
- A BMI between 25.0 and 29.9 falls within the *overweight* range.
- A BMI of 30.0 or higher falls within the *obese* range.

While obesity affects many people in the United States, being underweight is also a serious condition. Some people, particularly older adults, may become underweight and frail because they do not eat enough or their diet does not contain the nutrients they need. They may also have a poor appetite and a reduced sense of taste. Limited mobility, physical changes, tooth and mouth problems, poorly fitting dentures, and changes in the social environment can also decrease appetite and result in weight loss.

Normal weight loss can happen over time; however, sudden, rapid, unintentional, and unexplained weight loss is usually a sign of a disease and needs to be treated by a doctor. The significance or severity of weight loss is an important factor to be aware of for residents. *Significant weight loss* means the resident has lost 1–2 pounds in one week and 5 pounds in one month. Weight loss becomes *severe* when a resident loses even more weight in this time frame. For example, losing 3 pounds in one week is considered severe weight loss.

Ways to respond to residents who are overweight or underweight are discussed in the next section of this chapter.

Eating Disorders

Some people can become overly concerned about their weight. These people may not have an actual weight problem, but see themselves as overweight or even obese. They will usually have feelings of shame or

How to Calculate Body Mass Index

Measurement Units	Formula and Calculation
kilograms and meters (or centimeters)	**Formula:** weight (kg)/[height (m)]^2 In the metric system, the formula for BMI is weight in kilograms divided by height in meters squared. Since height is commonly measured in centimeters, divide height in centimeters by 100 to obtain height in meters. **Example:** Weight = 68 kg, Height = 165 cm (1.65 m) **Calculation:** $68 \div (1.65)^2 = 24.98$
pounds and inches	**Formula:** weight (lb)/[height (in.)]$^2 \times 703$ Calculate BMI by dividing weight in pounds (lb) by height in inches (in.) squared and multiplying by a conversion factor of 703. **Example:** Weight = 150 lb, Height = 5'5" (65") **Calculation:** $[150 \div (65)^2] \times 703 = 24.96$

Centers for Disease Control and Prevention

Figure 19.6 BMI determines the health of a person's weight based on weight compared to height.

HEALTHCARE SCENARIO

Obesity

The CDC recently released information that more than one-third (36.5 percent) of US adults are obese. Obesity is more common among middle-age adults ages 40–59 (40.2 percent) and older adults ages 60 or older (37.0 percent) than among younger adults ages 20–39 (32.3 percent). Approximately 17 percent (or 12.7 million) children and teens ages 2–19 are obese.

Apply It

1. Why do you think so many adults are obese? What might be one reason obesity is more common among middle-age and older adults?

2. If you were asked to help people who are obese, what would you suggest they do to decrease their weight?

anxiety about their body sizes and shapes. As a result, they may develop problematic eating behaviors as a way to deal with their views of their bodies. These behaviors can result in an *eating disorder*. Several factors can trigger an eating disorder, such as genetics; physical or sexual abuse; and personality characteristics, including perfectionism, high achievement, and low self-esteem. An eating disorder is not an eating preference, but is considered a serious illness.

Three common eating disorders are anorexia nervosa, binge-eating disorder (BED), and bulimia nervosa

- **Anorexia nervosa:** an intense fear of gaining weight or becoming fat leads to self-starvation. A person with anorexia nervosa might portion out food and eat very slowly, eat only small amounts of food, frequently check for weight gain, and deny that extreme weight loss is a serious problem. This eating disorder has many serious complications, including osteoporosis, low blood pressure, and heart malfunction, which may result in a heart attack or organ failure.

- **Binge-eating disorder (BED):** a condition in which a person loses control and excessively overeats. A person with BED may feel a need to eat that they cannot control, cannot stop eating even after the feeling of hunger is over, and is not satisfied after eating and goes back for more. Feelings of guilt or shame about bingeing are not dealt with in a healthy manner, but rather, cause more binge eating. People with BED are usually overweight or obese, increasing their risk for cardiovascular disease.

- **Bulimia nervosa:** a condition of recurring episodes of binge eating and purging (getting rid of) food to prevent weight gain. Purging can involve forced vomiting, the use of laxatives and enemas, the use of diuretics, fasting, excessive exercise, or a combination of these behaviors. Bingeing and purging can occur several times a day or week, are done in secret, and occur due to feelings of shame and disgust. When the cycle of bingeing and purging becomes chronic, symptoms such as worn tooth enamel and decaying teeth, severe dehydration, and electrolyte imbalance may occur.

Treatments for eating disorders are specific to individual issues and concerns. These may include counseling to ensure adequate nutrition (**Figure 19.7**), therapy (individual or family), medical supervision, and sometimes medications (for example, antidepressants). When an eating disorder is severe, hospitalization can provide the care needed to correct electrolyte imbalance and malnutrition. Eating may also be monitored and possibly supplemented to be sure a person is getting the nutrition he or she needs.

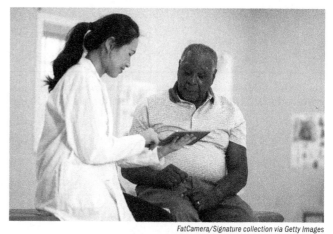

FatCamera/Signature collection via Getty Images

Figure 19.7 A dietitian can create a plan for residents with eating disorders to help make sure they get the nutrition they need.

SECTION **19.1** **Review and Assessment**

Key Terms Mini Glossary

calories units of energy.

carbohydrates the body's main source of energy; includes three types: starches, sugars, and fiber.

dehydration a lack of the necessary fluids in the body tissues.

dietary fats lipids; provide energy for and insulate the body; includes saturated fat, *trans* fat, and unsaturated fat.

eating disorder an abnormal pattern of eating that leads to serious and often fatal medical consequences.

electrolytes minerals in the blood and body fluids with an electrical charge that help balance fluids.

hydrated having sufficient fluids in the body tissues over a 24-hour period.

legumes plants with pods (long cases) that contain edible seeds.

malabsorption the reduced ability of the intestine to take in essential nutrients and fluids and transfer them to the bloodstream.

metabolism the chemical process by which nutrients are converted into energy in the body.

minerals inorganic substances in the body that regulate and assist in metabolism.

nutrition the ingestion of foods that provide nutrients to maintain the health of the body.

obesity a health condition in which body weight is much greater than what is considered healthy for a certain height.

proteins vital to cell structure, contribute to energy production, build body tissue, and promote growth and repair.

Recommended Dietary Allowances (RDAs) daily levels of nutritional intake needed to maintain good health.

vitamins organic compounds needed for cell development and growth; must be obtained from foods in a person's diet or from vitamin supplements.

Apply the Key Terms

An incorrect key term is used in each of the following statements. Identify the incorrect key term and then replace it with the correct term.

1. Malabsorption is the chemical process by which nutrients are converted into energy in the body.
2. Proteins are the body's main source of energy; these include three types: starches, sugars, and fiber.
3. Electrolytes are organic compounds needed for cell development and growth; must be in foods in a person's diet or obtained from vitamin supplements.
4. When residents have sufficient fluids in their body tissues over a 24-hour period, they have excellent nutrition.
5. Inorganic substances in the body that regulate and assist in metabolism are dietary fats.

Know and Understand the Facts

1. What are two factors that influence individual food preferences and selection?
2. Identify the food groups that should be part of a healthy diet.
3. List the six nutrients your body needs and explain why each nutrient is important.
4. What is the serving and portion size for grains?
5. Identify three eating disorders and describe the differences between them.

Analyze and Apply Concepts

1. Explain how MyPlate and the *Dietary Guidelines for Americans* impact your diet.
2. List three changes you might need to make to improve your diet.
3. Why is it important to read food labels?

4. Explain why someone might be overweight or underweight.
5. Describe how you might be able to tell if a person has bulimia nervosa.

Think Critically

Read the following care situation. Then answer the questions that follow.

Mrs. L is an active 79-year-old who has lived in the facility for several years. She has seemed more tired lately and has not been interested in activities she usually enjoys. The only activity she still seems interested in is swimming in the indoor pool. In the past, Mrs. L has been overweight and has always been self-conscious about it. She has tried many different diets. When she was a young woman, she tried fasting to keep her weight down. When her husband was alive he seemed happy with her weight, but he passed away six months ago after a long illness. Over the past three months, she has become thin—thinner than she should be. She has been refusing snacks and leaving food on her plate. She is now asking for smaller portions. Mrs. L has diabetes and is on medication for hypertension and osteoporosis.

1. What do you think happened that changed Mrs. L's current eating behaviors?
2. Do you think she might be developing an eating disorder? If so, which one? Why?
3. How will this change in eating affect Mrs. L's medical conditions?
4. What actions might you take to help Mrs. L?
5. What food groups and servings should Mrs. L be consuming to eat healthfully?

Therapeutic Diets and Nutritional Support

Objectives

To achieve the objectives for this section, you must successfully:

- **identify** environments and approaches that promote optimal eating.
- **explain** the reasons behind and care needed for selected diets, including therapeutic diets.
- **discuss** the responsibilities of nursing assistants in assisting residents who require alternative feeding therapies.
- **describe** challenges of eating and ways to help residents avoid or overcome them.
- **recognize** different types of adaptive eating equipment (assistive eating devices) and their functions.
- **demonstrate** how to assist with eating effectively and record food intake.

Key Terms

Learn these key terms to better understand the information presented in the section.

alternative feeding therapy	enteral
aspirate	parenteral
dysphagia	patent
	therapeutic diets

Questions to Consider

- Have you ever been on a special diet? Have you had to stay away from certain foods because they gave you a stomachache or because you were allergic to them? What did that feel like?
- How have the diets you have tried affected your daily eating patterns? Have you been able to stay on a diet for the length of time needed? If you were, what helped you stay on the diet? If you were not, what challenges did you face?

What Can Make Mealtimes Enjoyable?

Mealtimes should be special—not just with family and friends or when celebrating a holiday, but at *all* times. Eating does not just meet a resident's physical needs; it is also a significant part of each resident's day. Residents should enjoy both the act of eating and the opportunity to interact and socialize with others during mealtime. The dining experience, resident preparation, and the atmosphere all help make eating enjoyable (**Figure 19.8**).

The Dining Experience

In healthcare facilities, the dining experience is more structured than eating at home. Meals occur at specific times each day, and foods are often chosen by dietitians based on the ordered diet or to promote proper nutrition for older adults. The dietary department in a healthcare facility also includes several staff members in addition to dietitians who help cook and deliver food, drinks, and healthy supplements.

It is always important that the food prepared be appropriate for each resident. Some residents require *therapeutic diets* that promote healing. Other residents are able to select their meals from a buffet line or prepared menu. Long-term care facilities must provide meals that meet individual needs, follow special diets, contain all of the necessary nutrients, taste delicious with suitable seasoning, and are accompanied by a variety of beverages.

Preparation

Residents are prepared for their meals before eating and particularly during morning, or a.m., care. Preparation includes personal hygiene and oral and denture care (as discussed in Chapter 18). This preparation not only offers residents an opportunity

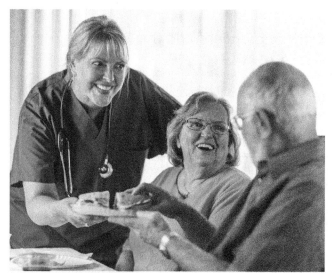

Andy Dean Photography/Shutterstock.com

Figure 19.8 As a holistic nursing assistant, you can help make eating enjoyable and healing for residents in your care.

to feel refreshed, but also gives nursing assistants a chance to see if residents have any problems with dentures or sores in the mouth that may prevent chewing or swallowing. If a resident is going to the dining room, he or she will need to dress appropriately. If a resident has eyeglasses or a hearing aid, be sure they are in place and working properly. Some residents may need time to pray before eating.

Atmosphere

In long-term care facilities, residents usually eat in dining rooms, as long as they are physically mobile, can ambulate using assistive devices, or can be transported by wheelchair. Residents may like to sit with certain people during mealtimes or may choose to sit alone. This is important information to learn, since holistic nursing assistants can use this information to make mealtime a pleasant experience. If a resident is bedridden, the meal is brought to his or her room and served on a tray. In any atmosphere, the resident should be encouraged to eat mindfully, or to pay attention during the meal (**Figure 19.9**).

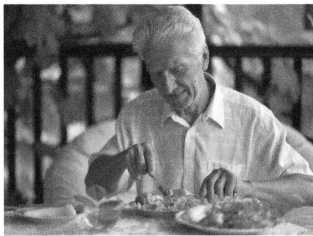

Ruslan Huzau/Shutterstock.com

Figure 19.9 Eating mindfully involves paying attention to your meal and surroundings while eating. Mindful eating makes meals more enjoyable and helps people make better food choices.

What Nutritional Support Is Available for Residents?

Licensed nursing staff members and dietitians usually conduct a *nutritional status assessment* to determine a resident's plan of care and evaluate how well a resident

---

eats and drinks. This assessment also identifies any eating and swallowing problems a resident has, any recent weight changes, and any complaints about meals and eating. Some residents, particularly those who are underweight or malnourished, may need nutritional support to make sure they are getting the nutrition they need.

As a holistic nursing assistant, you can follow the plan of care to help residents with nutritional support. You can also provide nutritional support by being aware of any special diets, recording weight on a daily basis, and maintaining skin integrity. You can provide small, frequent meals that are dense in calories; increase intake of appropriate beverages and snacks if the resident is not eating enough or needs more frequent meals (for example, a resident with diabetes); and add supplemental nutrition drinks as recommended by a doctor or dietitian.

Supplemental Nutrition Drinks

Supplemental nutrition drinks provide a balance of protein, carbohydrates, and fat. Supplemental nutrition drinks must not interfere with any medications the resident is taking. These drinks fall into two categories: shakes and formulas. *Shakes* are usually fortified (enhanced) with vitamins and sugar is used to improve taste. *Formulas* are typically given to those who have specific diseases, such as cancer or chronic obstructive pulmonary disease (COPD). Formulas can be drunk, but are often delivered through a feeding tube, and must be ordered by a doctor.

Another way to provide supplemental nutrition through a drink is a fruit smoothie, which is food based. Fruit smoothies tend to have fewer added sugars and are less processed than shakes or formula.

When a supplemental nutrition drink is ordered by the doctor and included in a resident's plan of care, it is important to be aware of its content. Read the food label. Supplemental nutrition drinks usually have 10–20 grams of protein and no more than 40 grams of carbohydrates in an 8-ounce drink. Pay attention to the number of calories in the drink. If the drink is a meal replacement, it should contain no more than 400 calories. Be careful about giving supplemental nutrition drinks after a full meal. A drink may be too filling for the resident and contain too many calories, making it difficult to reach specific nutritional goals. No matter which drink is used, know that supplements by themselves do not replace the nutrients provided by actual food sources (**Figure 19.10**).

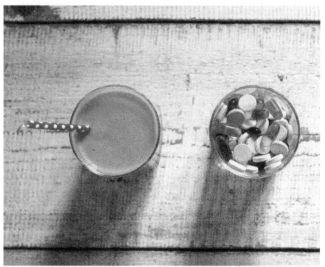

AndreaObzerova/Essentials collection via Getty Images

Figure 19.10 Supplementary nutrition drinks and vitamin and mineral supplements are two examples of supplementation used in healthcare facilities.

Therapeutic Diets

Therapeutic diets are commonly used in healthcare facilities. A resident may be admitted with a therapeutic diet, or a doctor may order a therapeutic diet during a resident's stay. The goal of therapeutic diets is to make sure residents get the nutrients they need while adjusting foods to be appropriate to a specific disease, condition, or procedure. When possible, a resident's cultural food preferences are considered.

Doctors and dietitians often use *liberalized diets* to find more creative ways of managing diseases. The goal is to encourage residents to follow the diet and increase their enjoyment. In a liberalized diet, the basics of a therapeutic diet are the same; however, providers explain why foods are chosen, and assistance is provided to help residents make smart food choices.

A variety of therapeutic diets are prescribed for different reasons. Each therapeutic diet has specific requirements.

Regular Diet

A *regular diet* is ordered when there are no food restrictions for a resident. This diet includes a variety of foods from all of the food groups. Regular diets may be adjusted by changing foods due to allergies or changing the consistency of food to make it pureed or soft.

Soft Diet

A *soft* or *mechanical soft diet* is ordered when a resident has difficulty chewing or swallowing due to weakness or dental difficulties from poorly fitting dentures; chemotherapy; radiation to the head or neck; radiation to the abdomen, which can cause digestive problems; or a sore mouth. Soft diets are sometimes used to relieve stomach or intestinal discomfort. They can also help determine residents' tolerance to transition from liquids to a regular diet.

Soft diets include foods that are easy to chew and swallow, such as tender, juicy meats; soup; eggs; pudding; custard; and smooth yogurt or ice cream. Soft diets limit or eliminate raw fruits and vegetables; chewy breads; and tough meats, which are hard to chew and swallow. Foods can be softened using machines or devices that cook or mash them. Canned or soft-cooked fruits and vegetables can be used. Foods should be varied according to taste preferences and ease of chewing and swallowing.

Full Liquid Diet

Residents transitioning from clear liquids to a soft diet or who have undergone special procedures or GI surgery usually follow a *full liquid diet*. This diet may also be ordered for residents who have certain chewing or swallowing problems.

A full liquid diet includes a variety of liquid foods, including cream soups (that have been strained), pureed meats, bland vegetables and white potatoes, custard-style yogurt, pudding, plain ice cream, sherbet, sorbet, coffee, tea, cream, carbonated beverages, fruit and vegetable juices, milk, milkshakes, cream of wheat or rice cereal, mild seasonings, margarine, sugar, syrup, jelly, and honey. No other foods are allowed on this diet. High-protein, high-calorie supplements with added vitamins and minerals may also be ordered. If a resident is lactose intolerant, then lactose-free liquid products may be used instead of milk products.

Clear Liquid Diet

A *clear liquid diet* is ordered before certain tests, medical procedures, or surgeries that require the gastrointestinal system to be free from food. This diet is also ordered for residents with certain digestive problems, such as nausea, vomiting, or diarrhea.

A clear liquid diet includes water (plain, carbonated, or flavored); fruit juices without pulp; lemonade; broth; plain gelatin; tea or coffee without milk or cream; strained tomato or vegetable juice; sports drinks; honey or sugar; hard candy, such as lemon drops or peppermint rounds; and ice pops without milk. Clear liquid diets do *not* provide all of the calories and nutrients the resident needs; therefore, they should be used for only a few days.

Bland Diet

A doctor may order a *bland diet* to help treat ulcers, heartburn, nausea, vomiting, diarrhea, and gas. It may also be ordered after stomach or intestinal surgery.

A bland diet includes foods that are soft, not spicy, and low in fiber. This may include milk and other dairy products (low-fat or fat-free only); cooked, canned, or frozen vegetables; fruit juices and vegetable juices; weak tea; breads, crackers, and pasta made with refined white flour; hot cereals, such as cream of wheat; lean, tender meats (such as poultry, whitefish, and shellfish) that are steamed, baked, or grilled with no added fat; creamy peanut butter; pudding and custard; eggs; tofu; and soup (broth).

A resident who is on a bland diet should not eat spicy, fried, or raw foods; strong cheeses; seeds; nuts; whole grains; cured or smoked meats; or drink alcohol or beverages with caffeine. A resident on a bland diet should also:

- eat small meals often during the day
- chew food slowly and well
- stop smoking cigarettes
- not eat within two hours of bedtime

Low-Sodium Diet

A *low-sodium diet* is ordered for residents who have kidney problems. This diet lowers the amount of salt consumed (to less than 1 teaspoon daily) because the kidneys cannot effectively filter sodium. Excess sodium causes fluid retention and swelling (edema). A low-sodium diet is also helpful for residents with heart diseases, as it reduces excess sodium and fluid buildup in the bloodstream and helps the heart pump more effectively.

A low-sodium diet includes reduced amounts of heavily processed foods such as hot dogs, sausage, ham, prepackaged meats, canned vegetables and soups, and frozen meals. Fresh or frozen beef, lamb, poultry, or fish; eggs or egg substitutes; milk, yogurt, or ice cream; fresh and frozen vegetables without sauces; and fresh potatoes are some of the foods that can be included in this diet.

Cardiac or Heart-Healthy Diet

A *cardiac* or *heart-healthy diet* is ordered for residents who have cardiovascular diseases or who are at risk for cardiac problems. Some people use this diet to promote overall health and weight loss.

A cardiac or heart-healthy diet includes heart-healthy foods such as whole grains, fiber, fruits, and vegetables. This diet does not allow some types of fat, sodium, cholesterol, and sometimes caffeine. Typically, this diet cuts out egg yolks, bacon, luncheon meats, cheese, high-fat milk, high-fat red meat, and bakery products. The diet usually restricts sodium intake to 2000–4000 mg daily. In this diet, snacks may consist of fruits, such as apples or grapes.

Diabetic or Carbohydrate-Controlled Diet

Residents with diabetes should follow a *diabetic* or *carbohydrate-controlled diet*. Residents on this diet eat three meals daily at regular times to keep blood sugar levels steady. This diet matches food intake with insulin needs by balancing healthy carbohydrates, such as fruits, vegetables, and grains; fiber-rich foods; proteins; and unsaturated fats. Saturated fats, *trans* fats, and cholesterol are avoided, and sodium is limited to less than 2,300 mg daily.

Diabetic diets are developed according to resident needs. Meal plans may be based on specific methods, such as preparing a plate with one-half nonstarchy vegetables (such as carrots); one-quarter protein (such as tuna); and one-quarter of a whole-grain item or starchy food. Another method involves counting carbohydrates and eating the same amount each day to control blood sugar. An exchange list system with categories based on carbohydrate, protein, and fat content may also be used. Each serving in a category has about the same amount of carbohydrates, proteins, fats, and calories. One other method is the *glycemic index*. This method ranks carbohydrate-containing foods by their effect on blood sugar levels.

Renal Diet

A *renal diet* is ordered for residents who have kidney damage or disease. Kidney function declines gradually, and the damage is permanent. Damage to the kidneys makes the kidneys less able to filter waste products, fluids, and nutrients (such as sodium, phosphorus, and potassium) from the blood. Excessive amounts of these substances can build up in the blood. The renal diet has to be carefully managed.

The renal diet limits consumption of the following four food and mineral-containing groups:

- **Proteins**: animal proteins, such as eggs, milk, meat, poultry, and fish
- **Phosphorus**: milk, cheese, yogurt, ice cream, pudding, custard, cocoa, dried beans, nuts, seeds, whole-grain breads and cereals, bran, chocolate, caramel, dried fruits, and beer
- **Potassium**: fruits and vegetables, milk products, meats, whole grains, dry beans, and salt substitutes
- **Sodium and fluid**: table salt, bouillon cubes, potato chips, salted nuts, bacon, hot dogs, cold cuts, cheese, canned soup and vegetables, pretzels, and fast food

High-Fiber Diet

Residents who have chronic constipation, irritable bowel syndrome, or an elevated risk for colon cancer may need a *high-fiber diet*. Foods that are high in fiber should also be part of a regular diet, as fiber is good for the colon and is also heart healthy.

A high-fiber diet includes approximately 20–25 grams of fiber daily. This amount can be reached by eating five or more servings of fruits and vegetables and between four and six servings of whole-grain breads or cereals. The AI for fluid intake is important and should also be consumed daily. Residents on this diet should limit restaurant meals and processed foods, which are low in fiber.

Low-Fiber Diet

A *low-fiber diet* is ordered when a resident is experiencing GI problems, such as abdominal pain, diarrhea, and diverticulitis. This diet is also ordered when a resident has an intestinal stricture or obstruction.

A low-fiber diet includes a fiber intake below 10 grams each day. This diet should only be used for the short term until GI problems are resolved.

Alternative Feeding Therapies

Some residents are not able to eat food through their mouths. These residents require nutrition to be delivered using an **alternative feeding therapy**. Alternative feeding therapies can be given by **parenteral** (by way of the veins) or **enteral** (by way of the gastrointestinal system) means.

Residents may be unable to eat food through their mouths due to a specific disease or condition such as cancer, surgery, oral trauma, eating disorders, frailness, or unconsciousness. Parenteral nutrition provides nutrients such as sugar, carbohydrates, proteins, and electrolytes, to the body via an IV (see Chapter 20). Enteral nutrition delivers a formula through feeding tubes. The formula contains proteins, carbohydrates, fats, vitamins, and minerals.

Feeding tubes are located at different places in the GI system (**Figure 19.11**). Some tubes are inserted, and others are placed surgically, depending on the doctor's order, the function of the GI system, and the length of time the tube will be used:

- **Nasogastric (NG) tubes**: are inserted through the nose and run down the esophagus into the stomach.
- **Nasoduodenal (ND) tubes**: are inserted through the nose and end in the first portion of the small intestine (duodenum). These tubes bypass the stomach, which can help residents who have stomachs that do not empty well, who experience chronic vomiting, or who *aspirate* (inhale) stomach contents into their lungs.
- **Nasojejunal (NJ) tubes**: are inserted through the nose and end in the second portion of the small intestine (jejunum).
- **Gastrostomy (G) tubes**: are surgically inserted through the abdominal wall into the stomach. These tubes are most commonly used for residents who receive enteral nutrition for a long period of time. A G tube may consist of a long tube, sometimes called a *percutaneous endoscopic gastronomy (PEG)* tube, and a skin-level button

device (**Figure 19.12**). When a button device is used, an extension tube is attached for feeding and removed when the feeding is complete.
- **Jejunostomy (J) tubes**: are surgically placed directly into the intestine.

Licensed nursing staff members regularly check a feeding tube's placement to be sure the feeding tube is *patent* (open) and to determine if the feeding tube has moved out of place or been tugged loose due to regular movement or care delivery. Licensed nursing staff members also check to see if the resident is restless, confused, or disoriented. As a holistic nursing assistant, it is important to always be observant and aware of the following information and guidelines about caring for residents receiving tube feedings:

- Tube feedings may be continuous or scheduled. If scheduled, tube feedings are usually given four times a day (8–12 ounces over 30 minutes). If a continuous pump is used, the feeding may be given slowly over a 24-hour period (with a certain amount being given each hour). If feedings are given on a continuous schedule, regularly check the level of the formula. The formula level should continually decrease as the feeding occurs. If this is not occurring, alert the licensed nursing staff.
- Formula is given at room temperature. Cold fluids can cause cramping. Open formula cans last only eight hours at room temperature.

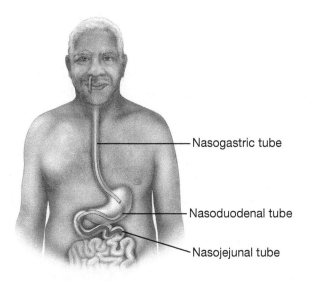

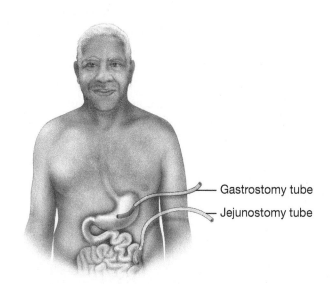

© Body Scientific International

Figure 19.11 The nasogastric, nasoduodenal, and nasojejunal feeding tubes are inserted through the nose. The gastrostomy and jejunostomy feeding tubes are surgically placed.

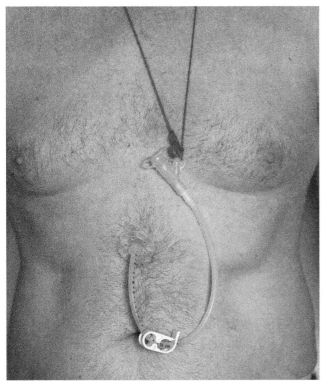

Lighthousebay/Signature collection via Getty Images

Figure 19.12 A lanyard or some other device is used to be sure the tube is not dislodged.

- Tube feedings may be given with a syringe or from a feeding bag (**Figure 19.13**).
- During tube feeding, the head of the resident's bed should be elevated at least 30–45°, or as specified in the care plan. If tube feedings are scheduled for certain times, make sure the head of the bed remains elevated for at least one hour after each feeding is completed.
- Regularly check the outer part of the feeding tube to be sure it is not bent or blocked in any way. Also note if it does not seem to be correctly placed. Let the licensed nursing staff know if there is a concern.
- Always check the area around the feeding tube and its insertion. Notify the licensed nursing staff if it seems to be pulled out or if there is any skin irritation.
- Check for redness, swelling, drainage, or odor around or from the tube insertion site.
- During tube feeding, notify the licensed nursing staff immediately if there is nausea or bloating; if the abdomen swells; complaints of pain or discomfort during the feeding; coughing, gagging, or vomiting during the feeding; respiratory distress; increased pulse rate; flatulence; diarrhea; or constipation.

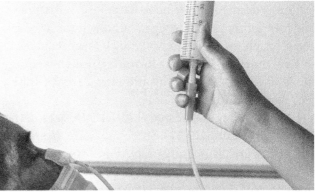

Srisakorn/iStock/Getty Images Plus via Getty Images

A

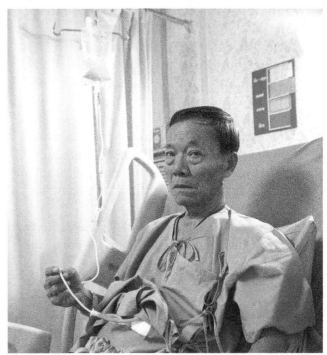

stockphoto mania/Shutterstock.com

B

Figure 19.13 Tube feedings can be delivered using a syringe (A) or a feeding bag (B).

- To improve a resident's comfort and hygiene, provide frequent oral and nasal care. Lubricate the lips often, as dryness is common. It is helpful to offer a mouth rinse every two hours. If appropriate, suggest that the resident suck on a lemon drop or chew sugarless gum.

Adaptive and Assistive Eating Equipment

Adaptive and *assistive eating equipment* includes devices and products that help residents remain as independent as possible during meals. These include

- adaptive and nonskid plates and bowls that prevent foods from slipping off or moving due to the force of eating utensils (**Figure 19.14A**);

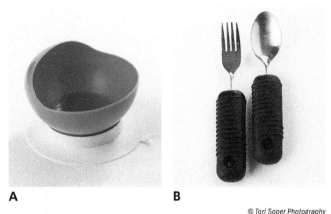

A   **B**

© Tori Soper Photography

Figure 19.14 This nonskid bowl (A) will not move while a resident is eating. Weighted utensils (B) are easier to grip than other utensils.

- weighted knives, forks, and spoons that help hands remain steady (**Figure 19.14B**);
- utensil holders (clips, straps, and foam handles) that help residents achieve better grip; and
- cup holders, weighted mugs, nonslip bases, and no-spill lids that help prevent spills.

Thickening fluids are helpful for residents who have *dysphagia* (difficulty swallowing). Signs of dysphagia include food spilling out of the mouth and coming up through the nose, coughing or choking during or after swallowing, complaining that food will not go down or feels stuck in the throat, and avoiding foods that require chewing or have a certain texture or temperature. Commercial thickening fluids help with safe swallowing and help prevent aspiration. Thicker liquids are easier to swallow and reduce the resident's risk of choking (**Figure 19.15**). These thickening products can be added to most hot and cold liquids without affecting taste.

Liquid Consistencies

Level of Consistency	Description
Extremely thick	Puddinglike; holds shape and can be served with a spoon
Moderately thick	Honeylike; will not flow freely, but will run off a spoon
Medium thick	Nectarlike; does not hold shape and will run off a spoon
Thin	Free-flowing liquids, such as water, soda, coffee, or juice

Goodheart-Willcox Publisher

Figure 19.15 The consistency of a liquid can influence the ease of swallowing.

What Are the Nursing Assistant's Responsibilities in Assisting Residents with Meals?

As a nursing assistant, you will assist residents with their meals. In some cases, you will assist by preparing residents for meals and helping residents to the dining room. In other cases, you will serve the meal tray, set it up at the bedside, and help feed the resident. Nursing assistants must also make sure that residents on therapeutic diets get the correct meal, that the resident eats enough of the required foods, and that residents with special diets or conditions eat on time.

When caring for residents, you should always practice good hygiene by washing your hands or using hand sanitizer, as appropriate. You must also make sure the resident remains safe throughout the meal. One of the most important aspects of caring for residents during mealtime is preventing aspiration. You can use the following guidelines to help prevent aspiration:

- Check to see if residents are on medications that may make them sleepy. Drowsiness may put residents at a higher risk for aspiration.
- Provide a 30-minute rest period prior to feeding time; a rested resident will likely have less difficulty swallowing.
- Sit the resident upright in a chair. If the resident is confined to bed, elevate the backrest to a sitting position.
- Slightly flex the resident's head to achieve a chin-down position. This is helpful for reducing aspiration and some types of dysphagia.
- Adjust the rate of feeding and the sizes of bites as needed for each resident. Do not force or rush the feeding.
- Provide small, bite-sized portions of food.
- Alternate between liquid and solid foods.
- Vary the placement of food in the mouth. Be aware if there is weakness on either side of the face. Always place food in the strongest side of the mouth.
- Check the thickness of food and liquid to be sure it can be tolerated without choking or gagging. For example, some residents best swallow thickened liquids.

Nursing assistants are also responsible for recording the resident's meal intake, or how much the resident ate. This information is recorded using a form provided by the healthcare facility or in the electronic record (**Figure 19.16**).

DIETARY INTAKE RECORD

Month	Year

Directions:

1. For each meal, record the **total percentage** of food the resident consumed in the **TOP** portion of the box.
2. For each meal, record the **total fluids (in milliliters)** the resident consumed in the **BOTTOM** portion of the box.
3. If resident was offered snacks, indicate **refusal** or **percentage consumed**.

DAY	1	2	3	4	5	6	7	8	9	10	11	12	13	14	15
BREAKFAST															
Snack AM															
LUNCH															
Snack PM															
DINNER															
Snack HS															

DAY	16	17	18	19	20	21	22	23	24	25	26	27	28	29	30	31
BREAKFAST																
Snack AM																
LUNCH																
Snack PM																
DINNER																
Snack HS																

FOOD INTAKE	FLUID INTAKE	SNACK INTAKE
0% = Consumed none or only bites (but less than 25%)	1 oz. Cup = 30 mL	R = Refused
25% = Consumed 1/4 of all item(s)	4 oz. Cup = 120 mL	0% = Consumed none or only bites (but less than 25%)
50% = Consumed 1/2 of all item(s)	5 oz. Cup = 150 mL	25% = Consumed 1/4 of all item(s)
75% = Consumed 3/4 of all item(s)	6 oz. Cup/Bowl = 180 mL	50% = Consumed 1/2 of all item(s)
100% = Consumed all item(s)	8 oz. Cup/Bowl = 240 mL	75% = Consumed 3/4 of all item(s)
		100% = Consumed all item(s)

Resident Name	ID#	Room #	Doctor

Figure 19.16 An intake form like this one is used to document the foods and fluids a resident consumes.

For the most part, keeping residents independent and self-reliant is always encouraged. Going to the dining room to eat meals is not only important for social interaction, but also helps promote and encourage better nutrition. The procedure that follows focuses on assisting residents who are eating in their rooms—in bed, by the bedside in a chair, or in a wheelchair. Many of the steps in the procedure also apply to assisting a resident in the dining room.

Procedure

Assisting with Meals in the Resident's Room

Rationale

Residents receive the nutrition they need when they consume the proper amounts of nutrients from a variety of food groups. Due to diseases or conditions, some residents require help to eat comfortably and eat sufficient amounts of their meals.

Preparation

1. Ask the licensed nursing staff if there are doctor's orders for the procedure, if there are any specific instructions listed in the plan of care, and if the resident can be moved into the positions required for this procedure.
2. Wash your hands or use hand sanitizer before entering the room.
3. Knock before entering the room.
4. Introduce yourself using your first or preferred name and title. Explain that you work with the licensed nursing staff and will be providing care.
5. Greet the resident and ask the resident to state his full name, if able. Then check the resident's identification bracelet.
6. Use Mr., Mrs., or Ms. and the resident's last name when conversing.
7. Explain the procedure in simple terms, even if the resident is not able to communicate or is disoriented. Ask permission to perform the procedure.

   Best Practice: To promote comfort during the meal, be sure the room is free from unpleasant odors.

8. Bring the necessary equipment into the room. Place the following items in an easy-to-reach place:
   - disposable gloves, if needed
   - a cloth or paper clothing protector to prevent soiling during the meal
   - adaptive and assistive eating devices, as needed
   - pen and pad, form, or digital device for recording meal intake
   - supplies for before-meal hygiene, if needed

   Best Practice: Always check to be sure adaptive and assistive eating devices are usable. If they are not, notify the licensed nursing staff immediately.

The Procedure

9. Provide privacy by closing the curtains, using a screen, or closing the door to the room.

   Best Practice: Before starting, ask the resident if he needs to use the toilet, bedpan, or urinal.

10. If the resident will be eating in bed and if you will be assisting, lock the bed wheels and then raise the bed to hip level. Raise the head of the bed and adjust for comfort in eating. Or, if appropriate, help the resident to a sitting position at the side of the bed or to a chair. If the resident is not dressed, help the resident put on a robe and slippers.
11. Maintain safety during the procedure. If there are side rails, raise and lock the rails on the opposite side of the bed from where you will be working. Lower the rail on the side where you are working.

    Best Practice: Wear disposable gloves only if required for infection prevention and control.

12. Provide before-meal hygiene. If the resident is ambulatory, hygiene can be performed in the bathroom. If the resident is not ambulatory, provide supplies for washing the hands and face, brushing teeth, or using mouth rinse. Assist the resident as needed.

(continued)

Assisting with Meals in the Resident's Room *(continued)*

Best Practice: Determine how well residents are able to eat by themselves. Also note if residents will be using adaptive and assistive eating devices. It is important to promote as much independence as possible, though you may need to assist fully or partially.

13. Check that the name on the meal tray matches the name of the resident.

14. Clear the overbed table before placing the meal tray. Check the meal tray to make sure that all appropriate foods are there and represent the correct diet. If any foods that should be on the tray are missing, get them or ask to have them brought in, if appropriate.

15. If the resident is in bed, place a cloth or paper clothing protector over the resident's chest to prevent the resident's clothing from becoming soiled with food during the meal.

16. Sit at eye level next to the resident.

Best Practice: Focus your attention on the resident during the meal. Always be alert for signs of choking or difficulty swallowing.

17. Prepare the meal tray. Depending on the situation, you may need to help with:
    - opening milk cartons
    - removing utensils from their wrappers
    - buttering bread
    - cutting up meat
    - seasoning food to the resident's taste (not to yours)

Best Practice: Serve the meal tray right away so that foods and liquids are at proper eating temperature. This will also ensure a pleasant room environment and eating experience.

18. If the resident can handle finger foods, arrange the plate so these are in reach.

19. If the resident has poor eyesight or limited vision, describe the foods being served. If the resident is feeding himself, help the resident locate the food on the plate by describing where foods are in terms of a clockface (**Figure 19.17**).

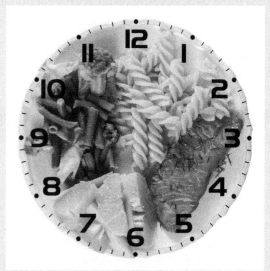

Figure 19.17

Oleksandra Naumenko/Shutterstock.com; GzP_Design/Shutterstock.com

20. If a resident cannot see the tray at all and needs assistance, name each mouthful of food as you offer it.

Best Practice: When feeding residents who are unable to feed themselves, use a spoon for safety. Fill the spoon until it is only half-full. Give food from the tip of the spoon, not from the side of the spoon. Put the food in one side of the resident's mouth so the food can be chewed more easily.

21. If a resident is weak or paralyzed on one side, feed the resident on the strong side, not on the side that is weak or paralyzed.

22. Alternate between solid foods and liquids. Offer liquids frequently between bites. Do not rush the feeding. Serve the food in order of resident preference.

23. Allow the resident enough time for chewing and swallowing. Encourage residents to swallow twice between each bite. Check the mouth to see if it is empty before offering more foods or fluids.

24. Provide a straw for liquids if the resident cannot drink from a cup or glass. Provide a different straw for each liquid. If the resident is weak, provide a short straw.

Best Practice: Residents with dysphagia usually do not use straws. They may take thickened liquids with a spoon.

25. Encourage the resident to eat as much as possible. Approaches or techniques you can use to help include:
    - using verbal cues, such as short and simple phrases, to prompt the resident
    - demonstrating or acting out what you want the resident to do
    - placing your hand over the resident's hand for guidance (**Figure 19.18**)
    - praising successes along the way

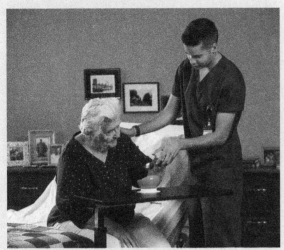

Figure 19.18   © Tori Soper Photography

26. Using a napkin, wipe the resident's hands, face, and mouth as needed during and at the end of the meal. Discard the napkin when done.
27. Once the resident has finished eating, remove the meal tray. Be sure to note how much was eaten and which foods the resident consumed. Identify which foods were not eaten. If a particular food was not eaten, ask the resident why.
28. Provide for privacy. Assist with hygiene by having the resident wash his hands and perform oral care. Assist as needed.

29. The amount of food eaten should be documented according to facility policy using a form provided by the healthcare facility or in the electronic record. Some policies require that you note the portion of the total meal consumed. Other policies require the percentage of the food eaten. Whatever method is used, the amount of food eaten will be converted into calories by the licensed nursing staff or a dietitian. Always inform the licensed nursing staff if less than 75 percent of a meal is eaten.
30. If the resident is in bed, check to be sure the bed wheels are locked. Then reposition the resident and lower the bed.
31. Follow the plan of care to determine if the side rails should be raised or lowered.
32. Take the used meal tray to the meal cart.
33. Remove, clean, and store equipment in the proper location. Remove soiled linens and discard disposable equipment.

Follow-Up

34. Wash your hands to ensure infection control.
35. Make sure the resident is safe and comfortable and place the call light and personal items within reach.
36. Conduct a safety check before leaving the room. The room should be clean and free from clutter or spills.
37. Wash your hands or use hand sanitizer before leaving the room.

Reporting and Documentation

38. Report any specific observations, complications, or unusual responses to the licensed nursing staff. Document this information, along with the care provided, in the chart or EMR.

SECTION 19.2 **Review and Assessment**

Key Terms Mini Glossary

alternative feeding therapy the practice of delivering food intravenously or through a gastrointestinal tube due to a resident's inability to ingest food through the mouth.

aspirate to inhale a foreign object or substance, such as food or liquid, when eating.

dysphagia difficulty or discomfort when swallowing.

enteral by way of the gastrointestinal system.

parenteral by way of the veins or intravenous infusion.

patent open.

therapeutic diets eating plans that promote healing.

Apply the Key Terms

Complete the following sentences using the key terms in this section.

1. When a nursing assistant was feeding Mr. T, he had difficulty swallowing, or _____.
2. When food is given through a gastrointestinal tube, the term used is _____.
3. When fluid is given by way of veins, the term used is _____.
4. The licensed nursing staff was checking the tube feeding for Mrs. A. She found that the tube was open, or _____.
5. It is important that residents not _____ their food or beverage when eating.

Know and Understand the Facts

1. Identify two factors that help make mealtimes enjoyable.
2. What is mindful eating and how can it be accomplished?
3. Describe two therapeutic diets and explain why they are ordered.
4. List three responsibilities nursing assistants have when they assist with alternative feeding therapies.
5. What are supplemental nutrition drinks and when are they used?
6. Identify two challenges residents may have when eating.
7. Describe two different adaptive or assistive eating devices and explain their functions.

Analyze and Apply Concepts

1. Identify three steps that should be taken to prepare a resident for a meal.

2. Identify one eating challenge a resident may face and describe two ways to avoid or overcome it.
3. Describe three important principles nursing assistants should keep in mind when assisting residents with meals.
4. Explain how to record food intake.

Think Critically

Read the following care situation. Then answer the questions that follow.

You are taking care of Mr. M today. Mr. M is a frail, 78-year-old man who was admitted last week to the long-term care facility where you work. Mr. M had been living at home with his sister for the last five years. Mr. M has been falling recently when ambulating, so he has several bruises on his arms. He is unstable when walking and has moderate-to-severe arthritis in his hands and hips. This is the first time you will be taking care of Mr. M. His EMR states that he is alert and communicative. When you entered Mr. M's room this morning, you found him sleepy, very weak, and unwilling to participate in his morning care. It is now time for Mr. M's noontime meal.

1. What is the first thing you should do before serving Mr. M's meal?
2. Mr. M will be eating lunch. How will you know whether Mr. M should go to the dining room, stay in his room to eat at his bedside, or stay in bed to eat?
3. What will you need to do to prepare Mr. M for his meal?
4. What should you do to prevent any eating challenges Mr. M may have (for example, choking on his food, since he seemed so tired and weak)?

19 Summary and Review

Key Points

Reviewing the key points for this chapter will help you practice more safely and competently as a holistic nursing assistant and will help you prepare for the competency certification examination.

- Calories provide the energy the body needs to function properly and build, maintain, and repair body tissues. Six nutrients are needed for a healthy diet: carbohydrates, dietary fats, proteins, vitamins, minerals, and water.
- MyPlate and the *Dietary Guidelines for Americans* provide guidance for what types of foods people should eat.
- Nursing assistants must understand the reasons for and importance of therapeutic diets.
- Residents may need assistance with eating, including feeding residents, providing adaptive and assistive eating devices, or preparing meal trays at the bedside or in the facility dining room. Some residents require alternative feeding therapies, such as tube feeding.

Action Steps to Holistic Care

Review the information in this chapter. Complete the following activities.

1. Select one set of guidelines or a procedure about assisting with meals in this chapter. Prepare a short paper or digital presentation that describes the top three most important practices for assisting with eating, including one that promotes comfort and one that assures safety.
2. With a partner, write a song or a poem about one nutrient. Include why the nutrient is important to body function and what foods contain it.
3. With a partner, prepare a poster that shows one eating disorder or condition. Include at least four facts that residents and the public should know about the disorder.
4. Research one therapeutic diet. Write a brief report that describes one new, science-based fact.

Building Math Skill

You have been asked to calculate how much Mr. H has consumed this morning. You know he had a full cup of coffee (6 ounces), a full glass of water (8 ounces), and a small cup of fruit juice (4 ounces). When you chart this you need to put the total in milliliters (mL). How many mL has he consumed?

Preparing for the Certification Competency Examination

To prepare for the nursing assistant certification competency examination, you will need to know content found in this chapter. This content may be tested in the knowledge (written or oral) and skills (hands-on demonstration) portions of the exam. The following areas will be emphasized:

- principles of nutrition
- essential nutrients and basic food groups
- serving and portion sizes
- personal, cultural, religious, and medical conditions requiring diet variations
- situational factors that influence or interfere with adequate intake
- contributory factors that influence age-related dietary problems
- therapeutic diets and their rationales
- alternate feeding methods
- care needed to assist in meeting dietary needs
- care for residents unable to obtain adequate nutrition independently
- the importance of observing and documenting food intake

These sample test questions are similar to ones you will find on the certification competency exam. See how well you can answer them. Be sure to select the *best* answer.

1. Which of the following is a fat-soluble vitamin?
   A. vitamin C
   B. vitamin A
   C. vitamin B_6
   D. vitamin B_{12}

2. Mr. U recently had a mild heart attack and is on dialysis. Which therapeutic diet would doctors most likely order for Mr. U?
   A. bland diet
   B. clear liquid diet
   C. soft diet
   D. renal diet

(Continued)

3. Which of the following is the major function of protein?
   A. storage in body tissue
   B. building of body tissue
   C. absorption of fats
   D. synthesis of minerals

4. A healthcare staff member is overweight and spends a lot of time eating snacks and food from home during her shift. Which of the following eating disorders might she have?
   A. cachexia nervosa
   B. dysphagia nervosa
   C. binge-eating disorder
   D. anorexia nervosa

5. Which of the following is an important responsibility holistic nursing assistants have when they provide care during enteral feeding?
   A. keeping the resident occupied during the feeding
   B. providing frequent oral and nasal care
   C. making sure the bed linens are not wrinkled
   D. letting the family know when the feeding occurs

6. A nursing assistant is taking care of Mrs. Q, who has become dehydrated after vomiting all morning from a mild stomach virus. Mrs. Q can now tolerate a clear liquid diet. To begin the process of hydration, how much liquid should the nursing assistant encourage Mrs. Q to drink today?
   A. 11 cups
   B. 8 cups
   C. 14 cups
   D. 10 cups

7. A nursing assistant wants to determine if a resident is underweight, at a healthy weight, overweight, or obese. She might use which of the following common methods?
   A. a balance scale
   B. the FDA
   C. a digital scale
   D. BMI

8. Which of the following help balance the amount of water in the body?
   A. electrolytes
   B. calories
   C. carbohydrates
   D. gluten

9. Units of energy that combine with oxygen to release energy the body needs are called
   A. carbohydrates
   B. vitamins
   C. calories
   D. minerals

10. A nursing assistant has been asked to assist Mrs. N with her eating. Mrs. N is independent, but her hands tremble when she holds her fork. What might the nursing assistant do to help?
    A. leave Mrs. N alone to eat
    B. go ahead and feed Mrs. N her main meal
    C. have Mrs. N wait until her family returns
    D. have Mrs. N try an assistive utensil

11. Which of the following are the three types of carbohydrates found in food?
    A. starch, sugars, and fiber
    B. minerals, fiber, and fats
    C. starch, fats, and sugars
    D. fiber, minerals, and water

12. Mrs. H is able to eat independently, but is not able to leave her bed. She sometimes has trouble swallowing. What position should Mrs. H be in during eating?
    A. on her left side
    B. on her back
    C. in a sitting position
    D. on her right side with her head raised

13. If a resident has dysphagia, which consistency of liquid is best to avoid choking?
    A. moderately thick
    B. extremely thick
    C. thin
    D. medium thick

14. MyPlate provides guidelines for selecting foods from the following five food groups:
    A. fruits, grains, gluten, protein, and lactose
    B. fruits, vegetables, grains, protein, and dairy
    C. fruits, vegetables, grains, vitamins, and dairy
    D. fruits, minerals, grains, vitamins, and dairy

15. Mr. X likes to eat a large breakfast early in the morning and is always upset when his meal tray comes late. This is an example of
    A. a therapeutic diet
    B. religious tradition
    C. food preferences
    D. alternative nutrition

Did you have difficulty with any of the questions? If you did, review the chapter to find the correct answer(s).

Welcome to the Chapter

As you learned in Chapters 9 and 10, regulating hydration and eliminating waste are functions of the urinary and gastrointestinal systems. As a nursing assistant, you will make sure residents are hydrated and help them with elimination needs. You may be asked to keep track of the fluids residents drink and lose through elimination. Maintaining hydration is important to promoting healing and achieving wellness, particularly for residents who are ill or frail. At times, residents do not drink enough fluids or have an illness or condition that prevents them from maintaining hydration. In these cases, fluids may be given through an IV.

Nursing assistants also assist residents with their elimination needs, including using a bedpan, urinal, bedside commode, or toilet. Nursing assistants provide catheter and ostomy care, empty urinary drainage bags, and change colostomy bags. Inserting suppositories and rectal tubes and administering soapsuds and commercial enemas may be additional responsibilities.

The information and procedures presented in this chapter will help you build the knowledge and skills needed to become a holistic nursing assistant. Check with your instructor to ensure these procedures are within your state's regulations for nursing assistant practice. The topics discussed in the chapter are highlighted on the Providing Holistic Care Framework.

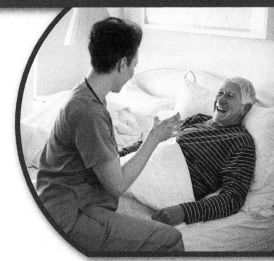

AJ_Watt/E+ via Getty Images

Chapter Outline

Section 20.1
Maintaining Hydration

Section 20.2
Assisting with Elimination

Providing Holistic Care Framework

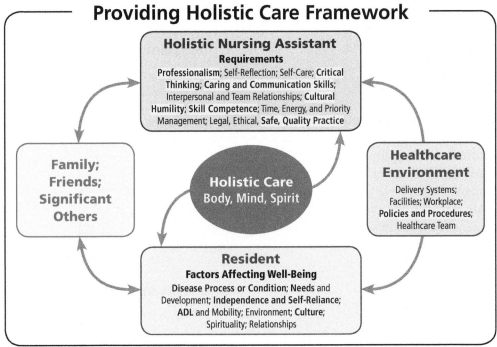

Holistic Nursing Assistant
Requirements
Professionalism; Self-Reflection; Self-Care; **Critical Thinking; Caring and Communication Skills;** Interpersonal and Team Relationships; **Cultural Humility; Skill Competence;** Time, Energy, and Priority Management; Legal, Ethical, **Safe, Quality Practice**

Family; Friends; Significant Others

Holistic Care
Body, Mind, Spirit

Healthcare Environment
Delivery Systems; Facilities; Workplace; **Policies and Procedures;** Healthcare Team

Resident
Factors Affecting Well-Being
Disease Process or Condition; **Needs** and Development; **Independence and Self-Reliance; ADL** and Mobility; Environment; **Culture;** Spirituality; Relationships

Goodheart-Willcox Publisher

Maintaining Hydration

Objectives

To achieve the objectives for this section, you must successfully:

- **discuss** the importance of hydration and the effects of dehydration.
- **describe** how nursing assistants care for residents receiving IV fluids.
- **demonstrate** how to empty urinary drainage bags.
- **measure** and **document** intake and output (I&O).

Key Terms

Learn these key terms to better understand the information presented in the section.

constipation   graduate

diarrhea   void

Questions to Consider

- Think about the last time you were extremely thirsty. Do you remember why you were thirsty?
- What were the physical signs of your thirst? How did you feel?
- What did you do to satisfy your thirst? How much did you have to drink to feel hydrated?

Why Is It Important to Stay Hydrated?

In Chapter 19, you learned about the importance of hydration. Having enough fluid in the body is necessary for the body systems to work properly. Fluids moisten tissues in the eyes, nose, and mouth; protect organs; control body temperature; lubricate joints; and get rid of toxins from the body. Too much fluid in the body, sometimes caused by a disease or condition, can lead to *edema*. Too little fluid can cause *dehydration*.

Some residents may be placed on *NPO*, which means "nothing by mouth." This means that the doctor has ordered the resident not eat or drink anything for a specific period of time. This order will be found in the resident's chart or EMR and plan of care. NPO notification will also be placed in an easily observed location on the door of the resident's room or in the resident's room. NPO orders typically last for a short period of time (from a few hours to 12 hours). NPO is usually ordered because the resident will be having a surgical or medical imaging procedure or is being prepared for surgery. This is done as a safety precaution to prevent aspiration (breathing stomach contents into the lungs) if the resident is

sedated. If there is concern that there may be possible dehydration, an IV may be ordered. NPO may also be ordered while the resident is receiving an IV.

Dehydration

Dehydration can happen very quickly. Even minor dehydration, such as a loss of two percent of body fluids, can decrease body function. This creates an imbalance in the body's systems and can become so severe it leads to death. Dehydration can occur due to unavailability of fluids, inability to drink fluids, dysphagia (difficulty swallowing), unconsciousness, exposure to long-lasting heat, exercise, high fever, constant vomiting, excessive *diarrhea* (frequent, watery stools), and burns.

The first signs of dehydration are increased thirst and a dry mouth. Some people may also feel dizzy, weak, or tired. Worsening dehydration may cause a swollen tongue, pounding heartbeat, headache, confusion, and fainting. Advanced dehydration can cause chest pain, difficulty breathing, inability to sweat, *constipation* (infrequent, hard, dry stools), and a decrease in urinary output. Urine becomes dark yellow or orange in color (**Figure 20.1**).

Increasing the amount and variety of fluids and offering fruits and vegetables that contain a lot of water—such as oranges, tomatoes, and pineapple—can prevent dehydration. Remind residents to drink plenty

Urine Color Chart

TRANSPARENT
You are drinking a lot of fluid

PALE STRAW COLOR
You are well hydrated

TRANSPARENT YELLOW
Normal

DARK YELLOW
Drink fluid soon

AMBER OR HONEY
Your body isn't getting enough fluid

SYRUP OR BROWN ALE
Drink a lot of fluid immediately

cbproject/Shutterstock.com

Figure 20.1 Urine color is a good way to determine a resident's level of hydration.

A doctor will determine the type, amount, and flow rate of the IV based on the resident's condition. The IV fluid drips at a prescribed flow rate from the bag through the tubing and catheter into the vein. Some residents may be able to drink fluids while receiving an IV, and others may be NPO.

Licensed nursing staff members make sure that the IV tubing is fully connected and all tubes remain open. They also keep the flow rate accurate, sometimes increasing or reducing the flow based on the doctor's orders. Licensed nursing staff also change the bag of fluid, monitor the insertion site, and maintain a record of IV fluid intake. There are dressings around the IV that keep the IV catheter in place. Many times, a bandage with a see-through top is placed over the catheter to keep it in place and provide a better view of the insertion. These are changed by licensed nursing staff. Residents are asked to avoid disturbing, twisting, or bending the tubing or dressing, which can prevent fluid from flowing into the vein. They are also asked to report any pain, burning, or swelling at the IV site or blood in the tubing. A resident receiving an IV should be monitored continuously for signs of dehydration, or for signs that they are getting too much fluid. These include elevated blood pressure, weight gain, edema, or difficulty breathing.

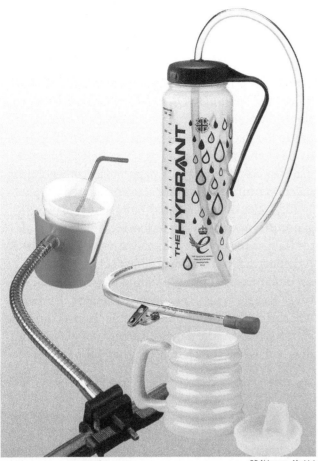

SP Ableware—Maddak

Figure 20.2 Assistive devices such as a clip-on drink holder, hand-to-hand mug, and hydrant water bottle make it easier for residents to maintain hydration.

of fluids during and between meals. Provide fresh drinking water at the bedside and offer a variety of beverages according to a resident's prescribed diet. Also remind residents to avoid caffeine because it has a *diuretic* effect that increases urine output. Assistive drinking devices such as cups with long spouts may help increase intake if the resident has problems drinking (**Figure 20.2**).

Residents with IVs

A doctor may order an IV for residents who are unable to drink liquids, need quick fluid replacement due to dehydration, or require specific medications by IV. IVs give fluid through a closed system made up of a bag of fluid, tubing, and a needle or *catheter* (**Figure 20.3**). The bag of fluid hangs above the resident's head. Gravity helps the fluid flow down. In some facilities, a medical device call an *IV pump* is used to control the flow of fluids through the IV. Catheters, or needles, are inserted into the resident's vein (usually in a hand, arm, leg, or foot) by the licensed nursing staff.

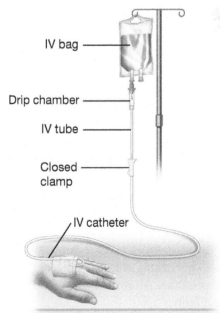

© *Body Scientific International*

Figure 20.3 The closed IV system consists of an IV bag, tubing, and catheter. Fluid flows through a clear, plastic drip chamber. This chamber prevents air from entering the IV tubing and regulates IV flow rate. The clamp is used to start and stop the IV solution and control the amount of fluids entering the vein.

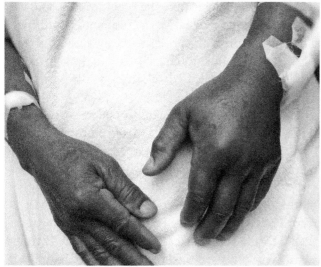

Arthit Premprayot/Shutterstock.com

Figure 20.4 Always observe around or at the IV site for possible signs of infiltration (swelling).

A nursing assistant can assist the licensed nursing staff with these responsibilities by:

- Frequently observe the IV site for possible signs of *infiltration* (swelling at or around the IV site due to IV fluid leaking into the body). Infiltration can occur at any time, but is more common one to two hours after the IV is inserted. Observe for puffiness or swelling, hot or cold skin, and pale or reddened skin at the site of the needle or catheter (**Figure 20.4**). Alert the licensed nursing staff immediately if you observe any of these.
- Regularly monitor the IV system to make sure the IV fluid bag remains above the resident's head and there is no fluid leaking or kinks in the tubing. Check for blood in the tubing and make sure there is enough fluid in the bag. Remind the resident to keep the arm with the IV lowered so blood does not flow into the tubing. If you observe any problems, let the licensed nursing staff know immediately.
- Respond if the resident complains of discomfort, such as pain or burning at or near the site. Other symptoms may affect the whole body—for example, fever, itching, shortness of breath, chest pain, irregular pulse, or a drop in blood pressure. Alert the licensed nursing staff immediately.
- Make sure the dressing remains in place and maintain the position of the tubing and the extremity in which the IV is inserted. This is very important during personal hygiene and ADLs.

How Are Intake and Output Documented?

Given the importance of hydration, you must be very careful when asked to measure and document fluid *intake and output (I&O)*. *Fluid intake* includes all oral fluids, IV fluids, and tube feedings. *Output* includes any urine that is **voided** (expelled from the body) and urine from a urinary drainage bag. Emesis (vomit), diarrhea, colostomy bag drainage, and any other drainage (such as from wounds) are also considered output.

I&O is measured on a 24-hour schedule using a **graduate**, or a container with a measurement scale for fluids and certain types of drainage (**Figure 20.5**). A urinary hat has a measurement scale and is also used to measure output. IV fluid bags and drainage bags often have their own measurement scales. Before measuring I&O, you should ask the licensed nursing staff for the standard measurements of glasses and dishes used by the facility (**Figure 20.6**). These

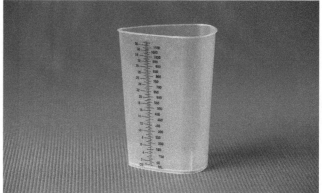

© Tori Soper Photography

Figure 20.5 A graduate measures urine and drainage output.

Standard Volumes for Intake and Output

Item	Volume in Ounces	Volume in Milliliters
Drinking glass	8 oz	240 mL
Cup	8 oz	240 mL
Teacup	6 oz	180 mL
Styrofoam cup	6 oz	180 mL
Juice cup	4 oz	120 mL
Popsicle	3 oz	90 mL
Ice cube	Melts to 1/2 the original volume	

Goodheart-Willcox Publisher

Figure 20.6 Standard measurements will help you accurately document fluid intake.

THINK ABOUT THIS

The *metric system* was developed in the late 1700s, and continues to be the primary system of measurement throughout the world. The metric system has three main units of measurement: the *meter* for length, the *gram* for weight or mass, and the *liter* for liquid volume. Prefixes are added to indicate their amounts based on measures of 10. For example, 1,000 meters is 1 kilometer. While the United States does use the metric system, it is not the official system of measurement. Instead, it uses *US customary units*. This measurement system includes inches and feet (for length); pounds and ounces (for weight); and pints, quarts, and gallons (for liquid volume). Both metric units and US customary units are used in healthcare. For example, metric units are typically used for measuring medication doses or for liquid measurement. The US customary unit of the pound is used for measuring a resident's weight. Because both systems are used, it is important to know each and the conversions between them (for example, 1 meter is equal to 3.28 feet). More information about the metric system and US customary units, and their conversions, can be found in Appendix B.

measurements may also be listed on the I&O form or can be obtained from the dietary department.

An *I&O form* can be paper or electronic and is used in facilities to document the intake and output amounts when ordered or in the plan of care (**Figure 20.7**).

I&O is documented throughout each shift. At the end of each shift, I&O is subtotaled. The next shift continues documenting I&O. All subtotals are added together for a total I&O at the end of the shift that completes the 24-hour period.

Intake & Output Form

Resident Name: _____   Room #: _____

Date: _____   Floor #: _____

	Intake			Output			
				Urine		Gastric	
	By mouth	Tube	Parenteral	Voided	Catheter	Emesis	Suction
Time 7–3							
Total							
Time 3–11							
Total							
Time 11–7							
Total							
24-Hour Total							
24-Hour Grand Total • Intake				24-Hour Grand Total • Output			

Figure 20.7 This sample I&O form documents total intake and output during a 24-hour period.

Procedure

Measuring and Documenting Fluid Intake and Urinary Output

Rationale

Careful and accurate measurement of intake and output (I&O) is needed to help maintain the body's fluid balance. This is very important for residents who may be dehydrated or who have a specific disease or condition.

Preparation

1. Ask the licensed nursing staff if there are doctor's orders for the procedure, if there are any specific instructions listed in the plan of care, and if the resident can be moved into the positions required for this procedure.
2. Wash your hands or use hand sanitizer before entering the room.
3. Knock before entering the room.
4. Introduce yourself using your first or preferred name and title. Explain that you work with the licensed nursing staff and will be providing care.
5. Greet the resident and ask the resident to state his or her full name, if able. Then check the resident's identification bracelet.
6. Use Mr., Mrs., or Ms. and the resident's last name when conversing.
7. Explain the procedure in simple terms, even if the resident is not able to communicate or is disoriented. Ask permission to perform the procedure.
8. Bring the necessary equipment into the room. Place the following items in an easy-to-reach place:
   - disposable gloves
   - pen and form or digital device for documenting the I&O
   - appropriate measuring containers and graduate
   - urinary hat, bedpan, or urinal
   - disposable protective pad
   - antiseptic swab(s)
   - paper towel

The Procedure: Measuring Oral Fluid Intake

9. Provide privacy by closing the curtains, using a screen, or closing the door to the room.
10. Wash your hands or use hand sanitizer to ensure infection control.

   Best Practice: Wear disposable gloves only if required for infection prevention and control.

11. Note the amount of liquid that the resident was served. Pour the liquid the resident did not drink into a measuring cup or graduate. Keep the graduate level. Measure the amount left in each container or glass at eye level.

Best Practice: Fluids are measured and documented in fluid ounces (oz.) or milliliters (mL): 1 fluid oz. = 30 mL. *Note:* You may see the notation "cc," which stands for "cubic centimeter." In the past, 1 cc was considered to equal 1 mL, and in many cases it does. However, because elevation and atmospheric pressure can change the amount of fluid that will "fit" in 1 cubic centimeter, preferred practice is to use milliliters, *not* cubic centimeters.

12. Subtract each amount measured from the full amount the resident was served. Note each amount. These are the amounts the resident actually drank.
13. Add all of the amounts together to get the total amount of liquid the resident drank. Immediately document this amount on the intake side of the I&O form.
14. All other intake, such as from IV fluids or liquids given by tube, will also need to be measured. Ask the licensed nursing staff who is responsible for this measurement.

The Procedure: Measuring Urinary Output

15. Provide privacy by closing the curtains, using a screen, or closing the door to the room.
16. Wash your hands or use hand sanitizer to ensure infection control.
17. Put on disposable gloves.
18. If the resident is ambulatory, place a urinary hat in the commode or toilet. Instruct the resident to urinate into the hat, not into the commode or toilet (**Figure 20.8**). Each resident will have his or her own personal urinary hat.

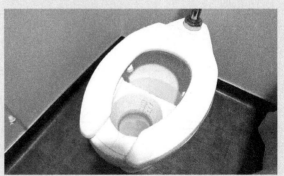

Figure 20.8   *Karin Hildebrand Lau/Shutterstock.com*

19. Ask the resident not to put toilet paper into the commode or toilet. Provide a bag or waste container for the toilet paper. Also instruct the resident *not* to remove the urinary hat. Ask the resident to use a call light to indicate if the urinary hat needs to be emptied.

20. If the resident is in bed, a bedpan, urinal, or urinary catheter with a drainage bag may be used to collect urine.

> **Best Practice:** Sometimes urine can remain in the handle of a urinal. Be sure this amount is poured out for measurement.

21. To empty a urinary drainage bag, place a disposable protective pad on the floor underneath the drainage bag and place a graduate on top of the protective pad. Clean the tubing with an antiseptic swab, open the drain at the bottom of the bag, and empty the urine into a graduate. When emptying the drainage bag, make sure that the urine does not splash and that the drainage tube does not touch the sides of the graduate (**Figure 20.9**).

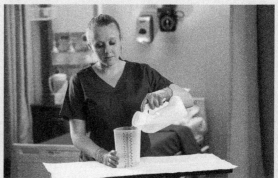

Figure 20.10   © Tori Soper Photography

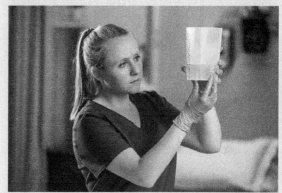

Figure 20.11   © Tori Soper Photography

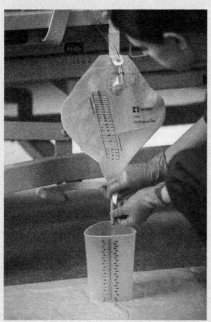

Figure 20.9   © Tori Soper Photography

22. Close the drain on the urinary drainage bag.
23. Wipe the drain on the urinary drainage bag with an antiseptic swab or according to facility policy. Replace the drain in the holder on the urinary drainage bag. Note the color, odor, clarity, or presence of any particles in the urine.
24. Place a paper towel on a level surface and put the graduate used to measure output on top of the paper towel. If a bedpan or urinal was used, carefully pour the urine into the graduate (**Figure 20.10**). Always measure the amount of urine at eye level (**Figure 20.11**). Make note of this amount.

25. Always dispose of urine in the toilet. Avoid splashes. Carefully rinse the graduate and pour the rinse water into the toilet as well.
26. All other output, such as the contents of a colostomy drainage bag, will also need to be measured. Ask the licensed nursing staff who is responsible for this measurement.
27. Remove, clean, and store equipment in the proper location. Remove soiled linens and discard disposable equipment.
28. Remove and discard your gloves.
29. Wash your hands to ensure infection control.
30. Document the urine output amount on the paper or electronic I&O form. At the end of your shift, or as ordered, document the total urine output amount on the output side of the I&O form.
31. Whether the resident ambulated to the bathroom or remained in bed, check to be sure the bed wheels are locked, then reposition the resident and lower the bed.
32. Follow the plan of care to determine if the side rails should be raised or lowered.

Follow-Up

33. Make sure the resident is comfortable and place the call light and personal items within reach.

(continued)

Measuring and Documenting Fluid Intake and Urinary Output *(continued)*

34. Conduct a safety check before leaving the room. The room should be clean and free from clutter or spills.
35. Wash your hands or use hand sanitizer before leaving the room.

Reporting and Documentation

36. Report any specific observations, complications, or unusual responses to the licensed nursing staff. Document this information, along with the care provided, in the chart or EMR.

SECTION 20.1 **Review and Assessment**

Key Terms Mini Glossary

constipation a condition in which bowel movements occur fewer than three times a week and contain hard, dry stools that are difficult to evacuate; can be an acute or chronic condition.

diarrhea a condition in which bowel movements have stools with excess water and occur frequently; can be an acute or chronic condition.

graduate a container used to measure intake and output.
void to expel from the body.

Apply the Key Terms

Complete the following sentences using the key terms in this section.

1. Several times today, Mrs. K's stools were very loose and there seemed to be lot of water in them. She has a condition called _____.
2. Another term for urinating, or expelling fluid from the body, is _____.
3. A resident who has hard, dry stools that are difficult to evacuate has a condition called _____.
4. Linda, an NA, needs a container to measure intake and output. She will look for a _____.

Know and Understand the Facts

1. Identify three reasons why hydration is important.
2. Describe two consequences of dehydration.
3. List three ways nursing assistants can assist the licensed nursing staff with IVs.

Analyze and Apply Concepts

1. What two actions must a nursing assistant take to measure input accurately?
2. Explain the steps needed to empty a urinary drainage bag.

3. A nursing assistant needs to document fluid intake for a resident who drank one full, 8-ounce glass of water. How many milliliters should she document on the I&O form?

Think Critically

Read the following care situation. Then answer the questions that follow.

Ms. A, who is 78 years old, just had hip-replacement surgery and has been transferred to the facility where you work. She is very restless. The doctor ordered an IV for the rest of the day and a full liquid diet when Ms. A asks to eat. Ms. A can drink beverages if she wants. She has a urinary catheter with a half-full urinary drainage bag. When you enter the room, it looks like she has had one-half of a glass of water.

1. Describe what you should check to make sure Ms. A's IV and urinary drainage bag are correctly placed.
2. You will need to measure Ms. A's I&O during your shift. List the steps you will take to measure her input.
3. You will be checking Ms. A's output at the end of your shift. Explain what you will need to do to take an accurate measurement.

Assisting with Elimination

Objectives

To achieve the objectives for this section, you must successfully:

- **discuss** the process of urinary and bowel elimination, including potential problems and related care needed.
- **explain** how to document bowel movements.
- **demonstrate** the ability to safely and effectively assist residents with elimination using a toilet, bedside commode, bedpan, or urinal.
- **perform** catheter and colostomy care.
- **show** how to insert a suppository or rectal tube and change a drainage bag.
- **describe** the process of bladder and bowel retraining.

Key Terms

Learn these key terms to better understand the information presented in the section.

defecate	motility
enema	ostomy
flatus	stoma
hernia	suppositories
impaction	

Questions to Consider

- Have you ever been constipated because of the food you ate or medications you took?
- If you have been constipated, was it uncomfortable? Were you hesitant to talk about your elimination problems because you felt self-conscious or embarrassed?
- Were you able to ease your level of discomfort? What did you do?

How Can Nursing Assistants Help with Urinary Elimination?

On average, a person urinates 800–2,000 mL every 24 hours, which requires six to eight trips to the bathroom. When a resident has limited mobility, nursing assistants may need to frequently assist him or her with elimination needs.

Residents with mobility challenges and who get up often during the night may need assistance getting to the toilet or bedside commode. Residents who are unable to ambulate may use bedpans for urinary and bowel elimination needs. There are two types of bedpans: a standard bedpan and a fracture bedpan (**Figure 20.12**). Both types are usually plastic. A *standard bedpan* fits the contour of the buttocks and has a shallow bowl that collects urine and stool.

A *fracture bedpan* is used when a resident has limited mobility, casts, traction, missing limbs, or spinal cord injuries or surgeries. It is flatter and has a lower collection pan to make placement under the buttocks easier and more comfortable. For women, bedpans should always be placed under the anus and urethra to prevent spillage onto the bed. Men will typically use a bedpan for bowel elimination and a urinal for urinary elimination (**Figure 20.13**). If a bedpan is used, it should be placed under the anus, and the penis should be placed so that urine streams directly into the bedpan. Bedpans can be

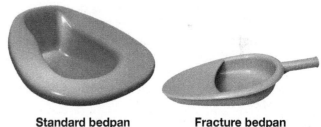

Standard bedpan   **Fracture bedpan**

Courtesy of Dynarex; ArtMari/Shutterstock.com

Figure 20.12 A regular bedpan is placed under the resident for the collection of urine and stool. A fracture bedpan is better for residents who have limited mobility.

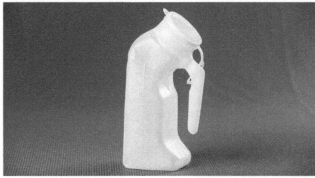

© *Tori Soper Photography*

Figure 20.13 A handheld urinal may be used while in bed. The penis is placed in the neck of the urinal and positioned so the urine goes directly into the bottle portion.

---

uncomfortable, so correctly positioning residents to reduce discomfort is important.

As a nursing assistant, your primary responsibility is to provide support and a safe process and environment for the resident. You should always be aware of any potential problems during urinary elimination and any abnormal conditions, such as a change in urine color, urgency, burning, painful or difficult urination (*dysuria*), and any abnormal amount of urine (small or large). Infection control and prevention procedures should always be followed, as urine and stool may contain pathogens.

Procedure

Assisting a Resident to a Toilet or Bedside Commode

Rationale
Residents who are ambulatory may need assistance to the toilet. A bedside commode is used for residents who have limited mobility.

Preparation
1. Ask the licensed nursing staff if there are doctor's orders for the procedure, if there are any specific instructions listed in the plan of care, and if the resident can be moved into the positions required for this procedure.
2. Wash your hands or use hand sanitizer before entering the room.
3. Knock before entering the room.
4. Introduce yourself using your first or preferred name and title. Explain that you work with the licensed nursing staff and will be providing care.
5. Greet the resident and ask the resident to state his full name, if able. Then check the resident's identification bracelet.
6. Use Mr., Mrs., or Ms. and the resident's last name when conversing.
7. Explain the procedure in simple terms, even if the resident is not able to communicate or is disoriented. Ask permission to perform the procedure.
8. Bring the necessary equipment into the room. Place the following items in an easy-to-reach place:
   - bedside commode with the container in place, if needed
   - toilet seat extension placed on the toilet, if needed
   - urinary hat, if needed
   - disposable gloves
   - bath blanket
   - resident's robe and slippers
   - gait belt, if appropriate
   - washbasin
   - soap
   - towels
   - disinfectant spray or wipes
   - toilet paper, if needed
   - pen and form or digital device for documenting the I&O

The Procedure: Assisting to the Toilet
9. Provide privacy by closing the curtains, using a screen, or closing the door to the room.

   > **Best Practice:** Make sure the bathroom has toilet paper and a clean hand towel or paper towels.

10. Lock the bed wheels. Raise the head of the bed and lower the bed, if needed.
11. Maintain safety during the procedure. If there are side rails, raise and lock the rails on the opposite side of the bed from where you will be working. Lower the rail on the side where you are working.
12. Wash your hands or use hand sanitizer to ensure infection control.
13. Put on disposable gloves.
14. Help the resident dangle at the edge of the bed and put on his robe and slippers, if needed or desired.
15. Help the resident stand and walk to the bathroom. Be safe. If appropriate, put on a gait belt for ambulation.
16. If the resident is on I&O, place a urinary hat in the toilet. Use a toilet seat extension, if needed.
17. Remove and adjust the resident's clothing so he can sit comfortably on the toilet. Ask the resident not to put toilet paper in the toilet. Provide a bag or waste container for the toilet paper. Ask the resident not to flush the toilet.
18. If the resident can be safely left alone, place the toilet paper and call light within his reach. Instruct him to use the call light when he is finished. Remove and discard your gloves. Wash your hands or use hand sanitizer before leaving the room.
19. If the resident cannot be left alone, stay in the bathroom to maintain safety.

20. If you left the room, return to the room when the resident uses the call light or within five minutes to check on the resident. Wash your hands or use hand sanitizer to ensure infection control. Put on disposable gloves.

21. Assist with wiping and with perineal care, as needed.

> **Best Practice:** Remember to wipe from front to back and use a new piece of toilet paper for each wipe.

22. Remove and discard your gloves.

23. Wash your hands or use hand sanitizer to ensure infection control.

24. Put on a new pair of disposable gloves.

25. Help the resident put on new briefs or undergarments, if worn. Change the resident's gown, if needed. Change gloves, if needed.

26. Help the resident wash his hands.

27. Help the resident back to bed and remove his robe and slippers, if worn.

28. Check to be sure the bed wheels are locked, then reposition the resident and make sure the bed is in its lowest position.

29. Follow the plan of care to determine if the side rails should be raised or lowered.

30. Return to the bathroom. Observe the urine for color, odor, and clarity. Check the stool for unusual appearance or odor.

31. If I&O is being monitored, measure the urinary output or the amount of liquid stool. Document the amount of output on the paper or electronic I&O form.

32. If there was a bowel movement, document it in the form provided by the healthcare facility or in the electronic record.

33. If a urinary hat was used, empty its contents into the toilet. Avoid splashes. Carefully rinse the urinary hat and pour the rinse water into the toilet as well. Then flush the toilet.

34. Using disinfectant spray or wipes, clean and then dry the urinary hat according to facility policy. Store the clean urinary hat in the proper location.

The Procedure: Assisting with a Bedside Commode

35. Provide privacy by closing the curtains, using a screen, or closing the door to the room.

36. Place the commode next to the bed (**Figure 20.14**). If the commode has wheels, lock them.

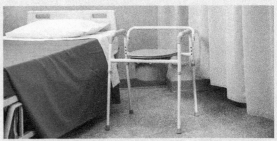

Figure 20.14   © Tori Soper Photography

37. Lock the bed wheels. Raise the head of the bed and lower the bed, if needed.

38. Maintain safety during the procedure. If there are side rails, raise and lock the rails on the opposite side of the bed from where you will be working. Lower the rail on the side where you are working.

39. Wash your hands or use hand sanitizer to ensure infection control.

40. Put on disposable gloves.

41. Remove the resident's undergarments or briefs. Help the resident dangle at the edge of the bed and put on his slippers.

42. Using proper body mechanics, assist the resident onto the bedside commode. Use a gait belt, if needed. Be sure the resident's gown or any clothing is out of the way.

> **Best Practice:** Cover the resident's lap and shoulders with bath blankets to maintain warmth and privacy.

43. If the resident is on I&O, ask him *not* to put toilet paper in the commode. Provide a bag or waste container for the toilet paper.

44. If the resident can be safely left alone, place the toilet paper and call light within his reach. Instruct him to use the call light when he is finished. Follow the plan of care to determine if the side rails should be raised or lowered. Remove and discard your gloves. Wash your hands or use hand sanitizer before leaving the room.

45. If the resident cannot be left alone, stay in the room to maintain safety.

46. If you left the room, return to the room when the resident uses the call light or within five minutes to check on the resident. Wash your hands or use hand sanitizer to ensure infection control. Put on disposable gloves.

47. Assist with wiping and with perineal care, as needed. Cover the commode.

> **Best Practice:** Remember to wipe from front to back and use a new piece of toilet paper for each wipe.

(continued)

Assisting a Resident to a Toilet or Bedside Commode (continued)

48. Remove and discard your gloves.
49. Wash your hands or use hand sanitizer to ensure infection control.
50. Put on a new pair of disposable gloves.

   Best Practice: Use appropriate products to get rid of odors, according to facility policy.

51. Help the resident back to bed. Remove the resident's slippers and help him put on new briefs or undergarments, if worn. Change the resident's gown, if needed. Position the resident safely in bed.
52. Fill the washbasin with enough warm water to cover the wrists. Check the water temperature. It should be 100–105°F. The water should feel comfortably warm to your elbow. You may also ask the resident to feel the water temperature, but always check it yourself first.
53. Place the washbasin and some towels on the bedside stand.
54. Help the resident wash his hands.
55. Remove the washbasin and used towels. Straighten or change the bed linens, as needed.
56. Check to be sure the bed wheels are locked, then reposition the resident and make sure the bed is in its lowest position.
57. Follow the plan of care to determine if the side rails should be raised or lowered.
58. Remove the container from the bedside commode. Take the container to the bathroom. Observe the resident's urine for color, odor, and clarity. Check the stool for unusual appearance or odor.

59. If I&O is being monitored, measure the urinary output or the amount of liquid stool. Document the amount of output on the paper or electronic I&O form.
60. If there was a bowel movement, document it in the form provided by the healthcare facility or in the electronic record.
61. Empty the contents of the container into the toilet. Avoid splashes. Carefully rinse the container and pour the rinse water into the toilet as well.
62. Using disinfectant spray or wipes, clean and then dry the container and the bedside commode according to facility policy.
63. Put the clean bedside commode back in the appropriate storage location.

Follow-Up

64. Remove and discard your gloves.
65. Wash your hands to ensure infection control.
66. Make sure the resident is comfortable and place the call light and personal items within reach.
67. Conduct a safety check before leaving the room. The room should be clean and free from clutter or spills.
68. Wash your hands or use hand sanitizer before leaving the room.

Reporting and Documentation

69. Report any specific observations, complications, or unusual responses to the licensed nursing staff. Document this information, along with the care provided, in the chart or EMR.

Procedure

Assisting with a Standard or Fracture Bedpan

Rationale

Proper bedpan use provides a safe means of urinary and bowel elimination for residents who are not able to ambulate to the bathroom.

Preparation

1. Ask the licensed nursing staff if there are doctor's orders for the procedure, if there are any specific instructions listed in the plan of care, and if the resident can be moved into the positions required for this procedure.
2. Wash your hands or use hand sanitizer before entering the room.
3. Knock before entering the room.
4. Introduce yourself using your first or preferred name and title. Explain that you work with the licensed nursing staff and will be providing care.
5. Greet the resident and ask the resident to state her full name, if able. Then check the resident's identification bracelet.
6. Use Mr., Mrs., or Ms. and the resident's last name when conversing.
7. Explain the procedure in simple terms, even if the resident is not able to communicate or is disoriented. Ask permission to perform the procedure.

8. Bring the necessary equipment into the room. Place the following items in an easy-to-reach place:
   - standard or fracture bedpan
   - toilet paper
   - bedpan cover, disposable pad, or towel
   - disposable protective pad
   - disposable gloves
   - washbasin
   - soap
   - washcloth(s)
   - towel(s)
   - bath blanket
   - waste container or plastic bag
   - laundry hamper
   - disinfectant spray or wipes
   - pen and form or digital device for documenting the I&O

The Procedure

9. Provide privacy by closing the curtains, using a screen, or closing the door to the room.
10. Lock the bed wheels and then raise the bed to hip level.
11. Maintain safety during the procedure. If there are side rails, raise and lock the rails on the opposite side of the bed from where you will be working. Lower the rail on the side where you are working.
12. Wash your hands or use hand sanitizer to ensure infection control.
13. Put on disposable gloves.
14. Fold the top linens back and raise the resident's gown. Keep it out of the way of the bedpan.
15. Ask the resident to bend her knees and put her feet flat on the mattress.
16. Ask the resident to raise her hips. If necessary, slip your hand under the lower part of the resident's back to help.
17. Put a disposable protective pad on the bed under the resident's hips. Then position the bedpan under the buttocks.
    A. **Standard bedpan:** position a standard bedpan like a regular toilet seat. The buttocks should be placed on the wide, rounded shelf, and the open end should point toward the foot of the bed.
    B. **Fracture bedpan:** position a fracture bedpan by having the resident lift her hips. The thin edge of the bedpan should face the head of the bed. Place the bedpan under the resident's buttocks (**Figure 20.15**).

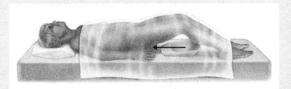

Figure 20.15   © Body Scientific International

18. If the resident is unable to lift her hips, roll her onto her side so she faces away from you. Place the bedpan against the resident's buttocks. Then have the resident roll to her back with the bedpan underneath her (**Figure 20.16**).

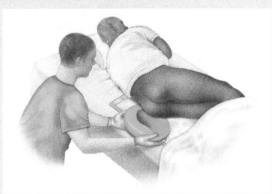

Figure 20.16   © Body Scientific International

Best Practice: For comfort and safety, properly position the bedpan under the resident.

19. Put a bath blanket over the resident. Raise the head of the bed or prop pillows behind the resident's back for comfort.
20. If I&O is being measured, ask the resident not to put toilet paper in the bedpan. Provide a bag or waste container for the toilet paper.
21. If the resident can be safely left alone, place the toilet paper and call light within her reach. Instruct her to use the call light when she is finished. Follow the plan of care to determine if the side rails should be raised or lowered. Remove and discard your gloves. Wash your hands or use hand sanitizer before leaving the room.
22. If the resident cannot be left alone, stay in the room to maintain safety.
23. If you left the room, return to the room when the resident uses the call light or within five minutes to check on the resident. Wash your hands or use hand sanitizer to ensure infection control. Put on disposable gloves.

Best Practice: To maintain skin integrity, do not allow a resident to sit on the bedpan for more than five minutes without checking on him or her.

(continued)

Assisting with a Standard or Fracture Bedpan *(continued)*

24. Assist with wiping and perineal care, as needed.

   Best Practice: Remember to wipe from front to back and use a new piece of toilet paper for each wipe.

25. Remove and discard your gloves.
26. Wash your hands or use hand sanitizer to ensure infection control.
27. Put on a new pair of disposable gloves.
28. Help the resident raise her hips or roll to the side so you can remove the bedpan. Also remove and discard the protective pad at this time. Practice safety and ask for assistance, if necessary.
29. Cover the bedpan immediately with a bedpan cover, disposable pad, or towel. Place the bedpan on top of a paper towel in a secure place.
30. Remove and discard your gloves.
31. Wash your hands or use hand sanitizer to ensure infection control.
32. Put on a new pair of disposable gloves.

   Best Practice: Use appropriate products to get rid of odors, according to facility policy.

33. Fill the washbasin with enough warm water to cover the wrists. Check the water temperature. It should be 100–105°F. The water should feel comfortably warm to your elbow. You may also ask the resident to feel the water temperature, but always check it yourself first.
34. Help the resident wash her hands.
35. Remove the washbasin and used towels. Place the used towels in the laundry hamper.
36. Help the resident put on clean briefs or other undergarments, if worn. Change the resident's gown, if needed.
37. Cover the resident with the top linens and remove the bath blanket, placing it in the laundry hamper. Straighten or change the bed linens, as needed.

38. Check to be sure the bed wheels are locked, then reposition the resident and lower the bed.
39. Follow the plan of care to determine if the side rails should be raised or lowered.
40. Take the bedpan to the bathroom. Check the stool and urine for unusual appearance or odor.
41. If I&O is being monitored, measure the urinary output or the amount of liquid stool. Document the amount of output on the paper or electronic I&O form.
42. If there was a bowel movement, document it in the form provided by the healthcare facility or in the electronic record.
43. Empty the contents of the bedpan into the toilet. Avoid splashes. Carefully rinse the bedpan and pour the rinse water into the toilet as well.
44. Using disinfectant spray or wipes, clean and then dry the bedpan and cover according to facility policy. Store the clean bedpan and cover in the appropriate storage location.
45. Remove and discard your gloves.
46. Wash your hands to ensure infection control.

Follow-Up

47. Make sure the resident is comfortable and place the call light and personal items within reach.
48. Conduct a safety check before leaving the room. The room should be clean and free from clutter or spills.
49. Wash your hands or use hand sanitizer before leaving the room.

Reporting and Documentation

50. Report any specific observations, complications, or unusual responses to the licensed nursing staff. Document this information, along with the care provided, in the chart or EMR.

Procedure

Assisting with a Urinal

Rationale

Proper urinal use provides a safe means of urinary elimination for residents who are not able to ambulate to the bathroom.

Preparation

1. Ask the licensed nursing staff if there are doctor's orders for the procedure, if there are any specific instructions listed in the plan of care, and if the resident can be moved into the positions required for this procedure.
2. Wash your hands or use hand sanitizer before entering the room.
3. Knock before entering the room.

4. Introduce yourself using your first or preferred name and title. Explain that you work with the licensed nursing staff and will be providing care.

5. Greet the resident and ask the resident to state his full name, if able. Then check the resident's identification bracelet.

6. Use Mr., Mrs., or Ms. and the resident's last name when conversing.

7. Explain the procedure in simple terms, even if the resident is not able to communicate or is disoriented. Ask permission to perform the procedure.

8. Bring the necessary equipment into the room. Place the following items in an easy-to-reach place:
   - handheld urinal and cover
   - disposable gloves
   - disposable protective pad, if needed
   - washbasin
   - soap
   - towel
   - disinfectant spray or wipes
   - pen and form or digital device for documenting the I&O

The Procedure

9. Provide privacy by closing the curtains, using a screen, or closing the door to the room.

10. Check to be sure the bed wheels are locked. Maintain safety during the procedure. If there are side rails, raise and lock the rails on the opposite side of the bed from where you will be working. Lower the rail on the side where you are working.

11. Wash your hands or use hand sanitizer to ensure infection control.

12. Put on disposable gloves.

13. Give the urinal to the resident. If assistance is needed, position the urinal so that the resident's penis is well inside the opening. Make sure the urinal does not spill. You may need to put a disposable protective pad under the resident.

14. If the resident can be safely left alone, place the call light within his reach. Instruct him to use the call light when he is finished. Ask the resident not to place the urinal on the overbed table or bedside stand when he is finished. This would contaminate those surfaces. Follow the plan of care to determine if the side rails should be raised or lowered. Remove and discard your gloves. Wash your hands or use hand sanitizer before leaving the room.

15. If the resident cannot be left alone, stay in the room to maintain safety.

> **Best Practice:** If the resident is in bed, do not leave the urinal in place longer than is needed. The hard plastic of the urinal could damage the soft flesh of the penis.

16. If you left the room, return to the room when the resident uses the call light. Wash your hands or use hand sanitizer to ensure infection control. Put on disposable gloves.

17. Remove the urinal and cover it. Place the urinal on top of a paper towel in a secure place.

18. Assist with any needed cleansing and with perineal care, as needed.

19. Remove and discard your gloves.

20. Wash your hands or use hand sanitizer to ensure infection control.

21. Put on a new pair of disposable gloves.

22. Fill the washbasin with enough warm water to cover the wrists. Check the water temperature. It should be 100–105°F. The water should feel comfortably warm to your elbow. You may also ask the resident to feel the water temperature, but always check it yourself first.

23. Help the resident wash his hands.

24. Remove the washbasin and used towels.

25. Help the resident put on clean briefs or other undergarments, if worn. Change the resident's gown, if needed.

26. Straighten or change the bed linens, as needed.

27. Check to be sure the bed wheels are locked and reposition the resident.

28. Follow the plan of care to determine if the side rails should be raised or lowered.

29. Take the urinal to the bathroom. Observe the urine for color, odor, and clarity.

30. If the resident is on I&O, measure the urinary output or the amount of liquid stool, if applicable. Document the amount of output on the paper or electronic I&O form.

31. Empty the contents of the urinal into the toilet. Avoid splashes. Carefully rinse the urinal and pour the rinse water into the toilet as well.

32. Using disinfectant spray or wipes, clean and then dry the urinal according to facility policy. Store the clean urinal and cover in the appropriate storage location.

Follow-Up

33. Remove and discard your gloves.

34. Wash your hands to ensure infection control.

35. Make sure the resident is comfortable and place the call light and personal items within reach.

36. Conduct a safety check before leaving the room. The room should be clean and free from clutter or spills.

37. Wash your hands or use hand sanitizer before leaving the room.

Reporting and Documentation

38. Report any specific observations, complications, or unusual responses to the licensed nursing staff. Document this information, along with the care provided, in the chart or EMR.

How Do Nursing Assistants Help Residents with Urinary Catheters?

Some residents need a *urinary catheter* to eliminate urine from the body. An *indwelling urinary catheter* (catheter left inside the bladder) is inserted into the urethra and passes into the urinary bladder. It is held in place by a balloon inflated after insertion. Some residents may require a *suprapubic catheter*, which is surgically inserted into the bladder through the abdominal wall just above the pubic area. This type of catheter is used when a resident has a urethral blockage or injury, or prostate cancer.

Gravity allows urine in the urinary bladder to flow into the catheter tubing and empty into a drainage bag outside the body. The urinary drainage bag should always be positioned below the bladder. This is important even when the resident is ambulating. When a resident is in bed, the urinary drainage bag can be attached to the lower bedframe of a resident's bed. The bag may also be attached to the side of a wheelchair or chair. The urinary drainage bag should not be attached to a movable part of the bed, should be clear of any wheels, and should never touch or rest on the floor.

Catheter Care

Nursing assistants are responsible for providing proper catheter care every eight hours, or as often as required by facility policy. Proper catheter care can help prevent *catheter-associated urinary tract infections*

(CAUTIs). Catheter care involves regularly cleansing the perineum and the area around the catheter, checking the catheter and drainage bag for leaks or kinks that can prevent the flow of urine, making sure the resident is not lying on the catheter, and observing any other problems related to the catheter.

Holistic nursing assistants should be aware of how catheter use affects residents physically and emotionally. Residents may worry about their body image, since an artificial device has been inserted to help them eliminate. They may also be embarrassed by having their urine visible in a bag. Many residents may also be experiencing pain. Offer residents your support and understanding. If residents are in pain, alert the licensed nursing staff.

Nursing assistants in many facilities use commercially prepared catheter care kits. A catheter care kit includes disposable gloves, a disposable protective pad, and applicators with antiseptic solution. In facilities that do not provide catheter care kits, nursing assistants use clean washcloths and mild soap in place of applicators and antiseptic. The same procedure is used whether or not a kit is available.

Procedure

Providing Catheter Care

Rationale
Proper catheter care provides consistent hygiene, maintains skin integrity, and helps prevent CAUTIs.

Preparation
1. Ask the licensed nursing staff if there are doctor's orders for the procedure, if there are any specific instructions listed in the plan of care, and if the resident can be moved into the positions required for this procedure.
2. Wash your hands or use hand sanitizer before entering the room.
3. Knock before entering the room.
4. Introduce yourself using your first or preferred name and title. Explain that you work with the licensed nursing staff and will be providing care.
5. Greet the resident and ask the resident to state his or her full name, if able. Then check the resident's identification bracelet.
6. Use Mr., Mrs., or Ms. and the resident's last name when conversing.
7. Explain the procedure in simple terms, even if the resident is not able to communicate or is disoriented. Ask permission to perform the procedure.

8. Bring the necessary equipment into the room. Place the following items in an easy-to-reach place:
   - catheter care kit, if available
   - disposable gloves
   - bath blanket
   - washcloths
   - soap
   - towels
   - washbasin, if used
   - disposable protective pad
   - plastic bag
   - laundry hamper

   | **Best Practice:** Always be sensitive to the resident's privacy, culture, and specific needs when performing catheter care.

The Procedure: Male Catheter Care

9. Provide privacy by closing the curtains, using a screen, or closing the door to the room.
10. Lock the bed wheels and then raise the bed to hip level.
11. Maintain safety during the procedure. If there are side rails, raise and lock the rails on the opposite side of the bed from where you will be working. Lower the rail on the side where you are working.
12. Wash your hands or use hand sanitizer to ensure infection control.
13. Put on disposable gloves.
14. Position the resident on his back, if possible.
15. Cover the resident with the bath blanket. Without exposing the resident, fanfold the top linens to the foot of the bed.

   | **Best Practice:** Catheter care is performed after providing perineal care. Remove and discard your gloves once perineal care is complete. Wash your hands to ensure infection control and put on a new pair of gloves before beginning catheter care.

16. Check the catheter insertion area for crusting, lesions, discharge, or anything abnormal. Notify the licensed nursing staff if you observe any of these conditions.
17. Open the catheter kit. Remove the disposable protective pad from the kit. If there is no kit, use the protective pad you brought into the room. Place the protective pad under the resident's buttocks.

18. Remove the applicators from the kit. The applicators are covered with an antiseptic solution. If there is no kit, fill the washbasin with warm water (between 100–105°F). The water should feel comfortably warm to your elbow. You may also ask the resident to feel the water temperature, but always check it yourself first. Instead of an applicator, you will use a washcloth and soap.
19. Using a circular motion, apply the antiseptic solution to the entire catheter insertion area. If there is no kit, use a clean part of the washcloth for each cleansing stroke.
20. If the male resident has not been circumcised, gently pull the foreskin of the penis back. Apply antiseptic solution to the area where the catheter is inserted into the penis or clean it using the washcloth and soap.

   | **Best Practice:** Work from the cleanest area of the penis to the dirtiest.

21. Hold the catheter tubing near the opening of the penis. This will help prevent pulling or tugging as you clean the catheter.
22. Using a circular motion, clean the catheter. Start near the penis and move down the catheter about four inches (**Figure 20.17**). If using a washcloth, use a clean part of the washcloth.

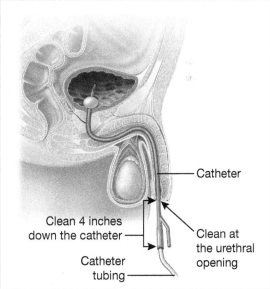

Catheter

Clean 4 inches down the catheter

Clean at the urethral opening

Catheter tubing

Figure 20.17   © Body Scientific International

23. Moving from front to back, pat the perineal area dry.
24. Secure the catheter and tubing to the resident's upper thigh as directed by the licensed nursing staff. Leave some slack in the catheter tubing. Coil the remaining tubing and be sure it is not under the resident, twisted, or bent.

(continued)

Providing Catheter Care *(continued)*

25. Secure the drainage bag to the bottom of the bedframe using the bag ties (**Figure 20.18**). The drainage bag should always be secured below the resident and should never be secured to a movable part of the bed or near the wheels.

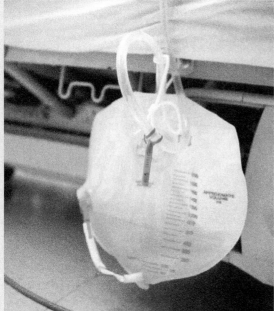

Figure 20.18   *P_Wei/Signature via Getty Images*

26. Remove the disposable protective pad. Cover the resident with the top linens. Remove the bath blanket.
27. Change the resident's gown or other clothing, as appropriate.
28. Check to be sure the bed wheels are locked, then reposition the resident and lower the bed.

    > **Best Practice:** If any part of the catheter comes apart, clean the catheter and tubing ends with an antiseptic pad and reconnect them. Alert the licensed nursing staff.

29. Follow the plan of care to determine if the side rails should be raised or lowered.
30. Remove, clean, and store equipment in the proper location. Remove soiled linens and discard disposable equipment.

The Procedure: Female Catheter Care

31. Provide privacy by closing the curtains, using a screen, or closing the door to the room.
32. Lock the bed wheels and then raise the bed to hip level.

33. Maintain safety during the procedure. If there are side rails, raise and lock the rails on the opposite side of the bed from where you will be working. Lower the rail on the side where you are working.
34. Wash your hands or use hand sanitizer to ensure infection control.
35. Put on disposable gloves.
36. Position the resident on her back, if possible.
37. Cover the resident with the bath blanket. Without exposing the resident, fanfold the top linens to the foot of the bed.

    > **Best Practice:** Catheter care is often performed after providing perineal care. Remove and discard your gloves once perineal care is complete. Wash your hands to ensure infection control and put on a new pair of gloves before beginning catheter care.

38. Check the catheter insertion area for crusting, lesions, discharge, or anything abnormal. Notify the licensed nursing staff if you observe any of these conditions.
39. Open the catheter kit. Remove the disposable protective pad from the kit. If there is no kit, use the protective pad you brought into the room. Place the protective pad under the resident's buttocks.
40. Remove the applicators from the kit. The applicators are covered with an antiseptic solution. If there is no kit, fill the washbasin with warm water (between 100–105°F). The water should feel comfortably warm to your elbow. You may also ask the resident to feel the water temperature, but always check it yourself first. Instead of an applicator, you will use a washcloth and soap.
41. Separate the labia with one gloved hand.
42. Use your other hand to pick up an applicator or washcloth. Cleanse the perineal area from front to back to prevent fecal matter or bacteria from moving upward into the vaginal canal or urethra.
43. Begin at the center of the perineal area and then cleanse each side. After each stroke, discard the used applicator in a plastic bag. If using a washcloth, use a clean part of the washcloth for each stroke.
44. Hold the catheter tubing near the opening of the urethra. This will help prevent pulling or tugging as you clean the catheter.
45. Clean the catheter in a circular motion from the meatus down the catheter about four inches (**Figure 20.19**). Do this two or three times. If using a washcloth, use different parts of the washcloth each time.

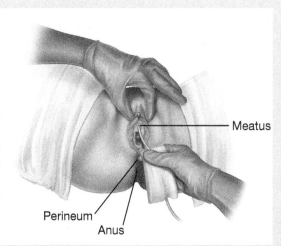

Figure 20.19   © Body Scientific International

Labels: Meatus, Perineum, Anus

46. Moving from front to back, pat the perineal area dry.
47. Secure the catheter and tubing to the resident's upper thigh as directed by the licensed nursing staff. Leave some slack in the catheter tubing. Coil the remaining tubing and be sure it is not under the resident, twisted, or bent.
48. Secure the drainage bag to the bottom of the bedframe using the bag ties. The drainage bag should always be secured below the resident and should never be secured to a movable part of the bed.
49. Remove the disposable protective pad. Cover the resident with the top linens. Remove the bath blanket.

50. Change the resident's gown or other clothing, as appropriate.
51. Check to be sure the bed wheels are locked, then reposition the resident and lower the bed.

> **Best Practice:** If any part of the catheter comes open or apart, clean the catheter and tubing ends with an antiseptic pad and reconnect them. Alert the licensed nursing staff.

52. Follow the plan of care to determine if the side rails should be raised or lowered.
53. Remove, clean, and store equipment in the proper location. Remove soiled linens and discard disposable equipment.

Follow-Up
54. Remove and discard your gloves.
55. Wash your hands to ensure infection control.
56. Make sure the resident is comfortable and place the call light and personal items within reach.
57. Conduct a safety check before leaving the room. The room should be clean and free from clutter or spills.
58. Wash your hands or use hand sanitizer before leaving the room.

Reporting and Documentation
59. Report any specific observations, complications, or unusual responses to the licensed nursing staff. Document this information, along with the care provided, in the chart or EMR.

Procedure

Changing a Urinary Drainage Bag

Rationale
Changing a resident's urinary drainage bag promotes cleanliness, prevents possible blockage, and helps maintain infection control.

Preparation
1. Ask the licensed nursing staff if there are doctor's orders for the procedure, if there are any specific instructions listed in the plan of care, and if the resident can be moved into the positions required for this procedure.
2. Wash your hands or use hand sanitizer before entering the room.
3. Knock before entering the room.
4. Introduce yourself using your first or preferred name and title. Explain that you work with the licensed nursing staff and will be providing care.
5. Greet the resident and ask the resident to state his full name, if able. Then check the resident's identification bracelet.
6. Use Mr., Mrs., or Ms. and the resident's last name when conversing.
7. Explain the procedure in simple terms, even if the resident is not able to communicate or is disoriented. Ask permission to perform the procedure.
8. Bring the necessary equipment into the room. Place a paper towel, towel, or disposable protective pad on the overbed table as an infection-control barrier before placing the following items:
   - new drainage bag and tubing
   - sterile package containing cap and plug
   - catheter clamp
   - disposable gloves
   - antiseptic wipes

(continued)

Changing a Urinary Drainage Bag *(continued)*

- 2 disposable protective pads
- paper towels
- graduate
- bedpan
- bath blanket
- pen and form or digital device for documenting the I&O

The Procedure

9. Provide privacy by closing the curtains, using a screen, or closing the door to the room.
10. Lock the bed wheels and then raise the bed to hip level.
11. Maintain safety during the procedure. If there are side rails, raise and lock the rails on the opposite side of the bed from where you will be working. Lower the rail on the side where you are working.
12. Wash your hands or use hand sanitizer to ensure infection control.
13. Put on disposable gloves.
14. Position the resident on his back, if possible. Place the disposable protective pad under the resident's buttocks.
15. Cover the resident with the bath blanket. Without exposing the resident, fanfold the top linens to the foot of the bed.
16. Fold the bath blanket to form a triangle on the side of the drainage bag. Turn the triangle up over the resident, exposing the catheter and drainage bag tubing.
17. Clamp the catheter to prevent urine from draining into the drainage tubing.
18. Let the urine below the clamp drain into the drainage bag.
19. Place a protective pad under the resident's leg at the site where the catheter and drainage bag tubing connect.
20. Open the antiseptic wipes and place them on the paper towels on the overbed table.
21. Open the package with the sterile cap and catheter plug. Do not let anything touch the sterile cap or catheter plug.
22. Attach the new drainage bag to the bedframe. Lay the end of the new drainage bag tubing on top of the protective pad on the bed.
23. Disconnect the catheter from the old drainage bag tubing. Do not allow anything to touch the end of the catheter.
24. Hold the sterile catheter plug, but do *not* touch the end that goes inside the catheter (**Figure 20.20A**).
25. Insert the sterile catheter plug into the end of the catheter. If the end of the catheter touches anything, wipe it with an antiseptic wipe before inserting the plug.

26. Place the sterile cap on the end of the old drainage bag tubing. Do *not* touch the end of the tubing.
27. Remove the cap from the end of the new drainage bag tubing.
28. Remove the sterile plug from the catheter.
29. Insert the end of the new drainage bag tubing into the catheter.
30. Remove the clamp from the catheter (**Figure 20.20B**).

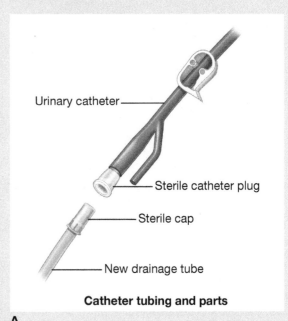

Urinary catheter

Sterile catheter plug

Sterile cap

New drainage tube

Catheter tubing and parts

A

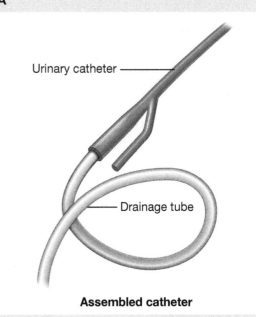

Urinary catheter

Drainage tube

Assembled catheter

B

© *Body Scientific International*

Figure 20.20

31. Coil and secure the remaining tubing. Be sure it is not twisted or bent.

32. Remove the old drainage bag from the bedframe and place it in the bedpan.
33. Remove and discard the protective pad.
34. Cover the resident with the top linens and remove the bath blanket.
35. Check to be sure the bed wheels are locked, then reposition the resident and lower the bed.
36. Follow the plan of care to determine if the side rails should be raised or lowered.
37. Take the old drainage bag and tubing to the bathroom.
38. Open the clamp at the bottom of the old drainage bag and allow the urine to drain into the graduate. After the bag is empty, close the clamp.
39. Measure the amount of urine in the graduate. Make note of this amount or document it on the I&O form.
40. Discard the old drainage bag and tubing according to facility policy.
41. Remove, clean, and store equipment in the proper location. Remove soiled linens and discard disposable equipment.

Follow-Up

42. Remove and discard your gloves.
43. Wash your hands to ensure infection control.
44. Make sure the resident is comfortable and place the call light and personal items within reach.
45. Conduct a safety check before leaving the room. The room should be clean and free from clutter or spills.
46. Wash your hands or use hand sanitizer before leaving the room.

Reporting and Documentation

47. Report any specific observations, complications, or unusual responses to the licensed nursing staff. Document this information, along with the care provided, in the chart or EMR.

Leg Bags

A *leg bag* may be used as an alternative to the urinary drainage bag when the resident is ambulatory (**Figure 20.21**). A leg bag is smaller than a drainage bag. It is attached with Velcro™ or elastic straps to the upper thigh, but is low enough on the thigh that gravity will help urine flow into the leg bag. Routinely alternating the thigh that holds the leg bag will help maintain skin integrity. Leg bags come in different sizes and can be hidden by clothing.

Attaching a Leg Bag

The procedure for attaching a leg bag is the same as the procedure for changing a urinary drainage bag. Once you have connected the new leg bag to the catheter, fasten the straps of the leg bag comfortably around the resident's thigh. Make sure the straps are not too tight. Secure the catheter to the thigh using a facility-approved product or as directed by the licensed nursing staff, and be careful not to pull or tug the catheter. Check the catheter and leg bag regularly to be sure the tubing is not twisted, bent, or pulled too tight.

Emptying a Leg Bag

Leg bags should be emptied when they are half-full or at least twice a day. Before emptying a leg bag, wash your hands and put on disposable gloves. The bag may be emptied into the toilet or another specified container, such as a graduate if I&O is being measured. Undo the straps or Velcro™ attaching the leg bag and be sure the catheter is not being pulled. Open the clamp on the leg bag to allow urine to drain. Never touch the tip of the bag while the urine is being emptied. When the bag is empty, close the clamp. Remove and discard your gloves and wash your hands.

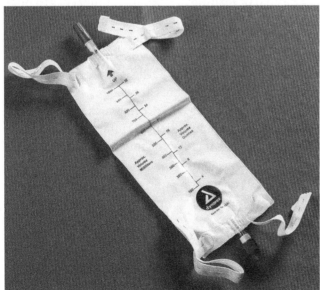

© *Tori Soper Photography*

Figure 20.21 Leg bags allow ambulatory residents more freedom and independence.

Replacing a Leg Bag with a Urinary Drainage Bag

When a resident will be staying in bed for a long period of time (for example, at night), the leg bag should be removed and replaced with the larger urinary drainage bag. To remove a leg bag and attach a new urinary drainage bag, bring a drainage bag, tubing, and sterile package containing a cap and plug into the room and follow these guidelines:

1. Practice proper hand hygiene. Wash your hands and wear disposable gloves during the procedure, as appropriate. Be sure there is bedpan available in which to place the leg bag.
2. Place a disposable protective pad on the bed. Attach a urinary drainage bag to the bedframe.
3. Safely help the resident lie on the bed. Keep the resident comfortable and covered, as appropriate.
4. Expose the catheter and leg bag. Clamp the catheter to prevent urine from draining into the tubing and let the urine drain from below the clamp into the leg bag.
5. Disconnect the catheter from the leg bag. If you touch the end of the catheter, use antiseptic wipes to clean it.
6. Hold the sterile catheter plug and do *not* touch the end that goes inside the catheter. Insert the sterile catheter plug into the end of the catheter. Place the sterile cap on the end of the old leg bag tubing and place the leg bag in a bedpan.
7. Remove the cap from the end of the new drainage bag tubing. Then remove the sterile plug from the catheter and insert the end of the drainage tubing into the catheter.
8. Remove the clamp from the catheter and coil the drainage tubing on the bed. Secure the tubing to the bottom bed linens.
9. Take the bedpan with the leg bag to the bathroom. Open the bottom of the leg bag and let the urine drain into the toilet or into a graduate if urine needs to be measured.
10. Clean and dry or discard equipment, according to facility policy.

How Should Nursing Assistants Help Residents with Incontinence?

Urinary incontinence is the loss of bladder control. Women are more likely than men to experience incontinence due to the stressors of pregnancy and childbirth and the structure of the female urinary tract. People over age 50 are also more likely to be incontinent due to age-related weakening of the bladder muscles. Incontinence may also be related to side effects from certain medications, chronic constipation and UTIs, kidney or bladder stones, an enlarged prostate, diabetes, stroke, Parkinson's disease, late-stage dementia, physical disabilities, or cancer.

Symptoms of incontinence range from mild to severe and may be temporary or permanent. There are three types of urinary incontinence:

- **Stress incontinence**: occurs when certain types of physical activity, such as coughing, sneezing, or laughing, stress a weak sphincter muscle that holds urine, causing urine to leak.
- **Urge incontinence**: also called an *overactive bladder (OAB)*, occurs when the bladder muscle contracts with enough force to weaken the urethral sphincter muscle's ability to contract, causing involuntary loss of urine.
- **Overflow incontinence**: occurs when the bladder is not completely emptied, causing the remaining urine to leak at a later time. This may be due to urinary blockages, weak sphincter muscles, or certain conditions or disorders. This is sometimes called *dribbling*.

People can reduce their risk of urinary incontinence by maintaining a healthy weight, eliminating spicy or acidic foods, taking part in regular physical activity, limiting caffeine and alcohol consumption, and avoiding smoking.

The goal of treating urinary incontinence is to help residents increase bladder control. This may include pelvic-floor muscle training, such as daily Kegel exercises; bladder retraining; adjusting diet and fluid intake; scheduling regular bathroom breaks; and using incontinence products as needed.

Caring for residents who are incontinent requires empathy, support, and patience. Guidelines for caring for these residents include the following:

- Reassure residents to help reduce feelings of embarrassment and guilt.
- Show respect and compassion for the resident's loss of dignity.
- Plan your care so you are not rushed for time, and ask for help when needed.
- To prevent embarrassment, do not use the term *diaper* when referring to incontinence briefs (**Figure 20.22**). Some residents may resist and feel angry about using incontinence briefs or other incontinence products.

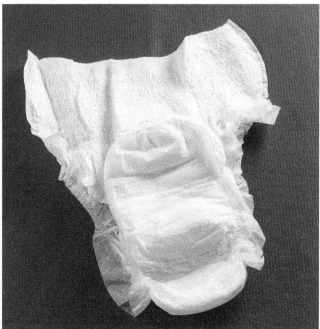

© Tori Soper Photography

Figure 20.22 Incontinence briefs can be used for residents with urinary incontinence to prevent them from soiling their clothes or bed linens.

- Learn to apply and remove incontinence briefs correctly to avoid skin breakdown due to rubbing. Ask the licensed nursing staff if you need clarification or further instruction.
- Perform careful perineal care after every episode of incontinence. Clean the skin with mild soap and water. Rinse the skin well and gently pat it dry. If residents have very dry skin, use soap-free skin cleansers that do not cause dryness or irritation.
- Maintain skin integrity by keeping the skin clean and dry. Frequently check for wetness or soiling and remove briefs whenever they are soiled. Check the skin daily for decubitus ulcers. Also look for blisters, sores, or lesions. Report any skin changes or issues to the licensed nursing staff.
- Change bed linens and clothing immediately after an incontinence episode.
- Use pillows or foam padding on any bony projections to prevent skin irritation.
- Use a skin sealant or moisture barrier, if ordered. These products can provide a protective barrier to the skin. Reapply the cream or ointment after you clean and dry the skin according to the plan of care. Do *not* use baby powder.

- If instructed by the licensed nursing staff, reduce the resident's intake of fluids in the late afternoon and evening to help prevent incontinence overnight. Residents should never be without fluids completely, unless they are NPO.

How Can Nursing Assistants Help with Bowel Elimination Needs?

Stool, or *feces*, is a waste product produced from digestion and metabolism. It is composed primarily of undigested food, and also contains bacteria, dead cells, and mucus.

Most people have their own definition of a regular bowel movement. Typical stool is brown in color because of the presence of *bilirubin* (found in bile). The Bristol Stool Chart shows some standard sizes, shapes, and consistencies (texture) of stool (**Figure 20.23**). Helpful bacteria found in the intestines give stool its normal odor. If stool has a fouler odor, this may be due to a change in diet, some vitamins, medications, food allergies, an infection, or a disease that causes malabsorption.

The number of bowel movements each day may vary. On average, most people **defecate** (have a bowel movement) once or twice a day.

Any change in stool or bowel habits (color, size, shape, smell, or frequency of bowel movements) is important and should be reported to the licensed nursing staff. A change in stool color can be the sign of a dietary change, the use of medications, or possible diseases or conditions:

- **Red stool**: can be caused by naturally or artificially colored foods or blood.
- **Orange stool**: can be caused by red or orange foods and some medications.
- **Green stool**: can be caused by green foods or iron supplements.
- **Black stool**: can be caused by vitamins that contain iron or other medications. Stool that is black, sticky (*tarry*), and foul smelling may mean there is blood in the stool, which is a serious condition.
- **Gray stool**: may also be clay colored or pale. It can be the result of some diagnostic tests, but may also be the sign of a blockage in the flow of bile or liver disease.

Bristol Stool Chart

Type	Appearance	Description
1	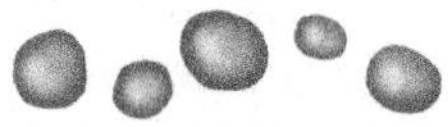	Separate, hard lumps like pellets; hard to pass
2	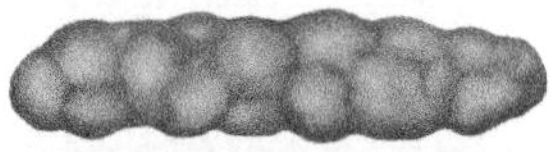	Sausage-shaped, but lumpy
3	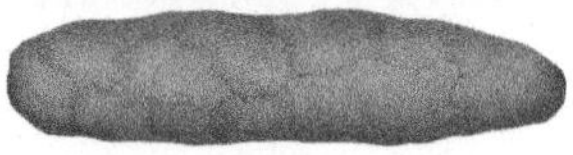	Like a sausage, but with cracks on the surface
4	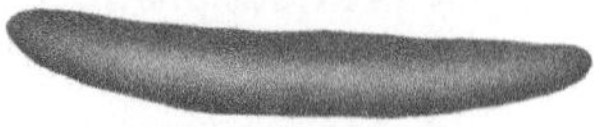	Like a sausage or snake, smooth and soft
5	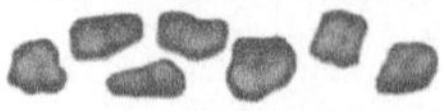	Soft blobs with clear-cut edges; easy to pass
6	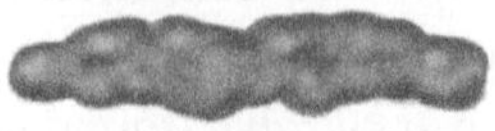	Fluffy pieces with ragged edges; a mushy stool
7	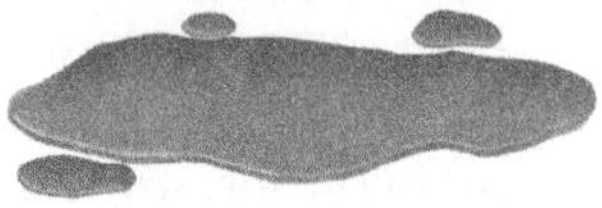	Watery with no solid pieces; entirely liquid

© Body Scientific International

Figure 20.23 The Bristol Stool Chart categorizes the consistency of stool. Stool consistency can be helpful in identifying gastrointestinal diseases or disorders. For example, watery stool over a long period may be a sign of a GI disease or disorder, or can be stress-related.

Documenting Bowel Movements

Careful observation and accuracy are important when documenting bowel movements. Nursing assistants measuring I&O must always wash their hands to ensure infection control and wear disposable gloves. If necessary, use a disposable stick or tongue blade to examine the stool more closely. The following observations, signs, and symptoms should be reported to the licensed nursing staff immediately:

- excessive *flatus* or *gas*
- diarrhea or constipation
- undigested food
- blood or mucus in the stool
- unusual color, particularly black or dark green
- foul-smelling stool

Caring for Residents with Bowel Elimination Problems

Your ability to provide comfort and understanding as you give care will be critical to the way residents respond. As you give care, maintain skin integrity, provide proper hygiene, and make sure the environment is odor-free. This approach will help promote healing and prevent infection.

CULTURE CUES

Toileting Practices

Bathroom practices, habits, and customs may vary among different cultures. For example, in many European countries (such as France and Germany), people must pay a fee to use a public bathroom. Some European homes have a *bidet*, which is used to wash after using the toilet. In Japan, high-tech toilets may feature bidet-like jet streams for cleaning, armrests, seat warmers, and deodorizers. Americans also have unique toileting practices. According to a recent survey, many Americans find the bathroom relaxing and use time on the toilet to read a book or magazine, talk on the phone, look at e-mails, or use their laptops.

Apply It

1. What are your toileting practices and habits? Do you also practice these in someone else's home or in a public restroom? If you do not, how does that make you feel? What do you do instead?
2. Are you aware of other people's toileting practices? How do they differ from your own?
3. How would knowing a resident's toileting practices help you give better care?

Residents with bowel elimination problems may need help easing pain caused by excessive flatus or from the need to evacuate their bowels if the resident has an **impaction** (blockage of hard stool in the rectum). Residents may be very anxious and fearful, so be patient and do not rush. Be positive and establish a calm, helpful environment.

Residents who experience significant discomfort due to elimination problems require special care. This may include inserting a rectal tube or suppository, or giving an enema. A rectal tube may be inserted to relieve flatus. Rectal suppositories may be used if the resident is having trouble eliminating or experiencing pain. An enema may be used to prepare residents for surgical or diagnostic procedures. Be sure to check whether giving this care is within your scope of practice.

Which Conditions Affect the Bowel?

Special attention and care may be required if residents experience acute or chronic diarrhea, constipation, or fecal incontinence. *Fecal* or *bowel incontinence* may be the result of diarrhea, constipation, or sometimes muscle or nerve damage. It is the accidental leaking or passing of solid or liquid stool or mucus, usually due to the inability to hold in a bowel movement. Some residents may not be aware if they have passed stool in their underwear. Age is a risk factor for fecal incontinence, as are diseases or conditions such as dementia. Fecal incontinence can be very embarrassing for residents, so special care and attention are needed. Excellent hygiene and the maintenance of skin integrity are particularly important.

Diarrhea

Diarrhea is frequent liquid stools, sometimes up to 20 or more per day. Diarrhea occurs when food and waste move so rapidly through the gastrointestinal system that the large intestine does not absorb fluids. Diarrhea may be caused by infection, parasites, contaminated food, some diseases and medications, and bowel and gastrointestinal **motility** (movement) disorders.

Symptoms of diarrhea may include fever of 102°F or higher, nausea, vomiting, and abdominal pain. Blood or pus may be present in the stool, depending on the cause of diarrhea. Complications of diarrhea may include mild to severe dehydration, lack of adequate nutrition, and extreme weight loss.

Residents with diarrhea should be observed for signs of dehydration and offered plenty of fluids. A doctor may order an IV, or medications to slow down or stop the diarrhea. Follow infection prevention and control practices carefully to prevent the spread of pathogens that may be in diarrheal stools.

Constipation

Constipation is difficult and infrequent bowel movements. Infrequent bowel movements can result in major or minor blockages in the intestines. Constipation can be short term or chronic. Risk factors for constipation include advancing age; a low-fiber diet; dehydration; limited physical activity; certain medications, and pain medications; or diseases such as multiple sclerosis, Parkinson's disease, or an eating disorder.

Symptoms of constipation may include a bloated feeling, swollen abdomen, feeling that there is a blockage in the rectum, or inability to empty the bowel. Straining during elimination, having lumpy or hard stool, and bleeding during a bowel movement may also occur. Constipation may also cause internal or external hemorrhoids (**Figure 20.24**), **hernia** (protrusion of an organ through the wall of the body cavity or structure that contains it), *anal fissure* (a break or tear in the lining of the anal canal), and *colitis* (inflammation of the large intestine). Bowel impaction, obstruction, and rectal prolapse (in which a small amount of the rectum protrudes from the anus) are other serious complications.

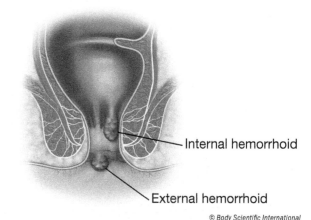

Internal hemorrhoid

External hemorrhoid

© Body Scientific International

Figure 20.24 Hemorrhoids are swollen veins in the tissue of the anus. Internal hemorrhoids form inside the anal canal. External hemorrhoids form around the opening of the anus.

In order to treat or avoid constipation, encourage residents to increase fiber intake, exercise, and take time on the toilet without being distracted or feeling rushed. A doctor may order laxatives, fiber supplements, stimulants, lubricants, stool softeners, *suppositories* (small, meltable cones that are inserted into a body passage), and enemas to help a resident with constipation.

Suppositories

A rectal suppository is used to stimulate bowel elimination (**Figure 20.25**). A suppository may also be used to administer medications that relieve pain and promote healing. Inserting a suppository may or may not be part of your scope of practice. If performing the procedure, always ask the licensed nursing staff if there are doctor's orders for the procedure, any special instructions, and if the resident can be moved into the positions required for this procedure.

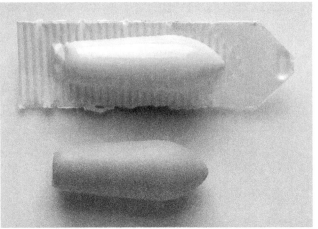

Lukasz Siekierski/Shutterstock.com

Figure 20.25 A suppository comes wrapped and is shaped to allow for easy insertion into the rectum. Once inserted in the rectum, a suppository dissolves, or melts.

Follow these guidelines to insert a rectal suppository:

1. After hand hygiene and putting on a pair of disposable gloves, cover the resident with a bath blanket, fanfold the linens to the foot of the bed, and place a disposable protective pad under the resident's buttocks.
2. Assist the resident into a Sims' position, lying on the left side with the right knee toward the chest. Expose the resident's buttocks by raising the lower corner of the bath blanket.
3. Unwrap the suppository. Then, use one hand to lift the upper buttock to expose the anus. Apply a small amount of lubricating gel to both the suppository and anus.
4. Gently insert the suppository into the rectum, about two inches beyond the anal sphincter (**Figure 20.26**). Wipe any excess lubricant from the anal area.
5. Encourage the resident to relax by taking slow, deep breaths until the resident feels the need to have a bowel movement (may take 5 to 20 minutes). Explain to the resident that his or her body heat will cause the suppository to melt and that this may feel unusual, but is expected.
6. Assist the resident to the bathroom or a bedside commode, or position the resident on the bedpan when the resident feels the need to have a bowel movement. Provide privacy and, when finished, assist the resident back into bed and provide personal hygiene, as needed.
7. Check the stool for any usual appearance. If you see anything abnormal, let the licensed nursing staff know immediately. Document the care provided in the resident's chart or EMR.

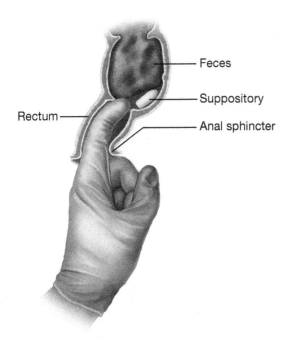

Figure 20.26 Insert the suppository gently and carefully.

© Body Scientific International

Enemas

Sometimes a suppository is not enough to stimulate a bowel movement. In this case, an **enema** may be needed. Different types of enemas include:

- *cleansing enemas*, which introduce tap water, water with soapsuds, or saline into the rectum and colon via the anus
- *retention enemas*, which use oil to soften and lubricate the stool for easy elimination
- commercial or small-volume disposable enemas

When giving an enema, nursing assistants usually use a disposable enema kit. The disposable enema kit contains an enema bag with tubing, clamp, and disposable protective pad (**Figure 20.27**).

Enemas can be uncomfortable for anyone, but especially for older adults. Residents may already be uncomfortable from constipation, and the positioning needed to effectively administer the enema can increase discomfort. Residents may also experience cramping when the enema solution flows into the rectum and colon. Working slowly and patiently and providing support by checking with the resident during the procedure can make the experience more comfortable and tolerable.

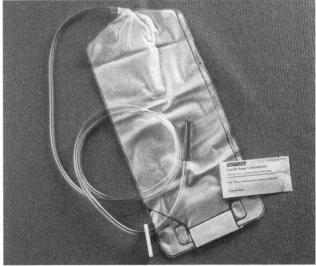

© Tori Soper Photography

Figure 20.27 The enema bag, tubing, lubricant, and clamp shown here are part of a disposable enema kit.

Procedure

Giving an Enema

Rationale

An enema is used to aid bowel elimination or to prepare the resident for certain procedures.

Preparation

1. Ask the licensed nursing staff if there are doctor's orders for the procedure, if there are any specific instructions listed in the plan of care, and if the resident can be moved into the positions required for this procedure.
2. Wash your hands or use hand sanitizer before entering the room.
3. Knock before entering the room.
4. Introduce yourself using your first or preferred name and title. Explain that you work with the licensed nursing staff and will be providing care.
5. Greet the resident and ask the resident to state her full name, if able. Then check the resident's identification bracelet.
6. Use Mr., Mrs., or Ms. and the resident's last name when conversing.
7. Explain the procedure in simple terms, even if the resident is not able to communicate or is disoriented. Ask permission to perform the procedure.

(continued)

Giving an Enema *(continued)*

8. Bring the necessary equipment into the room. Place the following items in an easy-to-reach place:
   - disposable enema kit or prepacked enema, as ordered
   - enema solution (1,000 mL for adults)
   - IV pole
   - disposable gloves
   - water-soluble lubricant
   - bath blanket
   - disposable protective pad

   Collect the following items, as needed:
   - bedpan and cover or bedside commode
   - urinal
   - nonskid slippers
   - toilet paper
   - paper towels
   - towels, soap, and washbasin

The Procedure: Cleansing Enema

9. Prepare the enema solution, as ordered, in the bathroom or utility room.
10. Close the clamp on the enema bag tubing. Fill the enema bag with the amount of enema solution ordered. Seal the enema bag.
11. Unclamp the enema tubing. Run a small amount of enema solution through the tubing to eliminate air and warm the tube. Check the temperature of the enema solution to be sure it is not too warm. Clamp the tubing. Bring the prepared enema bag into the room.
12. Hang the enema bag and tubing on the IV pole next to or on the bed. The enema bag should hang 18 inches above the mattress. Hanging the enema bag any higher could cause the resident pain.
13. Provide privacy by closing the curtains, using a screen, or closing the door to the room.
14. Lock the bed wheels and then raise the bed to hip level.
15. Maintain safety during the procedure. If there are side rails, raise and lock the rails on the opposite side of the bed from where you will be working. Lower the rail on the side where you are working.
16. Wash your hands or use hand sanitizer to ensure infection control.
17. Put on disposable gloves.
18. Cover the resident with a bath blanket. Fanfold the linens to the foot of the bed and place a disposable protective pad under the resident's buttocks.
19. Help the resident turn onto his left side. Bend the resident's right knee toward his chest to place him in Sims' position.
20. Expose the resident's buttocks by raising the lower corner of the blanket covering the anal area.

21. Lubricate the enema tubing 2–4 inches from the tip.
22. Expose the resident's anus by lifting the resident's upper buttock. Gently insert the enema tubing 2–4 inches into the rectum (**Figure 20.28**). Stop and immediately report to the licensed nursing staff if the resident complains of pain, if you meet resistance, or if there is bleeding.

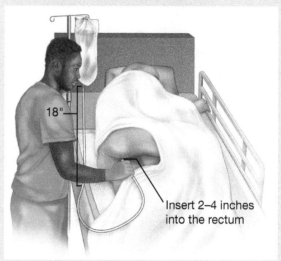

18"

Insert 2–4 inches into the rectum

Figure 20.28   *© Body Scientific International*

23. Unclamp the enema tubing and let the solution flow slowly. Ask the resident to take slow, deep breaths to relax. Explain that this will help relieve any cramps caused by the enema.
24. When most of the solution has flowed into the rectum, close the clamp before the enema bag is empty. This will prevent air from entering the bowel.
25. Hold toilet paper around the enema tubing and against the anus. Slowly withdraw the tubing. Wrap the tubing in paper towels and place it in the empty enema kit container.
26. Ask the resident to squeeze his buttocks so he holds the solution in the rectum for as long as possible.
27. When the resident is no longer able to hold the solution or when the urge to have a bowel movement is insistent, assist the resident to the bedpan, bedside commode, or bathroom. If the resident will be using a bedpan, reposition and raise the head of the bed. Put toilet paper where it can easily be reached. If the resident uses the bathroom, stay nearby to help, if needed, and ask the resident not to flush the toilet. Make sure the call light is within the resident's reach.
28. Remove and discard your gloves.
29. Wash your hands or use hand sanitizer to ensure infection control.
30. Check on the resident every few minutes.

31. While the resident is using the bedpan, bedside commode, or toilet, dispose of the enema equipment according to facility policy.

32. Wash your hands or use hand sanitizer to ensure infection control.

33. Put on a new pair of gloves.

> **Best Practice:** Check the stool for any unusual appearance or odor. If you see anything abnormal, immediately alert the licensed nursing staff.

34. When the resident has finished using the bedpan, bedside commode, or toilet, assist the resident back to bed, if needed. Assist with hygiene care.

35. If the resident is in bed, remove the disposable protective pad and bath blanket. Change any soiled linens and cover the resident with the top linens.

36. Check to be sure the bed wheels are locked, then reposition the resident and lower the bed.

37. Follow the plan of care to determine if the side rails should be raised or lowered.

38. Remove and discard your gloves.

39. Wash your hands or use hand sanitizer to ensure infection control.

40. Put on a new pair of gloves.

41. Remove, clean, and store equipment in the proper location. Remove soiled linens and discard disposable equipment.

The Procedure: Commercial Enema

42. Provide privacy by closing the curtains, using a screen, or closing the door to the room.

43. Lock the bed wheels and then raise the bed to hip level.

44. Maintain safety during the procedure. If there are side rails, raise and lock the rails on the opposite side of the bed from where you will be working. Lower the rail on the side where you are working.

45. Wash your hands or use hand sanitizer to ensure infection control.

46. Put on disposable gloves.

47. Cover the resident with a bath blanket. Fanfold the linens to the foot of the bed and place a disposable protective pad under the resident's buttocks.

48. Help the resident turn onto her left side. Bend the resident's right knee toward her chest to place her in Sims' position.

> **Best Practice:** Always read the package instructions before giving a commercial or small-volume enema.

49. Open the box and remove the enema. Place the solution container in warm water, if instructed.

50. Expose the resident's buttocks by moving linens away from the anal area.

51. Remove the cover from the prelubricated enema tip. Gently squeeze the container to make sure the container tip is open.

52. With one hand, raise the resident's upper buttock to expose the anus.

53. Ask the resident to take a deep breath through her mouth and let it out. As the resident lets out her breath, gently insert the enema tip 2 inches into the rectum (**Figure 20.29**).

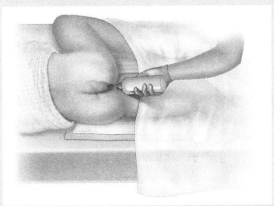

Figure 20.29   © Body Scientific International

54. Gently squeeze the bottom of the enema container and roll the container until almost all of the solution goes into the rectum. A small amount should remain in the container.

55. Remove the enema tip from the anus and place the container in the box.

56. Ask the resident to hold the solution in her rectum for 20 minutes, or as long as possible. Ask her to signal you when she has an insistent urge to defecate.

57. If the resident can be safely left alone, be sure she is positioned safely and place the call light within her reach.

58. If the resident cannot be left alone, stay in the room to maintain safety.

59. Discard the enema container. Remove and discard your gloves. Wash your hands or use hand sanitizer to ensure infection control.

60. If you left the room, return to the room when the resident uses the call light.

61. Help the resident to the bedpan, bedside commode, or bathroom. If the resident will be using the bedpan, reposition and raise the head of the bed. Put toilet paper where it can easily be reached. If the resident uses the bathroom, stay nearby to help, if needed, and ask the resident not to flush the toilet. Make sure the call light is within the resident's reach.

62. Check on the resident every few minutes.

(continued)

Giving an Enema *(continued)*

63. Wash your hands or use hand sanitizer to ensure infection control.
64. Put on a new pair of gloves.
65. When the resident has finished using the bedpan, bedside commode, or toilet, assist with hygiene care.
66. If the resident is in bed, remove the disposable protective pad and bath blanket. Change any soiled linens and cover the resident.
67. Check to be sure the bed wheels are locked, then reposition the resident and lower the bed.
68. Follow the plan of care to determine if the side rails should be raised or lowered.
69. Remove, clean, and store equipment in the proper location. Remove soiled linens and discard disposable equipment.

Follow-Up

70. Remove and discard your gloves.
71. Wash your hands to ensure infection control.
72. Make sure the resident is comfortable and place the call light and personal items within reach.
73. Conduct a safety check before leaving the room. The room should be clean and free from clutter or spills.
74. Wash your hands or use hand sanitizer before leaving the room.

Reporting and Documentation

75. Report any specific observations, complications, or unusual responses to the licensed nursing staff. Document this information, along with the care provided, in the chart or EMR.

Ostomies and Stoma Care

Bowel elimination problems can have a great effect on residents' lives, especially if the resident experiences problems related to colon cancer or an injury to the intestine. In some cases, a surgical procedure called an **ostomy** may be required. An ostomy procedure creates a **stoma**, or an artificial opening, between the surface of the abdomen and the intestine. This stoma allows waste to be eliminated (**Figure 20.30**). An *ostomy bag* is applied to the stoma to collect waste. If the stoma extends between the surface of the abdomen and the large intestine, the procedure is called a *colostomy*. If the stoma extends between the surface of the abdomen and the ileum of the small intestine, the procedure is called an *ileostomy*. A stoma may be permanent or temporary.

A colostomy or ileostomy can be very traumatic and embarrassing for residents. Residents may worry about soiling themselves or about odor. Being patient and supportive is an important responsibility for a holistic nursing assistant.

Nursing assistants are responsible for caring for the stoma and emptying and changing the ostomy bag. As part of hygiene, the stoma must be cleaned and the ostomy bag changed daily, if not more often.

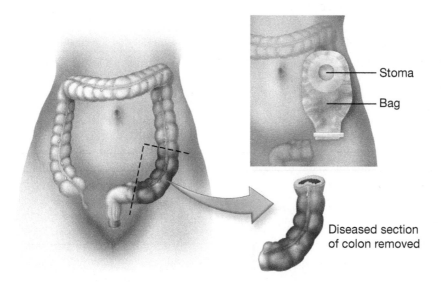

Stoma

Bag

Diseased section of colon removed

© *Body Scientific International*

Figure 20.30 An ostomy procedure creates a stoma, through which waste is eliminated. An ostomy bag is applied to the stoma to collect the waste.

The ostomy bag itself will need to be emptied during the day and should never be more than one-third full. Some residents may empty their bags themselves. Others may need assistance.

When providing ostomy care, you will need several pieces of equipment (**Figure 20.31**):

- correctly sized, clean ostomy bag (sometimes called an *appliance* or *pouch*)
- skin barrier that sticks to the stoma and protects the skin from stoma output
- clamp or clip to open and close the bag (may be attached to the bag)
- clean ostomy belt, if used (to secure the bag against the body)

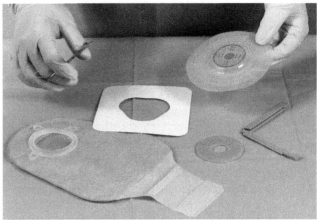

Sherry Yates Young/Shutterstock.com

Figure 20.31 When caring for a stoma, you will need an ostomy bag, skin barrier, and clamp, among other equipment.

Procedure

Providing Ostomy Care

Rationale

Regular care keeps the skin around a stoma clean and prevents irritation and breakdown from contact with stool.

Preparation

1. Ask the licensed nursing staff if there are doctor's orders for the procedure, if there are any specific instructions listed in the plan of care, and if the resident can be moved into the positions required for this procedure.
2. Wash your hands or use hand sanitizer before entering the room.
3. Knock before entering the room.
4. Introduce yourself using your first or preferred name and title. Explain that you work with the licensed nursing staff and will be providing care.
5. Greet the resident and ask the resident to state his full name, if able. Then check the resident's identification bracelet.
6. Use Mr., Mrs., or Ms. and the resident's last name when conversing.
7. Explain the procedure in simple terms, even if the resident is not able to communicate or is disoriented. Ask permission to perform the procedure.
8. Bring the necessary equipment into the room. Place a paper towel, towel, or disposable protective pad on the overbed table as an infection-control barrier before placing the following items:
   - correctly sized, clean ostomy bag with skin barrier
   - clamp or clip, if needed

- clean ostomy belt, if used
- adhesive remover, if needed
- antiseptic wipes
- disposable protective pads
- disposable gloves
- small trash bag
- bath blanket
- 4 × 4 gauze pads or toilet paper
- washcloths
- towels
- washbasin with warm water
- soap or cleaning agent, as ordered
- bedpan and cover
- graduate
- deodorant, if used

The Procedure

9. Provide privacy by closing the curtains, using a screen, or closing the door to the room.
10. Lock the bed wheels and then raise the bed to hip level.
11. Maintain safety during the procedure. If there are side rails, raise and lock the rails on the opposite side of the bed from where you will be working. Lower the rail on the side where you are working.
12. Wash your hands or use hand sanitizer to ensure infection control.
13. Put on disposable gloves.
14. Position the resident on his back, if possible. Place a disposable protective pad under the resident's buttocks and lower abdomen.
15. Cover the resident with a bath blanket. Without exposing the resident, fanfold the top linens and move clothing to expose the stoma.

(continued)

Providing Ostomy Care *(continued)*

16. Place another protective pad alongside the resident's body and cover the resident with the bath blanket from the waist down.
17. Remove the clamp at the bottom of the ostomy bag and let the stool drain into a graduate. Make sure the drain and the end of the bag do not touch the graduate. Avoid any splashing of the stool or drainage.
18. Wipe the open end of the ostomy bag with an antiseptic wipe, following facility policy. Fold the end of the ostomy bag and close it with the clamp.
19. Note the color, amount, consistency, and odor of the stool and measure the stool and drainage, if documenting I&O.
20. Empty the stool and drainage into the toilet or bedpan.
21. Remove and discard your gloves.
22. Wash your hands or use hand sanitizer to ensure infection control.
23. Put on a new pair of gloves.
24. Disconnect the ostomy bag from the ostomy belt, if used. Remove and inspect the belt. If the belt is soiled, dispose of it according to facility policy.
25. Remove the ostomy bag and skin barrier by gently stretching the skin and pulling the ostomy bag away from the skin. Use warm water or adhesive remover, if necessary.
26. Place the ostomy bag in the bedpan and cover the bedpan. Neutralize any odor, following facility policy.
27. Remove any stool or drainage by gently wiping the stoma with a 4 × 4 gauze pad or toilet paper (**Figure 20.32**). Discard the dirty gauze pads and your gloves in a disposable trash bag.

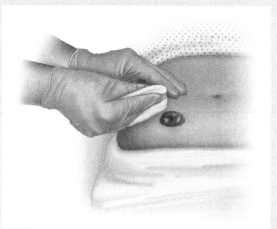

Figure 20.32   © *Body Scientific International*

28. Wash your hands or use hand sanitizer to ensure infection control.
29. Put on a new pair of gloves.
30. Wash the stoma and the skin around it using a 4 × 4 gauze pad or washcloth mitt, soap, and water or a cleansing agent (as ordered).
31. Rinse and thoroughly dry the skin around the stoma.
32. Observe the stoma and the skin around the stoma. Immediately report any skin irritation, breakdown, or bleeding to the licensed nursing staff.
33. Apply the correctly sized skin barrier, according to the manufacturer's instructions (**Figure 20.33**).

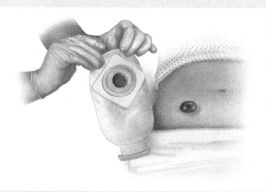

Figure 20.33   © *Body Scientific International*

34. Position the clean ostomy belt, if used.
35. Remove the adhesive backing from the ostomy bag. The opening of the ostomy bag should be the correct size for the stoma.
36. Make sure the drain or end of the bag is pointing downward and then center the bag over the stoma.
37. Gently press around the edges of the ostomy bag to seal it to the skin. If used, add deodorant to the bag.

   Best Practice: Make sure the skin around and under the ostomy bag is smooth and wrinkle free.

38. Close the ostomy bag at the bottom using the clamp or clip.
39. Attach the ostomy belt, if used, to the ostomy bag. Make sure the belt is not too tight. You should be able to slide two fingers underneath it.
40. Remove the protective pads and change any soiled linen. Remove the bath blanket and replace the top linens.
41. Check to be sure the bed wheels are locked, then reposition the resident and lower the bed.
42. Follow the plan of care to determine if the side rails should be raised or lowered.

43. Remove, clean, and store equipment in the proper location. Remove soiled linens and discard disposable equipment.

Follow-Up
44. Remove and discard your gloves.
45. Wash your hands to ensure infection control.
46. Make sure the resident is comfortable and place the call light and personal items within reach.
47. Conduct a safety check before leaving the room. The room should be clean and free from clutter or spills.

48. Wash your hands or use hand sanitizer before leaving the room.

Reporting and Documentation
49. Report any specific observations, complications, or unusual responses to the licensed nursing staff. Document this information, along with the care provided, in the chart or EMR.

What Are Bladder and Bowel Retraining?

Bladder or *bowel retraining* may be ordered by the doctor to help residents with elimination problems gain greater independence. Generally, retraining includes changing the diet, tracking elimination to determine individual patterns, scheduling toileting to increase the time between visits, determining any challenges to toileting, modifying any medications contributing to the issue, learning pelvic-floor exercises, and rehabilitating muscles when possible.

Successful bladder and bowel retraining requires residents to concentrate on the needed steps and keep trying. It may take up to three months or more before any progress is made. Retraining orders are written by the doctor, and guidance is given by the licensed nursing staff. A holistic nursing assistant may provide the resident assistance and support by following the guidelines in this section as the resident works on bladder or bowel retraining.

BECOMING A HOLISTIC NURSING ASSISTANT
Assisting with Elimination Needs

Residents who need assistance with elimination may feel uncomfortable and self-conscious about nursing assistants seeing and touching their genitals. They may also be embarrassed about what is happening and feel shame. Holistic nursing assistants can follow these guidelines to make this difficult time more pleasant, helpful, and comfortable:

- Be aware of your own feelings of comfort when assisting with elimination.
- Be sensitive to and compassionate about a resident's situation and feelings. Remind the resident that you are there to help.
- Some residents are more comfortable than others in expressing their feelings. Be sensitive to how open a resident is when you ask questions about the resident's feelings.
- Encourage the resident to ask questions and to share any changes he or she might be experiencing.

- Assure the resident with diarrhea or constipation that everyone has had these conditions at one time or another, so there is no reason to feel ashamed.
- Answer call lights immediately, particularly if a resident is having elimination problems such as diarrhea or incontinence.
- If a resident is having trouble urinating, put his or her hands in warm water or turn on the faucet so the resident can hear running water.
- Create a relaxing environment.
- Touch the resident gently and carefully when giving care.
- Never rush when giving care.

Apply It
1. Think about each of these guidelines. What are your feelings about elimination and elimination problems?
2. Are there any guidelines you might have trouble following as a holistic nursing assistant? Explain your answer.

Bladder Retraining Guidelines

Help residents maintain an ongoing toileting diary. The diary should include a log of how often they urinate, when they have the urge to urinate, and if and when they leak each day. This diary will be reviewed regularly with the doctor.

Remind residents to visit the toilet before they go to bed and to empty their bladder when they get up. Residents must remember the training schedule so that they can visit the toilet regularly. Add 15 minutes to the time between each bathroom visit. If the resident has been going to the bathroom every hour, she should wait until an hour and 15 minutes has passed before urinating again. Time between each toileting visit is increased by 15 minutes until there are three to four hours between each visit. Residents follow the schedule while they are awake. At night, they go to the toilet only if they awaken and find it necessary.

Another step is to wait five minutes every time residents feel an urge to urinate. This time is gradually increased by 10 minutes, until residents can delay urinating for at least three to four hours. Residents should visit the toilet only after they cannot wait any longer. Nursing assistants can help distract residents through conversation or an activity, using relaxation techniques, or deep breathing.

Kegel exercises can be used to strengthen the muscles that start and stop the flow of urine. To do a Kegel exercise, residents should squeeze, or *contract*, the muscles used to stop the flow of urine. Hold the contraction for 5 seconds and then relax for 5 seconds. Gradually increase to contract the muscles every 10 seconds, with 10 seconds of rest in between. Residents should work up to three sets of 10 contractions daily. If done daily, residents will be more successful. A diary can be used to keep track of daily Kegel exercises.

Encourage residents to limit beverages that increase urination. This includes caffeinated drinks such as sodas, coffee, and tea. Encourage them to drink less before bedtime.

Bowel Retraining Guidelines

Help residents set a regular time for daily bowel movements. The time should be convenient and fit with their daily schedule. The best time is 20 to 40 minutes after a meal because eating stimulates bowel activity.

A change in diet can help create soft, bulky stool. Eating high-fiber foods such as whole grains, fresh vegetables, and beans, and drinking 2–3 liters of fluid daily (unless it is not in the plan of care) can be helpful. If it is in the plan of care, residents may find drinking warm prune juice or fruit nectar helpful, as well as products that have *psyllium* (fiber made from husks of plant seeds), which adds bulk to the stool.

Digital stimulation to trigger a bowel movement may be a part of the training. The resident may be able to do this him or herself, or, the nursing assistant may be asked to provide assistance. Insert a lubricated finger into the anus. Move the finger in a circle until the sphincter muscle relaxes. This may take a few minutes. After stimulation, residents should sit in their normal position on the toilet, commode, or bedpan. Maintain privacy and help residents relax. Contracting the stomach muscles and bending forward while bearing down can help increase pressure to evacuate the bowel. If a bowel movement does not occur within 20 minutes, repeat the process.

The doctor may prescribe a suppository or an enema to help stimulate the bowels. Results usually take about 30 minutes.

Kegel exercises will also help strengthen the pelvic rectal muscles. See the bladder retraining guidelines for instructions for performing these exercises.

The doctor may also recommend *biofeedback*. A monitoring electrode is placed on the abdomen, and a plug is inserted into the rectum. This plug is attached to a computer that displays a graph of the rectal and abdominal muscle contractions as they are squeezed around the plug. The display provides feedback regarding the strength of these muscle contractions and will help the resident increase the intensity of his contractions.

To be most effective, many of these actions may be done together to make a total program. Know that residents will have both good and bad days. The key to success is to keep trying.

SECTION 20.2 **Review and Assessment**

Key Terms Mini Glossary

defecate to have a bowel movement.

enema a procedure in which liquid is inserted into the rectum to clean the lower intestine.

flatus gas or air in the gastrointestinal tract; is expelled via the anus.

hernia a bulge of an organ through the wall of the body cavity or structure that contains it.

impaction a blockage of hard stool in the rectum.

motility movement; in the gastrointestinal system, the contraction of muscles that moves substances through the gastrointestinal tract.

ostomy a surgical procedure that creates an opening in the abdominal wall so that stool can be eliminated from the intestines to the outside of the body.

stoma a surgically created abdominal opening, through which stool are eliminated.

suppositories small, meltable, solid cones or cylinders that may be medicated; inserted into a body passage such as the rectum or vagina.

Apply the Key Terms

Write a sentence using each key term properly.

1. defecate
2. flatus
3. impaction
4. motility
5. stoma

Know and Understand the Facts

1. Describe how the color of urine and stool can indicate the condition of the body.
2. Identify two problems residents can have with elimination and how nursing assistants can assist.
3. What are three guidelines for bladder retraining?
4. What are three guidelines for bowel retraining?
5. Discuss two reasons why performing catheter care is important.
6. What are the three differences in helping a resident use the toilet versus using a bedside commode?

Analyze and Apply Concepts

1. Explain how to document bowel movements.
2. Describe the steps needed to help a resident use a bedpan.
3. What steps would a nursing assistant follow to empty an ostomy bag?
4. Describe the steps for performing catheter care on a female.
5. Describe the steps for performing catheter care on a male.
6. What are two important guidelines when inserting a suppository?

Think Critically

Read the following care situation. Then answer the questions that follow.

Mr. P is 76 years old and was admitted to the long-term care facility two weeks ago. He has a permanent colostomy due to colon cancer. He also has a urinary catheter and is in the early stages of dementia. Mr. P is able to dangle on the side of the bed with assistance and is on a soft diet. He is on I&O. His wife visits daily and likes to help as much as she can. You are working the day shift, and Mr. P is one of five residents assigned to you today. He appears very agitated today and is not as cooperative in his care as he usually is.

1. What actions and approaches can you take to respond to Mr. P's agitation and uncooperative attitude?
2. Describe the procedure for caring for Mr. P's catheter. Identify two areas of special concern, given Mr. P's condition.
3. Describe the procedure for caring for Mr. P's stoma. Identify two areas of special concern, given Mr. P's condition.
4. Are there any specific safety or care problems you might need to respond to when taking care of Mr. P?
5. What actions can you take to include Mr. P's wife in his care?

Key Points

Reviewing the key points for this chapter will help you practice more safely and competently as a holistic nursing assistant and will help you prepare for the certification competency exam.

- Measuring and documenting a resident's intake and output (I&O) provides important measures of the amount of fluids consumed.
- Nursing assistants work closely with the licensed nursing staff to help monitor IVs.
- A urinary catheter may need to be inserted or a surgical procedure called an *ostomy* may be required to aid in elimination.
- Maintaining proper hygiene and skin integrity are very important while providing help during toileting, measuring and documenting bowel movements, providing catheter and colostomy care, changing drainage bags, and supporting bladder and bowel retraining.
- Elimination problems can be difficult, painful, and embarrassing. Holistic nursing assistants should try to make residents' experiences more pleasant and comfortable.

Action Steps to Holistic Care

Review the information in this chapter. Complete the following activities.

1. Select one procedure you learned in this chapter. Prepare a short paper or digital presentation that identifies and describes the three most important practices. Include one that promotes comfort and one that maintains safety.
2. Research current scientific information about incontinence. Write a brief report describing two current facts about incontinence treatments.
3. Create an instructional handout for residents discussing the guidelines for bladder and bowel retraining. Along with instructions for retraining, also include a section for fellow nursing assistants discussing strategies for assisting and supporting residents during these processes.

Building Math Skill

Shanice is taking care of Mrs. O, whose intake and output is being measured and recorded. Mrs. O has voided three times during the 7–3 shift. Each time, Shanice noted the amount on the I&O form:

9:00 a.m. – 350 mL
11:30 p.m. – 300 mL
2:30 p.m. – 300 mL
What is Mrs. O's total output for Shanice's shift?

Preparing for the Certification Competency Examination

To prepare for the nursing assistant certification competency examination, you will need to know content found in this chapter. This content may be tested in the knowledge (written or oral) and skills (hands-on demonstration) portions of the exam. The following areas will be emphasized:

- hydration, dehydration, and factors that influence adequate intake
- sources of fluid intake and output
- fluid restrictions
- calculations for accurate intake and output
- factors that contribute to elimination practices and problems
- care for residents who are incontinent
- catheter and ostomy care
- rectal tubes, suppositories, and enemas
- bladder and bowel retraining programs

These sample test questions are similar to ones you will find on the certification competency exam. See how well you can answer them. Be sure to select the *best* answer.

1. A nursing assistant is observing a resident who has an IV. To identify possible infiltration, she should observe the skin around the catheter for
   A. swelling
   B. dehydration
   C. warmth
   D. sweating

2. Which of the following describes frequent liquid stools?
   A. CAUTI
   B. constipation
   C. GERD
   D. diarrhea

3. Ms. U has had diarrhea all night, and a nursing assistant had to change her linens three times. When Ms. U has diarrhea again, what should the nursing assistant do first?
   A. sigh and quickly help her go to the toilet
   B. tell her he will be right back
   C. quietly change her linens and gown and help her wash
   D. assure her he understands and is happy to help

4. Mrs. O has a catheter. Why should the nursing assistant keep the urinary drainage bag secured to the bed below the resident?
   A. so that the weight of the bag can cause urine to drain
   B. so that the force of gravity can allow urine to drain
   C. to keep the drainage bag out of the way
   D. so the family does not see Mrs. O's urine

5. A nursing assistant is measuring intake for Mr. I. What should the nursing assistant do?
   A. monitor for dehydration
   B. measure for specific gravity
   C. keep the container at eye level
   D. check the pH of the urine

6. Kegel exercises are used to
   A. control excessive diarrhea
   B. retrain the bladder and bowels
   C. help close a stoma
   D. alleviate cramping and pain

7. When a nursing assistant is administering a cleansing enema, the bag should be
   A. below the resident for best drainage
   B. at the same height as the resident
   C. above the resident for best flow
   D. anywhere that is convenient

8. A new nursing assistant is providing catheter care for Mr. B. What should he do to help prevent a CAUTI?
   A. keep the tubes unkinked
   B. not pull on the tubes
   C. check for a foreskin
   D. keep the tubes coiled

9. A severe complication of constipation is
   A. impaction
   B. hernia
   C. diarrhea
   D. incontinence

10. A nursing assistant is taking care of Mr. E, who has had a colostomy. She will be providing ostomy care. When she removes his pouch, what is the first action she should take?
    A. gently cleanse the area around the stoma
    B. provide perineal care, if it is needed
    C. place a protective shield on the stoma
    D. measure the size of his stoma

11. Ms. X has not been feeling well. She refused her breakfast and lunch, and does not want to drink any fluids. Which of the following are the first signs of dehydration?
    A. dry mouth and increased thirst
    B. fainting and chest pains
    C. swollen tongue and headache
    D. confusion and heart palpitations

12. A nursing assistant was emptying the bedpan for Mrs. N. When she saw the color of Mrs. N's stool, she notified the licensed nursing staff immediately. Which of the following colors requires this response?
    A. orange
    B. yellow
    C. black
    D. gray

13. I&O is measured in
    A. liters
    B. milliliters
    C. grams
    D. milligrams

14. A new nursing assistant is aware that, when caring for residents with elimination problems, he should
    A. ignore the residents so they are not embarrassed
    B. put on residents' favorite music so they can relax
    C. be patient, reassuring, and supportive
    D. make sure residents wear double-padded briefs to prevent accidents

15. A nursing assistant observes that Mr. R's urine is amber. What might this mean?
    A. He is bleeding.
    B. He has a urinary tract infection.
    C. He is dehydrated.
    D. He has a kidney stone.

Did you have difficulty with any of the questions? If you did, review the chapter to find the correct answer(s).

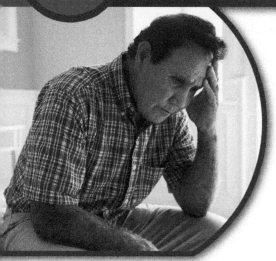

Monkey Business Images/Shutterstock.com

Chapter Outline

Section 21.1
Mental and Emotional Health and Related Health Conditions

Section 21.2
Disabilities, Delirium, and Dementia

Welcome to the Chapter

In this chapter, you will learn what mental and emotional health are and how they are influenced by developmental, social, and environmental factors. You will become familiar with emotional health concerns and mental health conditions, including anxiety disorders, trauma- and stress-related disorders, depressive disorders, substance-use disorders, personality disorders, and schizophrenia spectrum disorder. You will also learn about risk factors and responses to self-harm and suicide. This knowledge will help you understand the responsibilities holistic nursing assistants have when providing care.

As you read this chapter, you will also learn about disabilities, including vision, hearing, or speech impairments; congenital and genetic disorders; and disability caused by trauma or injury. You will also explore cognitive disorders such as delirium and dementia. You will examine how cognitive disorders impact daily living. Learning about these disabilities and disorders will help you understand how you can assist those affected.

The information presented in this chapter will help you build the knowledge and skills needed to become a holistic nursing assistant. The topics discussed in the chapter are highlighted on the Providing Holistic Care Framework.

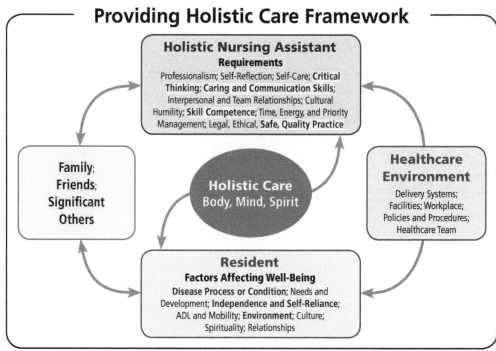

Providing Holistic Care Framework

Holistic Nursing Assistant
Requirements
Professionalism; Self-Reflection; Self-Care; **Critical Thinking; Caring and Communication Skills**; Interpersonal and Team Relationships; Cultural Humility; **Skill Competence**; Time, Energy, and Priority Management; Legal, Ethical, **Safe, Quality Practice**

Family; Friends; Significant Others

Holistic Care
Body, Mind, Spirit

Healthcare Environment
Delivery Systems; Facilities; Workplace; Policies and Procedures; Healthcare Team

Resident
Factors Affecting Well-Being
Disease Process or Condition; Needs and Development; **Independence and Self-Reliance**; ADL and Mobility; **Environment**; Culture; Spirituality; Relationships

Goodheart-Willcox Publisher

Mental and Emotional Health and Related Health Conditions

Objectives

To achieve the objectives for this section, you must successfully:

- **describe** the characteristics of mental and emotional health.
- **discuss** how mental health conditions are categorized.
- **explain** mental health conditions, including anxiety disorders, trauma- or stress-related disorders, substance-use disorders, depressive disorders, personality disorders, and schizophrenia spectrum disorder.
- **examine** issues related to self-harm and suicide.
- **identify** care needed for residents with mental health conditions.

Key Terms

Learn these key terms to better understand the information presented in the section.

bipolar disorder
post-traumatic stress
 disorder (PTSD)
schizophrenia spectrum
 disorder

self-harm
stigma
suicide

Questions to Consider

- What do you know about mental and emotional health? Do you believe you are mentally and emotionally healthy?
- Do you know someone diagnosed with a mental health condition? What symptoms does the person have, and how are these symptoms being treated?

THINK ABOUT THIS

It is important to know that the presence of a mental health condition does not mean a person is legally insane. *Insanity* is a legal term and is not used by healthcare professionals. It is defined as the inability to manage one's affairs or understand the consequences of one's actions. A determination of insanity is made by a judge and jury based on an expert witness, such as a qualified psychiatrist.

What Are Mental and Emotional Health?

Mental health involves a person's ability to function productively. People can store and use information, shape their environment to meet their needs, make voluntary choices, take action, have satisfying and meaningful relationships, engage in creative work, adapt to change, are flexible and resilient, and can cope with challenges. At any point in time, social, psychological, and biological factors can influence a person's mental health. Promoting mental health includes actions that can improve psychological well-being. These actions support a respectful environment and protect a person's civil, political, socioeconomic, and cultural rights.

Emotional health involves feeling good about and having respect for one's self and others, enjoying life, giving and receiving love, and positively expressing and managing emotions. Mental and emotional health interact with, and help promote, physical well-being. Mental and emotional health require a positive interaction among physical, social, family, psychological, and environmental factors throughout life.

There are times when mental and emotional health may be at risk. Life changes, aging, or limited coping mechanisms can lead to stress. These changes may include retirement from a well-liked and fulfilling position, the death of a loved one, or physical changes such as limited mobility. Stress is normal, but it affects each person differently and impacts a person's mental and emotional health. The signs and symptoms of stress, discussed in Chapter 7, can affect mental, emotional, physical, and behavioral health. Specific strategies for coping, managing stress, and achieving a life balance are also discussed in Chapter 7. These strategies can be applied to yourself and are also helpful guidelines for caring for others.

Some people experience more than just everyday stressors. Changes in their thinking, mood, or behavior interfere with daily functioning. When learning about mental health conditions, remember that health and wellness are still possible.

What Are Mental Health Conditions?

Mental health conditions are the most common cause of disability in the United States. They cause changes in thinking, emotions, or behaviors, and can result in distress and limited or impaired functioning. It is estimated that over 43 million or 18 percent of people in the United States have a diagnosed mental health condition. Risk factors for these conditions include stressful living conditions, abuse, negative experiences in childhood, learning disorders, congenital disorders, low birthweight, physical or mental trauma, and chronic illnesses such as dementia.

Differing Views of Mental Health Conditions

In the past, some cultures have viewed mental health conditions as forms of punishment, supernatural (existing outside scientific understanding or the laws of nature, such as a miracle), intervention, or religious or personal problems. These beliefs helped create a stigma that continues today. People with mental health conditions often feel different from others, leading to feelings of embarrassment, shame, and isolation. These differences may frighten others, causing them to stay away from the person. Families may decide not to talk about the condition or try to hide it. Those whose feelings and behaviors are hard to manage may see themselves as weak, avoid sharing their feelings, isolate themselves, and thus limit their ability to function productively on a daily basis.

Apply It

1. How do you react when someone acts differently in a public or family setting?
2. If you become uncomfortable when people act differently, what can you do to change this reaction?
3. How can your care help people who have experienced stigma?

Today, one in five US adults experience a mental health condition each year, and over half do not have access to mental healthcare. Many people with a mental health condition experience *stigma* (a negative perception from others), feel they are negatively labeled because of their conditions, and feel separated from others.

What Are the Different Types of Mental Health Conditions?

Mental health conditions are categorized in several different ways. The American Psychiatric Association's Diagnostic and Statistical Manual of Mental Disorders (DSM-5) is the source most often used by psychiatrists, psychologists, and researchers. Although mental health conditions are characterized by specific symptoms and risks, remember that each resident's experience is unique. Understanding the mental health conditions that follow will help you provide safe, quality care.

Anxiety Disorders

Anxiety disorders are more than normal anxiety. They cause continuing, excessive worry or fear of nonthreatening situations. Symptoms of anxiety disorders include tension, nervousness, irritability, a racing heart, shortness of breath, headaches, fatigue, an upset stomach, and diarrhea. Most people who have anxiety disorders develop them before age 21, and women experience anxiety disorders more often than men. Anxiety disorders are caused by genetics and by the environment (including stressful or traumatic events, such as abuse or violence).

Some anxiety disorders cause *panic attacks*, which are sudden feelings of terror that happen without warning. People with panic attacks have chest pain, heart palpitations, dizziness, shortness of breath, and stomach upset. Other anxiety disorders include *phobias*, which are strong, persistent (continuing), irrational fears. People can have phobias of many different things, such as animals, needles, thunderstorms, or flying. Some people have more than one phobia. People with phobias have difficulty functioning normally and do everything possible to avoid the item or situation that causes the fear.

Another common, chronic anxiety disorder is *obsessive-compulsive disorder (OCD)*, which can interfere with daily living. Uncontrollable, recurring, and interfering thoughts and urges (*obsessions*) result in repetitive behaviors (*compulsions*). Obsessions may range from a fear of germs to a fear that something bad will happen if everything is not in perfect order. Compulsions are the behaviors a person uses in response to an obsession. For example, a person may excessively clean or repeatedly arrange things in a particular way.

Trauma- and Stress-Related Disorders

Trauma- and *stress-related disorders* can develop after a person experiences or witnesses a traumatic or stressful event. One example of a stress-related disorder is *post-traumatic stress disorder (PTSD)*. Childhood neglect or physical abuse, sexual assault, physical attacks, or combat exposure can cause PTSD. People with PTSD have a variety of symptoms, which may begin within three months or even many years after the event. Symptoms of PTSD can vary in intensity over time, and may include the following:

- reliving the event with unpleasant and disturbing memories, dreams, nightmares, and flashbacks (even a certain smell, touch, or noise can trigger these symptoms)
- avoiding thinking or talking about the trauma, or visiting places associated with the trauma

- having intense, anxious feelings that disrupt daily living
- feeling emotionally numb and hopeless
- having negative feelings about yourself and others
- experiencing memory and concentration problems
- finding it difficult to maintain close relationships
- feeling angry and irritable
- participating in self-destructive behaviors such as drinking

Acute stress disorder (ASD) causes severe anxiety and dissociation (disconnection between thoughts, memories, feelings, and actions) within one month after a traumatic event, such as a death or serious accident. If ASD lasts longer than one month and if severe symptoms continue, the person may be diagnosed with PTSD.

Another short-term condition is *adjustment disorder,* or *stress-response syndrome.* This condition usually lasts no longer than six months. A person with this condition has extreme difficulty coping with or adjusting to a particular source of stress, such as a major life change, stressful workplace event, or loss of a job. Someone with this condition may become situationally depressed and be tearful, have feelings of hopelessness, and lose interest in daily activities.

Depressive Disorders

Depressive disorders are the most common type of mental health condition and include persistent depressive disorder (*dysthymia*), major or clinical depression, perinatal/postpartum depression, seasonal affective disorder (SAD), and bipolar disorder. Depression can develop at any age and is caused by a combination of biological, genetic, environmental, and psychological factors. Risk factors can include a family history of depression; a major life change; certain illnesses, such as cancer or heart disease; or a reaction to a medication.

Depressive disorders cause feelings of sadness, anxiety, hopelessness, helplessness, guilt, and worthlessness. Residents with a depressive disorder may also experience a sense of emptiness; irritability; and cognitive issues such as difficulty concentrating, memory loss, troubled sleep, and loss of interest in pleasurable activities (**Figure 21.1**). Physical symptoms of depressive disorders include decreased energy; fatigue; slow movements; appetite and weight changes; and pain, headaches, and GI upsets that do not come from physiological illness. Typically, not all symptoms will occur at any one time.

Depressive disorders vary in duration, symptoms, and causes; however, for depression to be diagnosed, symptoms must be present daily for a minimum of two weeks. One example of diagnosed depression is *major depression,* a serious mood disorder with severe symptoms that have a large effect on daily life activities. In SAD, symptoms are present during the winter months when there is less sunlight, but disappear during spring and summer (**Figure 21.2**).

Bipolar disorder is a serious mental health condition that causes episodes of mania and depression. A resident with bipolar disorder may swing from extreme happiness, increased energy, trouble sleeping, fast talking, agitation, and multitasking (mania) to sadness, fatigue, worry, memory loss, trouble concentrating, and confusion (depression). Some people experience mania and depression at the same time; other people are only manic and are not depressed. Some episodes may include hallucinations or delusions. There is no single cause of bipolar disorder, but risk factors may include family history and genetics. Women are more likely than men to develop bipolar disorder, and symptoms appear most often in the late teen years or early adulthood. People with bipolar disorder may also abuse substances such as alcohol or drugs.

Personality Disorders

Residents with *personality disorders* may have trouble sensing and relating to everyday situations and other people. These disorders can cause serious problems and limitations in relationships and social activities. Personality disorders usually develop during adolescence or early adulthood. There are different types of personality disorders with unique

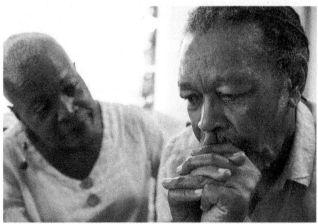

MBI/Shutterstock.com

Figure 21.1 A person with a depressive disorder has intense feelings of hopelessness, worthlessness, and helplessness.

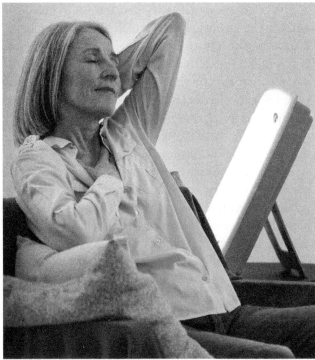

Figure 21.2 The use of light affects certain chemicals in the brain that influence mood and sleep, making light therapy an effective way to reduce the symptoms of SAD and other types of depression.

symptoms that can be mild or severe. Residents with personality disorders may have trouble realizing they have a problem.

Borderline personality disorder (BPD) is a personality disorder that affects how a person feels about himself or herself, relates to others, and behaves. BPD is a serious disorder that causes ongoing instability in moods, self-image, actions, and relationships. A resident with BPD may have extreme mood swings and be uncertain about his or her identity, leading to rapidly changing interests. Some signs and symptoms of BPD include an intense fear of abandonment; inappropriate anger; impulsive behavior, such as binge eating or quitting a good job; and a pattern of unstable and intense relationships. For example, a resident with BPD might feel extremely close and loving toward someone one moment and then suddenly believe the other person doesn't care enough about him or her.

Substance-Use Disorders

Substance-use disorders are excessive use of caffeine, alcohol, tobacco, cannabis (marijuana), hallucinogens, inhalants, opioids, sedatives, hypnotics (sleep medications), or stimulants such as cocaine. The most commonly used substances are alcohol, tobacco,

cannabis, stimulants, hallucinogens, and opioids. There are several common signs of these disorders. In general, they may include drastic changes in behavior and relationships; changes in performance and memory; lowered energy, concentration, coordination, and motivation; weight loss or gain; lack of interest in grooming; becoming secretive about their belongings; slurred speech; and changes in pupil size or red eyes.

Alcohol-Use Disorder

More than one-half of people in the United States ages 12 and older drink alcohol. *Binge drinking* is defined as consuming five or more alcoholic drinks for males or consuming four or more alcoholic drinks for females in a short period of time. *Excessive alcohol use* is considered five or more drinks at the same event on five or more days in the past 30 days.

Alcohol-use disorder (AUD) is more than just excessive drinking, although excessive drinking can lead to AUD. AUD is characterized by problems controlling alcohol intake, alcohol tolerance that leads to dangerous risks, withdrawal symptoms, and the continuation of drinking even with serious physical consequences. It is estimated that 16 million people in the United States (nearly 10 million adult men and over 5 million adult women) have AUD. A person's genetics influence the likelihood of developing AUD. AUD can be mild, moderate, or severe, depending on the number of symptoms displayed.

Stimulant-Use Disorder

People with a *stimulant-use disorder* consume amphetamines, methamphetamines, and cocaine orally, through nasal ingestion, or intravenously. Stimulants increase energy, alertness, attention, heart rate, blood pressure, and breathing. Stimulant use disorder is characterized by intense desire for a stimulant, the continuation of use even though it interferes with daily life, the use of larger amounts over time, and withdrawal symptoms.

Opioid-Use Disorder

Opioid-use disorder is characterized by the improper use or abuse of opioids and can have serious consequences. Opioids are a class of medications that includes the illegal drug heroin, synthetic opioids such as fentanyl, and other pain relievers available legally by prescription (for example, codeine and morphine). Opioids relieve pain and can also lead to a sense of *euphoria* (joy and excitement). Consuming more opioids intensifies the feeling; however, opioid overdose can depress respirations and cause death. Approximately 1.9 million people in the United States have an opioid use disorder.

Schizophrenia Spectrum Disorder

Schizophrenia spectrum disorder is a severe and chronic mental health condition that affects a person's entire life and ways of thinking, feeling, and behaving. Risk factors for schizophrenia spectrum disorder include genetics, the environment (including problems for a woman during pregnancy, such as increased stress, infections, and malnutrition), and possible chemical imbalances in the brain. Symptoms usually begin between the ages of 16 and 30. Most symptoms of schizophrenia spectrum disorder signify a loss of reality and include delusions such as persecution, hallucinations, thought disorders, and agitated body movements. Other symptoms interfere with emotions and behavior. For example, a symptom called the *flat affect* causes the lowering of emotions, lack of facial expression, and a dull tone of voice. The person might also have trouble with focus and attention, and an inability to make decisions.

What Should Nursing Assistants Know About Self-Harm and Suicide?

In addition to understanding mental health conditions, nursing assistants must also familiarize themselves with self-harm and suicide. Some people practice self-harm as a way to cope with emotional pain. Fatal, self-inflicted injuries, or suicide, may also be a sign of poor mental or emotional health. If a resident in your care practices self-harm or expresses suicidal thoughts, you must inform the licensed nursing staff immediately. Do not leave a resident who is considering suicide alone.

Self-Harm

When people inflict **self-harm**, they hurt themselves on purpose. Although practicing self-harm is not considered a mental health condition, it is a sign of emotional distress. For some people, self-harm is a coping mechanism used to lessen emotional pain or hard-to-express feelings. It is a way to provide emotional release or to create pain so the person feels something else.

Risk factors for self-harm include trauma, neglect, and abuse. A common method is skin cutting; however, some people burn themselves, pull out their hair, or pick at wounds to prevent healing.

When people harm themselves, they have feelings of shame. If that shame leads to intense negative feelings, people may hurt themselves again, creating a temporary but habitual cycle of self-harm. While self-harm is not the same as attempting suicide, it may increase the risk of suicide.

There are effective treatments for self-harm. Psychotherapy is important to any plan of care and helps the resident learn new coping mechanisms. Sometimes medications can also help.

Suicide

Suicide itself is not considered a mental health condition, but is a sign of poor mental and emotional health. **Suicide** is intentional death caused by fatal, self-inflicted injuries. Firearms are the most common method of suicide, accounting for almost one-half of suicide attempts. Suffocation and poisoning are also common methods, and poisoning is often used by females.

Some people may attempt suicide and inflict nonfatal injuries. Other people may have *suicidal ideation* and think about, consider, and plan suicide. Someone who survives a suicide attempt is likely to try again within the next three months and may succeed unless treated.

Risk factors for suicide include mental health conditions (such as depression), previous suicidal attempts, family history and violence, physical or sexual abuse, and chronic illness and pain. Traumatic life events may also lead to thoughts of suicide.

Be aware of the warning signs of suicide. These include hopelessness, increased anxiety, agitation, uncontrolled anger, dramatic mood changes, risky behaviors, feelings of being trapped, increased use of drugs or alcohol, and sudden withdrawal and isolation. The following are serious signs of an impending suicide attempt; this is an emergency:

- making threats of wanting to die or expressing a death wish
- looking for ways to die by suicide (such as taking risks or suddenly purchasing a firearm)
- talking or writing about suicide, putting affairs in order, or visiting or calling people to say goodbye

Always take suicide threats seriously. Never leave a resident who threatens suicide alone. Call for help and stay with the resident. If working outside a facility, help the person in danger seek assistance from a trained professional as quickly as possible or call a suicide hotline. Do not leave the person alone. Instead, immediately seek help from the nearest emergency room and call 9-1-1.

Some states have laws about mandatory reporting if a person intends to attempt suicide. Reporters must have reasonable cause to suspect a person will self-harm or attempt suicide. These reporters tend to be professionals such as teachers, social workers, healthcare providers, counselors or therapists, child care providers, or law enforcement officers. In some states, privileged communication that is considered confidential may complicate reporting. Privileged communication may include interactions between a doctor and resident, between an attorney and client, or with religious officials.

What Care Is Available for Residents with Mental Health Conditions?

Proper and accurate diagnosis is important for the care of a resident who has a mental health condition. Each resident will have his or her own response to the condition, set of symptoms, and plan of care for treatment. The goal of treatment is to improve quality of life. Plans of care will be individual, but will likely involve one or more of the following:

- **Psychotherapy**: usually includes talk therapy as an individual, in a group, or with the family. *Cognitive behavioral therapy (CBT)* helps a person develop mastery over thoughts and feelings (**Figure 21.3**). *Exposure therapy* treats phobias with gradual, repeated exposure so the person can learn to manage associated anxiety and feelings.

- **Selected medications**: may include antianxiety medications, antidepressants, sedatives, mood stabilizers, or antipsychotics. These will have side effects that need to be monitored.
- **Integrative medicine (IM) health approaches**: include stress relief, relaxation techniques, and supplements.

Holistic nursing assistants can take many actions to improve the daily lives of residents who have mental health conditions. Some of these actions include the following:

- Understand the symptoms of the mental health condition and recognize that they are very real to the resident.
- Never take a resident's behavior personally. Do, however, step back or stand away if a resident is physically aggressive.
- Respect the individuality of residents and focus on them as people, not on the behaviors they display. Use the plan of care as your guide and acknowledge that residents have rights.
- Be respectful, supportive, and caring. Understand that a mental health condition does not affect a resident's intelligence.
- Speak and act calmly to provide a peaceful and safe environment.
- Assist in providing proper nutrition and adequate exercise and activities.
- Observe, report, and document physical and behavioral changes, such as possible side effects of medications or alterations in behavior. These observations and reports are important to maintaining and ensuring an appropriate and effective plan of care.

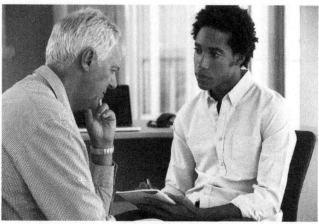

Figure 21.3 CBT is a type of therapy that involves mastering thoughts and feelings.

SECTION 21.1 **Review and Assessment**

Key Terms Mini Glossary

bipolar disorder a serious mental health condition characterized by changes in mood, energy, and activity levels; a person with bipolar disorder may swing from mania to depression.

post-traumatic stress disorder (PTSD) a stress-related mental health condition that develops after a person experiences or witnesses a traumatic or stressful event.

schizophrenia spectrum disorder a severe and chronic mental health condition in which a person experiences a loss of reality; has delusions, hallucinations, and thought disorders; and displays agitated body movements.

self-harm the act of hurting one's self on purpose.

stigma a negative perception that causes others to think less of an idea or person.

suicide the intentional self-infliction of fatal injuries.

Apply the Key Terms

Identify the key term used in each sentence.

1. Mrs. Z is having delusions and appears agitated. When you look at her EMR, you find that she has been diagnosed with schizophrenia spectrum disorder.
2. When residents commit self-harm they are hurting themselves on purpose.
3. People who experience or witness a traumatic or stressful event may develop post-traumatic stress disorder (PTSD).
4. Sometimes people with mental health conditions deal with negative perceptions where others think less of them. This is called a stigma.
5. Last night you read about an older adult you know who intentionally self-inflicted a fatal injury. You were very sad to hear about his suicide.

Know and Understand the Facts

1. Identify two similarities and two differences between mental and emotional health.
2. Describe how a mental health condition can affect a resident's daily life.
3. Choose one mental health condition and identify its risks and symptoms.
4. List three symptoms of PTSD.
5. Identify two signs that a person may be seriously considering suicide.
6. Describe two types of treatment for a mental health condition.

Analyze and Apply Concepts

1. Describe two important pieces of information you learned that will help you provide care for residents with mental health conditions.

2. List three guidelines for caring for residents with mental health conditions.
3. What should you do if a resident shares his or her suicidal thoughts?
4. What is one possible reason opioid use disorder is so common in the United States?

Think Critically

Read the following care situation. Then answer the questions that follow.

Mrs. O is a 75-year-old resident who was recently admitted to a long-term care facility. Mrs. O had a mild stroke, and her husband wants her to have full-time care while she is recovering. She has minimal physical disabilities from the stroke, has a slight limp that requires a cane, and has some slurred speech. Mrs. O was diagnosed with clinical depression five years ago and has attempted suicide twice. She is taking antidepressants and has tried individual and group therapy. Both have helped some. Mrs. O feels sad and anxious and is sometimes irritable. She often has difficulty concentrating and trouble sleeping. Mrs. O is very thin and seems fatigued. She said yesterday that she feels very hopeless that she will ever recover from the stroke.

1. What would you say to Mrs. O about her feelings of hopelessness?
2. In what specific areas should you be particularly observant when caring for Mrs. O?
3. What two approaches could you take to support Mrs. O during her recovery?
4. List three safety and comfort guidelines you could put in place when caring for Mrs. O.

Disabilities, Delirium, and Dementia

Objectives

To achieve the objectives for this section, you must successfully:

- **discuss** the difficulties residents may have due to vision, hearing, and speech impairments.
- **explain** the impact of congenital disorders, heredity, and developmental disorders.
- **identify** issues related to trauma, injury, and paralysis.
- **describe** the dimensions, behaviors, and challenges of delirium and dementia.
- **examine** the care required by residents who have disabilities and cognitive disorders.

Key Terms

Learn these key terms to better understand the information presented in the section.

cerebral palsy (CP)	paralysis
cues	paranoia
cystic fibrosis (CF)	perseveration
delusions	spina bifida (SB)
intoxication	sundowning
legal blindness	ventilator

Questions to Consider

- Think about a person you know who has experienced significant changes in his or her ability to walk, speak, hear, or see. Maybe this person had an accident and now needs to use crutches or a wheelchair. Maybe the person has a hard time hearing. How do you think these changes impact the person's daily life?
- What emotions and feelings do you think this person experiences? What did the person do to adjust? Were you able to help him or her?

What Are Disabilities and Cognitive Disorders?

In this section of the chapter, you will examine disabilities and cognitive disorders. A *disability* is a limitation of function. Disability can occur due to aging, disease, congenital or genetic disorders, developmental disorders, injury, or trauma. Disabilities affect one or more body systems, and people with disabilities may not be able to fully function in all activities.

THINK ABOUT THIS

The Americans with Disabilities Act (ADA) prohibits discrimination and guarantees equal opportunity for people with disabilities in employment, state and local government services, public accommodations, commercial facilities, and transportation. According to the ADA, a person with a disability has a physical or mental impairment that greatly limits one or more major life activities. ADA requirements affect public places such as restaurants, movie theaters, and schools. In these places, disability parking, wheelchair access, and specially constructed ramps and handrails aid people with disabilities. Employers also have to provide reasonable accommodations (adjustments or changes) to maintain equal employment opportunities for people with disabilities.

A *cognitive disorder* limits a person's ability to remember, learn, process and understand information, and behave appropriately in social settings. Cognitive disorders are the result of changes in the brain. Some cognitive disorders are reversible, and others are permanent. Reversible cognitive disorders are treatable and are usually called *delirium*. Delirium may be caused by a medical condition (such as electrolyte imbalance) or the overuse of a prescription medication or drug. Permanent cognitive disorders are called *dementia*. Types of dementia include Alzheimer's disease (AD), Lewy body dementia, and dementia caused by HIV/AIDS.

How Can Nursing Assistants Help Residents with Vision Impairment or Loss?

People who have *vision impairments* have difficulty seeing due to changes or conditions of the eye. Vision impairment is especially common among older adults. As a nursing assistant, you will care for residents with vision impairments ranging from refractive errors (eye conditions that cause changes in visual clarity)to **legal blindness** (a refractive error of 20/200 even after vision correction). A person who is legally blind must stand 20 feet from an object that a person with normal vision could see from 200 feet away. A resident with legal blindness may use *Braille*, a system of raised dots that is read with the fingers. Residents with legal blindness may also rely on a guide dog, if allowed by facility policy.

The most important parts of caring for a resident with vision impairment or loss are maintaining a safe environment and helping the resident retain self-esteem and have a life that still includes enjoyable activities. To correct vision impairment, residents may wear eyeglasses or contact lenses. Some residents may need an ocular prosthesis (artificial eye).

Caring for Eyeglasses

When residents wear eyeglasses, you will be responsible for helping them with their care. Eyeglasses should be washed at least once a day or whenever they are dirty. To wash eyeglasses, hold the frames by gripping the piece that crosses the bridge of the nose (**Figure 21.4**). Gently rub the lenses using warm, soapy water or use a specific spray or cleanser for eyeglasses. Let the lenses air-dry and then wipe them with a soft, clean, lint-free cloth. Never wipe dry lenses with paper towels, tissues, or napkins, as these can scratch the surface.

Be sure the eyeglasses are placed appropriately and ask residents if the glasses fit comfortably. Make sure that residents wear them when they get out of bed. When not in use, eyeglasses should be stored in a sturdy case or placed lens-side-up in a secure place. The resident must be able to reach his or her eyeglasses if they are not being worn.

Caring for Contact Lenses

Practice hand hygiene before handling contact lenses. When cleaning contact lenses, put the lenses in the palm of your hand, apply the appropriate cleaning solution, and gently rub each lens with the index finger of the other hand (**Figure 21.5**). Do not use

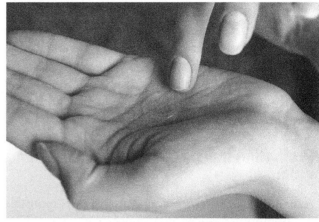
agrobacter/Signature collection via Getty Images

Figure 21.5 Contact lenses should be cleaned in the palm of your hand using the index finger of your other hand.

tap water directly on the lenses. Clean the lens case after each use with a sterile solution or hot tap water and let it air-dry. Replace the lens case every three months. Check with the licensed nursing staff regarding the placement of lenses in a resident's eyes. Always act according to facility policy and scope of practice.

Caring for Ocular Prostheses

An *ocular prosthesis*, or *prosthetic eye*, is fitted to the inner eye socket and is held in place by the upper and lower eyelids (**Figure 21.6**). An ocular prosthesis should be cleaned daily. Before inserting or removing an ocular prosthesis, check with the licensed nursing staff and be sure you are acting according to facility policy and scope of practice. When removing an ocular prosthesis, take care and place it in a plastic container filled with lukewarm water and padded with sterile gauze to prevent scratching. Rinse the eye socket

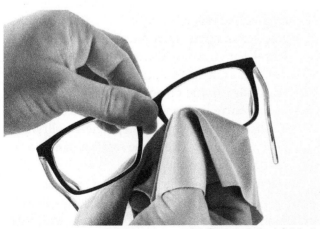
s-cphoto/Signature collection via Getty Images

Figure 21.4 When cleaning eyeglasses, be sure to hold them by the piece that crosses the bridge of the nose. Do not hold them by the arms or lenses.

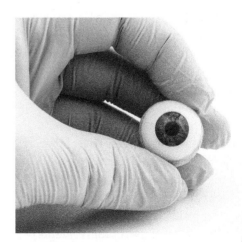
Shidlovski/Shutterstock.com

Figure 21.6 An ocular prosthesis is a false eye that is inserted into the eye socket.

with saline and warm water. To clean the ocular prosthesis, practice hand hygiene and use a soft brush with mild soap or the ordered cleaner and lukewarm water. Then rinse the prosthesis with clear water. If a resident does not wear the prosthesis overnight, the prosthesis should be cleaned; stored in a dry, closed container; and cleaned again before insertion.

Promoting Independence and Maintaining Safety

As a holistic nursing assistant, you will be responsible for promoting resident independence while making sure residents stay safe. Some residents who have vision impairments may not ask for help. Instead, they may stay in their rooms, be less active or social, or fall while trying to do something themselves. Residents may also be embarrassed, angry, or lonely. Recognize these feelings and be compassionate and patient. Encourage residents to participate in social activities and interact with others.

To promote safety, make sure residents who have vision impairment or loss feel comfortable and familiar in their surroundings. Help the resident become familiar with the environment by having him or her touch objects in the room. When ambulating or going up or down stairs, offer the resident your arm or hand, walk one step ahead of the resident, provide verbal directions, and let the resident know about any obstacles along the way. Encourage residents to use the handrails. Good lighting, a room that is neat and free from clutter, and an accessible call light also promote safety. Make sure that residents who have glasses wear them. Procedures and ADLs may take longer if the resident has vision impairments.

When helping a resident eat, identify each eating utensil and explain where it is placed. Also explain the position of the food on the plate. Use the hands of the clock to identify food locations. For example, you could say that the carrots are at 6:00. Cut up larger pieces of food so they are easier to manage. Do not overfill cups or glasses. When helping residents drink, tell them how full the glass is. Have residents use their index fingers to feel the glass and liquid level.

Large-print books and magazines, magnifying glasses, audio clocks and books, spoken computer programs, and writing aids (such as templates and bold-lined paper) may also be useful for residents with vision impairments.

How Should Nursing Assistants Assist Residents with Hearing Impairment or Loss?

Hearing impairments reduce a resident's ability to hear. A resident may have a *mild hearing impairment*, in which he or she has difficulty hearing every word in the presence of background noise. A resident with *moderate hearing impairment* needs words to be repeated during conversations and has a hard time keeping up without a hearing aid. *Severe hearing loss* makes it hard to hear a conversation without a powerful hearing aid and the use of lip reading. In *profound hearing impairment*, a resident is very hard of hearing and relies on lip reading and American Sign Language (ASL). ASL is the primary language of people who are deaf and uses hand signs combined with facial expressions and body postures.

Factors that can lead to hearing impairment include exposure to loud noise, certain medications, illnesses (such as hypertension or an ear infection), head trauma, heredity, and aging.

Hearing impairment can be permanent or reversible. Permanent hearing impairment occurs when there is damage to the inner ear or nerves. Reversible hearing impairment occurs when sound waves cannot reach the inner ear. An example of reversible hearing impairment is a punctured eardrum, which can be helped by treatment or surgery.

As a nursing assistant, you will care for many residents who have hearing impairments. You should use the following guidelines when taking care of these residents:

- Turn off background noise when conversing.
- Position yourself so you are facing the resident. Some residents will rely on lip reading when communicating.
- Never stand over the resident. If a resident is in a wheelchair, position yourself at the same level.
- Get the resident's attention before talking.
- Speak clearly and do not shout.
- Use assistive listening devices, such as TV-listening systems or telephone-amplifying devices. Internet telephone services can also help residents hear phone calls.

Residents with hearing impairments may use a *hearing aid*, which is a small, electronic device worn in or behind the ear (**Figure 21.7**). A hearing aid cannot restore hearing, but it can make sounds stronger and result in better hearing. The greater the hearing impairment is, the more amplification is needed.

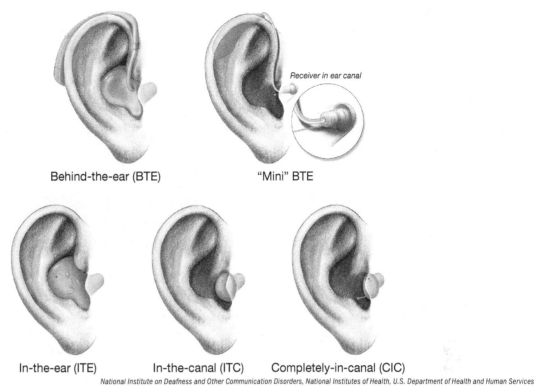

Behind-the-ear (BTE)

"Mini" BTE

Receiver in ear canal

In-the-ear (ITE)   In-the-canal (ITC)   Completely-in-canal (CIC)

National Institute on Deafness and Other Communication Disorders, National Institutes of Health, U.S. Department of Health and Human Services

Figure 21.7 Hearing aids can fit behind the ear, in the ear, or in the ear canal and are composed of a microphone, amplifier, and speaker.

Keep hearing aids away from heat and moisture, and clean them per the manufacturer's instruction. Advise residents to avoid hair-care products when wearing hearing aids. Turn off hearing aids when they are not in use and immediately replace dead batteries.

How Can Nursing Assistants Help Residents with Speech Impairment or Loss?

Speech impairments affect residents' abilities to communicate. Speech impairment or loss usually results from damage or injury to the part of the brain that controls language. One speech impairment you have already learned about is *aphasia*, which is an inability to understand and use words. Aphasia may be caused by a stroke, brain tumor, brain injury, infection, or dementia. Aphasia can be mild to severe, depending on the extent of damage and the area of the brain affected. There are four common types of aphasia:

- **Expressive aphasia (*nonfluent*)**: residents know what they want to say, but have difficulty communicating with others.
- **Receptive aphasia (*fluent*)**: residents can hear or read, but may not understand the meanings of words. Residents take language literally and do not understand meanings, which disrupts speech.

HEALTHCARE SCENARIO
Surgically Implantable Hearing Aids

It was recently announced that there are new, surgically implantable aids for hearing. A *middle ear implant (MEI)* is a small device attached to one of the bones in the middle ear. The MEI moves the bones directly instead of amplifying the sound to the eardrum. The *bone-anchored hearing aid (BAHA)* is a small device attached to the bone behind the ear. This device bypasses the middle ear and transmits sound vibrations directly into the inner ear through the skull.

Apply It

1. What do you think are the advantages of having an implantable hearing device?
2. What might be the disadvantages?

- **Anomic aphasia**: residents struggle to find the right words to speak or write.
- **Global aphasia**: residents have difficulty speaking and understanding words and are unable to read or write. This type of aphasia is the most severe and often occurs after a stroke.

Speech and language therapy can help residents improve their abilities to communicate, restore as much language as possible, and find other methods of communication. The recovery of language skills is often a slow process and starts early after impairment or loss.

As a holistic nursing assistant, the following guidelines will help you care for residents with speech impairments:

- Speak slowly and calmly.
- Use simple sentences.
- Use gestures and point to objects.
- Give the resident time to communicate.
- Do not finish the resident's sentences or correct errors.
- Check the resident's understanding and summarize what you have said.
- Eliminate any distracting noises.
- Make sure the resident has paper and pencils or pens, if needed and appropriate. For some residents, using written communication may be easier.
- Write one word or a short sentence, or use a gesture to help explain a procedure or direction.
- Help residents communicate more easily by asking them to select simple words and familiar images and photos from a personally created book or loose-leaf. You can help them develop this communication tool, or it can be something the family can help create (**Figure 21.8**).

Which Disabilities Are Due to Congenital and Genetic Disorders?

Some disabilities develop due to congenital or genetic disorders. *Congenital disorders* are caused by problems during fetal development prior to birth. Some of these disorders can be observed at birth. Others may be detected later in a person's life (for example, in the case of a congenital heart defect). *Genetic disorders* develop due to changes or mutations in the normal sequence of a person's DNA. A genetic disorder can be a mutation of one or multiple genes.

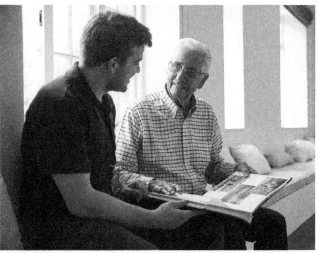

Monkey Business Images/Shutterstock.com

Figure 21.8 Books of words, illustrations, and photos can help residents communicate.

Examples of congenital and genetic disorders that can cause disability include Down syndrome; *spina bifida (SB)*, a congenital disorder that results in incomplete development of the spinal cord; and *cystic fibrosis (CF)*, a genetic disorder that changes how the body makes mucus and sweat.

Down syndrome is a genetic disorder in which a baby is born with an extra full or partial copy of chromosome 21. The presence of this extra genetic material results in developmental changes related to brain and body development. Life expectancy for people with Down syndrome has improved over the years, and today, a person with Down syndrome often lives to 60 years of age.

People who have Down syndrome have distinct facial and body features, including a flat face; small ears; slanted eyes; a small mouth; and a short neck, arms, and legs. Down syndrome may lead to physical disabilities related to poor muscle tone and loose joints. These disabilities can be improved with physical therapy. Down syndrome also causes intellectual disabilities and respiratory, cardiac, GI, and hearing problems. Adults who have Down syndrome experience premature aging and may

---

THINK ABOUT THIS

Thirty-six million people in the United States have at least one disability. The rights of people with disabilities are protected by federal and state laws and must be respected and protected. Examples of these rights include the right to life, equality before the law, freedom of expression, the right to education and work, and the right to self-determination.

show symptoms of early-onset Alzheimer's disease (occurring before age 65). Symptoms can include a decline in the ability to pay attention, less interest in social activities and interaction, changes in coordination, fearfulness, irritability, and memory loss.

What Are Developmental Disabilities?

Developmental disabilities are a group of conditions that occur during a child's development and result in physical, learning, language, or behavioral impairment. These disabilities affect people throughout their lifetimes. In this section, you will learn about the effects of several developmental disabilities, including cerebral palsy (CP), autism spectrum disorder (ASD), and fragile X syndrome (FXS). Knowing about these disabilities will help you understand how they affect residents who may have them.

Cerebral Palsy (CP)

Cerebral palsy (CP) is a disability that does not change over time and affects movement, muscle tone, and posture. It is typically caused by damage to the developing fetal brain or complications at birth, and is one of the most common causes of chronic childhood disability. Risk factors for CP include infections during pregnancy (such as rubella, or *German measles*); birth injuries; limited or poor oxygen supply to the baby's brain before, during, or immediately after birth; and prematurity. CP can also develop during early childhood as a result of brain injury due to severe illness (such as meningitis), extensive physical trauma, or serious dehydration. Life expectancy with CP depends on the severity of the disorder. People with mild CP have the same life expectancy as the general population.

The physical disabilities associated with CP vary. There may be some combination of abnormal posture, impaired mobility, muscle stiffness, abnormal reflexes and involuntary movements, and imbalance of the eye muscles (**Figure 21.9**). People with CP may also have swallowing problems, epilepsy, vision or hearing impairments, intellectual disabilities, or learning disorders.

The goal of CP treatment is to maximize abilities and physical strength, prevent complications, and improve quality of life. Specific treatments will vary depending on need, but usually include physical and

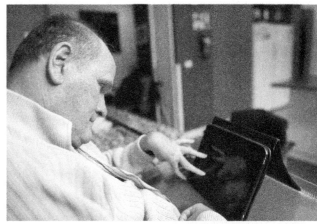

GaryRadler/Essentials collection via Getty Images

Figure 21.9 CP can result in impaired mobility and abnormal reflexes, depending on the severity of the disorder.

speech therapy; the use of assistive equipment, such as special shoes, crutches, *orthotics* (artificial devices such as splints and braces), casts, special seats, walkers, and wheelchairs; massage therapy; yoga and breathing exercises; biofeedback; medications; surgery; and pain relief. Some people with CP also benefit from behavioral therapy and occupational therapy, which promotes independent living.

Autism Spectrum Disorder (ASD)

Autism spectrum disorder (ASD) is a developmental disability that can cause considerable social, communication, and behavioral challenges. ASD includes a wide range, or *spectrum*, of symptoms and levels of disability.

ASD affects how a person communicates, behaves, and learns. There are often no distinguishing physical characteristics. The signs of ASD begin in early childhood and last throughout life. Signs and symptoms include:

- having trouble relating to or not having interest in others
- avoiding eye contact and wanting to be alone
- repeating or echoing communicated words or phrases
- repeating words or phrases in place of normal language
- repeating actions over and over again
- having trouble understanding other people's feelings or sharing feelings
- generally preferring not to be held or cuddled
- struggling to express needs using typical words or emotions

People with ASD have a wide range of skill levels. Some need a great deal of assistance to manage their lives, while others do not. Treatments for ASD include behavioral and communication approaches (such as auditory training); music, occupational, and physical therapy; dietary changes (such as removing certain foods from the diet or using vitamin or mineral supplements); and medications to manage symptoms such as lack of focus or possible depression.

Fragile X Syndrome (FXS)

Fragile X syndrome (FXS) is a genetic disorder caused by a change in the fragile X mental retardation 1 (FMR1) gene. This gene makes fragile X mental retardation protein (FMRP), which is needed for normal brain development. There is no cure for FXS, and males with FXS often have mild to severe intellectual disability. Females with FXS can have average intelligence, but may experience some degree of intellectual disability. ASD also occurs more frequently with people who have FXS.

Signs and symptoms of FXS may include developmental delays (such as missing a milestone for sitting or walking), trouble learning new skills, lack of eye contact, and difficulty paying attention. People with FXS may also be very active, flap their hands, and speak without thinking.

Treatment for FXS includes a variety of therapies that help with walking, talking, and other forms of communication. The goal is to help these residents achieve as much independence as possible. Medications may be used to help control behavioral issues, such as lack of focus or activity.

How Can Nursing Assistants Deliver Care After Trauma and Injury?

Trauma and injury can have a large impact on a person's physical and cognitive abilities. Many parts of the body can be damaged due to injury. Soft tissues and organs can be injured, and neurological and skeletal damage can lead to *amputation* (the loss of a portion or all of an arm or a leg). These injuries are considered emergencies, and the goal of treatment is restoration and rehabilitation of function.

Two types of serious injury you may see as a nursing assistant are traumatic brain injury (TBI) and spinal cord injury (SCI). These injuries can result in loss of consciousness or a coma, partial or total paralysis, and the need to use a mechanical **ventilator** to breathe.

Traumatic Brain Injury (TBI)

Traumatic brain injury (TBI) is an acute injury to the brain. TBI can be caused by a car accident, a bullet, a fall, assault, sports and combat injuries, tumors, infections, a stroke, and *deceleration injuries* (in which the brain hits the inside of the skull, causing contusion and swelling). Hypoxia can also cause TBI due to lack of oxygen in the brain.

After a TBI, the extent of brain injury may not be understood until several days, weeks, or months later. Brain injury can cause physical disabilities, mental and cognitive impairments, headaches, difficulty thinking, memory loss, changes in attention, mood swings, and personality changes. TBI can also result in a coma. It can lead to limited function or **paralysis** (loss of function and feeling) of the arms and legs, loss of cognition, and abnormal speech or language patterns. TBI can also cause secondary brain injuries due to bleeding in the skull, increased pressure and in the skull (**Figure 21.10**), swelling, and infection in the case of an open head injury.

TBIs range from mild to severe, depending on loss of consciousness and level of confusion. Treatment depends on the level and severity of TBI, and may require surgery. Recovery is usually long and challenging. The effects of TBI can be overwhelming for a resident and his or her family.

Spinal Cord Injury (SCI)

Spinal cord injury (SCI) is damage to any part of the spinal cord, vertebrae, discs, nerves, or the ligaments located at the end of the spine. SCI usually causes permanent changes, such as paralysis at the site of

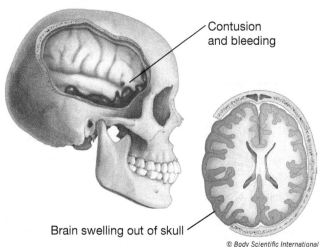

© Body Scientific International

Figure 21.10 Increased pressure and bleeding in the skull can increase the severity of a brain injury.

the injury. SCI often causes problems with body systems affected by that site (for example, loss of bladder or bowel control).

SCI can be caused by a fall, a blow to the back from a car accident or sports injury, a bullet, or a knife wound that severs, or cuts, the spinal cord. Changes in bone density or structure, cancer, or degeneration of the vertebral discs due to aging may cause SCI. Damage can also occur if there is inflammation, bleeding, or swelling from fluid around the spinal cord.

Extreme pain or pressure in the neck, head, or back; weakness; numbness; loss of movement and sensation; spasms; difficulty breathing or coughing; loss of bladder or bowel control; and changes in sexual function are all possible symptoms of SCI. The location and severity of the SCI determine how much arm or leg control is lost (**Figure 21.11**). If all movement and feeling are lost below the injury, the injury is considered complete. If only some function or sensation below the injury is lost, the SCI is incomplete.

Treatment for SCI starts with immediate emergency attention to the injury. A resident who has experienced SCI may be placed on a *mechanical ventilator* to support breathing (**Figure 21.12**). The mechanical ventilator is attached to an endotracheal (ET) tube inserted into the trachea through the mouth or a *tracheostomy* (surgical opening in the trachea). If the resident's breathing patterns change, a ventilator alarm will sound.

Licensed nursing staff members have total responsibility for caring for residents with SCI. Nursing assistants can assist by providing proper care, accurate observation, and immediate reports of any changes to the licensed nursing staff. The care given by nursing assistants may include:

- being alert to the ventilator alarm and reporting it immediately
- monitoring vital signs, as ordered, to make sure they remain stable
- assisting the licensed nursing staff with suctioning (removing secretions and mucus from) the ET tube and enteral feedings or IVs
- performing routine oral and skin care
- alerting the licensed nursing staff if the resident is or appears to be in pain
- following facility restraint procedures, if needed, to prevent the resident from pulling out or dislodging the tubes

- maintaining a safe environment
- providing positioning and range-of-motion (ROM) activities, as directed
- keeping all equipment clean

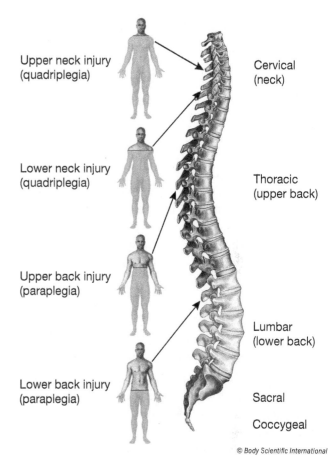

© Body Scientific International

Figure 21.11 Paralysis from SCI is classified according to the areas are affected. *Quadriplegia* (also called *tetraplegia*) is paralysis of the arms, trunk, legs, and pelvic organs. *Paraplegia* is paralysis of the trunk, legs, and pelvic organs.

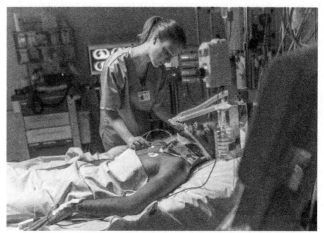

simonkr/Signature collection via Getty Images

Figure 21.12 Mechanical ventilators aid a resident's breathing. This aid can be extremely important for a resident who has experienced an SCI.

Residents on a mechanical ventilator are not able to speak. You may be able to communicate using lip reading, blinking the eyes when asked questions that require a yes or no (for example, one blink for yes and two blinks for no), pointing, using a picture board, or writing messages.

SCI cannot be reversed. After immediate intervention, longer-term treatment focuses on preventing further injury and helping people have full and active lives. Lifestyle changes after SCI might include changes in diet and fluids to prevent dehydration and weight loss, bladder and bowel retraining (discussed in Chapter 20), heightened attention to skin care to prevent decubitus ulcers, and pain relief. Residents who have experienced SCI may need assistance with mobility to prevent deep vein thrombosis (DVT) and muscle spasticity (uncontrolled tightening or movement) or flaccidity (lack of muscle tone). Changes in sexual function and depression due to impairment may also be a concern and require intervention.

Caring for Residents after TBI or SCI

As a nursing assistant, you will care for residents who have experienced TBI and SCI. These residents may need assistive equipment such as ramps, special sinks, and grab bars to help with mobility and ADLs. You may take vital signs; perform good skin and oral care; observe monitors, IVs, and tubes for possible changes or problems; provide wound care; and help with mobility to prevent DVT.

Be aware of and sensitive to the feelings of residents in your care. In just one day, one hour, or one minute, the TBI or SCI has changed the resident's life drastically. This is a difficult experience for everyone involved. The help you provide can aid the injured resident and his or her family with recovery. Usually, the injury is followed by feelings of denial and disbelief. These feelings are often followed by sadness and anger, and there may be a period of grief and mourning. The hoped-for outcome is acceptance.

Paralysis is a common result of TBI and SCI. As a holistic nursing assistant, you will care for residents who have varying levels of paralysis and who may be in a wheelchair. As you deliver care to these residents, follow these guidelines:

- Think about your own beliefs and assumptions about residents who are paralyzed and who need to use a wheelchair.

- Always focus on the resident in your care and not on the disability.
- Consider each resident's special needs, because residents will have different capabilities.
- Be respectful. Never talk down to a resident or pat him or her on the head. Speak to the resident directly, and if the conversation lasts longer than a few minutes, find a seat so you can have level eye contact with the resident (**Figure 21.13**).
- Always ask a resident if assistance is needed before attempting to help. Do not rob a resident of his or her independence.
- If a resident is not sitting in his or her wheelchair, be sure the wheelchair is nearby.
- Never hang or lean on a wheelchair. Remember that a wheelchair is an important part of a resident's personal life space.

What Is Delirium and What Are Its Challenges?

A *cognitive disorder* causes difficulty thinking, remembering, learning, processing and understanding information, and displaying appropriate behavior in public settings. Some cognitive disorders are treatable, and others are permanent. Treatable cognitive disorders are called *delirium*.

Delirium is usually caused by acute medical conditions, such as meningitis, urinary tract infections (UTIs), electrolyte imbalances, metabolic and endocrine disorders, and heatstroke. Delirium can also be caused by medications and **intoxication** (caused by overuse) or withdrawal from a substance. The change

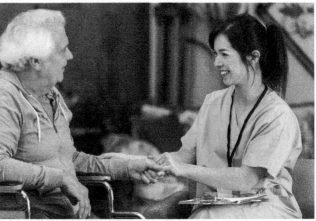

Steve Debenport/Signature via Getty Images
Figure 21.13 When talking with a resident in a wheelchair, sit down so you can maintain level eye contact.

BECOMING A HOLISTIC NURSING ASSISTANT

Caring for a Resident in a Coma

After a TBI, some residents may experience a *coma*, or a state of continuing unconsciousness. The length of the coma may vary; some residents will not regain consciousness. Whatever level of consciousness a resident has, it is important to provide safe, quality care and be aware of the following guidelines:

- **Learn how to effectively communicate with residents in a coma:** Establish a calm, supportive, and respectful environment. Remember that all resident rights apply to someone in a coma. Never talk about, around, or above someone in a coma. Rather, talk with the resident, even if you receive no response. Observe for small changes, such as a slight movement of a finger or toe, a quick noise, or the opening or closing of eyes. When the eyes are open, the resident may be able to see and follow movements.

- **Assume hearing is the last sense to go:** Always knock when entering the room and tell the resident who you are. Never leave a room without telling the resident you are leaving. Speak in a normal voice and tone, keep sentences short, and do not shout. You may read, sing, or play the resident's favorite music, as appropriate. Always ask for permission to do a procedure, even if the

resident cannot respond. Introduce yourself and let the resident know what you are doing step by step. If there is too much noise in the room (for example, a television), turn off the source of the noise. Touch can be helpful, but be sure to tell residents you are going to touch them. Hold residents' hands as you talk with them. If appropriate, massage their arms, legs, hands, and feet.

- **Know that residents in comas may feel pain:** Ask the comatose resident whether he or she is in pain. Residents may be able to answer using minimal communication. You can also observe for signs of pain, such as tears in the eyes.

Displaying personal photos in the room may help the resident. Keeping a comments book in the room for caregivers and family members to record any observed changes is another helpful approach. Remember that, during recovery, there is much to do and learn.

Apply It

1. What challenges would you face in providing holistic care to someone who is not conscious? How could you overcome these challenges?
2. What personal skills do you have that might help you effectively care for a resident in a coma?

---

in cognition is the result of an interruption in the brain's ability to create and use energy, or from altered chemical messengers in the brain and nervous system. One type of delirium, known as *delirium not otherwise specified (NOS)*, can result from sensory deprivation (decrease or removal of one or more of the senses, such as sight or sound) or follow the use of general anesthesia. Older adults are most at risk for delirium.

Delirium is dramatic because of its sudden appearance. A person with delirium is confused; is not clear about the time of day; and experiences severe attention, memory, language, and perception problems.

It can sometimes be difficult to recognize differences between delirium and dementia, since they have many of the same symptoms. The difference is that delirium, when treated effectively, will go away. If left untreated, delirium can cause more serious and permanent brain damage.

How Can Nursing Assistants Care for Residents with Dementia?

Dementia is not a specific disease, but describes a range of symptoms that begin slowly and gradually

get worse. The most common form of dementia is *Alzheimer's disease (AD)*. There is no direct cause for AD, but genetics, lifestyle, and other environmental factors contribute to its development. *Vascular dementia*, another form, occurs when blood flow to the brain is interrupted. This can be caused by a stroke or develop slowly over time due to very small blockages or the slowing of blood flow. Symptoms of vascular dementia appear more suddenly than symptoms of AD. Some dementias are linked to diseases and disorders such as TBI or Parkinson's disease.

Dementia is caused by damage to brain cells, which results in changes in thinking, behavior, and feelings. This damage can occur in different parts of the brain. For example, in AD, cells in the brain's center for learning and memory (hippocampus) are the first to be damaged. For that reason, memory loss is one of AD's earliest symptoms.

Signs and Symptoms of Dementia

The signs and symptoms of dementia vary greatly and include cognitive, psychological, and physical changes. As time passes, symptoms become more noticeable. For example, there are three stages

Think About This

According to the World Health Organization (WHO), 50 million people worldwide have dementia, and there are 10 million new cases annually. Alzheimer's disease (AD) is the most common form of dementia and may contribute to 60–70 percent of cases. In the United States, more than 5 million people are living with AD, and this number will likely triple by 2050.

of progressing symptoms for residents with AD (**Figure 21.14**). Residents with AD usually live four to eight years after diagnosis, though some can live up to 20 years. Residents who have dementia often do not recognize its symptoms. Instead, symptoms are noticed and pointed out by family members or significant others.

Cognitive Changes

Cognitive changes worsen over time. Some of these changes include:

- memory loss (shown by asking repeatedly for the same information, misplacing objects, and not remembering where one is)
- decreased ability to reason or problem-solve (shown by working with numbers incorrectly or taking much longer to complete tasks)
- difficulty reading or driving
- inability to plan and organize
- poor judgment (shown by overspending money or making unneeded purchases)
- confusion about time, dates, and location
- trouble communicating, finding appropriate words, and following or joining a conversation
- noticeable changes in coordination and motor function

Psychological Changes

Dementia may also cause changes in personality and mood that can lead to resistance, anxiety, agitation, ***delusions*** (irrational beliefs), hallucinations (false or distorted sensory experiences), and ***paranoia*** (unsupported or exaggerated distrust). Depression is another possible symptom. Other psychological changes may lead to rummaging (anxiously looking for a personal item that may or may not be there), hoarding items, and sundowning. ***Sundowning*** occurs at the end of the day and lasts into the evening. A resident experiencing sundowning may have increased confusion, inability to follow directions, and anxiety (shown by pacing or wandering). Residents may also become physically aggressive (shown by hitting, pinching, scratching, biting, or hair pulling) and verbally aggressive (shown by screaming, swearing, shouting, or making threats).

Stages of Alzheimer's Disease ***(AD)***

Stage	Symptoms
Early-stage or mild	The resident is able to function independently, but may have memory lapses (for example, may not remember new names or forget material just read). The resident may also have problems planning or organizing information.
Middle-stage or moderate	This stage is the longest. Continuing damage to brain cells causes difficulty doing daily activities, frustration, and anger. Memory loss, confusion, and restlessness continue, and the resident may wander and become lost. Personality and mood changes may lead to repetitive and compulsive behaviors such as hand wringing. During this stage, more aggressive behavior may occur such as biting, hitting, or swearing. This is also the stage where there may be sexual aggression. Physical changes include trouble controlling bladder and bowel functions and alterations in sleep patterns.
Late-stage or severe	The resident is no longer able to effectively interact with the environment, carry on a normal conversation, or control movements (sitting, walking, and eventually swallowing). The resident may still communicate at a very basic level, but experiences great memory and cognitive losses. The resident needs full-time care for all ADLs, including bathing, dressing, oral hygiene, and toileting. This stage can lead to coma and death, usually from a respiratory infection.

Goodheart-Willcox Publisher

Figure 21.14 The symptoms of AD progress through three stages.

As dementia worsens, so does the aggression. It may be caused by insufficient sleep; pain; side effects from medications; a distracting, disorganized environment; loud noises; confusion; and reaction to caregiver stress. ***Perseveration*** is another psychological change in which a resident has an uncontrollable need to repeat a word, phrase, or gesture for no apparent reason.

Psychological changes during dementia also affect sexual behavior. For many older adults, including those living in long-term care facilities, sexuality remains an important part of life. The effects of dementia, along with other issues such as physical discomfort, may cause less interest in sex; heightened sexual drive; or inappropriate sexual behavior such as disrobing, exposure, masturbation, and fondling. These inappropriate sexual behaviors often occur as a result of confusion or disorientation. A resident may think he or she is at home in the privacy of a bedroom rather than in a public setting. Lack of control can also cause residents to act out their sexual urges with unwilling and inappropriate partners. Inappropriate sexual behaviors such as these can be embarrassing, frightening, and disturbing for a resident's family members, other residents, and caregivers.

As a nursing assistant, you may find responding to inappropriate sexual behaviors difficult. If a resident displays an inappropriate sexual behavior, be respectful, understanding, calm, and patient. Firmly but gently inform the resident that the behavior is inappropriate and guide the resident to a private area. Use distraction or redirect the resident to more positive activities, such as taking a walk or eating a favorite snack. Be sure to report any inappropriate sexual behaviors to the licensed nursing staff. These behaviors are important symptoms and signal changes in the resident's condition.

As dementia progresses, more advanced psychological changes can develop. One of these advanced psychological changes is shadowing. *Shadowing* occurs when a resident follows a caregiver's every move due to increased dependency on the caregiver (**Figure 21.15**).

Physical Changes

Physical changes also happen as a result of dementia. Issues with nutrition can develop from residents' inability to chew and swallow. Residents may also experience problems breathing if they choke on or aspirate food while eating. Choking and aspiration affect the respiratory system and may result in pneumonia. Falling is another physical challenge

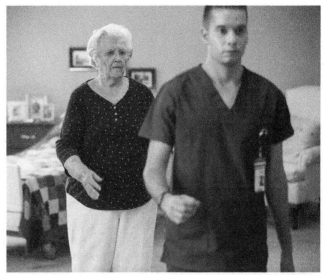

© Tori Soper Photography

Figure 21.15 As dementia progresses, residents may begin to shadow caregivers by following their every move. The resident believes that staying close to the caregiver will fulfill her need for comfort and safety.

that may happen as residents begin to lose their motor abilities. Maintaining a safe environment becomes a main focus of care.

Treatment for Dementia

Treatment for dementia focuses on managing symptoms; maintaining as many daily functions as possible; and providing relief and improving quality of life. The goal of care is to support the resident's current abilities. Many residents with dementia stay in long-term care facilities. Other residents are placed in special care or memory units, often during later stages.

Prescribed medications may improve some symptoms of dementia. These medications often have side effects that result in gastrointestinal problems or dizziness.

Physical activity to help with sleep and reduce agitation; massage therapy; light therapy (exposure to bright light) for depression and sleep disorders; doll, cuddle, or toy therapy to bring back happy memories; and music and art therapy (including dance, drawing, and painting) may also help. Integrative medicine (IM) approaches include the use of aromatherapy and dietary and herbal supplements, although scientific evidence is limited. Therapy animals have been shown to improve mood. The unconditional love expressed by a dog and the petting of its fur often helps to calm residents with dementia and promote appropriate behaviors (**Figure 21.16**).

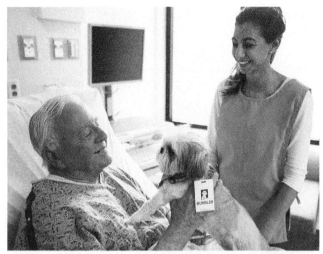

Figure 21.16 Contact with specially trained animals can help calm residents with dementia.

Caring for Residents with Dementia

The greatest ongoing benefit to residents with dementia is safe, quality care. As a holistic nursing assistant, you can help improve the daily life of a resident and help respond to symptoms and needs.

Understanding Symptoms

Dementia symptoms are caused by organic brain cell damage. Residents with dementia may also experience pain, infection, constipation, lack of sleep, and physical and psychological reactions to prescribed medications. They may display a variety of behaviors, which are often the result of unmet physical or social needs. Always try to identify and understand what might be causing these behaviors.

Residents with dementia may not know *why* they are doing or feeling something, but will always know *how* they are feeling. When caring for a resident with dementia, try to determine if pain is the cause of a behavior. If it is, alert the licensed nursing staff.

Never take the behavior of residents with dementia personally, but be sure to protect yourself from personal danger and step back or stand away if residents are physically aggressive.

Respecting Individuality

As a holistic nursing assistant, be sure to respect the individuality of residents and focus on them as people. Use the plan of care to guide activities and provide as much independence as is possible and safe. Using reasoning and logic likely will not affect residents' behaviors, as residents are no longer able to reason or use logic themselves.

Never try to restrain residents, even if they are physically aggressive. Instead, give them space and use distraction or redirection (for example, agreeing with what they are saying and suggesting a different activity). For example, a resident may shout and start to move others out of the way, saying, "I am late to work, so I need to hurry!" To affirm (or agree with), you can say, "I will drive you to work so you won't be late," and then use redirection by saying, "but let's eat breakfast first."

Staying Calm and Professional

Maintain a calm, professional attitude, and be positive and reassuring. Do not express anxiety, fear, or anger about a resident's behavior and keep an even tone of voice, because loud noises can cause aggressive responses. Maintain eye contact with residents and calmly explain why you are there and what is needed. Do not argue, criticize, or punish. Use proper body language to demonstrate respect and listen carefully, particularly when the resident is losing language skills. Smile, touch gently, and hug, when appropriate.

Keep instructions simple, break them down into steps, and wait between questions for answers. Never rush. Use closed-ended questions such as "Would you like to wear this sweater today?" This approach can keep confusion and stress to a minimum. However, if residents can still make independent decisions, offering choices is important.

Providing Cues

Use *cues*, or actions that invite responses. Verbal cues might be simple words such as "Roll to the right" or "Stand up," followed with praise such as "Great job." If verbal cues are not successful, use visual and manual cues, such as demonstrating a step or touching an item (**Figure 21.17**). For example, you could point to or tap a

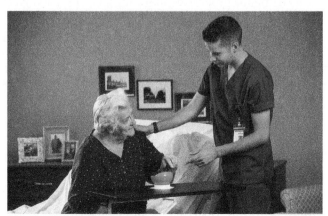

Figure 21.17 Using visual and manual cues can help residents with dementia understand you.

drinking glass that contains water you want a resident to drink. Be sure the resident is paying attention to and can see the cue. You can use a *hand-over-hand cue* to help with ADLs in later stages of dementia. For example, with a light touch, you could place your hand over the resident's hand while holding a utensil and begin the act of feeding (**Figure 21.18**). Always give praise to show the resident he or she is doing a good job.

Maintaining a Comfortable and Safe Environment

Maintaining a safe, familiar, comfortable, organized, clutter-free, simple, and quiet environment reduces overstimulation and helps prevent agitation or aggression. Make sure the resident's personal items are easy to find. Label drawers and cabinets with easy-to-use memory cues (such as an image of and the word *underwear*) to help residents find specific items. Pictures and words placed in clear sight can aid recognition and decrease agitation. Monitoring systems are used to alert caregivers when a resident is wandering away from their room and into areas that may be unsafe. Also, make sure any potentially hazardous personal care items are removed. This includes mouthwash, which contains alcohol. A confused resident might easily drink a bottle of mouthwash.

Maintain a routine schedule for ADLs to reduce confusion. Identify the time of day when the resident is most alert so you can more easily communicate and perform tasks during this time.

Incorporating Positive Activities

Activities that stimulate the mind and senses can improve memory, communication skills, and social interaction and decrease boredom, inactivity, and sensory deprivation. Activities should be based on a resident's changing abilities and interests. Relaxing activities, such as turning on favorite music, may be particularly helpful during the time of day a resident shows more aggressive behaviors. Residents who have delusions may benefit from a hand massage, since touch can be grounding and comforting.

Encouraging the resident to recall positive memories may help improve his or her mood. In dementia, long-term memories fade more slowly than short-term memories, so asking about past experiences can reduce stress. Conversations should be personal, positive, and important to the resident. Sometimes making a memory box of photographs and other familiar items or a life story book can be helpful. Residents can review these by themselves or with family members.

Some residents benefit from *validation therapy*. In validation therapy, a resident's values, beliefs, and reality are validated (confirmed). This approach focuses on agreeing with and then redirecting residents to reduce stress and maintain balance. Feelings and emotions should be addressed first, even if they do not make sense. For example, if a resident is afraid of losing a precious picture, you might provide a box to store the photo. If a resident states that she is angry after her deceased mother's visit last evening, you might say, "I understand why you might feel that way."

Communicating with Family Members and the Licensed Nursing Staff

As a nursing assistant, you will work closely with members of the licensed nursing staff and the resident's family to observe changes and understand the resident's condition. As dementia progresses, you can ask family members to assist with activities and approaches (**Figure 21.19**). Always observe, report, and document behavioral changes (such as increased aggression,

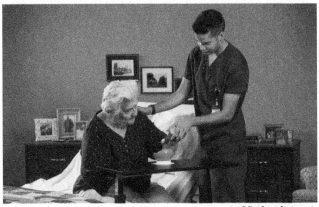

© Tori Soper Photography

Figure 21.18 Using the hand-over-hand cue can enable you to guide a resident's hand and promote eating.

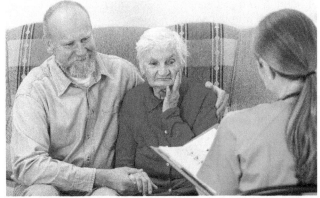

Ocskay Bence/Shutterstock.com

Figure 21.19 Reviewing the plan of care with the resident and his or her family involves the family to make sure their care is resident centered.

confusion, or wandering) and the effectiveness of actions taken. Observations and documentation are important to maintaining and ensuring an appropriate, effective, resident-centered plan of care.

Caring for residents with dementia is not easy, particularly when residents are in late stages.

Taking care of yourself is important. Use self-care approaches and strategies such as getting good nutrition and exercise, finding ways to relax at home, and talking about your feelings with appropriate people. This will help you have the energy and patience to care for others.

SECTION 21.2 **Review and Assessment**

Key Terms Mini Glossary

cerebral palsy (CP) a disability that affects movement, muscle tone, and posture; typically caused by damage to the developing fetal brain.

cues actions that invite a response; may be verbal or manual and can guide resident behavior.

cystic fibrosis (CF) a genetic disorder that changes how the body makes mucus and sweat; characterized by congestion, difficult digestion, and salty sweat.

delusions irrational belief that something is true, even when there is overwhelming proof that it is not.

intoxication a condition of reduced control caused by the overuse of a chemical substance.

legal blindness a refractive error of 20/200, even after vision correction.

paralysis the loss of function and feeling in one or more muscle groups.

paranoia an unsupported or exaggerated distrust of others.

perseveration uncontrollable need to repeat a word, phrase, or gesture for no apparent reason.

spina bifida (SB) a congenital disorder resulting in incomplete development of the spinal cord.

sundowning increased confusion, inability to follow directions, and anxiety (shown by pacing or wandering) that occurs at the end of the day and lasts into the evening.

ventilator a device used to mechanically aid breathing.

Apply the Key Terms

Describe the differences between each pair of key terms.

1. paranoia and delusions
2. cystic fibrosis and cerebral palsy
3. perseveration and sundowning
4. intoxication and ventilator
5. cues and paralysis

Know and Understand the Facts

1. Identify two types of vision impairment, hearing impairment, and speech impairment.
2. What is the difference between congenital and genetic disorders?
3. Explain three guidelines to follow when caring for residents with TBI or SCI.
4. Identify two guidelines to follow when caring for a resident who is paralyzed.
5. Compare and contrast delirium and dementia.
6. Discuss two cognitive, psychological, and physical changes that may occur in dementia.

Analyze and Apply Concepts

1. Give one example of a method you could use to communicate with a resident on a mechanical ventilator.
2. Explain three important ways to care for residents in a coma.
3. Describe four specific actions a holistic nursing assistant can take when caring for residents with dementia.

4. How can a nursing assistant practice self-care while caring for a resident with dementia?

Think Critically

Read the following care situation. Then answer the questions that follow.

Mrs. K, an 84-year-old widow with seven children who live nearby, has been in the long-term care facility in which you work for one year. She was diagnosed with Alzheimer's disease (AD) and has functioned fairly well over the time you have cared for her. Lately, Mrs. K's memory loss and confusion have been increasing, and she seems much more restless. Mrs. K has been incontinent the last few days, and is very embarrassed about it. She is also frustrated because she can't find things she is sure she put away. Mrs. K's children are very concerned and upset over the changes in their mother.

1. In what stage of AD do you think Mrs. K is?
2. How would you respond to Mrs. K's embarrassment?
3. What could you do to help with Mrs. K's continuing loss of memory and confusion?
4. What three actions could you take to care for and maintain Mrs. K's ADLs?
5. List three safety and comfort guidelines you could put in place when caring for Mrs. K.
6. In what ways might you support Mrs. K's children and help them be involved in her care?

Key Points

Reviewing the key points for this chapter will help you practice more safely and competently as a holistic nursing assistant and will help you prepare for the certification competency examination.

- Mental health conditions cause changes in thinking (cognition), mood (emotions), and behaviors and can cause distress and limited or difficult functioning.
- Proper support and safe, quality care can help improve quality of life for residents with disabilities or cognitive disorders.
- A disability is a limitation of function due to aging, a disease process, a congenital or genetic disorder, injury, or trauma.
- Cognitive disorders such as dementia cause trouble with thinking, remembering, learning, processing and understanding information, and displaying appropriate behavior in social settings.
- Observing, reporting, and documenting physical and behavioral changes is important to maintaining the plan of care.

Action Steps to Holistic Care

Review the information in this chapter. Complete the following activities.

1. Select one disability you learned about in this chapter. Prepare a short paper or digital presentation that identifies and describes the top three most important issues surrounding care. Include one that promotes comfort and one that maintains safety.
2. With a partner, select one emotional health concern or mental health condition discussed in the chapter. Prepare a poster that shows at least four facts that residents and the public should know.
3. Research current scientific information about one physical disability, emotional health concern, or mental health condition not discussed in this chapter. Write a brief report that describes two current facts about the disability, concern, or condition.
4. Prepare a poster or digital presentation about caring for residents with dementia. Include a description of the disease, treatment options, and important actions to take when caring for residents with dementia.

Building Math Skill

An estimated 17.3 million adults in the United States have had at least one major depressive episode. If there are 209,128,094 people over 18 in the United States, what percent of adults have had at least one major depressive episode?

Preparing for the Certification Competency Examination

To prepare for the nursing assistant certification competency examination, you will need to know content found in this chapter. This content may be tested in the knowledge (written or oral) and skills (hands-on demonstration) portions of the exam. The following areas will be emphasized:

- vision, hearing, and speech impairments or loss
- levels of consciousness
- communication with comatose residents and ventilator care
- needs and behaviors of residents with cognitive disorders
- appropriate responses to difficult behaviors
- appropriate and inappropriate expressions of sexual behavior
- interventions used to reduce the effects of cognitive disorders
- the differences between mental health and illness
- appropriate care for common mental health conditions
- physical and verbal aggression
- mental status and behavior changes

These sample test questions are similar to ones you will find on the certification competency exam. See how well you can answer them. Be sure to select the *best* answer.

1. Someone who has achieved good mental and emotional health is
   A. overconfident
   B. balanced
   C. inactive
   D. unsure

2. A reversible cognitive disorder is called
   A. bipolar disorder
   B. dementia
   C. delirium
   D. depression

(Continued)

3. A new nursing assistant will be taking care of Mr. X, who has a hearing impairment. Today he is not wearing his hearing aid. What is the best approach the nursing assistant can take?
   A. tell Mr. X he must wear his hearing aid
   B. talk as loudly as possible so Mr. X can hear her
   C. ask Mr. X's family to purchase him a new, more comfortable aid
   D. always face Mr. X when talking

4. While talking with Mr. R, you notice how depressed he has become. Mr. R asks you to call his daughter so she can see him. He wants to talk about his will and say goodbye to her. What should you do next?
   A. He wants to put his affairs in order, so you should call his daughter immediately.
   B. He may be thinking about suicide, so you should alert the licensed nursing staff.
   C. He is a very organized man and wants to be sure all is settled, so you should do nothing.
   D. He is feeling sad and wants to see his daughter, so you should call her.

5. Mr. T knows what he wants to say, but just can't get the words out. What type of aphasia does he have?
   A. receptive
   B. anomic
   C. global
   D. expressive

6. Which of the following happens during sundowning?
   A. A resident becomes more confused at the end of the day.
   B. A resident is very tired and lethargic at the end of the day.
   C. A resident has more clarity at the end of the day.
   D. A resident is happier at the end of the day.

7. Mr. E had a car accident and suffered a TBI. He is still unconscious after 30 minutes. He is likely
   A. paralyzed
   B. in a coma
   C. bleeding
   D. going to have an amputation

8. When caring for a resident with vision impairment, what should a holistic nursing assistant do?
   A. tell the resident to be careful when going to the toilet
   B. keep the bed linens and towels in their proper place
   C. practice safety by making sure there are no obstacles
   D. keep the room clean and tidy at all times

9. Mrs. M has false and distorted sensory experiences that seem real to her. These are called
   A. delusions
   B. hallucinations
   C. depression
   D. phobias

10. A nursing assistant is taking care of a resident in a coma for the first time. What is one guideline she should keep in mind?
    A. talk loudly in case the resident can still hear
    B. never sing or read to an unresponsive resident
    C. never talk about, around, or above the resident
    D. keep looking for the resident's eyes to open

11. Which of the following is a cognitive change in dementia?
    A. inability to chew or swallow
    B. physical or verbal aggression
    C. memory loss and confusion
    D. delusions and phobias

12. What is a mental health condition?
    A. changes in thinking, mood, or behaviors that limit or impair function
    B. reversible changes to cognition that do not affect function
    C. irreversible impairments that change function and daily activities
    D. changes in the body systems that limit or impair the senses

13. Which is the most common mental health condition?
    A. anxiety disorder
    B. depression
    C. bipolar disorder
    D. suicide

14. If someone has an SCI and can move his arms, but not his legs, he has
    A. omniplegia
    B. quadriplegia
    C. paraplegia
    D. tetraplegia

15. Mrs. B has bipolar disorder. What symptoms might you see?
    A. hallucinations and then delusions
    B. rage and then irritability
    C. sadness and then phobias
    D. increased energy and then fatigue

Did you have difficulty with any of the questions? If you did, review the chapter to find the correct answer(s).

22 End-of-Life Care

Welcome to the Chapter

This chapter will provide you with information about the views and attitudes people have about dying and death and about the decisions people make about the end of their life. Family traditions and spiritual and religious beliefs play an important role in these decisions. Think about your views of dying and death, and how these views will influence the care you give as a holistic nursing assistant. You must treat residents and their families with dignity, offer compassion, and provide resources that may be needed. In this chapter, you will also learn about the signs of dying and impending death, loss, the stages of grief, advance directives, and organ donation. You will learn how to provide personal care and support during the process of dying and after death (called *postmortem care*).

The information and procedures presented in this chapter will help you build the knowledge and skills needed to become a holistic nursing assistant. Check with your instructor to ensure these procedures are within your state's regulations for nursing assistant practice. The topics discussed in the chapter are highlighted on the Providing Holistic Care Framework.

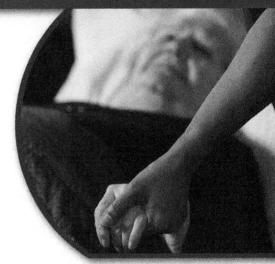

© Tori Soper Photography

Chapter Outline

Section 22.1
Dying, Death, and Grief

Section 22.2
Family Support and Postmortem Care

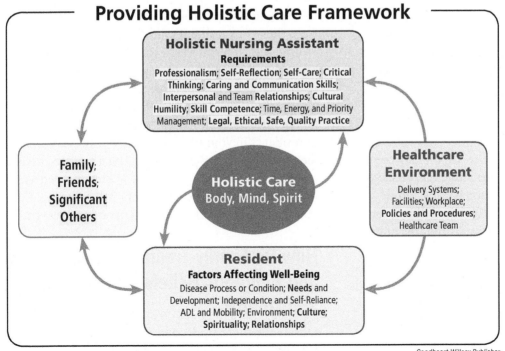

Providing Holistic Care Framework

Holistic Nursing Assistant
Requirements
Professionalism; Self-Reflection; Self-Care; Critical Thinking; Caring and Communication Skills; Interpersonal and Team Relationships; Cultural Humility; Skill Competence; Time, Energy, and Priority Management; Legal, Ethical, Safe, Quality Practice

Family; Friends; Significant Others

Holistic Care
Body, Mind, Spirit

Healthcare Environment
Delivery Systems; Facilities; Workplace; Policies and Procedures; Healthcare Team

Resident
Factors Affecting Well-Being
Disease Process or Condition; Needs and Development; Independence and Self-Reliance; ADL and Mobility; Environment; Culture; Spirituality; Relationships

Goodheart-Willcox Publisher

Dying, Death, and Grief

Objectives

To achieve the objectives for this section, you must successfully:

- **examine** your feelings and beliefs about dying and death.
- **describe** different traditions and beliefs about dying and death.
- **identify** behaviors related to loss and grief.
- **explain** the purpose and types of advance directives.
- **recognize** the changes that occur during the process of dying.
- **summarize** how to provide holistic care to residents who are dying.
- **examine** ways to support the family of the resident who is dying.
- **describe** how to pay attention to yourself as a caregiver of those who are dying.

Key Terms

Learn these key terms to better understand the information presented in the section.

advance directives	incapacitation
dignity	living will
do-not-resuscitate	mourn
(DNR) order	palliative care
grief	power of attorney

Questions to Consider

- Think about an experience you have had with dying and death. Has a family member, friend, or pet passed away? Was the death sudden or prolonged?
- What feelings did you have, and how did you express them? Was it difficult for you? What did you do to accept the death? Were any rituals, traditions, and decisions important to you or the deceased person?
- What resources provided comfort during this experience? Were the resources helpful, and in what ways?

We all experience the end of life. Death may come after an extended illness, after a long life, or suddenly. When death is nearing, a person is considered *terminally ill*. A person with a terminal illness can be reasonably expected to die in 24 months or less. Someone may be terminally ill due to an illness or condition such as end-stage cancer or kidney disease, heart failure, stroke, or chronic respiratory problems. Other people may die due to old age and organ system failure. Death is something we all have in common and all must face.

How Do You Feel About Dying and Death?

Examining your own feelings about dying and death will prepare you to assist others in their journeys at the end of life. Your feelings about dying and death are influenced by the experiences you had growing up, your family traditions, and spiritual or religious beliefs.

It can be helpful to write down the experiences you have had personally with dying and death. Do you feel comforted, or do you feel fearful or angry? Feelings of fear and anger are natural. We all have them.

If you do feel fear or anger, think about what might be causing these feelings. Maybe you believe it is not your time. Do you fear the unknown, dying alone, or severe pain? Or, perhaps you cannot bear the thought of leaving your loved ones.

It is important to reflect on your feelings about dying and death, because strong feelings can transfer to those in your care. If you are fearful, you may communicate fear to residents and their families through nonverbal behaviors such as not holding a resident's hand or avoiding the resident's room. You may also communicate these feelings verbally by not listening or not responding to residents and their families when they share *grief* (distress) about their impending (nearing) loss. As a result of your feelings, you may also have inappropriately strong responses to death and may not be able to separate your feelings from those of a resident's family (**Figure 22.1**).

One way to resolve feelings of fear and anger is to talk about them with someone you feel comfortable with, such as a friend or other healthcare staff member. Your feelings need to be resolved or managed so they do not influence or interfere with the lives and feelings of residents in your care. Another way to resolve these feelings is to learn more about the death-related beliefs and traditional practices of others. Your awareness of how others *mourn* (express grief) will help residents and their families feel better understood and respected.

How Do Family Traditions and Spiritual and Religious Beliefs Influence Dying and Death?

Different beliefs, traditions, and practices impact a person's experience of dying and death. They can

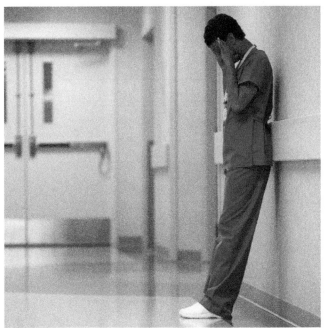

FangXiaNuo/Signature collection via Getty Images

Figure 22.1 If you have strong feelings about dying and death, these feelings could overwhelm you as you give care to residents who are terminally ill. Understanding and managing your feelings can help prevent this.

help those who are dying feel at peace and can also help mourners come to terms with death.

In Chapter 12, you learned about how different beliefs affect health and healthcare. Giving end-of-life care requires you to understand and respect the beliefs and traditional practices of different cultures and religious groups. Therefore, cultural humility and sensitivity are especially important.

The following sections provide an overview of some traditions, beliefs, and practices you may come across when delivering end-of-life care. These traditions, beliefs, and practices are discussed in a general way because individuals respond differently to dying and death and may interpret or follow traditional practices in their own ways.

Some residents' traditions, beliefs, and practices may be new to you, and you may not believe in them. It is still important that you respect these traditions, beliefs, and practices. The more you know about residents' beliefs, the better you will be able to provide support and care.

Family Traditions

Each family has unique traditions about dying and death. Often, these traditions are influenced by a family's cultural background and dynamics.

Following are some traditions you may observe in families facing dying and death:

- Some families do not discuss bad things such as death and believe that talking about bad things makes them happen.
- Some families believe that one should live intensely until death arrives. When people die, they move to a different phase of life, and the death should be accepted by all.
- In some families, a strong sense of community comes with loss. Extended family members gather at the time of death.
- In some families, females provide the majority of care for a person who is terminally ill.
- Some families believe that an older family member (sometimes the oldest son or closest relative) must be present at the time of death.
- Some families may resist leaving a loved one in a healthcare facility and prefer the person die at home with family members close.
- Some family members may cry and wail, while others may remain quiet and withdrawn.

Spiritual and Religious Beliefs

Many people rely on spirituality to understand death. For example, some people believe in the sacredness of life and consider the soul eternal. They may believe the souls of the dead pass into a spirit world. Thus, death is part of nature, is not to be feared, and is a journey to another world. Others believe the soul of the deceased travels safely, with the provisions it needs, to the afterlife. Spiritual beliefs and religious practices often influence decisions about burial, cremation, organ donation, and autopsy.

Every religion has its own unique practices and beliefs about death and dying. Some religions teach that there is an *afterlife*, or a life after death, potentially in another world. Other religions teach *reincarnation*, or the rebirth of the soul in another body. Residents who believe these teachings may find comfort in thinking they will continue to live in some way after death. Residents may seek comfort from a religious leader, complete specific predeath rituals, or find comfort in knowing loved ones will perform specific tasks after the moment of death. Prayers—either the resident's own or those of others—may also ease this difficult time.

Whatever a resident's religious beliefs may be, it is important to deliver respectful care. Special accommodations may be needed to help family members, friends, or religious leaders to complete religious practices

and rituals. Some religions also determine how the
body should be treated after death. There are many
resources that can help you understand the various
religious practices about death and dying. You may
also ask the resident, a family member, or a licensed
nursing staff member if you have any questions.

If you are ever uncomfortable discussing something
with a resident or find that your beliefs conflict with
what you are asked to do, you must discuss this with a
licensed nursing staff member to work out a solution.

How Are Loss and Grief Expressed?

We all experience loss and grief throughout life. Missing
an important event, losing a piece of jewelry, being
fired from a favorite job, ending a friendship, knowing
you are going to die soon, or experiencing the death
of a loved one may all cause frustration, sadness,
grief, or even anger. Loss is personal, causes change,
and brings feelings that need to be resolved. The
most important thing to remember about loss is that
it creates change in a person's life. What once was is
no longer, and when this occurs, most of us grieve.

Stages of Grief

According to Elisabeth Kübler-Ross, a Swiss-American
psychiatrist, all people experience five stages, or
patterns, of grief and mourning (**Figure 22.2**). These
stages are denial, anger, bargaining, depression, and
acceptance, and they are unique to each person. The
stages are not all experienced in the same order or
intensity. These five stages are the following:

1. **Denial**: people experience complete disbelief
   and describe themselves as being numb.
   They may become withdrawn, detached, and
   disoriented. This reaction helps people protect
   themselves from being completely overwhelmed.
   When the initial shock wears off, people may
   deny the reality of the situation or bad news by
   temporarily blocking it out or hiding from the
   facts. This allows people to push the news away
   and carries them through the first wave of pain.

Stages of Grief

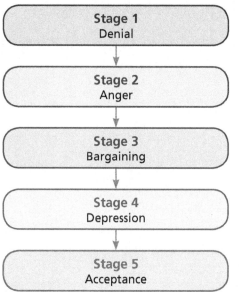

Goodheart-Willcox Publisher

Figure 22.2 The five stages of grief represent the way in which
residents may respond to dying and death.

2. **Anger**: pain is now expressed as anger. People
   may say, "Why me?" People may direct anger at
   themselves or at the person who is dying and
   leaving them.
3. **Bargaining:** as the person reacts to feelings of
   helplessness and vulnerability, he or she is trying
   to find a way to regain control. People may seek
   second and third medical opinions. They may
   try to make deals with a higher spiritual power to
   postpone death.
4. **Depression**: in this stage, the true extent of loss
   is realized, and feelings of depression develop.
   People understand that they or their loved ones
   won't get better, which brings feelings of sadness,
   despair, or regret. People may say, "I have not
   done all I wanted," or "I did not spend enough
   time with my family." People may also quietly
   prepare to say goodbye.
5. **Acceptance**: some people experience this stage
   faster than others. They may have come to peace
   with any concerns or issues about dying long
   ago. Others do not experience acceptance at all.
   Death may be sudden, or a person may never
   leave the denial or depression stage. When
   acceptance or hope does occur, time has passed,
   and the pain has lessened. People sense a new
   reality. What was can never be again, but there
   is a way to move forward. People who are dying
   can accept death, and those left behind can go on.

Holistic Care for Grieving Residents

Holistic nursing assistants can provide support through all five stages of grief. First, as a nursing assistant, recognize that residents' reactions are normal responses. Second, accept residents as they cope with the reality of the end of life. If a resident expresses anger toward you, do not take that anger personally. The resident is not angry at you, but with the situation. Reflect on the anger by saying, "Mrs. W, you seem very angry today." Then be prepared to talk with the resident about his or her anger.

When caring for grieving residents, use communication techniques such as mindfulness, active listening, open-ended questions, and reflection. These techniques will help support residents as they deal with grief. Also offer support by reassuring residents they will receive the care they need. Use gentle touch and silence to provide a sense of calmness and comfort, particularly during the depression stage (**Figure 22.3**). If a resident refuses food or medication, let the licensed nursing staff know so that guidance

can be provided. If appropriate, have the family bring in the resident's favorite foods.

Remember that, while all people experience dying and death, each person goes through the stages of grief in his or her own time and way. No two people or situations will be the same. For example, a younger person will respond differently to death than someone who is older and has experienced a long life.

Anticipatory Grief

Anticipatory grief is a reaction to *impending* (likely to happen) loss, as a person faces his or her own death or the death of a loved one. This type of grief is different from grief that occurs *after* death. Not everyone experiences anticipatory grief; however, anticipatory grief does provide the opportunity to resolve feelings before death and find closure. Anticipatory grief might include feelings of sadness, fear, anger, guilt, and denial. Feelings of anticipatory grief are difficult, but can help prepare a family for the grief that will come after a loved one dies.

Prolonged Grief

Prolonged grief, or *unresolved grief,* is grief that lasts more than one year after the death of a loved one and strongly influences a person's daily life and relationships. Prolonged grief may result from feelings of guilt about the loss. For example, a person may feel he or she did not do something important for the person or may believe it was his or her fault the person died. Prolonged grief may also result from a violent, traumatic loss. A person experiencing prolonged grief may refuse to talk about the loved one after death; become consumed by the memory of the person lost; be overly involved with work; show excessive concern about health; and start or increase addictive habits, such as drinking alcohol or smoking cigarettes. Children may express

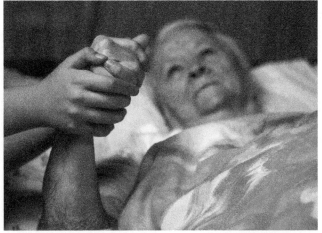

Volodymyr Baleha/Shutterstock.com

Figure 22.3 Gentle touch can help comfort a resident and provide a sense of calmness.

prolonged grief by having behavior problems or being afraid to be alone, particularly at night. People who experience prolonged grief may need help from a trained healthcare professional to break grief's cycle, move forward to acceptance, and resume life after the death of a loved one.

What Preparations Do People Make Before Death?

The *Patient Self-Determination Act (PSDA)* of 1990 gives people the control and autonomy to make decisions about end-of-life care. The PSDA also:

- requires that rights to control and autonomy be communicated in writing by the healthcare facility
- specifies that **advance directives** (legal documents containing medical and healthcare instructions) must be recognized and honored
- states that healthcare facilities must offer advance directives if residents do not have them
- requires that residents be told they have the right to refuse treatment

The PSDA does not usually affect doctors' offices, but does affect hospitals, long-term care facilities, and home healthcare agencies that receive Medicare and Medicaid reimbursement.

Advance directives are legal documents under the jurisdiction of state law. They provide instructions for medical treatment, healthcare, and preferences at the end of life. Advance directives may be handwritten or written and stored electronically. Some doctors and healthcare facilities provide advance directive forms that can be completed, sometimes with the help of an attorney.

Advance directives are legal documents that must follow specific requirements outlined in state law. For example, they must include the right to accept or refuse medical or surgical treatment. These documents should be kept in a safe, accessible place, and copies should be given to a doctor and to the agent or representative in case of **incapacitation** (lack of ability to make decisions). A copy of the advance directive should also be placed in the resident's health record.

Advance directives include a living will, a do-not-resuscitate (DNR) order, and power of attorney. These directives provide instructions about end-of-life care and identify a representative or agent to carry out the instructions if the resident who is dying is unable.

Living Will

A **living will** details the desired medical treatment in the event of incapacitation during a terminal illness or permanent unconsciousness (**Figure 22.4**). The living will specifies what types of *life-prolonging medical treatments* (treatments that extend life, such as tube feeding to maintain nutrition or measures that prolong dying) are desired. The living will does not become effective until the resident is certified by a doctor to be incapacitated and until recovery is not possible.

Common statements in a living will might be, "I direct all life-prolonging procedures be withheld or withdrawn," or "I do not want any of the following life-prolonging procedures," followed by specific information regarding treatment decisions. Treatment decisions might specify guidelines about the types of pain relief desired, the use of antibiotics and life-sustaining medications, enteral feeding, IVs, ventilator use, and organ and tissue donation.

Living wills must be dated and signed by the resident and two witnesses. If you are asked to be a witness as a nursing assistant, explain that witnessing this or any other similar document is not within your scope of practice.

Do-Not-Resuscitate (DNR) Order

A **do-not-resuscitate (DNR) order** is an advance directive that instructs healthcare providers not to attempt resuscitation if a resident's heart and breathing stop (for example, if the resident has a cardiac arrest or has an advanced stage of cancer). Performing CPR, applying an AED, inserting breathing tubes to open the airway, and giving rescue medications are not allowed if there is a DNR order. A doctor may write a DNR order, or a *No Code*. Another order is a *do-not-intubate order,*

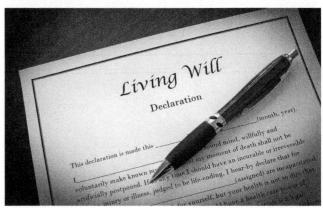

zimmytws/Shutterstock.com

Figure 22.4 A living will takes effect when a person is certified by a doctor to be incapacitated.

which makes sure an airway is not provided if breathing stops. The doctor writes the order only after talking with the resident (if possible), the healthcare proxy, or the family. DNR orders must be signed and dated.

Power of Attorney

A medical or healthcare *power of attorney* (also called a *healthcare proxy* or *durable power of attorney for healthcare*) is another advance directive. A power of attorney gives a designated person the authority to make healthcare decisions on behalf of the resident. This authority only takes effect if the resident becomes unable to make his or her own decisions.

Often, the person designated to receive authority is a spouse, family member, friend, lawyer, or member of a faith community. This person may be called an *agent, proxy, surrogate, representative,* or *advocate* and must meet the state's requirements. The agent selected may not be a member of the healthcare team delivering care. The agent must also make decisions that follow the resident's wishes and advocate if the healthcare provider disagrees with those wishes. According to the resident's wishes, the power of attorney must either follow all instructions in the advance medical directive or use them as guidance.

Five Wishes

The *Five Wishes* is another type of advance directive. This document meets the legal requirements for an advance directive in 42 states and the District of Columbia. In the other eight states, the Five Wishes can be attached to the state's required form.

The Five Wishes is unique because it addresses medical needs, personal needs, emotional needs, and spiritual needs. Unlike other advance directives, this document deals with how a resident wants to be treated and what the resident wants his or her loved ones to know.

What Care Is Available to Those Who Are Dying?

People who are in the process of dying can benefit from *palliative care*. The goal of palliative care is to relieve the symptoms of a disease or condition and improve quality of life for the person who is dying and his or her family. Palliative care does *not* aim to cure or treat a disease or condition, but rather provides support. Palliative care helps relieve symptoms such as pain, nausea, fatigue, breathing problems, and anxiety. It promotes comfort when an active treatment program is

---

> **THINK ABOUT THIS**
>
> Some cultures avoid discussing the end of life and resist completing advance directives. For example, some think advance directives violate their beliefs. Always be sensitive to differing beliefs when asking a resident or his or her family about advance directives.

no longer possible. This type of care should be provided holistically and should be specifically designed to meet the needs of the person.

Palliative care can be provided at any time during a person's illness, but is often provided through *hospice* during the last six months of life. Hospice is a model and philosophy for the quality, compassionate care given during terminal illnesses. Hospice care was first seen in the eleventh century during the Crusades, and its goal was to provide care and comfort for people with incurable diseases. This concept of specialized care for people with terminal illnesses has lasted for centuries and was fully established in the United States by the 1970s. Today, more than 1.3 million people in the United States receive care through hospice facilities and services each year. Ninety-four percent of those who receive hospice care are 65 years of age or older, and 27 percent have been diagnosed with cancer. In the United States, hospice services are a part of Medicare benefits and can be made available through a referral or request.

Hospice care can be delivered in the home, in a long-term care facility, in an inpatient hospice facility, or in an acute care hospital. The hospice team consists of staff members who provide medical and nursing services focused on pain relief, emotional support, counseling, and guidance. The hospice team also provides social services and spiritual resources.

In addition to supporting the person who is dying, hospice also helps family members deal with emotional and practical issues related to the death of a loved one, provides respite care to give family caregivers a break, and directs families to volunteer services that can help with preparing meals and running errands. As a nursing assistant, you will participate in hospice care by being familiar with the plan of care and assisting in any way appropriate.

How Do Nursing Assistants Provide Holistic Care for Those Who Are Dying?

Caring for residents at the ends of their lives is a special privilege and honor. As a holistic nursing assistant, you will be with residents during one of the most important times of their lives, and your actions will make a difference in residents' journeys.

Respecting the Dying Resident's Rights

Residents who are dying still have all the rights outlined in the Nursing Home Resident Rights. Additional rights are included in the *Dying Resident's Bill of Rights*, which is a useful guide to the expectations of those near death (**Figure 22.5**). As a nursing assistant, you will not be able to help in all of the areas described in these rights. If you come across areas where you cannot help, such as pain relief, you are responsible for letting the licensed nursing staff know.

Meeting Physical, Emotional, and Spiritual Needs

Except in the case of sudden death, the process of dying begins before death itself. Dying is a personal journey, and people approach death in their own ways. Specific symptoms are associated with the natural dying process, although people typically do not experience all the symptoms of dying. The process of dying may be very quick for some and slow for others.

Residents who are dying have specific physical, emotional, and spiritual needs. As a nursing assistant, you must be aware of these needs and respond appropriately and effectively. The goal of care will not be to promote recovery, and treatment procedures may be stopped. Instead, care focuses on promoting comfort for the resident. When providing this care, be gentle, use appropriate touch and communication, and treat the resident with **dignity** (worthy of honor or respect) at all times. Pay attention to the safety of the resident and of the environment. Always follow the plan of care and facility policy.

Responding to Physical Needs

The process of dying is a response to specific changes in the body. When someone begins to die, certain signs of impending death appear. As a nursing assistant, you will provide care that focuses on the physical changes in the resident's body:

- **Respiratory changes:** breathing may be more difficult and rapid. Congestion may cause a rattling sound and cough. Pay attention to and document breathing patterns. Oxygen therapy may be used to improve breathlessness. If not contraindicated, a Fowler's position can be helpful and lower the risk of the possible aspiration of phlegm.

Dying Resident's Bill of Rights

I have the right to be treated as a living human being until I die.
I have the right to maintain a sense of hopefulness, however changing its focus may be.
I have the right to be cared for by those who maintain a sense of hopefulness, however changing its focus may be.
I have the right to express my feelings and emotions about approaching death in my own way.
I have the right to participate in decisions concerning my care.
I have the right to expect continuing medical and nursing attention, even though *cure* goals must be changed to *comfort* goals.
I have the right not to die alone.
I have the right to be free from pain.
I have the right to have my questions answered honestly.
I have the right not to be deceived.
I have the right to receive help accepting my death from and for my family.
I have the right to die in peace and dignity.
I have the right to retain my individuality and not to be judged for my decisions, even if they are contrary to the beliefs of others.
I have the right to discuss and enlarge my religious and spiritual experiences, no matter what they mean to others.
I have the right to expect that my body will be respected after death.
I have the right to be cared for by caring, sensitive, and knowledgeable people who will attempt to understand my needs and will gain some satisfaction in helping me face my death.

Created at a workshop, "The Terminally Ill Patient and the Helping Person," in Lansing, Michigan, sponsored by the Southwestern Michigan Inservice Education Council and conducted by Amelia Barbus (1975), Associate Professor of Nursing, Wayne State University

Figure 22.5 Even when residents are dying, they still have rights that need to be respected.

- **Cardiovascular changes:** the nose, lips, fingers, nail beds, and extremities may become pale, gray, or blue due to slowed blood circulation. The legs and ankles may swell, and wounds and infections may not heal well. Check the body's extremities for discoloration (**Figure 22.6**). When you take the resident's vital signs, blood pressure will likely be lower than normal, and pulse may be irregular.
- **Temperature changes and increased sweating:** body temperature often lowers by one degree or more and may be accompanied by sweating. Keep the resident's body dry and change linens, if needed. Pay attention to the room environment, maintaining a comfortable temperature. Sometimes the resident who is dying has a high temperature due to a primary or secondary disease or condition (such as pneumonia caused by limited mobility in the advanced stages of cancer). If the resident has a high temperature, use cold compresses on the forehead and neck according to the plan of care.
- **Decreased appetite:** the need for food declines. A resident may refuse meals and beverages or consume only small amounts. Even favorite foods may be refused. Residents who are dying may experience weight loss as their bodies begin to slow down. Continue to offer a variety of soft foods as long as the resident is conscious. Never force-feed a resident. The resident may experience nausea and vomiting due to bowel blockage, constipation, and certain medications. Offer the resident ice chips or sips of water, if tolerated.
- **Dry mouth and nose:** gently wipe a moistened washcloth around the mouth and nose. Lubricate the lips and nose with lip swabs or balm to prevent cracking (**Figure 22.7**). Moisten the mouth with a few drops of water from a straw or wet toothette.

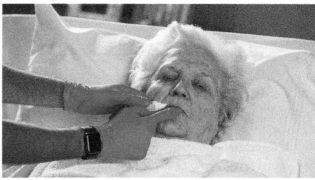
© Tori Soper Photography
Figure 22.7 Lubricating the lips can help prevent them from cracking.

- **Fatigue and increased sleep:** residents who are dying tend to sleep more, sometimes for a good portion of the day. Fatigue is usually the result of limited food intake and possible dehydration, which cause the metabolism to slow down. Residents may not seem to enjoy or desire activities due to fatigue. Let residents sleep. Always avoid shaking a resident to awaken him or her. Due to increased sleep, the resident's eyes may not blink as often, causing the eyes to become dry. Mucus may crust on the eyelids. Use a warm, wet washcloth to cleanse the eyes and eyelids.
- **Decubitus ulcers:** residents who are dying often have limited mobility, increasing their risk for decubitus ulcers. Check the skin often and provide skin care (see Chapter 18). Gently reposition the resident every two hours (see Chapter 14). Provide needed padding around bony parts of the body and use pillows and other positioning devices to maintain comfort and protect the skin.
- **Changes in elimination:** constipation is common due to immobility, poor diet, dehydration, and weakness. Stool softeners and medications may be given by the licensed nursing staff.
- **Pain:** check on and report a resident's pain levels. If the resident sleeps a great deal or is semiconscious, observe for signs such as grimacing, moaning, guarding an area, and having an increased heart and respiratory rate. Pain-relief medications do not shorten the life span, and can make the resident more comfortable during the process of dying. Sometimes a back rub can be comforting (see Chapter 17).

As you provide care, remember that the resident can still hear, even if he or she is not communicating with you. Always assume that everything you say can be heard clearly.

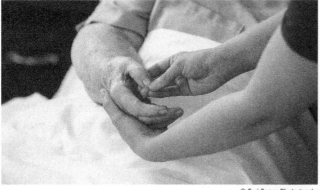
© Tori Soper Photography
Figure 22.6 Checking the body's extremities for discoloration can help you determine a resident's level of blood circulation.

Responding to Emotional and Spiritual Needs

Physical changes in the body affect a resident's emotional health, and residents will have emotional and spiritual needs that need to be met during dying. Many of these needs are related to the emotional changes that accompany dying:

- **Concerns:** conscious residents may fear death or be worried about dying and things they have not done or said. They may know they are dying or want to start the process of saying goodbye. You can ask residents if anything is worrying them. Listen actively and carefully, and encourage residents to share their worries with their families. It is not your role to give advice; however, you can ask if a resident would like to talk with a licensed nursing staff member or spiritual leader. Be sure to report any information you gain to the licensed nursing staff.
- **Restlessness, confusion, and anxiety:** residents may feel restless, confused, or anxious due to an inability to relax and staying in one position. Change residents' positions frequently. Some residents may try to climb out of bed. Maintain safety precautions for these residents.
- **Hallucinations or visions:** do not be alarmed if a resident who is dying starts speaking with someone who is not there. Many times, the resident is talking with someone dear who is already dead. Hallucinations may be caused by medications, changes in metabolism, an infection, or the disease itself.
- **Withdrawal from active participation in social activities:** as residents who are dying start to accept their mortality, they may separate themselves from their surroundings. They may desire visits from significant people in their lives, but not show an interest or willingness to talk. Continue to speak to the resident while giving care, even if the resident does not respond. Do not try to make the resident talk with you or with the family.

Providing Family Support

The family is an important part of a resident's care. As a holistic nursing assistant, you can help with communication between the family and resident, the doctor, and the healthcare staff by making sure questions or concerns are answered, particularly as the resident nears death. Families may become frightened when they see their loved one's condition worsen. They may be upset by the changes in breathing, confusion, or extreme drowsiness associated with dying. Provide comfort by assuring the family you are there to help care for the resident and keep him or her safe and comfortable. Always alert a licensed nursing staff member to any changes.

Many family members will want to stay with their loved one and provide care. The family's presence and touch can help the resident who is dying feel calmer and more at peace. Remind the family that their loved one may be able to hear them up until the moment of death.

Maintain a calm and comfortable environment. Keep lights dim, and be slow and patient when giving care. Be sure to give family members an opportunity to help with care if they want to and are able.

Help make family members and visitors feel welcome and comfortable and provide them with information about the facility, facility policy regarding meals, and areas of rest outside the room.

Caring for Yourself and Your Coworkers

The time of dying is challenging and is filled with emotion. As a holistic nursing assistant, you can use the following guidelines to manage your own emotions as a caregiver:

- Keep in touch with your emotions so they do not influence the care you give.
- If you are ever uncomfortable caring for a resident, let a licensed nursing staff member know.
- Talk about your feelings with other appropriate staff.
- Always use your resources. Consult with the licensed nursing staff about any care issues and ask for assistance from the palliative care team, if appropriate.

Just as the time of dying and death is filled with emotion for you, your coworkers may also be experiencing and struggling with emotions. As a holistic nursing assistant, you can help your coworkers by:

- providing support by talking about the emotions being felt
- being empathetic and actively listening
- suggesting that methods such as deep breathing can be useful when they are feeling stressed or anxious
- asking them if they have family, friends, or spiritual advisors who may be helpful
- recommending that they talk with the licensed nursing staff about how they are feeling; facility resources such as support groups may also be of assistance

Always maintain professional boundaries and understand what is and is not within your scope of practice. Choose your words carefully when talking to the resident and his or her family. If you are doing any of the following, you may be crossing boundaries:

- You begin to think a lot about the resident when you are not at work.
- You visit or spend extra time with a resident who is not part of your work assignment.
- You take sides with the resident against his or her family or other staff members.
- You share inappropriate personal information.
- You act in a verbally or physically abusive way or use touch inappropriately.
- You accept personal gifts from the resident or family.

SECTION 22.1 **Review and Assessment**

Key Terms Mini Glossary

advance directives written legal documents signed by a living, competent person; describe that person's medical and healthcare instructions in the event of incapacitation.

dignity worthy of honor and respect.

do-not-resuscitate (DNR) order a medical and legal request that lifesaving measures such as CPR not be administered if a person's heart or breathing stops.

grief an emotional response to or distress about a physical or personal loss.

incapacitation the lack of ability to make decisions.

living will an advance directive that details the life-prolonging treatments a person desires in the event of incapacitation during a terminal illness or permanent unconsciousness.

mourn to express feelings and behaviors that show grief.

palliative care care that provides relief from the symptoms of a disease or condition; does not aim to cure the disease or condition.

power of attorney an advance directive that gives a designated person the authority to make healthcare decisions on behalf of another person; authority only takes effect if the person who writes the power of attorney becomes unable to make his or her own decisions; also called a *healthcare proxy* or *durable power of attorney for healthcare*.

Apply the Key Terms

An incorrect key term is used in each of the following statements. Identify the incorrect key term and then replace it with the correct term.

1. Mr. K wrote a living will to provide a medical and legal request to avoid lifesaving measures if his heart or breathing stop.
2. The resident you are caring for is mourning; that is, she is not able to make decisions.
3. An advance directive is care that provides relief from symptoms of a disease or condition.
4. Ms. P has a power of attorney—a legal document signed by a living, competent person that describes her medical and healthcare instructions in the event of incapacitation.
5. Palliative care is an advance directive that details life-prolonging treatments in the event of incapacitation during a terminal illness or permanent unconsciousness.

Know and Understand the Facts

1. Explain three actions nursing assistants can take to provide holistic care for grieving residents.
2. Briefly describe the five stages of grief.
3. Identify three physical changes often encountered by someone who is dying and explain how a nursing assistant can deliver care that addresses each change.
4. Describe two different types of advance directives.

Analyze and Apply Concepts

1. Describe the behaviors that occur during the five stages of grief.
2. Explain how nursing assistants can give care that meets the emotional and spiritual needs of a resident who is dying.
3. Identify two ways nursing assistants can perform self-care when caring for residents who are dying.

Think Critically

Read the following care situation. Then answer the questions that follow.

You have been assigned to care for Mr. O, an 80-year-old Hispanic man. Mr. O has end-stage kidney disease and had been receiving hospice care at home. He was admitted to the inpatient hospice unit one week ago due to a serious bladder infection and pneumonia. Mr. O has been sleeping a great deal and is irritable when awakened for meals. He usually refuses meals and does not have an IV or feeding tube. He says he hates being in this facility and would rather go home. His large family visits regularly. Mr. O has advance directives, and his oldest daughter is his agent. By the end of the week, Mr. O is more inactive and withdrawn. He does not want to eat or drink anything.

1. What are Mr. O's signs of impending death?
2. How can you support Mr. O's family?
3. How might Mr. O's advance directives affect his care?

Objectives

To achieve the objectives for this section, you must successfully:

- **recognize** signs of death.
- **describe** ways to provide holistic family support at the time of death.
- **explain** decisions residents may make before death concerning organ donation, cremation, and burial.
- **identify** the steps in performing postmortem care.

Key Terms

Learn these key terms to better understand the information presented in the section.

Cheyne-Stokes respiration	postmortem care
moribund	rigor mortis
pathologist	transplants

Questions to Consider

- How do you feel when you think about caring for people who are dying or near death? Do you feel uncomfortable, frightened, or distressed?
- How can you deal with or overcome any negative feelings you may have about death?
- How might your care be affected if you do not feel comfortable providing care for those who are dying or near death?

What Are the Signs of Approaching Death?

Certain changes in the body signal that death will happen soon and that a resident is **moribund**, or near death. There are two phases of dying: the *pre-active phase* of dying and the *active phase* of dying. Most residents are in the pre-active phase for approximately two weeks, while others last a month or longer in this phase.

The active phase of dying typically lasts approximately three days, although some residents are in this phase for two weeks or longer. The exact length of the dying process will vary from resident to resident, as will the signs of death. Signs of death can be seen in the respiratory, cardiovascular, nervous, musculoskeletal, gastrointestinal, and urinary systems.

Respiratory System

The breathing of the resident who is dying becomes irregular and slow. The resident breathes in a pattern called **Cheyne-Stokes respiration**, which is a period of rapid breathing followed by periods of *apnea*, or no breathing (**Figure 22.8**). Secretions collect in the throat, causing congestion and a loud, rattling sound during breathing. Toward the end of the dying process, a resident will experience much longer periods of apnea and other abnormal breathing patterns, such as breathing that is very slow, speeds up, and then slows again and breathing that is very fast and becomes very slow. At the very end, the resident breathes through a wide-open mouth and can no longer speak, even if awake. Providing comfort and care during approaching death is very important.

Cardiovascular System

Because blood circulation decreases, the skin of a resident who is dying becomes pale and cool to the touch. The resident's hands and feet may appear blotchy and purplish (*mottled*) and feel numb. Discoloration may affect the arms and legs as well. The resident's lips and nail beds will become bluish or purple, and due to the decrease in blood circulation, blood pressure will drop 20–30 points from the resident's normal range.

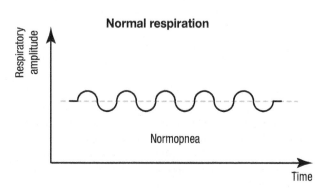

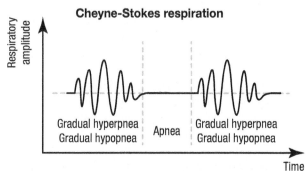

Goodheart-Willcox Publisher

Figure 22.8 Cheyne-Stokes respiration includes periods of rapid breathing (hyperpnea), slow breathing (hypopnea), and no breathing (apnea).

Nervous System

As a resident dies, less blood circulates through the brain, and the resident may drift in and out of consciousness. The resident's eyes may be open or semiopen but will not focus on the surroundings. The resident may become agitated or restless due to cognitive impairment (called *terminal delirium*). The resident will eventually become unresponsive and move into a coma.

Musculoskeletal System

A resident who is dying may experience a short burst of energy. As death approaches, however, the resident will not move his or her extremities as much, and the body will start to become more rigid. The jaw will no longer be held straight and may droop to the side.

Gastrointestinal System

A resident who is dying will not eat and typically will be unable to swallow. Lack of eating during the dying process is actually protective and causes chemical changes that lead to a sense of well-being. The resident will experience bowel incontinence.

Urinary System

As the body slows down and the resident stops drinking fluids, urine output decreases, and urine darkens (to red or brown). Like lack of eating, lack of fluids and dehydration also cause chemical changes that increase a sense of well-being. The resident will experience urinary incontinence.

At Death

At the moment of death, breathing will cease, and the heart will stop (leading to no heartbeat or pulse). The pupils will be fixed and dilated, and the eyes will remain open unless the resident was sleeping. The skin will be pale, bluish, and cool to the touch, and the jaw will become slack and drop open. These signs will be used to determine death.

When a resident dies, all of his or her muscles relax completely and then stiffen. The stiffening of muscles after death is called **rigor mortis**. Rigor mortis's onset depends on age, gender, physical condition, and muscular build, but typically begins two to six hours after death and starts with the eyelids, neck, and jaw. After four to six hours, rigor mortis spreads to all other muscles.

The pronouncement of death can be made by a variety of healthcare providers, including doctors, coroners, medical examiners or deputy medical examiners, or licensed nursing staff members. Each state has its own laws regarding who can pronounce death. The termination of vital signs must be documented and can be included in the resident's

---

BECOMING A HOLISTIC NURSING ASSISTANT

Caring for the Family of the Deceased

One of your most important roles as a holistic nursing assistant is providing support and assistance to the family of the resident who is dying or deceased. Pay attention to the family's needs, be compassionate, and provide holistic nursing care using the following guidelines:

- Make sure that the family has privacy at the time of death and when viewing the body.
- Provide adequate space and chairs in the room if there is a large family.
- Be respectful of the family's response to death and of any family traditions or religious practices.
- Prepare the room for any religious practices the family has requested.
- Listen to what the family says and respond as best as you can to provide comfort and any needed resources. If family members start crying or acting out, give them the space they need to express their feelings. Do not say, "This will pass," or "You will get over it."

- If the family becomes angry and starts blaming or complaining about the healthcare staff, do not respond. Instead, refer the family to a member of the licensed nursing staff.
- Use touch, if appropriate, by holding hands or touching a family member's arm.
- If appropriate, share positive memories and feelings about the resident who has died.
- Let the family know how the resident's body will be prepared. Be aware of any special preparation based on religious practices or the plan of care.
- If the family is not already aware of transport decisions, help facilitate communication with healthcare staff members who can best provide this information.

Apply It

1. Which actions would you find difficult or challenging to perform as a holistic nursing assistant? Explain.
2. What can you do to overcome any difficulties or challenges identified?

health record. Once death occurs, the focus of your care should shift from the deceased resident to the family (**Figure 22.9**).

What Decisions Affect Care After Death?

When a resident dies, the care you deliver will depend on arrangements in several areas. For example, a resident may have volunteered for organ or tissue donation or may require an autopsy. The resident or family will also have made decisions about burial and cremation.

- **Organ donation:** a resident can become an organ or tissue donor by registering with a state donor agency or placing the decision on a driver's license. It is important that the donor lets his or her family or a significant individual know about this decision. After a resident has been declared dead by an approved healthcare provider who is not connected to the donation or transplant recovery team, action is taken to make sure organs and tissues are removed quickly.
- **Autopsy:** an autopsy is a specialized procedure performed on the deceased's body by a *pathologist* (disease specialist) to determine cause of death. It may be done for legal or medical reasons. If an autopsy has been ordered, a healthcare facility, doctor, or licensed nursing staff member will provide instructions prior to and upon death so that special arrangements can be made.
- **Burial and cremation:** when a resident is dying, he or she must decide whether to be buried or cremated. This decision is often made with the input of the resident's family. If the resident chooses to be buried, the burial can be in-ground, using a casket, or above-ground in a building called a mausoleum. If cremation is chosen, the body is burned, creating ashes, or *remains*. The remains are placed in a container and given to the family or responsible party, who will carry out the resident's wishes to have his or her remains buried or scattered.

How Do Nursing Assistants Assist with Postmortem Care?

Care provided after the death of a resident is *postmortem care*. The purposes of postmortem care include:

- preparing the resident's body for viewing by the family

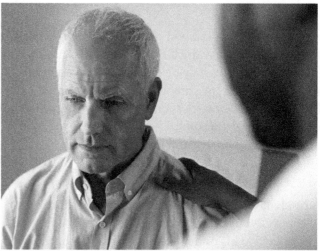
MBI/Shutterstock.com

Figure 22.9 As a nursing assistant, you should provide holistic care to the family of the deceased after a person's passing.

- providing appropriate care
- gathering the resident's personal belongings according to facility policy
- properly identifying the resident's body before transport to the morgue or funeral home

The nursing assistant's most important responsibility in postmortem care is preparing the resident to make sure there is a clean, peaceful, and comforting environment for family members who want to say goodbye before transport. Caring for the resident's body shows the family that you have empathy and concern for the deceased.

Respond to any requested religious or cultural practices. These might affect how the body is washed and dressed. For example, upon death, body openings may be filled with gauze or cotton, and the deceased may be dressed in his or her finest clothes. According to some religions, the body should not be left unattended. A family member, designated person, or religious official may stay in the room.

The death of a loved one is a challenging and emotional time for a family. If appropriate, you may invite the family to participate in the preparation of the body and provide instructions.

When delivering postmortem care, you can use a *postmortem kit*, which includes a shroud or body bag for transport, identification tags, gauze squares, ties to hold the hands together, safety pins, and tape to secure the shroud (**Figure 22.10**). Some kits have a chin strap to secure the jaw.

Keep in mind that rigor mortis and other bodily changes after death can impact the postmortem procedure. Because of this, postmortem care should

Organ Donation

According to a recent publication, more than 116,000 men, women, and children in the United States currently need lifesaving organ *transplants*. A transplant is the surgical removal of an organ or tissue from one body so that it can be transferred into another body. The publication identified that, during one year, there were 15,947 organ donors in the United States, and 33,612 organ transplants were performed. Although 95 percent of US adults supported organ donation, only 54 percent were signed up as donors. Decisions about donating organs or tissues were often made many years prior to death or during the dying process. In some cases, a person's family members decided if the person's organs could be donated. The following

organs and tissues can be donated: heart, liver, pancreas, lungs, kidneys, intestines, corneas, skin, heart valves, bone, blood vessels, and connective tissues such as tendons. A person can choose which organs or tissues to offer for donation.

Apply It

1. Why do you think some people do not want to donate their organs or tissues?
2. Why do you think some people choose to donate their organs?
3. How can you know if someone is an organ donor?
4. What experiences have you had with organ and tissue donation?

be completed as soon as possible after death. When you are delivering postmortem care, a resident's body may make unexpected sounds or movements. Do not be alarmed. Bodies hold air, and when the body relaxes at death, air often escapes through the mouth or anus. Sometimes a resident's body may appear to be breathing again, as air trapped in the lungs leaves the body and makes a noise like a moan or cry. The bowels and bladder also relax, so stool and urine may be expelled. Remember that these sounds and actions are normal after death. Respect and dignity should be maintained at all times.

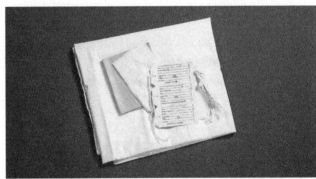

© *Tori Soper Photography*

Figure 22.10 A postmortem kit contains the supplies necessary for delivering postmortem care.

Procedure

Providing Postmortem Care

Rationale

Postmortem care must be provided as soon as possible after death to keep the resident's body in proper alignment (before rigor mortis) and prevent skin damage. Postmortem care also prepares the resident's body for family viewing, if appropriate, and transport.

Preparation

1. Ask the licensed nursing staff if there are doctor's orders for the procedure, and if there are any specific instructions listed in the plan of care (such as organ donation or autopsy). A licensed nursing staff member will provide instructions about the maintenance or removal of equipment such as IVs or urinary catheters.

2. Wash your hands or use hand sanitizer before entering the room.
3. Knock before entering the room if the deceased resident's family is in the room.
4. Introduce yourself to the deceased resident's family using your first or preferred name and title. Explain that you work with the licensed nursing staff and will be providing care.
5. Check the deceased resident's identification bracelet.
6. Use Mr., Mrs., or Ms. and the family members' last names when conversing.
7. Determine whether the family will be staying in the room for the procedure. If the family wants to stay, explain the procedure in simple terms.

(continued)

Providing Postmortem Care *(continued)*

8. Bring the necessary equipment into the room. Place the following items in an easy-to-reach place:
   - postmortem kit
   - an envelope or bag for personal belongings and valuables
   - several pairs of disposable gloves
   - several washcloths
   - several towels
   - disposable protective pad
   - bath blanket
   - cotton balls
   - gauze bandages and tape
   - clean gown
   - washbasin
   - labeled denture cup, if needed

The Procedure

9. Provide privacy by closing the curtains, using a screen, or closing the door to the room.

   Best Practice: If instructed by the licensed nursing staff, turn off all medical equipment.

10. Lock the bed wheels and then raise the bed to hip level.

11. Maintain safety during the procedure. If there are side rails, raise and lock the rails on the opposite side of the bed from where you will be working. Lower the rail on the side where you are working.

   Best Practice: Always follow facility policy and consider your own safety during and after the postmortem procedure.

12. Wash your hands or use hand sanitizer to ensure infection control.

13. Put on disposable gloves.

14. Make sure the bed is flat. Place a pillow under the resident's head and shoulders to keep the body aligned.

15. Fanfold the linens to the foot of the bed.

16. Straighten the resident's arms and legs and place the arms at the side of the body.

17. Undress the resident and cover the resident with a bath blanket.

   Best Practice: Always show an attitude of respect while quickly and calmly providing care.

18. Gently close the resident's eyes if they are open by grasping the eyelashes and pulling the eyelids down. Hold the eyes shut for a few seconds. Place moistened cotton balls over the eyelids if the eyelids will not stay closed over the eyes.

19. If appropriate, clean and insert dentures into the resident's mouth to maintain a normal appearance. If dentures are not to be worn, clean and place them in a labeled denture cup.

20. Close the resident's mouth. If the mouth will not stay closed, ask the licensed nursing staff for instructions. A rolled washcloth under the chin can help keep the mouth closed.

21. Remove all jewelry, except for a wedding ring, unless instructed to do otherwise. If a ring is left in place, put a cotton ball over it and tape it in place.

22. Place the resident's jewelry and personal belongings (such as eyeglasses) into an envelope or bag designated for valuables. Attach an identification tag to the envelope or bag. All valuables should remain in the facility safe until they are claimed and signed for by an approved relative or other designated person.

23. Empty and replace any drainage bags, such as a colostomy bag. If instructed, remove tubing and appliances. Ask for guidance from the licensed nursing staff if the resident is wearing a prosthetic.

24. Remove and discard your gloves.

25. Wash your hands or use hand sanitizer to ensure infection control.

26. Put on a new pair of disposable gloves.

27. Fill the washbasin with warm water. Place the washbasin on the overbed table.

28. Wash the resident's body. Dry the body thoroughly. Place and tape gauze bandages on areas that may need drainage absorbed.

29. Change any wet or soiled linens on the bed.

   Best Practice: Always ask for help if you need it. This may be necessary if you are caring for overweight residents.

30. Place a disposable protective pad under the resident's buttocks.

31. If the family did not stay for the procedure but has asked to view the resident, put a clean gown or other clothing, as appropriate, on the resident's body. Comb or brush the hair as needed.

32. Keep a pillow behind the resident's head and raise the bed to a supine or low Fowler's position. Cover the resident's body up to the shoulders with a sheet. *Never* cover the resident's face.

33. Before the family arrives, dispose of any soiled linens, dressings, and tubing. Straighten the room, lower the lights, and provide chairs for the family.

34. Remove and discard your gloves.

35. Wash your hands or use hand sanitizer to ensure infection control.

   Best Practice: Maintain the family's privacy and provide time for the viewing.

36. When the family leaves, close the door and remove the sheet covering the resident's body.

37. Put on disposable gloves.

38. Fill out the identification tags. Tie one identification tag on the resident's ankle or right big toe.

39. Position the shroud or body bag under the resident's body.

40. If using a shroud, bring the top of the shroud over the resident's head and fold the bottom of the shroud up over the resident's feet. Fold the sides of the shroud over the resident's body and pin or tape the shroud in place.

41. Attach one identification tag to the shroud.

42. Gather all personal belongings and the denture cup, if used. List and label these items, as they will stay with the resident's body.

43. Ask the licensed nursing staff if the resident's body should stay in the room until transport to the funeral home or if the resident's body should be moved to the morgue. If the resident's body should be transported, check facility transport policy.

44. Remove, clean, and store equipment in the proper location. Remove soiled linens and discard disposable equipment.

45. If the resident's body is still in the room, pull the privacy curtain around the bed or close the door.

Follow-Up

46. Remove and discard your gloves.

47. Wash your hands or use hand sanitizer before leaving the room.

48. After the resident's body has been removed from the room, clean the room according to facility policy.

Reporting and Documentation

49. Report the date and time the resident's body was transported to the funeral home or moved to the morgue to the licensed nursing staff. Also report how the resident's personal belongings and valuables were handled and secured and if dentures and any other artificial body parts accompanied the resident. Document this information, along with the care provided, in the chart or EMR.

SECTION 22.2 **Review and Assessment**

Key Terms Mini Glossary

Cheyne-Stokes respiration a pattern of breathing that indicates death is near; causes hyperpnea (rapid breathing) followed by periods of no breathing (apnea).

moribund about to die.

pathologist a doctor who specializes in studying diseases; conducts autopsies to determine causes of death.

postmortem care care performed shortly after death; prepares the body for burial or cremation, puts the body in alignment, and prevents skin damage.

rigor mortis the stiffening of the body's muscles several hours after death.

transplants surgeries in which organs or body tissues are removed from one person and transferred into another.

Apply the Key Terms

Write a sentence using each key term properly.

1. transplants
2. postmortem care
3. moribund
4. pathologist
5. rigor mortis

Know and Understand the Facts

1. Identify four signs that death may be approaching.
2. Explain how a nursing assistant's caregiving role changes at the time of death.
3. Which actions have to occur for organ donation to take place?
4. Name two ways a person can be buried.

Analyze and Apply Concepts

1. Identify three ways a nursing assistant can provide holistic family support.

2. Describe the purposes of postmortem care.
3. List the steps needed to perform postmortem care.

Think Critically

Read the following care situation. Then answer the questions that follow.

Janie, a new nursing assistant, has just witnessed the death of Mrs. Y and was asked to provide postmortem care. Janie became close with Mrs. Y, her husband, and son while caring for Mrs. Y. When Mrs. Y passed, her family cried, and now they do not want to leave Mrs. Y's body. Janie knows she has to provide postmortem care quickly but also does not want to cause the family more grief.

1. What can Janie do to support Mrs. Y's family at this difficult time?
2. What three postmortem care steps should Janie be sure to complete when preparing Mrs. Y's body?

Key Points

Reviewing the key points for this chapter will help you practice more safely and competently as a holistic nursing assistant and will help you prepare for the certification competency examination.

- Examining your own feelings about dying and death can help you deliver effective and appropriate end-of-life care. Strong feelings about dying and death can be transferred to those in your care.
- The five stages of grief are denial, anger, bargaining, depression, and acceptance.
- Providing holistic family support is an important responsibility.
- Advance directives are legal documents that provide instructions about treatment and care preferences at the end of life.
- People who are dying and their families often face difficult decisions about organ donation, autopsy, and burial or cremation.
- Postmortem care must be performed as soon as possible after death to keep the resident in proper alignment and prevent skin damage. Postmortem care prepares a resident's body for family viewing, if appropriate, and transport.

Action Steps to Holistic Care

Review the information in this chapter. Complete the following activities.

1. Prepare a short paper or digital presentation that identifies and describes the three most important practices of postmortem care. Include one that promotes comfort for the family and one that maintains safety.
2. With a partner, prepare a poster that shows at least four facts about advance directives that residents and the public should know. Include the legal requirements for these documents in your state.
3. Research current scientific information about the dying process. Write a brief report that describes two current facts you did not know.
4. Create a poster or digital presentation that discusses the emotional challenges associated with dying and death. Discuss how to provide emotional support for a resident who is dying, strategies to support a grieving family, and self-care techniques to help other nursing assistants deal with their own feelings during this time.

Building Math Skill

Recent statistics on deaths from pancreatic cancer include the following:

- In 2015, 40,560 people died from pancreatic cancer.
- In 2020, 47,050 people died from pancreatic cancer.

What is the percentage increase in deaths in that 5-year period?

Preparing for the Certification Competency Examination

To prepare for the nursing assistant certification competency examination, you will need to know content found in this chapter. This content may be tested in the knowledge (written or oral) and skills (hands-on demonstration) portions of the exam. The following areas will be emphasized:

- the impact of death on self and others
- influence of attitudes, beliefs, and cultural and spiritual practices on dying and death
- signs of impending death, stages of grief, and the dying process
- care of the dying resident and support for family members
- the role of the nursing assistant in hospice care
- legal and ethical standards in end-of-life care
- requirements of advance directives
- postmortem personal care

These sample test questions are similar to ones you will find on the certification competency exam. See how well you can answer them. Be sure to select the *best* answer.

1. Which of the following is an advance directive?
   A. cremation
   B. patient rights
   C. living will
   D. PSDA

2. A person who says, "If only I had had those tests done sooner," is in the stage of grief known as
   A. denial
   B. anger
   C. acceptance
   D. depression

3. Which of the following may be a sign that death will happen soon?
   A. increased activity
   B. bluish tinge of the nail beds
   C. increased appetite
   D. increased urine output

4. A nursing assistant is assigned to care for Mr. B, who is dying. Which symptom is Mr. B most likely to have?
   A. increased activity
   B. hunger and thirst
   C. fatigue and sleep
   D. decreased pain

5. Palliative care focuses on
   A. treatments that cure
   B. aggressive action
   C. no medications
   D. the relief of symptoms

6. A physical sign of impending death is
   A. depression
   B. withdrawal from family and friends
   C. increased appetite
   D. difficult and rapid breathing

7. A nursing assistant has been asked by Mrs. U's doctor to witness a DNR order. The nursing assistant should respond by saying,
   A. "Of course. I would be happy to."
   B. "I am not able. It is not in my scope of practice."
   C. "Let me ask the nurse if it is okay."
   D. "Did you check with the family to see if it is okay?"

8. When a resident is dying, a nursing assistant should
   A. help the resident ambulate to prevent constipation
   B. help the resident eat as much as possible
   C. observe and record breathing patterns, as they will change
   D. encourage the resident to talk with family as much as possible

9. When providing postmortem care, how should a nursing assistant handle valuables?
   A. place them in a labeled bag and give them to a family member
   B. place them in a labeled bag and give them to the licensed nurse
   C. place them in a labeled bag and put them in the facility safe
   D. place them in a labeled bag and give them to the unit clerk

10. A nursing assistant who recently lost his mother to cancer has been asked to take care of Mrs. R, who has end-stage cancer. What might the nursing assistant do to be sure he does not overstep his boundaries?
    A. use Mrs. R's experience to process his mother's death
    B. never talk with Mrs. R about her feelings about dying
    C. share his experience with Mrs. R
    D. talk with the licensed nurse about his feelings

11. During the last viewing of Mrs. V's body, Mrs. V's daughter tells the nursing assistant that her mother would not have died if the nurses had taken better care of her. What should the nursing assistant do?
    A. tell the daughter the licensed nurse will talk with her
    B. apologize to the daughter
    C. ignore the daughter and console other members of the family
    D. tell the daughter there is nothing more to do

12. Which stage of grief is described as someone asking, "Why me?"
    A. acceptance
    B. anger
    C. denial
    D. depression

13. Which of the following is true of organ donation by a deceased resident?
    A. It can only occur after death is pronounced by an approved healthcare provider.
    B. It does not affect the care given during or after death.
    C. Everyone has to make a decision about it before death.
    D. Only the licensed nursing staff needs to know about it.

14. Mr. F's family has decided to request hospice services. Why might they make this decision?
    A. Mr. F needs to increase his mobility and activity.
    B. Mr. F has withdrawn and needs companionship.
    C. Mr. F has a special diet and needs guidance.
    D. Mr. F has a terminal illness and needs special care.

15. How can a nursing assistant best deal with her own feelings about dying and death?
    A. exercise as a way to be more active
    B. spend more time with family and friends
    C. hold feelings in so they don't interfere with her work
    D. talk with someone with whom she is comfortable

Did you have difficulty with any of the questions? If you did, review the chapter to find the correct answer(s).

23 Certification, Employment, the Workplace, and Lifelong Learning

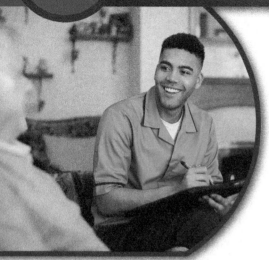

sturti/Signature collection via Getty Images

Welcome to the Chapter

You are now ready to prepare for and take the nursing assistant certification competency examination. This chapter provides information about studying for the exam and using test-taking strategies. You will also explore ways to search for employment as a nursing assistant and learn how to best interview for a position. This chapter emphasizes beginning and advancing your nursing career and becoming a lifelong learner.

What you learn in this chapter will help you build the knowledge and skills needed to become a holistic nursing assistant. The topics discussed in the chapter are highlighted on the Providing Holistic Care Framework.

Chapter Outline

Section 23.1
The Certification
Competency Examination

Section 23.2
Your Nursing Career

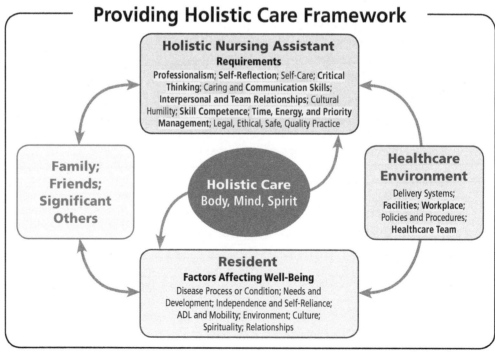

Providing Holistic Care Framework

Holistic Nursing Assistant
Requirements
Professionalism; Self-Reflection; Self-Care; Critical Thinking; Caring and Communication Skills; Interpersonal and Team Relationships; Cultural Humility; Skill Competence; Time, Energy, and Priority Management; Legal, Ethical, Safe, Quality Practice

Family; Friends; Significant Others

Holistic Care
Body, Mind, Spirit

Healthcare Environment
Delivery Systems; Facilities; Workplace; Policies and Procedures; Healthcare Team

Resident
Factors Affecting Well-Being
Disease Process or Condition; Needs and Development; Independence and Self-Reliance; ADL and Mobility; Environment; Culture; Spirituality; Relationships

Goodheart-Willcox Publisher

The Certification Competency Examination

Objectives

To achieve the objectives for this section, you must successfully:

- **describe** the skills needed to study effectively and prepare for the certification competency examination.
- **demonstrate** successful test-taking strategies.

Key Terms

Learn these key terms to better understand the information presented in the section.

auditory
concentration
cramming

flash cards
procrastination

Questions to Consider

- Describe your experience with taking tests. Do you know how to prepare for tests? Are you calm when getting ready for a test?
- How do you feel when you are taking a test? Do you feel relaxed? anxious? nervous?
- How well do you score on tests? If you do not score well, what areas of studying and preparation can you strengthen? If you do score well, what actions do you take to get a good score?

What Is the Certification Competency Examination?

As you learned in Chapter 1, the *certification competency examination* is a test that nursing assistants must take and pass to become certified. Each state is responsible for making sure nursing assistant education and training programs meet the OBRA (*Omnibus Reconciliation Act*) standards set by the federal government and for establishing the minimum age at which people can enter a program. States also determine how nursing assistant certification is given, which certification competency examination will be used, and when and where the exam will occur. Each state has different fees for taking the exam, requirements for application, and exam schedules. Each state also determines how many times a person can take the exam if he or she does not pass.

The length of instruction in a training program ranges from a minimum of 75 hours to more than 150 hours. Programs also require supervised clinical training of 24 hours or more in long-term care facilities. Some programs also include hospital and other related clinical experiences.

After completing a state-approved nursing assistant education and training program, graduates take the certification competency examination required by their state. The certification competency exam tests knowledge (in a written or oral exam) and skills (in a hands-on demonstration). The written exam may be completed electronically or by hand. The written exam usually consists of 50 or more multiple-choice questions covering such areas as safety, infection control, personal care, communication, and basic nursing skills. Information about a state's exam may be found in a handbook on the state's board of nursing website, on the Department of Health and Human Services website, or through the state's exam administrator.

The skills demonstration portion of the exam requires applicants to perform specified procedures on a model in front of a test observer or evaluator. Skills demonstrations are timed, and skills must be performed (not explained) to count. The list of required skills is often provided ahead of time. Some states provide specific procedures for performing each skill. Other states randomly draw skills to test from the list of skills provided. Examples of skills that may be tested include hand washing, providing oral care or perineal care, dressing a resident, performing a partial bed bath, and providing range-of-motion exercises.

To become certified as a nursing assistant, a person must meet the exam application requirements, verify completion of a state-approved training program, pay the fees, schedule the exam, and pass both parts with a state-determined score. Other requirements might include photo identification, documentation that shows legal presence in the United States, and a fingerprint background check. Some states use an online process to apply for certification, and others use a paper application.

It is often best to take the exam right after completing the training program, while your knowledge and skills are most current. Check your state's standards regarding test-taking requirements and time lines.

How Can You Prepare for the Certification Competency Exam?

Knowing what to expect is an important part of successfully taking the certification competency exam. Reviewing your state's certification competency exam handbook will provide information about how to apply for the exam, and what to prepare for and bring on the day of the exam.

Start by focusing on what you need to know. Read your state's handbook and review the end of each chapter in this textbook to find a list of topics that might be covered on the exam. You can also complete the practice test questions at the end of each chapter.

Developing good *test-taking skills* is another important part of preparing for the exam. For some people, test taking causes a lot of anxiety. Other people are not nervous at all. Often, what makes the difference is the amount of test preparation and past test-taking experiences.

Learning how to study and prepare for the exam can make a difference in the outcome (**Figure 23.1**). The more prepared and comfortable you feel with the exam content and process, the more likely you will succeed. Building excellent study habits and skills is important.

Do you know how to study to your best advantage? Think about how you study now as you read these helpful study habits and skills. Determine which habits or skills you already have. Keep using these skills. Then select new habits or skills you want to try as you study for the certification competency exam.

Know Your Learning Style

How do you learn best? The way you learn best is your *learning style*. For example, if you are a *visual learner*, you must see material to learn it best. If you are an **auditory** learner, you may prefer to listen to material. *Kinesthetic learners* need to feel or experience material to learn it best.

Instead of being one type of learner, you may use a combination of these styles. Even so, you probably tend to use one style more than others. When you know your learning style, you can use it to your advantage. For example, if you are a visual learner, you can use **flash cards** for studying. By taking notes on and reviewing the flash cards, you will see the important information you want to learn and remember.

Concentrate

Once you know your learning style, identify the best place to study. Some people like to study at a desk or table; others prefer to study outside, rather than indoors. Wherever you choose to study, make sure you can use the same place every time. You will want this place to be used only for studying so your brain switches into study mode as soon as you sit down. This will help with your **concentration**, or ability to direct your complete attention toward a particular object or task.

Your selected study place should be quiet, well lit, and devoted to studying (**Figure 23.2**). An easy chair and your bed are not the best places for serious studying. While studying, avoid distractions such as your phone, video games, or other activities you like to do. Let others know you are studying so they do not disturb you. Be sure your study area is clutter free, is organized, and has the resources you need. Getting up to get additional supplies will distract you from your main purpose: studying.

Schedule Study Time and Breaks

How motivated are you to study? Are you willing to sacrifice time for other activities in your life to learn what you need to know? One way to help maintain

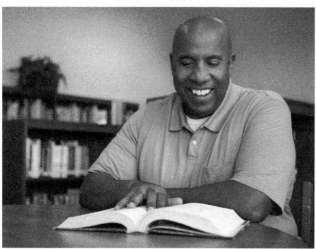

Figure 23.1 Study skills and exam preparation can improve your chances of passing the certification competency exam.

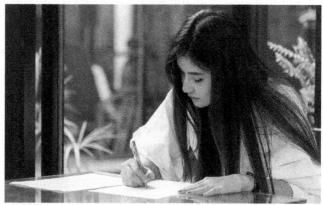

Figure 23.2 A good study location is well lit and quiet. It is devoted to studying and has needed supplies.

motivation is to set a realistic study schedule that includes both study time and activities you like to do. This can help you avoid **procrastination** (the purposeful postponement of a task) and **cramming** (studying a lot of material in a short amount of time) before a test.

The study time you schedule does not need to be long. In fact, it is good to start with a shorter amount of time and slowly increase the amount of time spent studying. First, schedule 15 minutes to study one subject or content area in which you are having difficulty. You can then add time from there. As you increase your study time, be sure to include breaks. This will help you divide the material into smaller portions that are more manageable. Do not waste your time. If you are not able to concentrate, are tired, or do not want to study, stop. Schedule another study time during that same day.

Scheduling time to study is important, but using your time wisely is even more critical. How well do you concentrate when you are studying? Concentration is a learned skill and develops over time. The time between when you start studying and when your mind wanders is called your *concentration span*. To determine your concentration span, identify how long it takes for your mind to wander when you are reading something you do not find interesting. This is your *minimum concentration span*. Then read something of interest. Again, identify how long it takes for your mind to wander. This is your *maximum concentration span*. Concentration spans can range between 10 and 20 minutes. Once you know your concentration span, do not study beyond it. Instead, take a break. Watch a video, take a walk, or have a snack, but keep thinking about what you were studying. This gives your brain time to organize the information. When you return to studying, you will find the information clearer and easier to recall.

Build Short- and Long-Term Memories

Concentration is related to how the brain stores information for memory. Two types of memory are short-term memory and long-term memory. *Short-term memory* allows you to remember information for a brief period of time. If this information is not stored, it is forgotten. For example, if you cram right before a test, the information may be recorded in your short-term memory and remembered for the test but will disappear quickly after that. To be retained (kept) on a permanent basis, information must pass into long-term memory. *Long-term memories* are formed through rehearsal, repetition, and association with information. Committing information to long-term memory actually requires physical changes in the brain. Long-term memory allows you to easily recall information, such as the steps for performing your nursing assistant skills. To improve your long-term memory, you can do the following:

- Focus your studying on one section at a time (for example, only vital signs or only infection control). Study these topics on different days.
- Practice active reading by asking yourself questions such as "What does this term mean?" or "Why is this important?" while you read. Look for answers to these questions while you are reading (**Figure 23.3**). Make sure all of your questions have been answered when you finish reading.

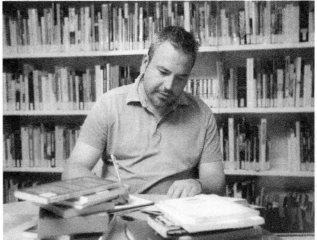

Maica/Signature Collection via Getty Images

Figure 23.3 Reading to answer your questions will help you focus on what you are learning.

- Keep your notes short and focus on the main points. Write the main points in your own words so you can remember them later. Review your notes often.
- Use acronyms to help recall the information you need to memorize. For example, when you need to determine a resident's pain, you can use the acronym *ELR* to remember to consider how the resident **E**xpresses pain, the **L**evel of pain, and any specific aspects of pain you should **R**eport.
- Draw, find, or imagine a picture of a topic you are studying. Mentally refer to the picture when you are studying or taking a test.
- Use certain smells to improve memory. Rosemary, lemon, lavender, and peppermint are scents that provide a calming effect and increase memory. You can put one drop of essential oils of these scents on a cotton ball and place it where you can smell it, such as in your pocket.
- Use flash cards to remember specific information. Each card may have a question on one side and the answer on the other side. Flash cards can also be helpful when reviewing vocabulary. You can write the key term on one side and the definition on the other. Use flash cards to quiz yourself or ask someone to quiz you.
- Form a study group with students who are as motivated as you (**Figure 23.4**). Practice skills with your group, taking turns as the nursing assistant, resident, and evaluator. Use the information provided in your state's handbook to guide the steps and evaluation.

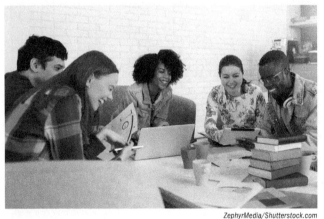

ZephyrMedia/Shutterstock.com

Figure 23.4 Study groups can help you review information and practice important skills.

- Reward yourself for your studying efforts. When you reach a studying milestone, such as learning a particularly difficult concept, reward yourself by spending time with friends or playing a video game. If you set rewards for yourself, you will be more motivated to continue studying.

What Should You Do on the Day of the Exam?

There are several steps you can take to prepare shortly before an exam. The night before the exam, quickly review the material and make a checklist of items to bring with you the next day. For example, many states require that you bring a watch with a second hand. Organize the needed items so you will remember to collect them the next morning. If there are specific instructions about the exam, review them. Go to bed early and try to get your normal amount of sleep. Remember that cramming will not help. If you have been studying consistently, you have learned what you need to know. It is important to give your brain and body the rest they need to function well during the exam.

On the day of the exam, set your alarm so you get up early enough to eat a healthy breakfast. Have a meal that includes starch from cereal, waffles, or any kind of bread. This type of breakfast will release a steady supply of sugar to your brain during the exam. Avoid candy, soda, or fruit juice, which will cause your sugar levels to rise too quickly and then drop so you feel sleepy. If you exercise regularly, do so before the exam. You might consider quickly reviewing any materials you still find challenging.

When you go to the exam, take all of the items and materials you will need, such as sharpened No. 2 pencils to complete the test answer sheet. If you are asked to dress in a particular way (wearing scrubs or some other type of clothing), make sure your clothes are clean and neat. Exam sites typically do not permit personal belongings, such as your cell phone, extra books, backpacks, or study materials. Arrive at the exam site early so you do not feel rushed. Late arrivals are not admitted to the exam. Go to the bathroom before walking into the exam room. Imagine yourself as being successful, and it will be easier to achieve success (**Figure 23.5**).

Successfully Preparing for Your Exam

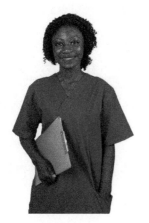

Review material the night before.

Make a list of items to bring to the exam.

Go to bed early.

Eat a healthy breakfast.

Quickly review any challenging materials.

Dress appropriately for the exam.

Gather all items you need for the exam.

Arrive at the exam early.

Use the restroom before the exam.

Visualize yourself as being successful.

vystekimages/Shutterstock.com

Figure 23.5 Successful preparation can help you do your best on the exam.

What Are Successful Test-Taking Strategies?

When taking the nursing assistant certification competency exam, you want to be successful. One of the first issues you may need to overcome to be successful is test anxiety. *Test anxiety* is an exaggerated worry about doing well. Anxiety can negatively influence your performance and can cause extreme nervousness and memory lapses during the exam. The following strategies can help you reduce or overcome test anxiety and be successful:

- Be familiar with specific instructions found in your state's handbook.
- Make sure you have everything you need at hand.
- Listen closely to verbal directions, and read instructions slowly and carefully.
- Ask for explanations of any instructions you do not understand.
- Stay relaxed. If you feel nervous, take two or three slow, deep breaths to relax yourself. Do this as often as you need to.
- Be positive. Imagine yourself completing the exam successfully.

The following are test-taking strategies specific to the written portion of the certification competency exam:

- Budget your time so you don't have to rush. If taking a paper test, quickly scan the questions to determine how you will spend your time. If taking an electronic test, know how long you have to complete the exam and the number of test items (**Figure 23.6**). Wear a watch to help pace yourself.

- Focus on your own test and on each question. Do not let your mind wander and don't be concerned if others finish before you do.
- If possible, answer all of the questions you are sure about first. This will help build your confidence.
- If you don't know the answer to a question, reread it. If you still cannot answer it, move on and come back to it later. You don't have to answer every question correctly to do well on the written exam.

The written exam is made up of multiple-choice questions. When answering multiple-choice questions, use the following strategies:

- Read the whole question.
- Think of the answer before looking at the options listed.
- Read all of the answer options and choose the one that most closely matches your answer.
- If you are unsure of the answer, eliminate any answer options that appear totally wrong. Select the option that seems like the best choice.
- If you are forced to guess, choose the longest, most detailed answer.
- Don't keep changing your answer. Your first choice is usually the correct answer.
- If you finish with time left, review your answers. Be sure you answered all of the questions you can. Review questions you were not sure of, but only change an answer if you did not correctly interpret the question or misread it.

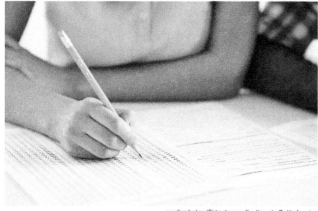

A

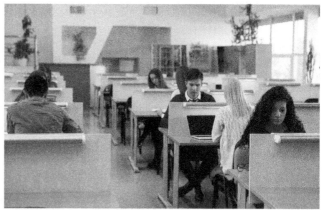

B

Figure 23.6 The written exam may be a paper test (A) or a computerized test (B).

SECTION 23.1 **Review and Assessment**

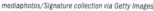

Key Terms Mini Glossary

auditory related to the sense of hearing.

concentration complete attention directed toward a particular object or task.

cramming studying large amounts of information in a short period of time.

flash cards a set of cards used for studying; cards typically have a question on one side and an answer on the other.

procrastination the act of purposely postponing a task.

Apply the Key Terms

Identify the key term used in each sentence.

1. Because you are a visual learner, you like using flash cards for studying because they have a question on one side and the answer on the other.
2. It has been difficult to study every day, and even though it is not a good idea, you spend the weekend cramming so you can study large amounts of information in a short period of time.
3. Procrastination seems to be a part of your friend Jane's life. She seems to postpone every task she needs to complete.
4. You have learned that your concentration has improved since you found a place to study where you can have your complete attention directed toward learning new information.
5. Edward's learning style is auditory because he likes to read his assignments out loud.

Know and Understand the Facts

1. Identify three skills needed to study effectively.
2. What types of testing are part of the certification competency exam?
3. Describe two ways to prepare for taking the certification competency exam.
4. List three ways to increase your concentration span.
5. Explain two ways you can improve your memory.

Analyze and Apply Concepts

1. In what two ways can people reduce test-taking anxiety?
2. What are three actions you can take to be successful when answering multiple-choice questions?
3. Identify three actions you can take to prepare yourself to be successful on the skills portion of the certification competency exam.

Think Critically

Read the following situation. Then answer the questions that follow.

Mario is ready to take his nursing assistant certification competency exam. He has done well in school, but is always nervous before taking exams. Sometimes he does well, and other times he gets so anxious that he feels physically ill. When this happens, his grades are lower than usual. He does not want this to happen when he takes the certification competency exam.

1. What can Mario do to study for the exam?
2. What actions can Mario take before the exam to remain calm?
3. If Mario does start to get anxious, what strategies can he use during the exam to decrease these feelings?

Your Nursing Career

Objectives

To achieve the objectives for this section, you must successfully:

- **identify** the steps and strategies for finding nursing assistant positions.
- **develop** a cover letter and résumé.
- **complete** employment applications.
- **demonstrate** successful employment interview skills.
- **design** a nursing or healthcare career plan.
- **explain** strategies for becoming a lifelong learner.

Key Terms

Learn these key terms to better understand the information presented in the section.

bullying   network
cover letter   résumé
job campaign

Questions to Consider

- What has been your experience with looking for and getting a job? Have you had an easy time finding and applying for the perfect job, or was the process challenging? Did you get the job or were you turned down? How did that feel?
- If you got the job, what was it like? Was it what you expected, or did it not turn out as you had hoped? What did you do about that?

What Are the Best Ways to Find a Nursing Assistant Position?

Finding your first nursing assistant position can be exciting, but it does require work. As a soon-to-be nursing assistant, you will want to explore which facilities you are most interested in and where you might want to apply. You may have the opportunity to get a position in the facility where you did your clinical training. You will have experienced the culture and organization of the facility, the types of residents, and the delivery of care. The facility staff members there will have also had the chance to observe your professional behaviors and attitudes, skills, abilities, and approach to care. If staff members like what they see, they may offer you a position.

If this does not occur or if you would rather work in another facility, you will need to develop and implement a *job campaign*, or organized activities needed to find a desired job. A job campaign can include the following strategies:

- Visit school or college job-placement centers and job fairs.
- Look for open position ads in newspapers, online, and on job boards.
- Search the websites of federal, state, and local government offices, job career centers, community organizations, and schools and colleges (posted ads and placement offices).
- Search websites of local healthcare facilities, or visit or call facilities' human resources departments.
- *Network*, or communicate, with friends, relatives, members of religious institutions, and participants in social activities to ask if anyone is aware of job openings (**Figure 23.7**).
- Identify facilities in which you would like to work and contact them about a position. You can ask to talk with the human resources department to find out if there are any open positions. Career opportunities may also be posted on the facility's website.
- If you identify a facility in which you would like to work, ask to talk with the supervisor of the department in which you are interested, even if there are no open positions. You can ask the supervisor about his or her expectations of nursing assistants and about the experience of working in the facility and on that unit.
- Review the descriptions of jobs to be sure they fit your interests and qualifications. Job descriptions can usually be found on a facility's website or by contacting the human resources department.

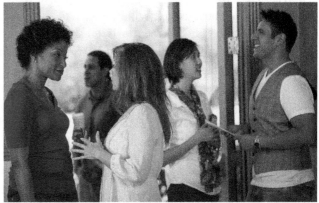

pixelheadphoto digitalskillet/Shutterstock.com

Figure 23.7 Networking allows you to connect with people who have similar interests and aspirations. It can help you learn about job openings and opportunities.

Applying directly to a facility, networking, and answering employment ads are the most common strategies for finding nursing assistant positions. You might also ask friends about opportunities or use school placement offices to find a position.

What Tools Are Needed to Find and Obtain a Position?

To obtain a position as a nursing assistant, you first need to develop a cover letter and résumé. Once you have identified a position of interest, you will likely also be required to complete an employment application.

A cover letter and résumé provide an opportunity for you to show a potential employer your education, skills, experience, and abilities. Each document should be a factual representation of you and should give enough information that the employer can decide if you are a good fit.

Cover Letter

A *cover letter* precedes a résumé and introduces you, your capabilities, and your skills to a prospective employer. If written in letter format, a cover letter should include your return address, the current date, and the mailing address of the employer. The greeting should be directed at the person responsible for hiring. In large facilities, this person might be the human resources manager. In small facilities, this person might be the director of nursing. Often, the information of the person responsible can be found on the facility website. You can also call the facility to ask who should receive this material. Many facilities request hiring information electronically and require that a cover letter be inputted or uploaded.

When writing a cover letter, start with a greeting such as "Dear Mrs. Jones" or the correct contact in the facility. If you do not have a specific name, use "To Whom It May Concern." The body of the letter should have an opening paragraph, in which you identify the position you are applying for and how you heard about it. The next paragraph should briefly describe why you believe your education, skills, and experience relate to the position. For example, you could write "I just completed a nursing assistant program and received my certification. I am enclosing my résumé, which provides more information about my experiences in helping others." The final paragraph should request a personal interview to discuss the position and your qualifications. Always thank the recipient for his or her time, and let him or her know that you look forward to hearing back soon.

If using a letter format, use the closing of *Sincerely*, and sign your name. Be sure to also print or type your name below the signature so the recipient can see the spelling of your name. If you are submitting the cover letter electronically, a signature is usually not necessary.

A cover letter should always be formal, clear, and to the point (**Figure 23.8**). If printed, it should appear on letter-size white or off-white paper.

Résumé

The *résumé* follows a cover letter. A résumé goes into more detail and should be brief (one page, if possible). Great résumés quickly grab the reader's attention and sell the applicant's accomplishments and strengths. They show why the applicant is a good fit and match for the position (**Figure 23.9**). A well-crafted résumé will take you to your desired next step: a personal interview for the position.

There is no best way to write a résumé; however, several important items should always be included:

- **Personal information:** list your full name, address, telephone number, and e-mail address.
- **A brief employment objective or goal:** in one or two sentences, state what you would like to do at the facility or accomplish in your nursing career. For example, you could write "My goal is to provide the best possible care for older adults," "My passion is to help others be as healthy as possible," or "I would like to begin my nursing career as a nursing assistant so I can someday be an RN."
- **Work experience:** start with the most recent experience and include dates employed, position title, organization, and address. You may want to provide a short sentence describing your primary responsibilities.
- **Education:** include the school, college, and program; time attended; and diploma, degree, or certificates earned. In some résumés, education precedes work experience.
- **Additional information:** this section can include licenses and certifications earned (with their identification numbers), organizations to which you belong, and volunteer experiences.
- **References:** you can simply say "Furnished upon request" or you can list no more than three *references*, or people who can comment on your skills and abilities. Include each reference's name, address, job title, and telephone number or e-mail address. Do not put a reference on your résumé without the reference's permission.

Jamelle Thompson
765 State Street
Lansing, Michigan 48906
555-555-5555
jthomp2@e-mail.com

January 8, 20XX

Natalie Smith
Manager
Briar Senior Living Center
533 Pat Street
Lansing, Michigan 48906

Dear Ms. Smith,

I am writing to express my interest in the opening your facility has for a certified nursing assistant. I found out about this position when I contacted your human resources department.

I am eager to work at your facility because of my interest in and experience with working with older adults. I discovered through weekend and summer volunteer work at the Community Senior Citizen Center that I have a special ability to motivate others to become more active and independent. I also enjoy assisting others. I am responsible for helping my two great-aunts, who need transportation to and from their doctors and extra help shopping. I always enjoy the times I spend with them.

I just completed a nursing assistant program and received my certification. My plans are to go back to school and become a registered nurse. My career goal is another reason I am interested in this position. My research about your facility has shown that there are many opportunities for motivated people such as I.

I am enclosing my résumé, which provides more information about my experiences helping others. I look forward to talking with you further about my experience and interest in the position. Thank you for your time and consideration.

Sincerely,

Jamelle Thompson

Figure 23.8 A good cover letter has an introduction, body paragraphs that highlight your interests and skills, and a closing that requests a desired next step.

The cover letter and résumé should always have correct spelling, grammar, and sentence structure. Carefully proofread these documents to make sure they are free from errors. Use a 12-point font. If printed, the résumé should be letter size on white or off-white paper. It should *not* include a photo.

Employment Application

Most positions require you to fill out and submit an *employment application* (**Figure 23.10**). A paper copy of the application may be filled out in person, or the application may be available to complete and submit online. The following information will likely be needed to complete the application:

- **Your address and phone number:** include your current address and the number of a phone you will answer.
- **Work experience:** include organization names, addresses, dates of employment, positions, and contact information. If you have limited work experience, you can include part-time positions, summer jobs, and volunteer work.
- **Education:** include the names and addresses of schools and dates attended.
- **References:** list the names, addresses, and phone numbers of people who can speak to your knowledge and skills. You should usually include three references. Be sure you have asked these references for permission.

Jamelle Thompson
765 State Street
Lansing, Michigan 48906
Cell Phone: 555-555-5555
E-mail: jthomp2@e-mail.com

Employment Goal:

My goal is to help older adults be as healthy, active, and independent as possible.

Work Experience:

Call Desk Representative, June 2019 to August 2021

Basic Credit Card Company, 17 Broadway, Lansing, Michigan 48909

My primary job responsibility was to gather basic customer information and direct the call to the appropriate department.

Clerk, June 2018 to May 2019

City Pharmacy, 4 Main Avenue, Lansing, Michigan 48909

My primary job responsibility was to help customers with their desired purchases. I also helped stock inventory.

Education:

Michigan Community College, Fall 2021

Completed Nurse Assisting Program

East Lansing Community College, Spring 2020

Completed Anatomy and Physiology and Chemistry courses

Lansing High School, 2014 to 2018

College preparatory program

Additional Information:

Nursing Assistant Certification, Michigan, #75443

Volunteer Experiences:

Volunteer, Arts and Music Program, during high school (summers and weekends)
Community Senior Citizen Center, 17 Lakewood Avenue, Lansing, Michigan 48906
Helped older adults become involved with arts, music, and reading programs.

References:

Jade Johnson, supervisor

Community Senior Citizen Center, 17 Lakewood Avenue, Lansing, Michigan 48906

Phone: 517-776-2323

Jim Sims, supervisor

Basic Credit Card Company, 17 Broadway, Lansing, Michigan 48909

Phone: 517-798-5421

John Lane, pharmacy manager

City Pharmacy, 4 Main Avenue, Lansing, Michigan 48909

Phone: 517-798-6655

Figure 23.9 A résumé should always have correct spelling, grammar, and sentence structure. Carefully proofread before sending it out.

Employment Application

Date

January 8, 20XX 📅

Which position(s) are you applying for?

○ RN   ○ Speech Therapist   ○ Physical Therapist

○ LPN   ○ Administrative Staff   ○ Occupational Therapist

○ Home Health Aide   ○ Social Worker   ○ Data Entry

◉ CNA

Name

First

Jamelle

Last

Thompson

Type/License #

Certified Nursing Assistant, License #75443

Issued by the State of

Michigan ▼

Expiration

November 30, 20XX 📅

Address

Street Address

765 State Street

City

Lansing

State

Michigan ▼

Zip Code

48906

Phone Number

555-555-5555

E-mail

jthomp2@e-mail.com

Do you have a valid driver's license?

◉ Yes   ○ No

Have you ever been convicted of a criminal offense other than a traffic violation?

○ Yes   ◉ No

What days are you available to work?

◉ Sunday   ◉ Thursday

◉ Monday   ○ Friday

◉ Tuesday   ◉ Saturday

◉ Wednesday

Please tell us about any experience you feel may qualify you for this position.

When I was in high school, I volunteered during the summers and weekends at the Community Senior Citizen Center. I helped with arts, music, and reading programs. I also worked for two years as a call desk representative for a credit card company. My primary responsibility was to gather basic customer information and direct the call to the appropriate department. I also spent one year working as a clerk in a local pharmacy. There, I helped customers with their desired purchases. For the past five years, I have assisted two of my older family members who have chronic illnesses. I transport them to the doctor, help them with their meals, accompany them to the store and church, and often read to them.

Figure 23.10 Always answer the questions on an employment application completely and honestly.

- **Salary expectations:** provide the minimum salary you require or let them know you are open to negotiations (a two-way discussion to come to an agreement).
- **Reason for applying:** provide an answer that shows how you are a good fit for the position and facility.

Answer all of the questions on the application. If you do not answer a question, have a reason why, as you will likely be asked about unanswered questions at the interview.

How Can You Be Successful When Interviewing for a Position?

After reviewing your cover letter, résumé, and employment application, the hiring manager will decide whether or not to ask you for a phone or in-person interview. The purpose of an interview is for the facility to find the right person for a position, but the interview is also an opportunity for you to decide if the position and facility are good fits for you. The outcome of a successful interview is an offer of a position from the facility.

A *phone interview* is often conducted before an in-person interview. A phone interview is a screening tool that allows the hiring manager to determine which candidates to meet in person. During a phone interview, speak clearly and confidently and be prepared to answer questions about your skills and experience.

Several skills can help you have a successful in-person interview. It is often helpful to practice your interviewing skills with a friend or family member. Follow these guidelines to be prepared and professional during an in-person interview:

- Be on time and come alone. Do not bring family members or friends.
- Enter the interview prepared and with a positive attitude. Research the facility before the interview. Know the facility's leadership, mission, and values. You may want to determine how the facility is unique compared to others.
- Wear clothing that shows you are a professional person (**Figure 23.11**). Dress in clean, neat business attire. Be sure that you have bathed and that your hair is groomed. Do not wear cologne or perfume. Remove body jewelry, such as lip, nose, and eyebrow rings and studs. Cover body art, if possible.
- Turn off your cell phone.

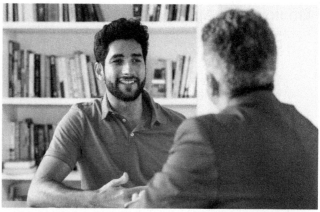
Daniel M Ernst/Shutterstock.com

Figure 23.11 When attending an interview, wear professional clothes that are clean and neat.

- Politely greet the interviewer(s). There may be more than one interviewer. An interviewer may be a supervisor from the area in which you would be working, a person from the human resources department, or another supervisor or director.
- Establish eye contact and smile. Try to be as relaxed as possible without slouching in the chair.
- Actively listen and be friendly.
- Speak clearly and with respect.
- Do not chew gum or communicate nonverbally that you are nervous or disinterested.
- Answer questions honestly to the best of your ability. If you do not understand a question, politely ask the interviewer to repeat it or ask it in another way. If you do not have an answer for a question, say you don't know the answer.
- Be prepared to answer several different kinds of questions related to your work history, relationships with coworkers, conflicts and resolutions at work, desire for a position in the facility, career goals, strengths, and areas or skills that need development. You will also be asked questions related to being a nursing assistant in the facility (**Figure 23.12**).

THINK ABOUT THIS

As you look for a position, have your driver's license and copies of your certifications or licenses on hand. Once you are employed, you may need to complete an I-9 (Employment Eligibility Verification), which will ask you to certify your identity using a combination of items (such as your driver's license, Social Security card, US passport, or birth certificate). You may also need to complete a background check and fingerprinting. You will likely be required to show evidence of specific immunizations (such as for hepatitis B) and have signed documentation from a healthcare provider that you have no communicable diseases and are able to perform the required job duties.

Commonly Asked Interview Questions and Prompts

- Why have you chosen nurse assisting as a career?
- What do you like and dislike about being a nursing assistant?
- What motivates you to work in healthcare and with residents?
- Describe a time you were very satisfied in a job you were doing.
- What are your strengths, and what areas do you think you need to develop?
- What do you find most stressful in a workplace? How do you handle your stress?
- With what type of manager do you work best?
- Talk about a difficult person you worked with and how you handled the situation.
- If you noticed a nurse, doctor, or nursing assistant not doing his or her job properly, what would you do?
- What would you do if a resident became agitated?
- What would you do if a resident refused care?
- How would you spend your time if all of your work was done and you had a few minutes to spare before completing your shift?
- What are your nursing career goals?

Goodheart-Willcox Publisher

Figure 23.12 Coming up with answers to questions and prompts like these before the interview can help you feel more prepared.

- When answering questions, emphasize your strengths. Explain why you think you are the best person for the position.
- Do not prolong the interview, but do ask questions, if appropriate. Ask questions that will help you understand and make a decision about the position. You can ask such questions as "What are you looking for in a successful nursing assistant?" or "What is the best thing about working in this facility?"
- Do not bring up salary yourself, but if the interviewer mentions it, you can ask about the salary and benefits of the position.

At the close of the interview, emphasize your accomplishments and ask if you can provide any additional information to show your abilities and interest in the position. Also ask when you will be notified about the position.

After the interview, send a thank-you message to the interviewer. The thank-you message should be brief and express appreciation for the interviewer's time and consideration. Offer again to provide any further information, and tell him or her that you are excited about the possibility of working at the facility.

After the interview, you may receive a job offer immediately or after several weeks. Generally, you should contact the facility about the position two weeks after the interview if you have not heard back. A job offer may come from the human resources department, the hiring manager, or some other administrative staff member. If you receive a job offer, always request it in writing. If salary, wages, and benefits (such as health insurance) were not discussed at the interview, be sure they are outlined and agreed to in the job offer. You should also know your start date, any other requirements (such as a physical examination), the location where you will be working, and the name of your supervisor. When you receive a job offer, express your appreciation and ask any remaining questions you have. If you are not sure whether you want to accept the offer, ask for time (usually 24 hours) to think it over before accepting.

What Will Your Work Environment Be Like?

Starting your first position as a nursing assistant can be very exciting and motivating. When you begin your job, you will be oriented to the facility and learn what is expected of you. You will be provided with on-the-job training, usually an employee handbook, and guidance from the licensed nursing staff. The first few weeks will be a learning experience, and as time passes, the environment and care will become more familiar.

Determining If a Job Is Right for You

Most facilities have a 60–90 day *probationary period*, during which time an employee is evaluated for fit in the facility. The employee is evaluated on whether he or she demonstrates the behaviors, attitudes, skills, and capabilities needed to provide safe, quality care. When you start a new position, pay attention to whether the position is a good fit for you, too. You may not know

---

THINK ABOUT THIS

State and federal equal employment opportunity (EEO) laws help prevent discrimination against an applicant or employee based on race, color, religion, sex (including pregnancy, gender identity, and sexual orientation), national origin, age (40 or older), disability, or genetic information. As a result, only job-related questions may be asked during an interview. For example, an interviewer may not ask an applicant about his or her marital status or children. Any questions about family status must be about any responsibilities or commitments that may prevent the applicant (regardless of sex) from meeting a work schedule.

this until you are well into the position, but you can start by considering whether you are excited to come to work each day, enjoy the people you work with, can take advantage of the educational programs provided, and feel supported in providing safe, quality care. If you feel supported, you will be able to help others feel supported and motivated.

Workplace Environment, Attitudes, and Behaviors

There are many different types of workplace environments. The environment is usually determined by the organization/unit culture, the types of residents being cared for, and the facility's leadership. While these are influential environmental factors, you are also a contributor to the workplace environment. You contribute through the attitudes and behaviors you bring with you every day as a nursing assistant who is eager and ready to care for residents. The following are eight positive and successful workplace attitudes and behaviors. Remember that possessing these attitudes and behaviors can make a difference in how well you engage with residents, coworkers, and the licensed nursing staff. How many of these attitudes and behaviors do you already demonstrate? Which might you need to work on?

- Being enthusiastic and positive about the position you have and the care you give as a nursing assistant.
- Being respectful to and appreciating the diverse people you work with and the residents you care for.

- Showing up to work on time and effectively managing your time during your shift. This is an important contribution you make to those you care for, but it is also essential to your coworkers' time management.
- Being conscientious, organized, dependable, and achievement-oriented.
- Being friendly, cooperative, and helping others. Know that the more helpful you are to others, the more your coworkers will be willing to work with and help you.
- Being aware of your own actions and their consequences. Take responsibility for any errors you make, and learn from them.
- Balancing your work and life so that each supports and positively contributes to the other.
- Being open to new experiences and believing you will be/are successful.

While possessing these attitudes and demonstrating these behaviors will certainly make a positive difference in your work environment, you will also experience problems and issues at work. Some problems you may bring to work, some may be organizational, others may be due to communication issues and gossip (private or secret stories that are repeated and spread about others), or they may be due to ineffective leadership, interaction with your coworkers, such as dealing with their lack of motivation or being in conflict with them, and, finally, some work problems and issues are due to an ongoing stressful work environment.

HEALTHCARE SCENARIO
Career Development Opportunities

A recent study found a strong relationship between a person's job satisfaction, career development, and retention (keeping the same employees) in the workplace. Another study found that, after salary, the reason most often given for employees leaving a facility was lack of career development opportunities. Based on the results of both studies, a local community hospital's leadership decided to provide employees with a full range of career planning opportunities. This year, the hospital increased staff development programs and provided time for employees to attend these programs. The hospital developed formal career opportunities between different positions and within positions. In addition, the hospital

is financing career advancement by offering tuition reimbursement and scholarships for employees who would like to earn certificates and degrees or attend conferences. To make sure these opportunities are used well, the hospital hired a career counselor who works full time in human resources to meet with employees and help them plan their careers at the hospital.

Apply It

1. What career planning opportunities might you use to advance your career? Explain.
2. If you were to meet with a career counselor, what specifically would you want the counselor to know about your career plan?

BECOMING A HOLISTIC NURSING ASSISTANT

Lifelong Learning

Several strategies can be used to strengthen your ability to become a lifelong learner. These strategies include the following:

- Make self-improvement and an awareness of new things to learn your priorities.
- Find time each day to learn something new.
- Read books and articles about professional and personal areas of interest.
- Reflect on your practice by journaling and discussing your awarenesses with other nursing assistants.
- Keep a list of things you want to learn.

- Spend time with people who have similar professional interests.
- Attend conferences and educational programs.
- Teach others.
- Work in facilities that challenge you.

Apply It

1. Which of these strategies are already part of your daily life?
2. Which strategies might you add to ensure you continue to be a lifelong learner?

Managing Stress and Dealing with Workplace Violence

For a nursing assistant, the goal of each and every day at work is to provide safe, quality care. Healthcare today, however, is very fast paced, and those in your care will have needs and demands that can create a great deal of stress. Sometimes this stress can lead residents, family members, other healthcare providers, and coworkers to act aggressively. Aggressive acts may range from violent or physical acts (such as assault) to verbal abuse, threats, hostility, *bullying* (repeated and harmful verbal, physical, social, or psychological behavior), or harassment. The Occupational Safety and Health Administration (OSHA) reports that incidents of serious workplace violence (incidents requiring days off work for the injured worker) are four times more common in healthcare than in other industries. Residents may act aggressively toward healthcare workers, and worker-to-worker violence may also occur.

Being aware of violence in the workplace is important. Some strategies to deal with workplace violence include the following:

- Understand the facility's workplace violence policy and safety and security procedures.
- Immediately report incidents.
- Recognize the warning signs of possible violence. Verbal cues include speaking loudly or yelling, swearing, or using a threatening tone of voice. Nonverbal cues include holding the arms tight across the chest, clenching the fists, or pacing with agitation.
- Remember to use effective communication techniques and skills to resolve conflicts (see Chapter 11).

- Use stress-management and relaxation techniques (see Chapter 7).
- Be aware that fatigue can lower your alertness and ability to respond appropriately to a challenging situation.
- Practice personal security measures. Dress for safety, keep long hair tucked away so it cannot be grabbed, and avoid wearing earrings or necklaces that can be pulled. Avoid overly tight clothing that can restrict movement and overly loose clothing or scarves that can be caught. Do not leave anything dangling from cords or chains, and use breakaway safety cords or lanyards.

Successfully Leaving a Position

The goal of every professional should be to make the work and work environment as positive as possible. Remember, however, that if a position is not a good fit, it is best to look for another. If you wait to look for another position, you may become frustrated, depressed, or angry, and this can affect the care being delivered. It is helpful to talk with your supervisor first. Give a brief explanation about why you are leaving. If you want to stay in the facility, but not on the unit, ask if there may be another position available. If you decide to leave the facility, be professional by thanking your supervisor for the opportunity and share how much you have learned. Give at least two weeks' notice and stay for the entire two weeks unless you are asked to leave sooner. You may also be asked to stay longer until a replacement is hired. If you can, try to honor that request. Remember that during your last two weeks you should continue to complete your assignments, follow all policies and procedures, and train others who may take your place, with the same commitment as if you were not leaving.

Leave on good terms by communicating to others the same brief explanation about why you are leaving as you did when talking with your supervisor. Do not blame others for your leaving or say negative things about the organization, your supervisor, or coworkers. You may want to return to the facility in the future.

Before you leave, you may want to meet with the human resources department or the person who handles this area to find out what benefits and compensation you are entitled to. You should also provide a letter of resignation. It can be as brief as including the date you are leaving and that you are leaving for another opportunity.

When you leave, do not take anything that does not belong to you. If you are not offered a reference from your supervisor, know that you can still ask for one at a later time.

How Do You Advance Your Nursing or Healthcare Career?

In addition to career development, advancing your career also means gaining further education, training, and experience. In nursing, advancement might mean becoming a registered nurse. If you are interested in another field in healthcare, you might become a dietitian, physical therapist, or doctor. Thinking about your future career now is helpful and gives you a chance to identify your short- and long-term career goals. There are four stages in career planning for advancement:

1. **Examination:** determine your present values, skills, and abilities. You might complete career or job strength assessments or talk with a counselor. Recognizing your strengths and preferences will help you choose a future career.

2. **Exploration and preparation:** research careers of interest to find out what each requires. Learn about the career's education, training, certification, experience, salaries and benefits, employment possibilities, and career advancement. You might interview someone who has this career or ask to spend a day observing to see what an average day in the career is like. If possible, you might volunteer with an organization or facility related to your career of interest.

3. **Commitment to career:** you know what you want to do and feel confident about your chosen career. Commitment requires setting goals, focusing on the expectations of the career, and fulfilling the career's requirements. If you wish to pursue a nursing career, completing a nursing assistant training program is an effective first step.

4. **Transformation:** occurs after an initial career has been launched. Many times, a person decides to advance further in a career (for example, by going from a staff nurse to a nurse manager or nurse practitioner) or pursue a related career. Changes usually require further education, training, certification, and experience.

The way to implement career planning is to establish an action plan that helps guide you through each stage. Your action plan should include all four stages and identify your goals.

CULTURE CUES
A Culture of Lifelong Learning

A nursing assistant's chances of becoming a lifelong learner increase when he or she works in a facility that values lifelong learning. In this type of facility, the organization and leadership create a culture of lifelong learning. To find such a facility, look for one that prioritizes the professional growth and self-development of employees; supports innovation, clinical quality, and excellence; is comfortable with change; financially invests in employee education and training; and promotes the well-being of a community and its people.

Apply It

1. Have you ever worked in a lifelong learning culture? What was it like?

2. If you have not, what could you do to create a lifelong learning culture for yourself?

How Can You Become a Lifelong Learner?

An important part of developing as a nursing assistant and building your healthcare career is becoming a person who desires and seeks learning. Further learning improves competence throughout life and makes a lifelong learner. Qualities and characteristics of lifelong learners include:

- curiosity
- flexibility, adaptability, and comfort with change
- accountability and self-reliance
- innovation and creativity in problem-solving
- quality and excellence
- education to promote self-development, well-being, and care
- workplaces that promote lifelong learning

SECTION 23.2 Review and Assessment

Key Terms Mini Glossary

bullying repeated and harmful verbal, physical, social, or psychological behavior toward others.

cover letter a formal, written introduction that outlines a person's capabilities and skills to a prospective employer.

job campaign a series of organized activities needed to find a desired job.

network to communicate with an informal, interconnected group of people.

résumé a formal, written representation of a person's experience, skills, and credentials.

Apply the Key Terms

Complete the following sentences using the key terms in this section.

1. You have decided that you would like to look for a nursing assistant position. The first step will be to develop a _____, which will include organized activities to find your desired job.
2. Another strategy will be to informally _____ with people you know to see if they know of any available positions.
3. Once you find a position of interest, you will need to write a _____ that will include a written introduction outlining your capabilities.
4. You will also need a written _____ that shows your experience, skills, and credentials.
5. In your exploration for a job, you hear about a facility that you do not want to apply to. You were told that there is repeated and harmful verbal, physical, social, and psychological behavior directed toward healthcare staff. This is called _____.

Know and Understand the Facts

1. Identify two different methods of finding a nursing assistant position.
2. List two important items to include in a cover letter.
3. List two important items to include in a résumé.
4. Identify two important pieces of information to include on an employment application.
5. Describe four successful interviewing skills.
6. Identify two follow-up actions to take after an interview.

Analyze and Apply Concepts

1. How can you best determine if a nursing assistant position will be a good or bad fit for you?
2. Complete a career planning action plan for your future career.
3. List two strategies for becoming a lifelong learner.

Think Critically

Read the following situation. Then answer the questions that follow.

LoriAnne has just completed her nursing assistant training program and has successfully passed the nursing assistant certification competency exam. She applied for a position at the facility in which she did her clinical training. LoriAnne was asked to submit a cover letter and résumé and complete the employment application. She was told the director of nursing would like to interview her next week. She really wants this position.

1. What type of information should LoriAnne include in her cover letter and résumé to best represent her qualifications?
2. What advice would you give LoriAnne about conducting herself during the interview?
3. What questions should LoriAnne ask during the interview?
4. List four attitudes and behaviors LoriAnne can demonstrate to help her get this position.

Key Points

Reviewing the key points for this chapter will help you practice more safely and competently as a holistic nursing assistant and will help you prepare for the certification competency examination.

- Using excellent study habits and skills can help you pass the nursing assistant certification competency exam.
- Prevent test anxiety by listening closely to instructions and breathing deeply if nervous. Budget your time, answer the questions you know first, and eliminate incorrect options.
- To find a nursing assistant position, search online, network, and apply to desired facilities.
- A cover letter and résumé are opportunities to show a potential employer your education, skills, experience, and abilities.
- An employment application is a requirement for all positions, and each facility will have its own form for completion.
- When interviewing, be prepared, be professional, answer questions honestly and fully, and ask questions to better understand the position and facility.
- Being a lifelong learner means desiring and seeking learning to improve competence throughout your life.

Action Steps to Holistic Care

Review the information in this chapter. Complete the following activities.

1. Prepare a short paper or digital presentation that identifies your three most effective test-taking strategies. Explain why these strategies work for you.
2. With a partner, prepare a poster that lists at least eight actions you can take to effectively prepare for the certification competency exam.
3. Write a song or a poem about short- and long-term memories. Discuss why this information is important.
4. Research current scientific information about how people concentrate. Write a brief report describing two current facts you did not know.
5. Prepare a one-page résumé that outlines your employment objective, education, work experience, and any additional information you think wise to include. Identify three references and seek permission to use them on your résumé. Carefully proofread and format your résumé. Then exchange résumés with a partner. Review his or her résumé, offering constructive criticism. Review your partner's feedback on your résumé and implement any appropriate changes.

Building Math Skill

Harry is getting ready to take the certification competency exam. He decides to take a practice written test. The test has 60 multiple-choice test questions. When Harry finishes the test, he finds that he has 45 correct answers. What percent of questions did Harry answer correctly?

Preparing for the Certification Competency Examination

This chapter provides information to help you prepare for the nursing assistant certification competency exam and find your first position as a nursing assistant. As you get ready to accomplish these tasks, reflect on and answer the following questions about preparing for the certification competency exam and finding your first nursing assistant position.

Consider the following questions about preparing for the certification competency exam:

1. Describe where you study best.
2. What changes can you make to your study space to improve the quality and time of your studying?
3. How do you handle distractions when studying?
4. What is the length of your concentration span?
5. What have you done to improve your memory skills in the past?
6. After reading this chapter, do you want to use any new skills to improve your memory? Explain.
7. Draft a plan of action you can use to prepare the night before and the day of the certification competency exam.
8. Which of the test-taking strategies discussed in this chapter do you think you will use? Why?

Consider the following questions about pursuing your first nursing assistant position:

9. How will you go about getting your first nursing assistant position? What specific strategies will you use in your job campaign?
10. What information should you include in a cover letter and résumé to secure your first nursing assistant position?
11. Are any parts of the employment application unclear? If so, what can you do to clarify these questions?
12. Describe the most important steps in having a successful interview.

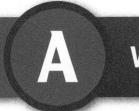

A Word Parts

Word Parts

Combining Forms			
Combining Form (Root Word Plus Combining Vowel)	**Meaning**	**Combining Form (Root Word Plus Combining Vowel)**	**Meaning**
anter/o	front	infer/o	below
arthr/o	joint	later/o	side
bi/o	life	lip/o	fat
cardi/o; card/o	heart	log/o	study
caud/o	tail	medi/o	middle
cephal/o	head	my/o	muscle
cervic/o	neck; cervix (neck of uterus)	neur/o	nerve
col/o; colon/o	colon; large intestine	path/o	disease
cost/o	rib	pneum/o	lung; air; gas
cyt/o	cell	poster/o	back; behind
dist/o	away from the point of origin	proxim/o	near the point of origin; close
dors/o	back of the body	sarc/o	connective tissue
enter/o	intestine (small)	super/o	above
gastr/o	stomach	thorac/o	chest
glyc/o	sugar	ventr/o	front side of the body
hepat/o	liver	viscer/o	internal organ
hist/o	tissue		

Prefixes			
Prefix	**Meaning**	**Prefix**	**Meaning**
a-; an-	not; without	dis-	apart; abnormal
ab-	away from	dorsi-	back
ad-	toward	dys-	bad; difficult; painful
ante-	before	ec-	outside
anti-	against	echo-	reflected sound
auto-	self	en-; em-	in; within
bi-	two; both	endo-	in; within
brady-	slow	epi-	on; over; upon
circum-	around	eso-	inward
con-	together	eu-	good
dia-	through; complete	exo-	outward

(continued)

Word Parts (continued)

Prefixes			
Prefix	**Meaning**	**Prefix**	**Meaning**
hemi-	half	pan-	all
hetero-	different	para-	near; beside
homo-	same	per-	through
hyper-	above normal; excessive	peri-	around; surrounding
hypo-	below normal; less than	poly-	many
in-	into	post-	after; behind
infra-	beneath; below; under	pro-	forward; in front of
inter-	between	quadri-	four
intra-	within; into	sub-	below; under
macro-	large	supra-	above; over
mega-	big	syn-	together; with
meta-	change; after	tachy-	fast
micro-	small	trans-	across
mono-	one	tri-	three
neo-	new	ultra-	beyond; excess
non-	not		

Suffixes			
Suffix	**Meaning**	**Suffix**	**Meaning**
-ac; -al; -ar; -ary; -atic; -iac; -ial; -ic; -ical; -ior; -ory; -ous; -tic	pertaining to	-cusis	hearing
-algesia	pain; sensitivity	-cyte	cell
-algia	pain	-dipsia	thirst
-ant	substance that promotes	-dynia	pain
-arche	beginning	-ectasis	dilation; expansion
-ase	enzyme	-ectomy	surgical removal
-assay	analyze; analysis	-edema	swelling
-asthenia	weakness	-ema	condition
-ation	process	-emesis	vomiting
-blast	developing cell	-emia	blood condition
-capnia	carbon dioxide	-emic	pertaining to blood condition
-cele	swelling; protrusion	-esthesia	condition of feeling or sensation
-centesis	procedure to remove fluid	-fusion	to pour
-chezia	defecation	-gen	substance that produces
-clysis	irrigation; washing	-genesis	formation
-crit	to separate	-genic	produced by; in

Word Parts *(continued)*

Suffixes			
Suffix	**Meaning**	**Suffix**	**Meaning**
-gram	record; image	**-pheresis**	removal
-graphy	process of recording	**-phoresis**	transmission
-gravida	pregnant	**-plasia**	development; formation
-ia; -ism	condition	**-plasm**	formation; structure
-in; -ine	chemical	**-plasty**	surgical repair
-ion	process	**-plegia**	paralysis
-ist	specialist	**-plegic**	pertaining to paralysis
-itis	inflammation	**-pnea**	breathing
-lepsy	seizure or sudden attack	**-poiesis**	formation
-logist	one who specializes in the study	**-porosis**	condition of small holes
-logy	study of	**-prandial**	meal
-lysis	breaking down	**-ptosis**	droop; sag
-lytic	pertaining to breakdown or destruction	**-rrhage**	rupture
-malacia	softening	**-rrhaphy**	suture
-megaly	enlargement	**-rrhea**	flow
-meter	measure	**-salpinx**	fallopian tube
-metry	process of measuring	**-sclerosis**	hardening
-oid	like; resembling	**-scope**	instrument used to view
-oma	tumor	**-scopy**	visual examination with a scope
-opia	vision condition	**-sis**	state; condition
-opsy	view of	**-spasm**	muscle contraction
-orexia	appetite	**-stalsis**	contraction
-osis	abnormal condition	**-stasis**	stoppage of flow
-osmia	smell	**-stenosis**	narrowing
-otia	ear condition	**-stitial**	standing; positioned
-paresis	weakness	**-stomy**	new opening
-partum	childbirth	**-taxia**	muscle coordination
-pathy	disease	**-tension**	pressure
-penia	decrease; deficiency	**-therapy**	treatment
-pepsia	digestion	**-thorax**	chest
-pexy	surgical fixation	**-tomy**	incision
-phagia	eating; swallowing	**-trophy**	condition of growth
-phasia	speech	**-tropic**	turning

(continued)

Word Parts *(continued)*

Suffixes			
Suffix	**Meaning**	**Suffix**	**Meaning**
-tropin	hormone	**-uria**	condition of urine; containing urine
-tripsy	process of crushing	**-version**	to turn
-um; -us	structure; thing; membrane	**-y**	process of

Conversion Table: US Customary to SI Metric*

When You Know ⬇	Multiply By ⬇	To Find ⬇
Length		
inches	25.4	millimeters
inches	2.54	centimeters
feet	0.3048	meters
feet	30.48	centimeters
yards	0.9	meters
miles	1.6	kilometers
Weight		
ounces	28.0	grams
ounces	0.028	kilograms
pounds	0.45	kilograms
short tons	0.9	tonnes
Volume		
teaspoons	5.0	milliliters
tablespoons	15.0	milliliters
fluid ounces	30.0	milliliters
cups	0.24	liters
pints	0.47	liters
quarts	0.95	liters
gallons	3.8	liters
cubic inches	0.02	liters
cubic feet	0.03	cubic meters
cubic yards	0.76	cubic meters
Area		
square inches	6.5	square centimeters
square feet	0.09	square meters
square yards	0.8	square meters
square miles	2.6	square kilometers
acres	0.4	hectares
Temperature		
Fahrenheit	$5/9 \times (F - 32)$	Celsius
Celsius	$(9/5 \times C) + 32$	Fahrenheit

*Note: For all but temperature, when you know the metric measurement, divide by the same numbers given above to determine the US customary measurement.

BMI Calculation

US Customary	SI Metric
$BMI = \dfrac{wt\ (lb)}{ht\ (in^2)} \times 703$	$BMI = \dfrac{wt\ (kg)}{ht\ (m^2)}$

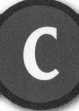
Sexually Transmitted Infections (STIs)

Infection	Cause	Signs and Symptoms	Treatment
Chlamydia	• Caused by bacteria (*Chlamydia trachomatis*) • Spread during vaginal and anal intercourse	• Symptoms begin 5–10 days after exposure. • Symptoms are often mild, particularly for men. • In women, symptoms include abdominal pain, abnormal vaginal discharge, bleeding between menstrual periods and after intercourse, low-grade fever, painful intercourse, burning during urination, swelling in vagina, and itching and swelling around anus. • In men, symptoms include pain or burning during urination, pus or watery/milky discharge from the penis, swollen or tender testicles, and itching and swelling around the anus.	• Antibiotics are taken to resolve the infection. • Both partners must be treated and remain abstinent until treatment is completed. • Condoms should be used to prevent future infection.
Gonorrhea	• Caused by bacteria (*Neisseria gonorrhoeae*) transmitted during sexual contact • Spread by vaginal and anal intercourse and oral sex • May also be passed from a woman to her fetus during childbirth • Cannot be spread by kissing or hugging • Often accompanied by chlamydia	• Some people do not show symptoms or only have minor symptoms. • Symptoms begin 1–14 days after exposure. • In women, symptoms include abdominal pain, bleeding between menstrual periods, menstrual irregularities, fever, painful intercourse, painful or frequent urination, swelling or tenderness of the vulva, vomiting, and yellow or yellow-green vaginal discharge. • In men, symptoms include puslike discharge from the penis, pain or burning during urination, and frequent urination. • In both sexes, symptoms include anus itchiness, discharge and pain during bowel movements, and itching and soreness of the throat (with trouble swallowing if the infection is oral).	• Antibiotics are used to treat infection. All of the antibiotics must be taken, even if symptoms clear up early. • Pregnant women and teens should not be given certain antibiotics. • Both partners must be treated and remain abstinent until treatment is completed. • Untreated gonorrhea in pregnant women can cause premature labor and stillbirth. • Condoms should be used to prevent future infection.

Sexually Transmitted Infections (STIs) *(continued)*

Infection	Cause	Signs and Symptoms	Treatment
Herpes	• Caused by herpes simplex virus type 1 (HSV-1) and herpes simplex virus type 2 (HSV-2) • Spread by touching, kissing, and sexual contact (including vaginal, anal, and oral sex) • Can also be spread from a woman to her fetus during childbirth • Is most contagious when sores are open, moist, or leaking, but can be spread when no symptoms are present	• Some people do not show symptoms or only have minor symptoms. • Symptoms may last several weeks and then go away for weeks, months, or years. The initial outbreak has the worst symptoms. • Symptoms typically begin 2–20 days after exposure, but may take years. • Symptoms include a cluster of blistery sores on the vagina, vulva, cervix, penis, buttocks, or anus; a burning feeling if urine flows over sores; inability to urinate if severe swelling blocks the urethra; and itching and pain in the infected area. • During the initial outbreak, symptoms include swollen, tender glands in the pelvic area, throat, and underarms; fever or chills; headache; general rundown feelings; and achy, flulike feelings.	• There is no cure, but certain medications help manage the infection. Treatment is usually very effective in speeding the healing of sores and preventing them from returning frequently. • Warm baths give some pain relief, as do cold compresses or ice packs. • Pain medications such as aspirin, acetaminophen, or ibuprofen may help relieve discomfort and fever. • Partners must stop all sexual activity as soon as they feel warning signs of an outbreak. • A small, daily dose of antiherpes medication (called *suppressive therapy*) can reduce the risk of transmission and the frequency and duration of outbreaks. • Other antiherpes medications treat individual outbreaks. • Good diet, adequate rest and sleep, and effective stress management may help prevent herpes outbreaks.
Human immunodeficiency virus (HIV)	(See discussion in Chapter 10.)		
Human papillomavirus (HPV)	• Transferred through skin-to-skin contact, usually during vaginal, anal, or oral sex	• Some types of HPV do not cause any noticeable signs or symptoms. • One possible symptom is genital warts. • Some types of HPV cause cell changes that may lead to cervical cancer and other genital and throat cancers.	• There is currently no cure for HPV. • Some HPV infections are harmless, do not require treatment, and go away within 8–13 months. • Colposcopy, cryotherapy, and LEEP procedures may be used to remove abnormal cells from the cervix. • Condoms reduce the risk of transmitting HPV during vaginal or anal intercourse, but are not as effective as against other STIs.

(continued)

Sexually Transmitted Infections (STIs) *(continued)*

Infection	Cause	Signs and Symptoms	Treatment
Pelvic inflammatory disease (PID)	• Usually caused by bacteria from other STIs such as chlamydia or gonorrhea • Sometimes caused by normal bacteria found in the vagina	• The early stages of PID may not produce noticeable symptoms. • Later stages are characterized by unusually long or painful periods, unusual vaginal discharge, spotting and pain between menstrual periods or during urination, pain in the lower abdomen and back, fever, chills, nausea, vomiting, and pain during vaginal intercourse.	• Infections are treated with antibiotics, bed rest, and lots of fluids. • Surgery may be needed to repair or remove reproductive organs in advanced cases. • Pain medications such as aspirin, acetaminophen, or ibuprofen may help relieve discomfort. • A heating pad on the stomach may reduce discomfort. • Both partners must be treated and remain abstinent until treatment is completed.
Syphilis	• Caused by bacteria (*Treponema pallidum*) introduced through direct contact with a syphilis sore (during unprotected vaginal, anal, or oral sex) • Can be transferred from an infected mother to her unborn baby	• The primary stage causes a single or multiple firm, round, painless sores at the location bacteria entered the body. The sore lasts three to six weeks. • The secondary stage starts with a rough and red, itch-free body rash on the palms or soles of the feet. Other symptoms are mucous membrane lesions, fever, swollen lymph glands, sore throat, muscle aches, and fatigue. • The late stage causes numbness, blindness, difficult coordination, and dementia. The stage may result in death.	• A single dose of penicillin will usually treat syphilis in the first year of infection. • Additional doses may be required for those who have had untreated syphilis for longer than one year.

Glossary

12-hour clock: a method of indicating time that splits the day into two 12-hour periods: the 12 hours from midnight to noon (called *a.m. hours*) and the 12 hours from noon to midnight (called *p.m. hours*); each hour is numbered consecutively and labeled as *a.m.* or *p.m.* (13)

24-hour clock: a method of indicating time that divides the day into 24 hours, from midnight to midnight and numbered from 0 to 24; does not use *a.m.* or *p.m.* designations; also called *military time*. (13)

A

abrasions: scraping of the outer layer of skin. (8)

abuse: a deliberate action (physical, verbal, financial, or sexual) that causes harm. (3)

accountable: responsible; able to explain any actions taken. (6)

accreditation: an official determination that a healthcare facility meets professional and community standards that promote safety and quality. (3)

acronyms: words formed from the first letters or groups of letters in a phrase. (9)

active listening: the process of showing interest in what a person is saying; includes paying attention, making eye contact, clarifying, summarizing, and reflecting on what a person has said. (11)

activities of daily living (ADLs): actions that residents take during a typical day; includes bathing, walking, eating, dressing, and toileting. (1)

acute care: serious, critical, or surgical care; typically delivered in hospitals. (2)

acute disease: a short-term disease or condition that usually starts suddenly. (10)

acute pain: an intense discomfort, often the result of trauma, that goes away within six months with treatment. (10)

addendum: a type of amendment in which an item is added to a health record to correct an error. (13)

addictive: causing a psychological and physical inability to control or stop taking a medication. (10)

advance directives: written legal documents signed by a living, competent person; describe that person's medical and healthcare instructions in the event of incapacitation. (22)

alcohol-based hand sanitizer: a liquid, gel, or foam preparation containing alcohol; kills most bacteria and fungi and destroys some viruses found on the skin. (8)

alimentary canal: a muscular tube of organs that starts in the mouth and leads down to the anus; a part of the gastrointestinal system; also called the *gastrointestinal (GI) tract*. (9)

allergen: any substance that the body perceives as a threat, causing an allergic reaction. (5)

alternative feeding therapy: the practice of delivering food intravenously or through a gastrointestinal tube due to a resident's inability to ingest food through the mouth. (19)

always events: routine activities and processes that are so important they must be performed consistently and without error. (4)

Alzheimer's disease (AD): a degenerative brain disease and the most common form of dementia; results in progressive memory loss, confusion, disorientation, and changes in personality and mood; advanced cases lead to decline in cognitive and physical functioning. (4)

ambulating: moving about or walking. (1)

amendments: corrections to a health record. (13)

analgesic: a type of pain medication that does not cause loss of consciousness. (10)

anaphylaxis: a severe allergic reaction that can affect the whole body; may cause skin reactions, swelling, trouble breathing, rapid pulse, nausea, and dizziness. (5)

anatomy: the study of the body's structure and parts. (9)

anesthetic: a medication that produces a loss of sensation. (10)

aneurysm: a distended and weak area in the wall of an artery supplying blood to the brain. (10)

anger: a strong feeling or emotion that develops from frustration, displeasure, or a threat. (11)

angina: chest pain or discomfort; there may be a sensation of squeezing, pressure, heaviness, or tightness in the center of the chest. (5)

ankylosis: the stiffening or immobility of a joint. (14)

antibodies: proteins in the blood that attach themselves to antigens and mark them for destruction by the immune system. (8)

antigens: substances foreign to the body that trigger the production of antibodies. (8)

anxiety: a feeling of worry, uneasiness, or nervousness. (2)

aphasia: a condition in which a resident cannot understand or use words. (10)

apical pulse: a measurement of heartbeat taken by listening to the apex of the heart (to the left of the sternum slightly under the left breast) with a stethoscope. (15)

apnea: a lack of breathing. (15)

appendicular skeleton: the skeletal structure that enables the body to move; includes bones in the body's appendages (arms and legs). (9)

arrhythmias: abnormal heart rhythms. (10)

arteriosclerosis: a condition in which arteries thicken, harden, and lose elasticity. (10)

asepsis: the absence of infection or infectious material; also called *sterile*. (8)

asphyxia: a lack of oxygen in the body; may be caused when breathing stops due to a blockage or swelling in the trachea. (5)

Note: The number in parentheses following each definition indicates the chapter in which the term can be found.

aspirate: to inhale a foreign object or substance, such as food or liquid, when eating. (19)

assault: any words or actions that a person finds threatening or that cause a person to fear harm. (3)

assertive: bold and clear. (11)

assessing: examining a situation so it can be evaluated. (6)

assistive devices: used for support during ambulation because residents can bear only a limited amount of weight on their legs and feet; includes canes, crutches, and walkers. (14)

atherosclerosis: a condition in which arteries narrow due to plaque buildup. (10)

atony: a lack of sufficient muscular strength. (14)

atrophy: to shrink or decrease in size. (9)

attitudes: ways of thinking or feeling about a person, situation, or object. (1)

auditory: related to the sense of hearing. (23)

aural: relating to the ear or the sense of hearing. (15)

automated external defibrillator (AED): a medical device that gives an electric shock to the heart to stop irregular heart rhythm and allow normal heart rhythm to begin. (5)

autonomic nervous system (ANS): the part of the peripheral nervous system that controls involuntary, unconscious body functions. (9)

autonomy: the personal independence and freedom to determine one's own actions and behavior. (7)

axial skeleton: the skeletal structure that provides stability for the body; includes bones in the body's trunk. (9)

axilla: the armpit. (14)

axillary temperature: a measurement of body temperature taken by placing a thermometer under the axilla. (15)

B

bacteria: single-celled, microscopic pathogens that can cause infection. (8)

basic life support (BLS): care given to a person experiencing respiratory arrest, cardiac arrest, or airway blockage; includes giving cardiopulmonary resuscitation (CPR), using an automated external defibrillator (AED), and relieving a blocked airway. (5)

bath blanket: a blanket, usually made from cotton or another absorbent material, that keeps a resident warm during a bed bath; may also be used as a protective covering to maintain resident modesty and warmth during various procedures. (17)

battery: the act of touching a person without his or her permission. (3)

behavior: a manner of acting; the way a person responds to stimulation. (7)

beliefs: ideas that a person or group of people accepts to be true. (12)

beneficence: the moral obligation to do good. (3)

benign: not cancerous. (10)

bias: an unfair belief that some people, objects, or situations are better than others. (2)

biopsy: the removal of a small piece of tissue from a tumor using a special needle; the sample is tested for cancer cells. (10)

bioterrorism: the use of harmful agents and products with biological origins (including pathogens or toxins) as weapons. (5)

bipolar disorder: a serious mental health condition characterized by changes in mood, energy, and activity levels; a person with bipolar disorder may swing from mania to depression. (21)

bloodborne pathogens: infectious microorganisms in the blood; can cause disease. (4)

body alignment: the optimal placement of all body parts such that bones are in their proper places and muscles are used efficiently. (14)

body cavities: spaces in the human body that contain organs. (9)

body language: gestures, posture, and movements that communicate a person's thoughts and feelings. (11)

body mass index (BMI): a number that uses height and weight to determine whether a person is a healthy weight, overweight, or underweight; is determined by dividing weight in kilograms (kg) by height in meters (m) squared. (15)

body mechanics: actions that promote safe, efficient movement without straining any muscles or joints. (4)

boundaries: accepted and expected limits on behavior or actions. (1)

bradycardia: an abnormally slow pulse (fewer than 60 beats per minute). (15)

bradypnea: abnormally slow breathing. (15)

bullying: repeated and harmful verbal, physical, social, or psychological behavior toward others. (23)

C

calories: units of energy. (19)

carbohydrates: the body's main source of energy; includes three types: starches, sugars, and fiber. (19)

cardiopulmonary resuscitation (CPR): an emergency procedure in which air is breathed into a person's mouth or nose to provide ventilation; external chest compressions help oxygenated blood flow to the brain and heart. (5)

care conferences: routinely scheduled meetings that bring together all members of the healthcare staff who deliver care to a particular resident; during the meeting, the resident's plan of care is discussed. (13)

caring: providing assistance and comfort to affect the health and well-being of a resident positively. (11)

carotid pulse: a measurement of heartbeat taken by feeling the carotid artery, which is located on the neck by the trachea below the angle of the jaw. (15)

catheter: a flexible tube that is inserted through a narrow opening into the body. (8)

cell: the smallest and most basic structural and functional unit of the human body. (8)

Celsius (C): a temperature measurement scale in which the freezing point of water is 0° and the boiling point is 100° under normal atmospheric pressure; also called *centigrade*. (15)

census: the number of patients or residents on a nursing unit. (2)

Centers for Disease Control and Prevention (CDC): a US federal agency responsible for preventing and controlling the spread of infectious diseases and responding to health threats; also provides information and research to the healthcare community. (1)

central nervous system (CNS): the part of the nervous system that consists of the brain and spinal cord. (9)

cerebral palsy (CP): a disability that affects movement, muscle tone, and posture; is typically caused by damage to the developing fetal brain. (21)

certification: a credential earned when a person has completed the designated education, training, and testing that prepares him or her for a specific field, discipline, or professional advancement. (1)

certified nursing assistant (CNA): a person who has successfully completed the education and training needed to take and pass the CNA state certification competency examination; scope of practice is regulated by the state, and CNAs are supervised by registered nurses (RNs) or licensed practical/vocational nurses (LPNs/LVNs); in some states, CNAs are called *nurse aides, licensed nursing assistants,* or *registered nursing assistants*. (1)

chain of command: the levels of staff in a facility with regard to authority; from top to bottom, staff members at each level have direct authority over staff members below them. (2)

change-of-shift report: a verbal report that transfers essential information about residents from one shift to the next. (13)

Cheyne-Stokes respiration: a pattern of breathing that indicates death is near; causes hyperpnea (rapid breathing) followed by periods of no breathing (apnea). (22)

chlorophyll: a green substance found in plants; absorbs light and transfers it through the plant during photosynthesis. (8)

chronic care: care given to those who have long-term diseases or illnesses; is given in a variety of healthcare facilities, including doctors' offices, outpatient clinics, rehabilitation centers, or long-term care facilities. (2)

chronic disease: a long-term or recurring disease or condition. (10)

chronic pain: a persistent, uncomfortable feeling that does not go away over time. (10)

civil law: a type of law that deals with disagreements between individuals and organizations; money is awarded to the victim for injuries or damages. (3)

clarification: the process of restating what you believe was said to make sure you heard the message correctly. (11)

clinically adverse events: medical errors. (4)

closed-ended question: a question that requires only a one-word answer, such as *yes* or *no*. (11)

cognitive status: the ability to understand, think clearly, and remember. (6)

collaboration: the process by which people work together to resolve conflict in a way that satisfies everyone. (11)

coma: a state of deep and prolonged unconsciousness. (10)

commode: a chair that contains a place to go to the bathroom; can be used as a toilet by residents with mobility challenges. (4)

communicable diseases: diseases that can be transmitted between people and animals, and to objects; also called *contagious diseases* or *infectious diseases*. (8)

communication barriers: any actions, behaviors, or situations that block or interfere with a person's ability to successfully send and receive communication messages. (11)

compassion: the desire to help another person who is suffering or in pain. (1)

competence: having the knowledge and skills needed to do something well. (1)

compresses: pads of material; can be warm, cold, dry, or moist. (18)

compromise: the process by which two sides of a conflict give and take to find the best resolution. (11)

concentration: complete attention directed toward a particular object or task. (23)

confidentiality: the act of keeping personal information that has been shared with the healthcare staff private. (3)

conflict: a disagreement between two or more people. (11)

connective tissue: a type of body tissue that connects or supports other body tissues, structures, and organs; is composed of collagen fibers that provide strength and elastic fibers that enable flexibility. (4)

conscious: aware of feelings, actions, and outside surroundings. (7)

constipation: a condition in which bowel movements occur fewer than three times a week and contain hard, dry stools that are difficult to evacuate; can be an acute or chronic condition. (20)

consultations: meetings with a healthcare expert; the expert gives advice or information. (13)

contaminated: soiled or dirty as a result of contact or mixture with something that is not clean. (1)

continuity: an uninterrupted connection or sequence of events. (6)

contracture: the tightening or shortening of a body part (such as a muscle, a tendon, or the skin) due to lack of movement. (14)

contusions: bruises caused by damaged or broken blood vessels; may cause swelling. (8)

conventional medicine: symptoms and diseases are treated using prescription medications, clinical procedures, radiation, or surgery; also called *Western medicine* or *allopathic medicine*. (10)

co-payment: a fixed fee for specific medical services covered partially by health insurance; the patient is required to pay this fee. (2)

cover letter: a formal, written introduction that outlines a person's capabilities and skills to a prospective employer. (23)

covert: not shown openly; hidden. (7)

cramming: studying large amounts of information in a short period of time. (23)

criminal law: a type of law that punishes criminal offenses; includes imposing a fine or a prison sentence to keep offenders and others from acting unlawfully again. (3)

critical observation: the appropriate use of both objective and subjective observation. (13)

cross-cultural communication: the use of practices and approaches that promote and improve relationships between people from different cultures. (12)

cryotherapy: the use of cold applications to reduce swelling and ease pain. (18)

cues: actions that invite a response; may be verbal or manual and can guide resident behavior. (21)

cultural humility: awareness and understanding of one's own culture, as well as the cultures of others; includes knowledge of personal limitations, barriers, and gaps in knowledge and provides the openness needed to be sensitive to and respectful of other cultures. (12)

culture: (1) a set of traditions, beliefs, rituals, customs, and values that are learned over time and are specific to a group of people; (2) the process of cultivating (growing) living tissue cells in a substance favorable to their growth. (1, 8)

culture of safety: the shared commitment of a healthcare facility's leadership and staff to ensure a safe work environment. (4)

customs: established practices and beliefs that are followed by a group of people over multiple generations. (12)

cyanotic: discolored and bluish due to insufficient oxygen. (18)

cyberattacks: illegal attempts to gain access to a digital device or network to cause harm. (5)

cystic fibrosis (CF): a genetic disorder that changes how the body makes mucus and sweat; is characterized by congestion, difficult digestion, and salty sweat. (21)

D

decubitus ulcer: a skin condition caused when continuous pressure on the skin and on bony areas restricts blood flow and creates a sore; also called a *bedsore* or *pressure ulcer*. (4)

deductible: the amount of money that a health insurer, program, or employer requires people to pay out of pocket as their share of the cost for health insurance coverage. (2)

deduction: the use of specific information to reach a conclusion. (2)

defamation of character: false statements made about a person that damage his or her reputation. (3)

defecate: to have a bowel movement. (20)

defense mechanisms: unconscious behaviors that enable people to ignore or forget situations or thoughts that cause fear, anxiety, and stress. (11)

deformity: the distortion of a body part. (13)

dehydration: a lack of adequate fluids in the body tissues. (19)

delegate: to transfer duties to another competent person; the person who delegates the responsibility is still accountable for the proper completion of the tasks involved. (6)

delusions: irrational beliefs that something is true, even when there is overwhelming proof that it is not. (21)

dementia: a progressive, permanent, severe loss of mental capacity that interferes with a person's ability to lead a normal life. (2)

deoxyribonucleic acid (DNA): a chemical compound that contains instructions for developing and directing the growth and activities of living organisms. (9)

diabetes mellitus: a disorder in which there are excessive amounts of glucose (sugar) in a person's blood due to insufficient production of insulin (the hormone that regulates glucose) or insulin resistance; commonly referred to as *diabetes*. (5)

dialysis: the process of removing waste products and excess fluid from the body. (10)

diarrhea: a condition in which bowel movements have stools with excess water and occur frequently; can be an acute or chronic condition. (20)

diastolic blood pressure: the pressure of blood against the arteries when the heart muscle relaxes. (15)

dietary fats: lipids; provide energy for and insulate the body; include saturated fat, *trans* fat, and unsaturated fat. (19)

dignity: worthy of honor and respect. (22)

dilemma: a choice between two difficult options; options may be desirable or undesirable. (3)

discharge plan: a set of instructions given at the time of discharge; may include the doctor's instructions about activity level, medications, continued treatment, important changes in condition, and follow-up appointments with the doctor. (6)

disease: a condition in which an organ or body system functions incorrectly and exhibits particular signs and symptoms. (10)

disposable protective pad: a pad that is small, often multilayered, leakproof, and highly absorbent; can be placed under the buttocks of incontinent residents, used to absorb drainage, or used during procedures to prevent the bed from becoming soiled; also called an *incontinence pad*. (17)

distress: bad stress; causes bodily symptoms that can lead to disease and poor coping and decision-making. (7)

diversity: the presence of differences among people. (12)

do-not-resuscitate (DNR) order: a medical and legal request that lifesaving measures such as CPR not be administered if a person's heart or breathing stops. (22)

dormant: having slowed or stopped functions. (8)

draw sheet: a small, flat sheet or a regular-size flat sheet folded in half and placed lengthwise over the middle of the bottom sheet of the bed; is used to help turn a resident in bed; also called a *pull sheet*, *turning sheet*, or *lift sheet*. (17)

dressing: a protective material placed on a wound; also called a *bandage*. (8)

ducts: tubes for conveying substances in the body. (9)

dysphagia: difficulty or discomfort when swallowing. (19)

dyspnea: difficult breathing or shortness of breath. (15)

dysrhythmia: an irregular or abnormal heart rhythm. (17)

E

eating disorder: an abnormal pattern of eating that leads to serious and often fatal medical consequences. (19)

edema: the retention of fluid in body tissues. (10)

elder abuse: a deliberate action (physical, verbal, financial, or sexual) that causes harm to an older adult. (3)

electrolytes: minerals in the blood and body fluids with an electrical charge that help balance fluids. (19)

electronic health record (EHR): an electronic record that includes information about a person's entire medical history and all healthcare experiences. (13)

electronic medical record (EMR): a component of an EHR that includes administrative and clinical information about a single stay in a healthcare facility. (13)

embolus: a mass (most commonly a blood clot) that travels through the blood and can become trapped in a blood vessel and obstruct blood flow. (14)

emesis basin: a small, kidney-shaped bowl often used for oral care or if the resident needs to vomit. (18)

empathy: understanding for another person's feelings and emotions. (7)

empower: to give a person the power to control his or her own destiny and decision-making. (1)

endocrine glands: ductless glands that secrete hormones directly into the bloodstream. (9)

enema: a procedure in which liquid is inserted into the rectum to clean the lower intestine. (20)

energy: the power and drive to make decisions and complete tasks. (7)

engagement: the practice of being fully involved and committed to the task at hand. (2)

enteral: by way of the gastrointestinal system. (19)

entrapment: a harmful event in which a resident falls between the bed and side rails. (4)

enzymes: chemical agents that can cause specific biochemical reactions. (8)

epidermis: the outermost layer of the skin; contains keratin and melanin. (8)

ethics: principles that guide behavior with respect to what is right and wrong. (3)

ethnicity: identification with common social, cultural, and traditional practices that are shared within a group. (12)

ethnocentrism: an outlook in which one judges another culture based on the beliefs and standards of one's own culture. (12)

eustress: good stress; helps people become motivated and productive. (7)

evacuation: the intentional removal of people or objects from a dangerous area. (5)

evidence-based practice: the process of locating and using research findings to guide decisions made about care delivery. (6)

excretions: waste products expelled from the body. (8)

exocrine glands: glands with ducts that transport hormones to other organs or to the surface of the skin. (9)

exudate: a liquid or semisolid discharge from body tissues or a blood vessel; drains from a wound and is caused by tissue damage. (8)

F

Fahrenheit (F): a temperature measurement scale in which the freezing point of water is 32° and the boiling point is 212° under normal atmospheric pressure. (15)

false imprisonment: illegal confinement in which a person is held against his or her will by another, resulting in restraint of movement; the person can be confined using force or threats. (3)

fatigue: a feeling of extreme tiredness or exhaustion. (17)

fear: an unpleasant feeling or emotion resulting from the threat or presence of danger. (11)

fibrillation: an irregular heart rhythm. (5)

fidelity: the quality of being faithful and not abandoning those who need care. (3)

fire triangle: the three elements—fuel, oxygen, and heat—needed to start a fire. (4)

flash cards: a set of cards used for studying; cards typically have a question on one side and an answer on the other. (23)

flatus: gas or air in the gastrointestinal tract; is expelled via the anus. (20)

flow meter: a medical device used to make sure a resident receives the prescribed amount of oxygen. (4)

foot drop: a condition of paralysis or weakness in the front muscles of the foot and ankle; results in the dragging of the foot and toes. (14)

Fowler's position: a body position in which a resident lies with legs extended on an examining table or bed; the head of the bed is raised to a 45° angle. (9)

friction: the resistance between two objects or surfaces rubbing against each other. (8)

frostbite: a condition in which extremely cold temperatures cause freezing and damage to body tissues, such as the skin on the fingers, toes, nose, ears, cheeks, and chin. (8)

G

gait: a manner of walking. (4)

gait belt: a belt worn around a resident's waist that serves as a safety device when a resident stands and ambulates; also called a *transfer belt* when used for moving a resident. (4)

gangrene: a condition characterized by the death and decay of body tissue due to lack of blood supply. (18)

generation: a group of people who are born and who live during the same time. (7)

generation gap: a lack of communication between one generation and another; is often due to differences in customs, attitudes, and beliefs. (7)

genuine: honest, open, and sincere in communication and relationships. (7)

giving of self: the quality of putting a resident's health and wellness needs before one's own needs as a caregiver. (11)

gland: a group of specialized cells that secrete substances. (9)

glucometer: a medical device that measures blood sugar levels. (16)

graduate: a container used to measure intake and output. (20)

grand mal seizure: a generalized seizure in which a person may experience loss of consciousness and violent muscle contractions; is caused by abnormal electrical activity in the brain. (5)

grief: an emotional response to or distress about a physical or personal loss. (22)

guaiac test: a diagnostic procedure used to detect fecal occult blood. (16)

H

hallucinations: visual, verbal, or physical perceptions of objects that are not real, but are mistaken for reality. (17)

Hands-Only™ CPR: an emergency procedure in which uninterrupted chest compressions restore heartbeat and promote blood circulation; is a procedure for those not trained in conventional CPR. (5)

harm: unintended physical injury that requires additional monitoring, treatment, or hospitalization; may result in death. (4)

health: the condition of a person's physical, mental, social, and spiritual self. (10)

healthcare: the prevention, diagnosis, and treatment of diseases; the management of acute and chronic illnesses; and the promotion of wellness. (2)

healthcare services: screening, diagnostic, and evaluation activities that assist and support the restoration, maintenance, or improvement of health. (2)

health literacy: a person's ability to understand fully and use information about health, diseases, conditions, or treatments. (11)

Heimlich maneuver: an emergency procedure in which a person places his or her fist just above the navel of a choking person, covers his or her fist with the other hand, and performs quick inward and upward abdominal thrusts. (5)

hemiplegia: a condition of paralysis on one side of the body. (10)

hemorrhage: the excessive loss of blood over a short period of time due to internal or external injury. (5)

hemorrhoids: swollen, inflamed veins found under the skin around the anus (external) or inside the rectum (internal); are caused by pressure from straining during bowel movements; may be itchy or painful at times and can cause rectal bleeding. (18)

hernia: a bulge of an organ through the wall of the body cavity or structure that contains it. (20)

holistic care: care that is sensitive to a person's values and desires and that integrates a person's physical (body), emotional (mind), and spiritual (spirit) needs to help achieve the highest level of well-being possible. (1)

homeostasis: an internal balance of the human body. (7)

hormones: chemical substances that are produced in the body and that control and regulate specific body processes. (7)

hospice: a healthcare facility or service that provides supportive care for those who are terminally ill and their families; is available on-site at healthcare facilities or in private homes. (1)

humility: modesty; the quality of not putting one's self first. (2)

hydrated: having sufficient fluids in the body tissues over a 24-hour period. (19)

hydration: a sufficient amount of fluid in the body tissues. (18)

hygiene: routine actions such as bathing that promote and maintain cleanliness and health. (18)

hypertension: high blood pressure. (10)

hyperventilation: deep, rapid breathing. (15)

hypotension: low blood pressure. (15)

hypothermia: a condition of abnormally low body temperature. (4)

hypoventilation: slow, shallow breathing. (15)

hypoxia: a lack of adequate oxygen supply in the body. (15)

I

ideal body weight (IBW): the healthiest weight for an individual; is determined primarily by height, but also takes gender, age, build, and muscular development into account using adjusted statistical tables. (15)

illness: a feeling of poor health; is not always caused by a disease. (10)

immunization: a method of providing protection against diseases such as influenza, pneumonia, measles, tetanus, and polio; a weakened or killed antigen is introduced to cause the body to develop antibodies specific to that antigen; usually given by injection. (2)

impaction: a blockage of hard stool in the rectum. (20)

incapacitation: the lack of ability to make decisions. (22)

incident report: a document that records information about an unusual event, such as a resident injury; also called an *accident report* or *occurrence report*. (4)

incontinence: a lack of bowel or bladder control. (10)

infection: the invasion and growth of harmful pathogens in the body; leads to disease. (8)

infection control: policies and procedures used to lessen the risk of spreading diseases and infections. (1)

inflammation: the protective response of body tissue to irritation, injury, or infection; is characterized by swelling and redness. (8)

informed consent: the legal process of getting written permission prior to giving care or conducting procedures. (3)

inspection: the visual examination of a body part. (16)

integrative medicine (IM): alternative approaches that are used along with, or in place of, conventional medicine. (10)

integrity: strong moral principles and professional standards. (1)

interpersonal relationships: relationships between two or more people who share similar interests or goals; meet physical and emotional needs. (11)

interpreter: a person who translates written or spoken words into another language. (11)

intimate relationships: relationships between two people who have romantic feelings of love for each other. (11)

intoxication: a condition of reduced control caused by the overuse of a chemical substance. (21)

intuitive: perceptive about a situation; having insight. (2)

isolation: specific preventive measures that limit or eliminate the spread of pathogens from an infected person to others. (8)

J

jargon: words, phrases, and language used by a specific group of people or culture. (11)

job campaign: a series of organized activities needed to find a desired job. (23)

job description: a written document that describes the duties, responsibilities, and qualifications required for a particular position. (1)

joints: locations where two or more bones connect. (4)

journal: a written record of observations and experiences. (2)

K

kinship: a feeling of being close or of having an association or connection. (12)

L

labeling: describing someone using a specific word or phrase. (11)

lacerations: wounds that tear body tissue and result in ragged edges. (8)

laryngeal mirror: a medical instrument used to examine the mouth, tongue, and teeth. (16)

lateral position: a body position in which a resident lies on his or her side with arms free and knees slightly bent. (9)

legal blindness: a refractive error of 20/200, even after vision correction. (21)

legumes: plants with pods (long cases) that contain edible seeds. (19)

level of care: the type of care needed for a particular patient or resident; is typically higher for a patient with a serious illness and lower for a resident who needs assistance only with ADLs. (2)

liability: legal responsibility. (3)

libel: false written statements made about a person that damage his or her reputation; a type of defamation of character. (3)

licensed nursing staff: nursing staff members who have passed state licensing examinations that allow them to perform healthcare tasks within their scope of practice; RNs and LPNs/LVNs. (1)

licensed practical/vocational nurse (LPN/LVN): a person who has successfully completed the education and training needed to take and pass an LPN/LVN state licensing examination; scope of practice is regulated by the state, and LPNs/LVNs provide care under the supervision of an RN; care can include monitoring and reporting, preparing and giving medications, inserting catheters, and performing wound care. (1)

licensure: official permission given to a person or facility to deliver care; is based on meeting standards set by law. (3)

ligaments: fibrous cords of tissue that attach bone to bone and support organs. (9)

living will: an advance directive that details the life-prolonging treatments a person desires in the event of incapacitation during a terminal illness or permanent unconsciousness. (22)

M

malabsorption: the reduced ability of the intestine to take in essential nutrients and fluids and transfer them to the bloodstream. (19)

malignant: cancerous. (10)

malnutrition: lack of proper nourishment due to inadequate or unbalanced intake of vitamins, minerals, and other nutrients or due to the body's inability to use nutrients. (15)

malpractice: a form of negligence in which a caregiver does not comply with the standards expected and set by his or her discipline's regulatory body, resulting in resident injury. (3)

managed care: a form of insurance in which there are contracts with specific healthcare providers who will deliver care at a reduced cost. (2)

manually: by hand. (13)

Medicaid: a US law passed in 1965 that provides a combination of federal and state financing to offer healthcare at the state level for those with low incomes; participants must meet certain income requirements to qualify. (2)

medical terminology: the standard way to communicate structure, processes, functions, diseases, and conditions of the human body; the language used in healthcare. (9)

Medicare: a US law passed in 1965 that supplies federal funds to deliver healthcare to people who are 65 years of age or older, who are under 65 years and have disabilities, or who have end-stage renal disease. (2)

meditation: the practice of emptying the mind of thoughts, feelings, and emotions to reach a state of relaxation through concentration. (2)

membranes: thin, soft, flexible structures that cover, line, or act as boundaries for cells or organs. (9)

metabolism: the chemical process by which nutrients are converted into energy in the body. (19)

metastasis: the spread of cancer cells to other locations in the body. (10)

microorganisms: living things, or *organisms*, that are so small they can only be seen through a microscope. (8)

mindfulness: the practice of being aware and mentally present in every situation by focusing on what is being said, what is being done, or what is happening in the environment; requires a nonjudgmental attitude. (2)

minimum data set (MDS): complete assessment by licensed nursing staff of residents' mobility, transfer skills, and ADLs to identify health problems. (4)

minerals: inorganic substances in the body that regulate and assist in metabolism. (19)

moribund: about to die. (22)

motility: movement; in the gastrointestinal system, the contraction of muscles that moves substances through the gastrointestinal tract. (20)

motivation: choosing to act on something a person wants. (7)

mourn: to express feelings and behaviors that show grief. (22)

mucus: a thick, slippery fluid that moistens and protects parts of the body. (8)

myocardial infarction: a sudden medical emergency that occurs when blood flow to part of the heart muscle is blocked, causing the heart muscle to become severely damaged and die; can cause loss of heart function, or cardiac arrest; also known as a *heart attack*. (5)

N

nasal cannula: a narrow, flexible, plastic tube used to deliver oxygen through the nostrils. (4)

near misses: unplanned health outcomes that do not cause harm, even though they have the potential to; considered *close calls*. (4)

necrosis: the death of body tissue. (10)

needlesticks: puncture wounds caused by needles. (4)

neglect: the failure to provide necessary care that meets a resident's daily needs. (3)

negligence: the unintentional failure to act or provide care that a sensible person would; can result in injury. (3)

network: to communicate with an informal, interconnected group of people. (23)

neurons: cells of the nervous system that transmit information throughout the body in the form of electrochemical messages (neural impulses); each neuron is composed of a cell body, dendrites, and axons. (9)

never events: actions or errors that result in harm, death, or significant disability; are usually preventable. (4)

nodules: small, round lumps of body tissue; can be felt by touch. (10)

noncommunicable diseases: diseases that are not contagious and cannot be transmitted between people and animals or to objects. (8)

nonmaleficence: the moral obligation to avoid harm. (3)

nonpenetrating wounds: wounds that do not enter into or through the skin; are caused by rubbing or friction on the surface of the skin. (8)

nonpharmacological: without the use of medication. (10)

nonverbal communication: the use of gestures, facial expressions, tone of voice, or body movements to convey a message. (2)

numbness: an inability to feel sensations due to changes in nerve function. (13)

nursing diagnosis: the identification of a health problem or the cause of a health problem; does not identify a specific disease. (6)

nursing orders: instructions outlining the actions that should be taken to achieve stated goals of care; written by the RN. (13)

nursing process: assessing, identifying problems, planning implementing, and evaluating to deliver safe, quality care. (6)

nursing unit: an area in a healthcare facility in which care is delivered; is typically designated by a floor name, area, or type of illness (as in an *Alzheimer's* or *surgical unit*). (2)

nutrients: substances the body needs to function normally; include water, protein, carbohydrates, fats, minerals, and vitamins. (9)

nutrition: the ingestion of foods that provide nutrients to maintain the health of the body. (19)

O

obesity: a health condition in which body weight is much greater than what is considered healthy for a certain height. (19)

objective observations: descriptions of the facts about a situation. (13)

occult blood: the presence of very small amounts of blood in the stool. (16)

open-ended question: a question that requires more than a one-word answer. (11)

ophthalmoscope: a medical instrument used to examine the eyes. (16)

organs: collections of tissues that have specific structures and functions. (9)

orthostatic hypotension: a condition in which blood pressure falls when a person stands. (14)

orthotic: a device that supports, aligns, or corrects a weakened, immobile, injured, or deformed part of the body. (14)

osteoporosis: a condition of porous bones; characterized by low bone density. (4)

ostomy: a surgical procedure that creates an opening in the abdominal wall so that stool can be eliminated from the intestines to the outside of the body. (20)

otoscope: a medical instrument used to examine the ears. (16)

overt: open to view; observable. (7)

P

pain scales: devices used to measure a person's perception of the severity of pain. (10)

palliative care: care that provides relief from the symptoms of a disease or condition; does not aim to cure the disease or condition. (22)

pallor: an unusually pale color of the skin. (18)

palpation: the use of the hands to feel an object, such as a lump or mass in the body, to determine its size, location, shape, or hardness. (16)

pandemic: worldwide spread of a disease among people who have no immunity. (5)

paralysis: the loss of function and feeling in one or more muscle groups. (21)

paranoia: an unsupported or exaggerated distrust of others. (21)

parasympathetic nervous system (PNS): part of the body's nervous system that controls the automatic daily functions of the cardiovascular, respiratory, and gastrointestinal systems; helps the body return to a homeostatic state after experiencing pain or stress. (7)

parenteral: by way of the veins or intravenous infusion. (19)

patent: open. (19)

pathogens: disease-causing microorganisms. (4, 8)

pathologist: a doctor who specializes in studying diseases; conducts autopsies to determine causes of death. (22)

pathology: a collection of changes to the body's tissues or organs; can trigger a disease or can be caused by a disease. (10)

patients: people who visit a healthcare facility, such as a hospital, for a physical examination or for the treatment of an illness or disease. (1)

penetrating wounds: wounds that enter into or through the skin. (8)

perineal care: hygiene care that involves cleansing the area between the thighs (the coccyx, pubis, anus, urethra, and external genitals). (18)

perineum: the area between the thighs; includes the coccyx, pubis, anus, urethra, and external genitals. (18)

peripheral nervous system (PNS): the part of the nervous system that consists of 12 pairs of cranial nerves and 31 pairs of spinal nerves. (9)

perseveration: uncontrollable need to repeat a word, phrase, or gesture for no apparent reason. (21)

personal protective equipment (PPE): specialized clothing and accessories, such as gloves, gowns, masks, goggles, and other pieces of equipment, that are worn to protect against infection or injury. (4)

petit mal seizure: a generalized seizure in which a person has no or lessened awareness and responsiveness and may lose consciousness; is caused by abnormal electrical activity in the brain. (5)

phagocytosis: the process by which a white blood cell engulfs (surrounds) and destroys foreign antigens. (8)

phobias: unsupported, exaggerated fears that sometimes interfere with daily life. (11)

photosynthesis: the process by which plants and other organisms convert light energy from the sun into chemical energy; allows plants and other organisms to function. (8)

physiology: the study of how the body functions. (9)

plan of care: a written plan that provides directions and guides delivery of individualized, holistic care; also called a *service plan*. (4, 6)

plaques: superficial, solid, elevated lesions. (10)

plasma: the liquid component of blood; composed of water, hormones, protein, sugar, and waste products. (9)

platelets: flat, circular cells in the blood that assist in the clotting process. (9)

podiatrist: a doctor who specializes in diagnosing and treating diseases and conditions that affect the feet. (18)

point-of-care testing (POCT): specimen collection at the place in which a resident is receiving care. (16)

positive regard: an attitude that is supportive and accepting of others. (1)

postmortem care: care performed shortly after death; prepares the body for burial or cremation, puts the body in alignment, and prevents skin damage. (22)

post-traumatic stress disorder (PTSD): a stress-related mental health condition that develops after a person experiences or witnesses a traumatic or stressful event. (21)

posture: the way in which a person holds his or her body; the manner in which the body remains upright against gravity when sitting down, lying down, or standing up. (4)

power of attorney: an advance directive that gives a designated person the authority to make healthcare decisions on behalf of another person; authority only takes effect if the person who writes the power of attorney becomes unable to make his or her own decisions; also called a *healthcare proxy* or *durable power of attorney for healthcare*. (22)

prejudice: an opinion or feeling that is formed without facts and that often leads to unfair feelings of dislike for a person or group because of race, sex, or religion. (11)

premium: the amount of money paid, usually on a schedule, to an insurance company for a specific insurance policy. (2)

primary care provider (PCP): a doctor, nurse practitioner, or physician assistant whose legal scope of practice allows him or her to be the first contact for a person's healthcare needs; is responsible for monitoring a person's overall healthcare needs and coordinates care across healthcare services when necessary. (2)

priorities: items or actions of high importance. (6)

prioritizing: organizing responsibilities or tasks so that the most important tasks are completed first. (7)

private insurance: a plan for the payment of healthcare services; may be purchased by an employer on the employee's behalf or by an individual. (2)

probe: a long, thin, medical instrument used to measure temperature. (15)

procrastination: the act of purposely postponing a task. (23)

professional: demonstrating an expected level of excellence and competence. (1)

prognosis: a projection of the likely course and outcome of a disease and the potential for recovery. (3)

prone position: a body position in which a resident lies on his or her abdomen with arms and hands at each side, feet comfortably positioned, and head turned to the side. (9)

prosthetic: an artificial device designed to replace a missing body part. (14)

proteins: vital to cell structure, contribute to energy production, build body tissue, and promote growth and repair. (19)

pulse: the beat of the heart measured through the walls of a peripheral artery. (5)

pulse oximeter: a medical device, usually applied to the end of a finger, that indirectly measures the amount of oxygen in the blood; oxygen content is recorded as a percentage. (6)

Q

quarantine: an action taken to separate and restrict exposed people from those who have not been exposed to prevent the spread of a communicable disease. (8)

R

race: a set of inherited physical characteristics, such as skin, eye, and hair color. (12)

RACE system: an acronym for the process of responding to a fire; stands for *rescue*, *activate alarm*, *confine the fire*, and *extinguish*. (4)

racism: intolerance, discrimination, or prejudice based on race. (12)

radial pulse: a measurement of heartbeat taken by feeling the radial artery, which is located on the inside of the thumb side of the wrist. (15)

range of motion (ROM): the amount that a person can move a joint voluntarily. (4)

rapport: mutual understanding in a relationship. (7)

ratio: the number of patients or residents in a healthcare facility or unit assigned to each member of the healthcare staff. (2)

rational: having the ability to think clearly and make decisions based on facts. (2)

receptors: sensory nerve endings on or within a cell that react to various stimuli and produce an effect. (9)

Recommended Dietary Allowances (RDAs): daily levels of nutritional intake needed to maintain good health. (19)

red blood cells: the components of the blood that contain hemoglobin; responsible for oxygen and carbon dioxide exchange; also called *erythrocytes*. (9)

registered nurse (RN): a person who has successfully completed the education and training needed to take and pass an RN state licensing examination; delivers nursing care, assesses residents, and provides nursing diagnoses; also plans, implements, and evaluates care. (1)

regulation: in healthcare, a rule or requirement that healthcare facilities and staff members must follow; is usually enforced by an authority, such as the federal or state government. (3)

rehabilitation: a period of recovery in which healthcare staff members help residents regain their strength and mobility with the goal of learning to function independently. (3)

residents: people staying in a long-term care facility due to age, illness, or inability to care for themselves at home. (1)

resilience: the ability to recover from or easily adjust to difficulties or change. (1)

respect: a feeling of appreciation and admiration for another person. (7)

restorative care: care that assists with any adjustments and improvements that help residents live as independently as possible. (14)

restraint: any physical equipment or chemical substance that prevents a resident from moving freely. (4)

résumé: a formal, written representation of a person's experience, skills, and credentials. (23)

rigor mortis: the stiffening of the body's muscles several hours after death. (22)

rituals: actions that are always done in the same way, often for religious purposes or as part of a ceremony. (12)

rounds: opportunities to monitor and discuss the status of a resident's condition or disease; conducted inside or right outside the resident's room. (13)

rule of nines: a method of determining the surface area of the body affected by burns. (5)

S

safety data sheet (SDS): a document found in the facility safety plan; contains information about the potential hazards of a chemical product and use, storage, handling, and emergency procedures; also called a *material safety data sheet (MSDS)*. (4)

schizophrenia spectrum disorder: a severe and chronic mental health condition in which a person experiences a loss of reality; has delusions, hallucinations, and thought disorders; and displays agitated body movements. (21)

sclerosis: the thickening or hardening of a body part. (10)

scope of practice: the specific responsibilities, procedures, and actions of a healthcare provider, as permitted by state regulations; actions within the scope of practice are allowed only when special educational requirements have been met and when knowledge and skill competency are demonstrated. (1)

secretions: substances produced and released by cells or organs. (8)

seizures: sudden changes in the brain's normal electrical activity; causes change in or loss of consciousness. (5)

self-actualization: a person's belief that he or she has fully developed to full potential. (7)

self-determination: the process of making choices and decisions based on a person's own preferences and interests. (3)

self-esteem: a person's confidence and regard for himself or herself. (7)

self-harm: the act of hurting one's self on purpose. (21)

self-image: the way a person thinks about himself or herself, abilities, and appearance. (7)

self-reflection: the practice of looking at one's self in an honest and truthful way and being open to any changes that may be needed. (2)

self-respect: a person's appreciation and acceptance of himself or herself. (7)

sharps: objects such as needles, razors, broken glass, and scalpels that can penetrate the skin. (4)

shock: a condition in which the organs and tissues of the body do not have sufficient oxygen. (5)

sign: a piece of objective or factual information about a disease or condition. (10)

sitz bath: a type of therapeutic bath that soaks a person's perineum, buttocks, and sometimes hips in warm water. (18)

skin integrity: the condition of the skin; healthy skin is whole or intact without irritation, inflammation, or damage. (18)

slander: false spoken statements made about a person that damage his or her reputation; a type of defamation of character. (3)

sleep deprivation: a loss or deficiency of the recommended hours of sleep. (17)

Social Security: a US law in 1935 that provides retirement benefits, disability coverage, dependent coverage, and survivor benefits; is funded by mandatory payments by employers and employees. (2)

somatic nervous system: the part of the peripheral nervous system that controls voluntary body functions and the movement of skeletal muscle. (9)

specimens: samples of a body substance. (16)

speculum: a medical instrument used to examine the vagina or other body cavities. (16)

sperm: the male reproductive cell; fertilizes the ovum during reproduction. (9)

sphincter: a circular muscle that can open or close; found in the heart and gastrointestinal system. (9)

sphygmomanometer: a medical device used to measure blood pressure; includes a cuff that wraps around a person's upper arm and a measuring device. (6)

spina bifida (SB): a congenital disorder resulting in incomplete development of the spinal cord. (21)

sputum: a blend of saliva and mucus; also called *phlegm*. (16)

staffing: the process of determining the numbers and types of healthcare staff needed to take care of a group of patients or residents on a nursing unit. (2)

staffing plan: a formal document that outlines the mix and types of healthcare staff members who will work on each shift in the nursing unit; changes are based on the needs of the facility and the care requirements of particular patients or residents. (2)

standards of care: methods, processes, and actions healthcare providers follow. (6)

stereotypes: simplifications or biases about a group that shape the treatment of all group members. (7)

sterile: free of living microorganisms. (8)

sterile field: an area that is free from living pathogenic microorganisms. (8)

stertorous breathing: a type of breathing that sounds like snoring. (15)

stethoscope: a medical device used to listen to body sounds such as breathing, heartbeat, and lung and bowel sounds; has two earpieces connected by flexible tubing and a diaphragm and bell at the end. (15)

stigma: a negative perception that causes others to think less of an idea or person. (21)

stoic: detached from emotion or feeling. (10)

stoma: a surgically created abdominal opening, through which stool are eliminated. (20)

stress: a physical or psychological response to a situation that causes worry or tension. (2)

stress management: the process of taking actions to lessen or remove reactions to stress and stressful events. (7)

stroke: a sudden blockage or rupture of a blood vessel in the brain; can cause a loss of consciousness, partial loss of movement, and speech impairment; also called a *cerebrovascular accident (CVA)*. (5)

subacute care: care provided to a person who has a moderate-to-severe illness, injury, or recurrence of a disease, but who does not require acute care in a hospital. (2)

subconscious: not fully aware of feelings, actions, and outside surroundings. (7)

subjective observations: descriptions based on feelings or opinions about a situation. (13)

suicide: the intentional self-infliction of fatal injuries. (21)

supine position: a body position in which a patient lies flat on his or her back with the arms at each side. (9)

suppositories: small, meltable, solid cones or cylinders that may be medicated; inserted into a body passage such as the rectum or vagina. (20)

sundowning: increased confusion, inability to follow directions, and anxiety (shown by pacing or wandering) that occurs at the end of the day and lasts into the evening. (21)

sympathetic nervous system (SNS): part of the body's nervous system; sets off the fight-or-flight response. (7)

symptom: a piece of subjective information about a disease or condition; is based on a person's feelings or opinions. (10)

syncope: temporary unconsciousness; fainting. (14)

systematic: using a specific method; orderly. (2)

systolic blood pressure: the pressure of blood against the arteries when the heart muscle contracts and pushes blood out to the body. (15)

T

tachycardia: an abnormally fast pulse (more than 100 beats per minute). (15)

tachypnea: rapid, shallow breathing. (15)

temporal arteries: arteries located on each side of the head. (15)

tendons: bands of fibrous tissue that connect muscle to bone. (9)

tepid: slightly warm. (18)

The Joint Commission (TJC): a private regulatory agency that accredits various healthcare facilities, such as hospitals, behavioral health agencies, home healthcare services, and nursing and rehabilitation centers; facilities that pursue accreditation by TJC must meet specific guidelines and standards for safety and quality. (3)

therapeutic: having a healing effect on the body and mind. (18)

therapeutic diets: eating plans that promote healing. (19)

thermotherapy: the use of heat applications to increase circulation and ease pain. (18)

thrombus: a blood clot that forms within a blood vessel and does not travel through the blood. (14)

tingling: a sensation that feels like sharp points digging into the skin due to changes in nerve function. (13)

tissue: a collection of specialized cells that act together to perform specific functions. (8)

toxins: poisons. (8)

tracheostomy: a surgical opening in the trachea; a tube is inserted into the opening to help people who have difficulty breathing. (6)

traction: weights, pulleys, and tape used to exert a slow, gentle pull; used to treat a muscular or skeletal disorder, such as a fracture, and to bring displaced bones back into place. (17)

traditions: behaviors or practices that have special meanings or symbolism and that are handed down from one generation to another. (12)

trait: a distinctive physical quality or characteristic. (12)

transparency: lack of secretive or hidden information; honesty. (4)

transplants: surgeries in which organs or body tissues are removed from one person and transferred into another. (22)

trochanter rolls: soft rolls that are placed along the body and that span from above the hip to above the knee; prevent external (outer) rotation of the hips; are usually premade or made from a towel or bath blanket and are usually 12–14 inches long. (14)

tumor: an abnormal growth of tissue that has no function in the body; can be benign (noncancerous) or malignant (cancerous). (9)

tympanic temperature: a measurement of body temperature taken by placing a thermometer into the ear. (15)

U

unethical: not in line with accepted rules of conduct. (1)

V

vaccine: a mixture that is given by injection or taken orally to protect a person against a specific disease; contains a weakened or killed antigen, which causes the body to develop antibodies specific to that antigen, increasing immunity. (2)

values: beliefs or ideals; set a standard for what is good or bad and significantly influence attitude and behavior; may be shared by people of the same culture. (1)

ventilator: a device used to mechanically aid breathing. (21)

veracity: honesty; the act of providing full disclosure to enable residents to make informed decisions. (3)

verbal communication: the use of spoken words to convey a message. (2)

viruses: the smallest microorganisms; viruses cannot grow or multiply by themselves; instead, they take over another living or host cell. (8)

vital signs: the rates or values of a person's body temperature, pulse, respirations, and blood pressure. (1)

vitamins: organic compounds needed for cell development and growth; must be obtained from foods in a person's diet or from vitamin supplements. (19)

void: to expel from the body. (20)

W

well-being: the state of a person's health; influenced by balancing one's diet, exercise, relationships, financial resources, work, education, and leisure. (10)

wellness: a feeling of good health. (10)

whirlpool: a type of bathtub used for therapeutic purposes; has small spray jets that swirl water. (18)

white blood cells: components of the blood that fight infection and provide protection; also called *leukocytes*. (9)

work ethic: a belief in the importance of work; can strengthen a person's character. (1)

work-life balance: the state of a person's time and energy contributions to career, work, and family commitments. (7)

World Health Organization (WHO): an agency of the United Nations that focuses on international public health. (8)

wound: an injury to body tissue; can be caused by a cut, blow, or other force. (8)

Index

Note: Page numbers followed by f indicate figures.